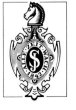

Gerd Plewig · Albert M. Kligman

ACNE and ROSACEA

Second, Completely Revised and Enlarged Edition

With a Contribution by Ch. Bluhm and J. Hollmann

With 207 Mostly Colored Plates

Springer-Verlag
Berlin Heidelberg New York
London Paris Tokyo
Hong Kong Barcelona
Budapest

Gerd Plewig, Prof. Dr.
Dermatologische Klinik und Poliklinik
der Universität München
Frauenlobstrasse 9–11
W-8000 München 2, FRG

Albert M. Kligman, M.D., Ph.D.
University of Pennsylvania
School of Medicine
Philadelphia, PA 19104, USA

ISBN 3-540-52277-8 Springer-Verlag Berlin Heidelberg New York
ISBN 0-387-52277-8 Springer-Verlag New York Berlin Heidelberg

ISBN 3-540-07212-8 1. Auflage Springer-Verlag Berlin Heidelberg New York
ISBN 0-387-07212-8 1st edition Springer-Verlag New York Heidelberg Berlin

Layout and Production Supervision: W. Bischoff, Heidelberg. Cover Design: Struwe & Partner, Heidelberg.
Typesetting, Printing and Bookbinding: Universitätsdruckerei H. Stürtz AG, Würzburg
27/3130-5 4 3 2 1 0 - Printed on acid-free paper

To Helga and Lori,
two exceptional women

Foreword to the First Edition

Acne vulgaris is an extraordinarily common, worldwide disease. Some see the disorder as merely cosmetic. Nonetheless, few skin diseases cause as much physical and psychological misery as this scourge of adolescence.

Dermatologists of course have more than a passing familiarity with acne vulgaris. Recognition is easy but there is still an extraordinary amount of controversy concerning causative factors and the best modes of treatment. Recent studies have brought forth some important findings about which practicing physicians know too little.

This volume is a surprising book. What features make it so unique? This is the first complete account of the great diversity of clinical manifestations. Moreover, gross morphology is coordinated with a thorough microscopic analysis of evolution of the disease. The material is presented in a readable and stimulating way. References are limited because they have been carefully selected.

The authors emphasize that this richly illustrated work is intended for physicians who care for acne patients. Accordingly, this is above all a practical treatise to assist doctors to diagnose and treat acne, and not only acne vulgaris but all the species of acne.

This work is an overview of the entire acne problem with contributions from bacteriology, endocrinology, physiology, anatomy, immunology, cellular kinetics, and experimental acne. Above all it concludes with an optimistic presentation of therapeutic strategies which make it possible for the informed physician to control the abominable effects of this distressing disorder.

O. Braun-Falco
Munich, Germany
1975

Preface to the First Edition

The material on which this account is based derives from observations of several thousand of adolescents with acne. All have been treated; many hundreds have been biopsied and have participated in various tests. These constitute our bona fides. Our plan and intentions are as follows:

Firstly, we have sought to create a portfolio of still-life pictures of the gross and microscopic anatomy of acne. This will be a photographic record of what acne looks like, of its usual and unusual features, its archtypical as well as of its recondite visages. Secondly, we wish to create a moving picture of acne rather than an atlas. We hope the reader will have the feeling of being in a theater watching an unusual drama. Since anatomy can only come to life when animated by physiology, a vigorous attempt has been made to collate function with structure. It is the eye that observes but it is the mind that sees.

Finally, this book is intended for those who wish to understand and treat acne more effectively. The themes are programmed for the clinician. This book will be chiefly a didactic account and not a detailed report of research. We present ourselves as teachers, not as investigators. We conceive it to be the prime mission of medical research to learn how to identify, prevent, and treat the disease. We shall present our personal therapeutic strategies, the ones we use to treat acne patients.

The vision displayed herein is our own and not a mélange constructed from the works of scholars. Our biases and prejudices will appear as plain as birthmarks and will not be concealed under a cosmetic concoction of literary paste. This work will not follow the format of a review. We shall be parsimonious with references, furnishing only those which we think are required to illuminate the subject. We have, of course, drawn extensively on the knowledge gathered by others. The most important sources will be listed. However, authors will not be mentioned in the text so as not to interfere with the telling of the story.

Our depictions will appear to many be overly simplified, too speculative, and too subjective. Such are the risks of rendering a personal account of a mercurial and strange disease.

A picture of pathogenesis is emerging which is not so misty as a decade ago. We reveal herewith our full-length portrait of acne, a bewitching lady whom we have pursued with more passion than intelligence and whose tantalizing qualities have kept us stimulated, even though our attentions have frequently been unrequited.

GERD PLEWIG, Munich
ALBERT M. KLIGMAN, Philadelphia
1975

Preface

The first edition of this book was published more than 15 years ago. Since then there have been considerable advances in the understanding of the etiopathogenesis and in the ability to treat the diverse disorders that comprise the family of acnes. Acne vulgaris and its related forms, as well as acneiform eruptions and rosacea, are now eminently treatable, and sometimes preventable and even curable. With proper diagnosis, the informed physician possesses a multitude of therapeutic options to help patients who suffer from these distressing diseases.

Acne is not life-threatening but rather life-spoiling. In our beauty- and health-conscious world, disfiguring diseases have profound psychologic and social effects. In our high visibility culture, even a few intermittently recurring lesions can lead to social isolation and depression. Acne is long-lasting and ravages the psyche as well as leaving ugly skin scars which last for the patient's lifetime. There are still too many physicians who regard acne as a cosmetic problem which time will take care of: in fact, some forms of acne can persist for decades with hapless patients futilely running from one specialist to the next. More than a few fall prey to charlatans.

Acne is a serious disorder and deserves meticulous attention. Sadly, general practitioners are poorly educated with regard to the diagnosis and treatment of skin diseases. In fact, accurate diagnosis of acne and acne-like disorders is often quite difficult even for the expert. A number of unrelated disorders have features in common with acne. For example, acne is often confused with rosacea, which is a serious diagnostic error since its medical management is so different. What works well in acne will often be harmful in rosacea. To the inexperienced, almost any eruption on the face of a young person is likely to be perfunctorily labeled acne; the result is inappropriate therapy at least, and harmful interventions at worst. Accordingly, differential diagnosis has been a primary concern throughout this volume.

Myths and fictions invariably grow up around chronic, stubborn disorders. As regards the causes and treatment of the acnes, these are plentiful. Patients commonly entertain notions which are wrong and even ridiculous. A remarkable collection of folkloristic beliefs have been passed on to us regarding the role of diet, sex, and emotions. These are matched by a long list of therapeutic nostrums which are not only useless, but even harmful. The first interview should broadly cover the patient's beliefs and past practices. Doctors who are in a hurry should not treat acne, since sympathetic counseling after careful history taking markedly influences the therapeutic outcome, and a caring attitude promotes trust and compliance. Unlike many infectious disorders such as syphilis, acne cannot be cured by an injection or a short course of antibiotics. The doctor has to make a convincing effort to become a therapeutic partner. Too few patients and physicians are fully aware of the tremendous advances in acne treatment at all stages of the disease. Experienced surgeons can routinely bring about dramatic improvements in the most horridly scarred and disfigured patients. Patients need to be told about these wonderful resources to overcome despair and resignation. Before and after photos will generally excite the most skeptical patients.

It is our intention to cover acne and acne-type disorders thoroughly, with an emphasis on clinical practice. Contention and controversy is a notable feature of acne literature. The reader will find that we often disagree with the orthodox concepts enshrined in textbooks. We express our own views firmly, while acknowledging different opinions. This text is not intended to be a manual for researchers. Our central goal is to teach physicians how to treat the various forms of acne more effectively. There is hardly ever a case which lies beyond therapeutic reach. Getting acne under control is one of the great satisfactions of medical practice.

The reader will note that we are therapeutic optimists and naturally biased towards our own management strategies. The last word on acne has not yet been written. We proffer here instead the good word, the good news, which we hope will find its way into common practice. Finally, we wish to emphasize that the references we have cited have been carefully selected. We apologize for unwitting omisssions of important works. Those who wish a complete review of the literature must make use of other sources of information.

GERD PLEWIG, Munich
ALBERT M. KLIGMAN, Philadelphia
1993

Contents

The Acnes

Acneiform Diseases

XIV

Acknowledgments

Many highly skilled professionals have generously helped us to create this book. Our gratitude for their superb collaboration is acknowledged herewith. Our thanks are small recompense for their indispensable contributions. We are especially grateful to those who have enriched this volume with their technical expertise:

Mr. WILFRIED NEUSE, photodesigner and enthusiastic photographer, Department of Dermatology, Heinrich-Heine-University of Düsseldorf.

Mr. PETER BILEK, a master of photography, Department of Dermatology, Ludwig-Maximilians-University of Munich.

Dr. med. THOMAS JANSEN, Department of Dermatology, Ludwig-Maximilians-University of Munich, meticulously supervised with enthusiastic endorsement the composition of this book, including typing, language editing, literature research, and reviewing of many chapters. Without his expert advice, the publication of this book would not have been possible.

Cand. med. JULIANE HABIG, student of the Ludwig-Maximilians-University of Munich, generously gave up her time and provided outstanding editorial help.

Dr. rer. nat. CHRISTEL BLUHM, Düsseldorf, carefully assisted with typing, language editing, references, and proofreading. She contributed parts of the chapter on epidermal lipids and sebaceous glands.

Dr. med. JOHANNES HOLLMANN, Department of Dermatology, Ludwig-Maximilians-University of Munich, also contributed parts of the chapter on epidermal lipids and sebaceous glands.

Cand. med. MARTIN FLUER and cand. med. WIDO BARNSTORF, students of the Heinrich-Heine-University of Düsseldorf, painstakingly put text and references into the computers, enduring the authors' seemingly endless corrections.

Miss ELFRIEDE JANUSCHKE, Department of Dermatology, Ludwig-Maximilians-University of Munich, a very experienced medical technician, who made available to us the powers of the electron microscope.

Mrs. GUDRUN KUTTER, Munich, a freelance graphic designer, who has been very helpful since the 1975 and 1978 editions of this book in regard to the artwork and reproduction of all illustrations. She contributed some beautiful illustrations.

THE DEUTSCHE FORSCHUNGSGEMEINSCHAFT has generously supported dermatologic investigations on which we have drawn heavily in presenting this account.

Mr. LES RILEY, President of Ortho Pharmaceutical Corporation, Rantan, New Jersey, USA, provided financial support without which we could not have achieved such a richly illustrated volume. His help was unstinting.

The clinical photographs and the electron microscopic pictures were superbly reproduced by BROS. CZECH and PARTNERS, a Munich offset company.

The histopathology plates were superbly set by REPRO TEAM PLC, a Munich lithographic studio.

Most of the microphotography was done on an OLYMPUS AH-2 autofocus photomicroscope, the remaining microphotographs on ZEISS LUMINAR equipment.

Dr. J. WIECZOREK, Dr.Dr. V. GEBHARDT, Mr. W. BISCHOFF, and Ms. A. HEPPER, Springer-Verlag Heidelberg, once again expertly handled the publication of this book.

Many friends and colleagues throughout the world lent us some of their illustrations; they are acknowledged in the legends to the plates.

Finally, we acknowledge our indebtedness to a corps of collaborators who shared their thoughts and feelings with us on innumerable occasions. They are too numerous to name. We shall have to be content with mentioning the members of our immediate family: JAMES J. LEYDEN, Professor of Dermatology and KENNETH J. MCGINLEY, both of the Department of Dermatology, University of Pennsylvania, USA.

GERD PLEWIG, Munich
ALBERT M. KLIGMAN, Philadelphia
1993

ACNE

A Précis of Pathogenesis

Acne is the pleomorphic disease par excellence. Its expressions are multifarious and eloquent. Students dispute its causation, histopathology, pathophysiology – in fact, everything but its existence.

Acne flourishes in adolescence, beginning in prepuberty and dying away when the threshold of early adulthood is crossed. Almost no individual makes the transit through adolescence without a few comedones or pustules. The prevalence is, therefore, close to 100%, individuals differing only in severity of expression. Only 10% of adults recall having acne, but surveys among adolescents show more than an 80% incidence of manifest disease. Most commonly, therefore, acne is rather trivial, though a single "pimple" may be irksome and four may precipitate panic on important occasions.

Causation

Acne has no cause in the sense that tuberculosis or phenylketonuria has a cause. No single feature is present or absent that distinguishes the acne patient. Acne is universal in adolescents though remains unnoticed in most; therefore differences are merely quantitative, not qualitative. All members of the adolescent population can be distributed along a continuum according to the severity of their acne. Severity is the result of many intrinsic factors acting in concert. The sum of the individual strengths of these factors determines whether the individual will have acne *minor* or acne *major*. Each factor is an absolute prerequisite, without which the process sinks below clinical visibility. Extrinsic factors merely modify the expression of the disease.

Sebum

Sebum fuels the acne flame. Adult levels of sebum output are an absolute prerequisite for the development of the disease. Castrates do not get acne. Measures which reduce sebum production – estrogens, X-rays, and antiandrogens – invariably moderate the disease. No other factor can be so convincingly correlated with severity. Severe acne is always associated with intense seborrhea; conversely, when sebum production is very low, the disease has a correspondingly low profile.

Hormones

Acne vulgaris is not an endocrine disorder. The general belief is that there are neither deficiencies, excesses, nor imbalances. However, normal circulating levels of androgens from the gonads and adrenals are absolute requirements. Without a source of androgens, the sebaceous glands remain small.

In addition, adrenal glucocorticosteroids play a collaborative role. They potentiate the effects of androgens and in particular they influence "end-organ" sensitivity. They influence the capacity of the follicle to form comedones.

Bacteria

Only one organism, *Propionibacterium acnes*, can be implicated, and that only indirectly. It is not virulent in the same sense that *Staphylococcus aureus* causes furunculosis. It does not invade living tissue. It multiplies only within the follicular canal. Its products, however, mediate the formation of comedones and contribute to their rupture.

Heredity

Heredity plays an important role in determining the size and activity of sebaceous glands. When both parents have scarred faces, one can predict trouble for the offspring. In identical twins, concordance for acne is very high, including distribution and severity. While formal epidemiologic studies are lacking, acne bears all the hallmarks of a polygenic disease, that is to say, simple Mendelian ratios are not found, and the expressions are variable and are influenced by external factors.

Reactivity

The predisposition to acne, the "X" factor so to speak, resides in the skin itself. The anatomical and physiological characteristics of the target organ, the sebaceous follicle, is the most important determinant of severity. Acne-bearing skin is more permeable. The pilosebaceous units are larger, and substances can gain ingress more easily through follicular shunts. Chemicals which cause follicular reactions have greater effects in acne patients. Pustules are easily provoked by croton oil topically and potassium iodide topically or orally.

The follicular epithelium is more reactive to all agencies, chemical and physical. It is sensitively programmed to respond to various comedogenic substances, of which sebum is the natural prototype.

Cunliffe WJ (1989) Acne. Dunitz, London

Frank SB (ed) (1979) Acne. Update for the practitioner. Yorke Medical Books, New York

Kligman AM (1974) An overview of acne. J Invest Dermatol 62:268–287

Plewig G, Kligman AM (1975) Acne. Morphogenesis and treatment. Springer, Berlin Heidelberg New York

Randazzo SD (1991) Acne in the history of dermatology. J Appl Cosmetol 9:43–53

Stern RS (1992) The prevalence of acne on the basis of physical examination. J Am Acad Dermatol 26:931–935

Strauss JS, Pochi PE, Downing DT (1974) Acne: perspectives. J Invest Detmatol 62:321–325

The Anatomy of Follicles

Acne is a dermatosis that is strictly confined to hair follicles. It cannot be understood without a detailed knowledge of the structure of the *pilosebaceous unit*.

Three kinds of follicles occur on the face: vellus, sebaceous, and terminal. The drama of acne unfolds entirely in sebaceous follicles. These are limited to the face, ear lobes, neck, shoulders, upper V-shaped areas of the chest and back, and the lateral parts of the upper arms. It is this above all which determines the distribution of acne to these very regions. Sebaceous follicles are most numerous and largest on the face and are more elaborately structured there than elsewhere. Therefore, acne is chiefly a facial disease though some of the worst expressions of the disorder occur on the back. It will be instructive to see just how facial follicles differ. Acne in its full expression is a disorder peculiar to humans since comparable sebaceous follicles do not exist in animals.

Beard follicles on the face of men are typical terminals follicles. The hair is stiff, thick, and long. Its diameter is wide enough to occupy almost the entire lumen of the canal. Because of its stiffness and its steady growth, the hair can keep the canal free of horny debris, hence acne does not occur in terminal follicles. The only one exception to this is acne inversa, which originates from terminal follicles.

In terminal follicles, sebaceous glands empty their contents into the follicular canal via short ducts. The region above their insertion is called the *infundibulum*. It is lined by an epithelium which produces sturdy, well-differentiated horny cells similar to those of the adjacent epidermis. Consequently, the horny layer of the infundibulum possesses barrier properties. Substances cannot readily diffuse across this membrane except at the thinnest portion below. The horny cells desquamate continuously and invisibly through the orifice.

Vellus follicles are miniatures of terminal ones with disproportionately large sebaceous glands. On the face, they are about three to four times more numerous than sebaceous follicles and accordingly contribute appreciably to the pool of surface lipids. The hairs and orifices of vellus follicles are very tiny and can scarcely be seen with the naked eye. Vellus follicles are not targets for acne lesions.

Sebaceous follicles have special characteristics which make them specifically vulnerable to acne. The canal is deep and cavernous. The pilary unit is tiny and inconspicuous. It produces a wispy hair whose width is less than one-fifth to one-tenth that of the internal diameter of the canal. It is virtually lost in the huge lumen. The sebaceous glands are exceptionally large, multilobulated and enter via short ducts into the bottom of the canal. These features, large, multilobulated glands, deep, cavernous canals, and puny hairs give the sebaceous follicle its individuality.

But it is the peculiar qualities of the infundibulum which provide insight for understanding the structural events in the pathogenesis of acne. Their terminal portion, for which we have created the term *acro*infundibulum, is similar to the infundibulum of terminal follicles, extending downwards about 200 µm. It keratinizes like the contiguous epidermis and functions as a barrier. Below this the epithelium has exceptional properties. We have called this portion the *infra*infundibulum. It makes up the greatest part of the epithelial lining of the sebaceous follicle. It keratinizes, too, but produces only a thin, inconsequential, horny layer whose cells soon slough. The desquamated corneocytes are fragile and imperfect; many break open and lose part of their contents. They stain poorly, the cell outlines are ill defined, and they are not well organized or are actually in disarray. In consequence, a loose mass of horny detritus occupies the canal. The sturdy laminae of a true stratum corneum are lacking in the infrainfundibulum. The granular layer can barely be made out, being generally one cell layer thick with tiny granules. Unlike normal epidermis periodic acid-Schiff (PAS) staining discloses glycogen granules in many of the Malpighian cells.

The epithelium of the sebaceous ducts keratinizes in much the same way, producing empty-looking, flimsy, horny cells which float up into the canal in a stream of sebum. In this way, separate streams of keratinized cells are created which correspond to the number of sebaceous ducts. These are more evident in horizontal sections and help explain some easily overlooked features of the internal structure of comedones. The canal itself contains chiefly a mixture of sloughed corneocytes and sebum. When frozen or fixed thick sections are stained for bacteria, a variable number of follicles show masses of gram-positive diphtheroids, which can be visualized histologically only when colonization is very dense. These bacteria-rich follicles comprise sebaceous filaments (seborrheic filaments, follicular casts). When the contents of such follicles are expelled by pressure, cheesy, waxy, whitish, worm-like structures emerge. Culture and smears identify them as virtually pure colonies of *Propionibacterium acnes*.

The sebaceous filament contains a core of lipid and bacteria encased in a cylinder of coherent horny cells.

Kligman AM (1974) An overview of acne. J Invest Dermatol 62:268–287

Cunliffe WJ, Perera WDH, Thackray P, Williams M, Forster RA, Williams SM (1976) Pilo-sebaceous duct physiology. III. Observations on the number and size of pilo-sebaceous ducts in acne vulgaris. Br J Dermatol 95:153–156

Lavker RM, Leyden JJ, McGinley KJ (1981) The relationship between bacteria and the abnormal follicular keratinization in acne vulgaris. J Invest Dermatol 77:325–330

Plewig G (1974) Follicular keratinization. J Invest Dermatol 62:308–315

Facial Pores

Ordinarily only the orifices of the sebaceous follicles are visible. The more numerous vellus follicles are too small to be seen. The diameter of the pore is roughly proportionate to the size of the pilosebaceous unit; hence people with oily skin and large glands tend to have larger pores. Wide orifices contribute to a coarse appearance and texture.

Above   Cheek of a young man who had moderate acne. The pores are conspicuous. The larger irregular depressions are small scars. The skin is obviously oily

Below   Cheek of a young woman without acne. One can barely make out the pores. The skin is nonoily

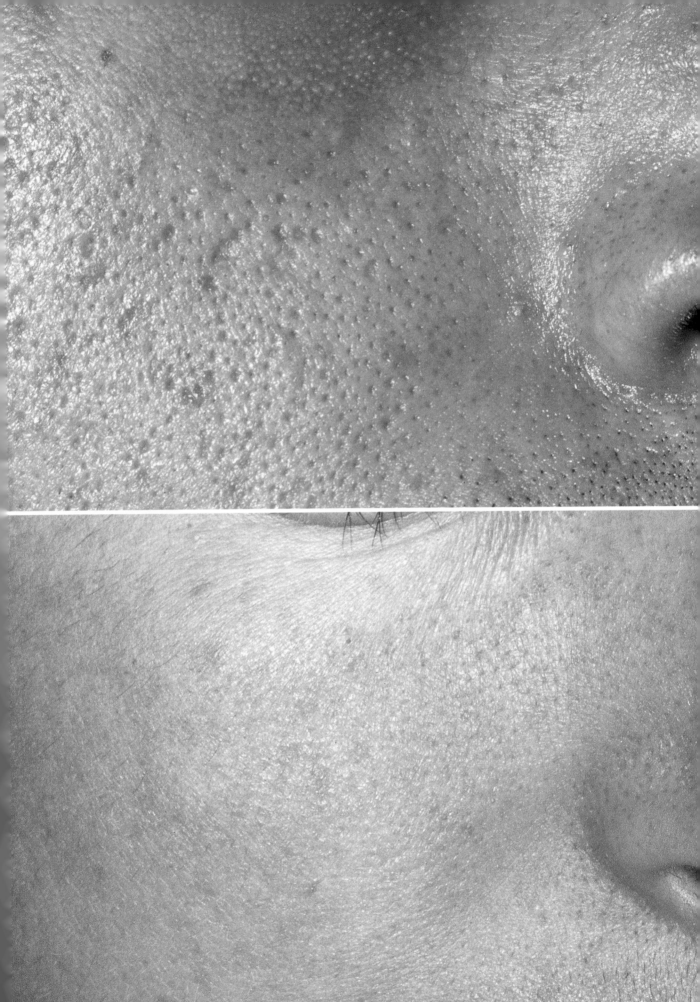

The Pilosebaceous Unit: The Stage Setting

These sketches illustrate the architecture and size differences of the three types of facial follicles.

Left   Vellus follicle. These are very numerous. Their sebaceous lipids contribute to the surface lipids but are mere bystanders in acne

Middle   Sebaceous follicle. This is the theater where the drama of acne is performed. The sebaceous glands are large and multilobular. The puny hair is a flimsy thread in the huge canal which is filled with loose keratinized cells. The sketch shows an anagen follicle

Right   Terminal beard hair. The stiff, thick hair fills up the canal. Acne ignores these follicles, except in acne inversa

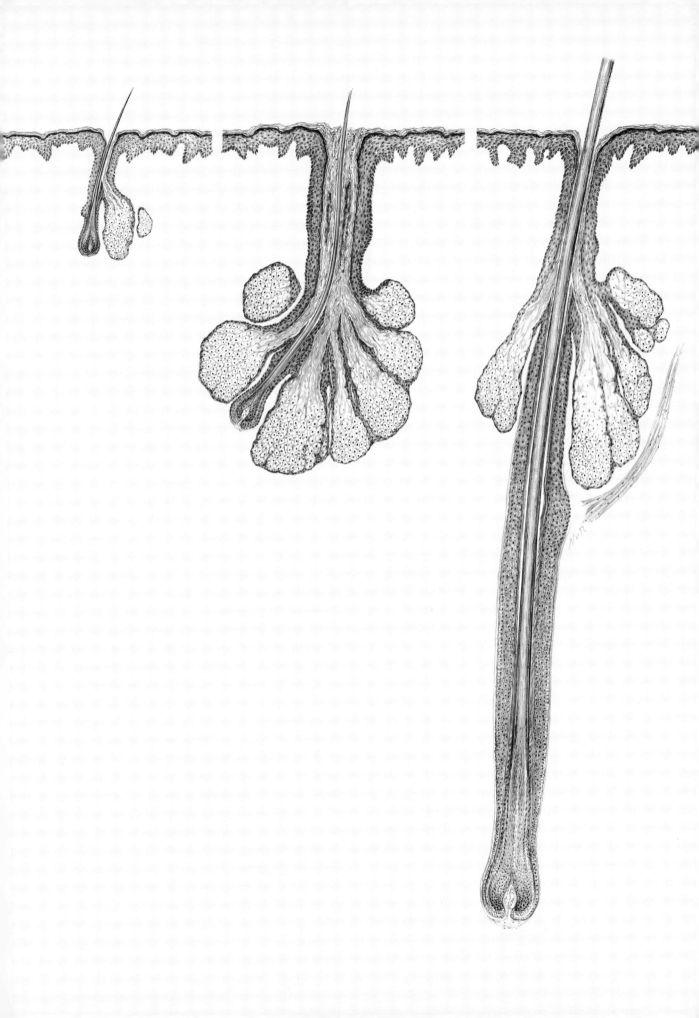

Sebaceous Follicles of Back and Face

No single sebaceous follicle seems to be identical to the next one. Furthermore sebaceous follicles of the back differ from those of the face.

Above   Sebaceous follicles of the back

Left   One normal sebaceous follicle with an acroinfundibulum containing *Pityrosporum ovale* yeasts, the infrainfundibulum, the pilary portion (peripherally cut in this section), and two large sebaceous acini draining sebum through sebaceous ducts

Right   Sebaceous follicles have one hair apparatus. The thin brownish hair seems to be lost in the spacious infundibulum. Most of the corneocytes from the follicular canal got lost during sectioning

Below   Sebaceous follicles of the face

Left   The follicular canal is wide and filled with horny cells. The epithelium has a well-pronounced granular layer. The puny hair is cut tangentially twice. The sebaceous acini are numerous, and all lobules shown here drain into this follicle

Right   A tortuous sebaceous follicle. Melanin pigment is produced in the epidermis and in the acroinfundibulum, but not below it. The tiny hair is cut once. Five sebaceous lobules belong to this unit, some of which are located above the draining sebaceous ducts. The contents of the follicular canal corresponds to the waxy worms that can be squeezed out from facial skin

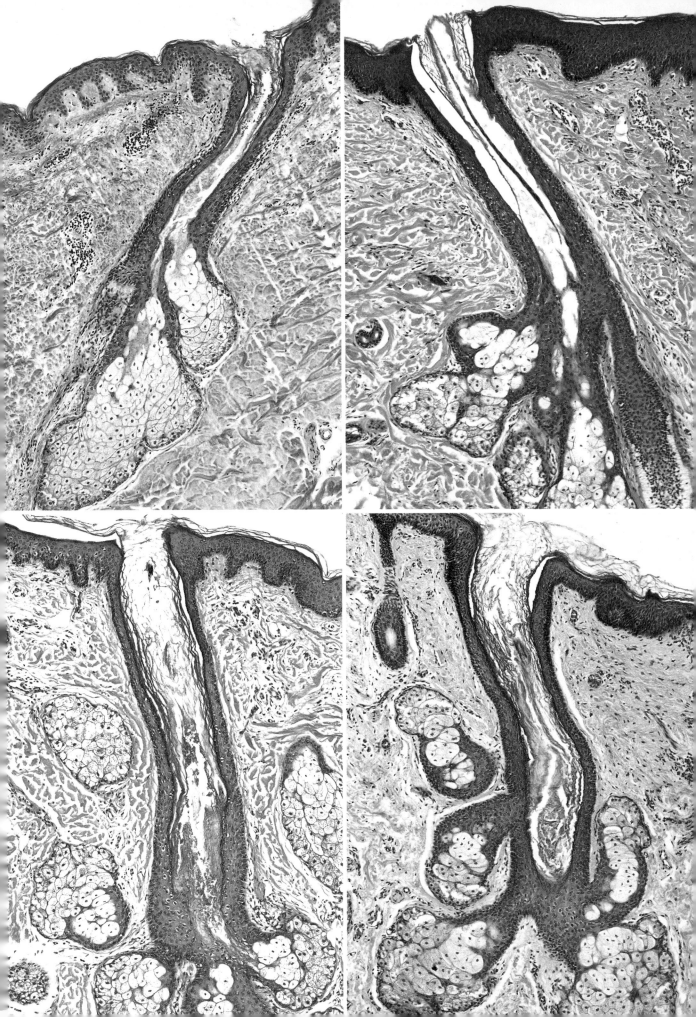

A Descent into Follicles

Normal-appearing skin from a young man with ongoing mild acne (a–c), and a man without acne (d–f) was serially cut in a horizontal fashion.

a Close to the skin surface

An acroinfundibulum of a sebaceous follicle with pigment in the basal cell layer, a sebaceous filament and one hair (→). To the left is a vellus follicle with its tiny sebaceous gland

b Midinfundibulum

The follicular canal is distended by a well-developed sebaceous filament with a central chamber full of bacteria. The sebaceous duct (✱), partly keratinized, is about to merge with the follicular canal. The hair (→) also joins at this triangular point

c Level of sebaceous glands

Two sebaceous acini belong to this follicle, one showing its sebaceous duct. The pilary unit (→) is still outside the sebaceous duct and infundibulum

d Close to the skin surface

An acroinfundibulum with some melanin pigment in the basal cell layer. A sebaceous filament, two hairs (→), and a bacteria-filled cavity are seen. The two hairs are from one pilary unit (trichostasis). To the right is a much smaller vellus follicle with one hair

e Midinfundibulum

The follicular canal contains a filament with two cavernas filled with bacteria. The hair (→) is just joining the canal. A sebaceous acinus is to the right

f Level of sebaceous gland

One sebaceous lobule with multiple trabeculae and undifferentiated cells (o→) in close association with the pilary structure (→)

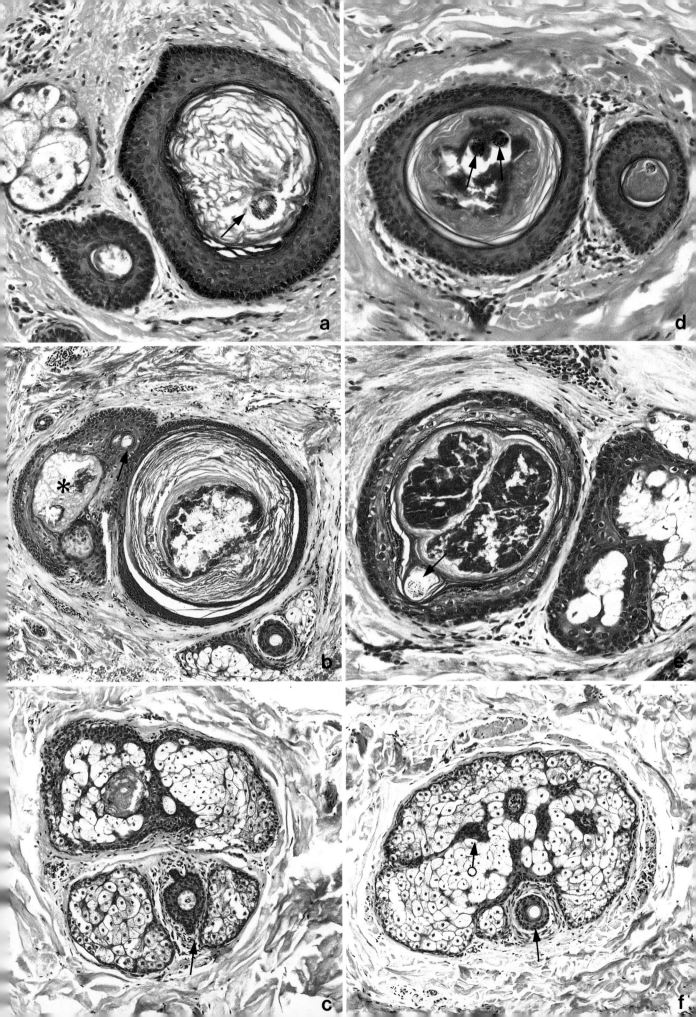

Comparative Anatomy of Adnexa from Face and Upper Back

The sections are approximately 0.5 mm below the skin surface. The photographs were taken at the same magnification.

Above   Forehead. Abundant vellus follicles (→) and sebaceous follicles (→). The latter have a spacious follicular canal and larger sebaceous glands. The small vellus hair follicles are about five times more numerous than the sebaceous follicles

Below   Lower back. Sebaceous follicles are very few in numbers, only one unit with the pilary portion above and the sebaceous acinus below is seen in this cut. Considering the number of skin adnexa, the face can be compared to an oasis, the back to a desert. Therefore the face is often oily, the back rarely

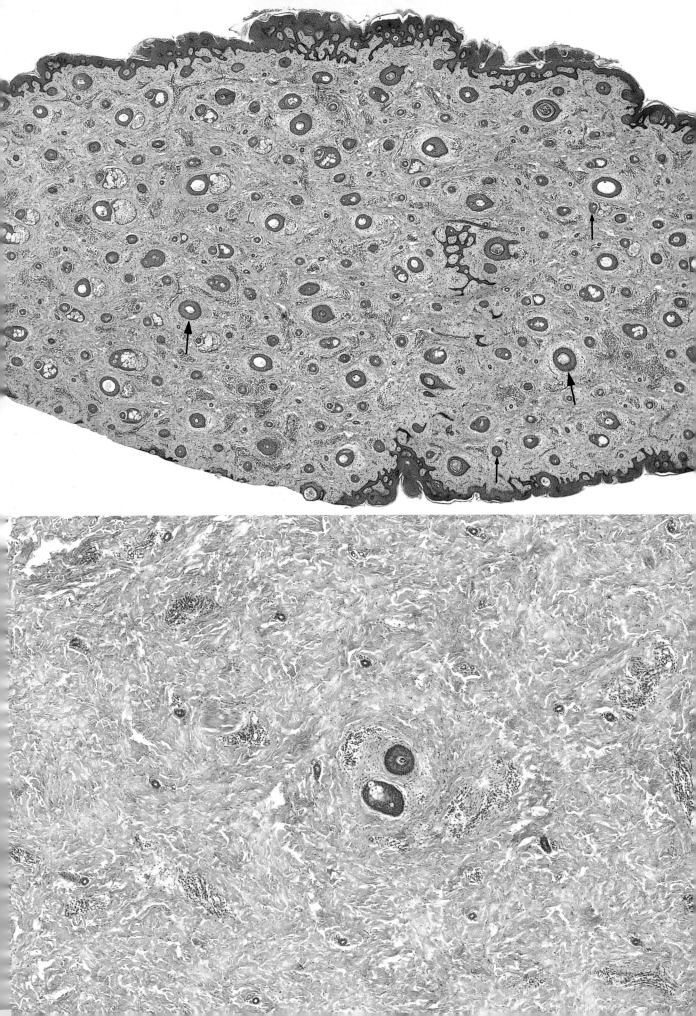

Follicular Filaments and Microcomedones

Follicular filaments (sebaceous filaments, follicular casts) are physiological elements and not part of the acne spectrum, whereas microcomedones present incipient acne lesions.

Above   Follicular filaments

Left   A sebaceous follicle from the back filled with a cocoon of corneocytes. The sebaceous glands below constantly soak the filament with sebum

Right   The follicular filament consists of about 30 layers of corneocytes, encompassing a matrix of sebum and dense colonies of *Propionibacterium acnes*. The follicular epithelium has a well-developed stratum granulosum. This is not a microcomedo as the accumulation of corneocytes is not large enough. A perpetuous self-cleaning mechanism keeps this follicle well-balanced

Below

Left   A microcomedo. This type of lesion is clinically not visible. The epithelium is acanthotic, with hypergranulosis, and rapidly producing coherent corneocytes, which are no longer discharged through the orifice above. The proliferation-retention hyperkeratosis distends the infundibulum. Usually dense colonies of *Propionibacterium acnes* are present, not seen in this particular section. One sebaceous acinus is attached to the lower left

Right   Horizontal cut through a follicular filament. This could be the horizontal counterpart to the vertical section above right. The follicular epithelium shows a stratum granulosum and encases a filament of corneocytes. The chambers are full of *Propionibacterium acnes*; one tiny brownish hair is below

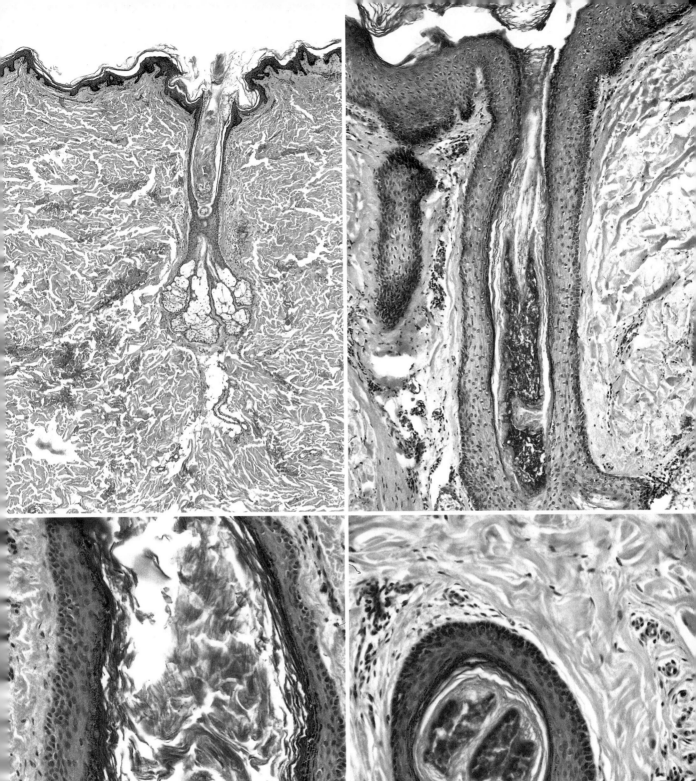
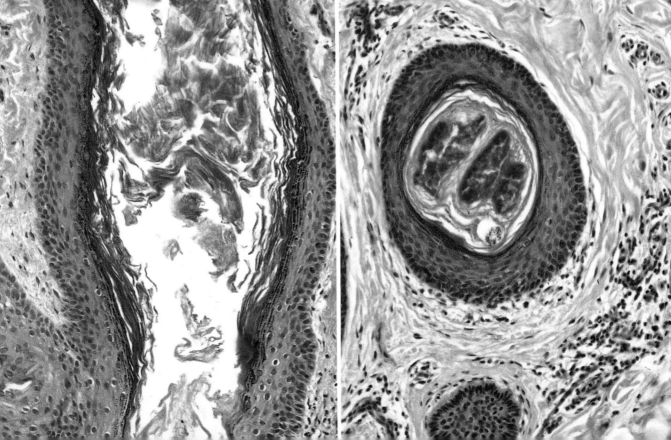

Scanning Electron-Microscopic Overview
of a Sebaceous Follicle

Rarely can one see the full architectural pattern of a sebaceous follicle. Sections of this extent are not easily obtained. This in the midportion of a normal sebaceous follicle from the back of a young man. The follicular epithelium is in the upper right and lower left corners. The hair with its cuticule is in the center. About 15 layers of corneocytes line the epithelium; the outermost layers detach and desquamate in an amalgam of sebum. One cannot see bacteria in this section, although present elsewhere in the follicle. (Electron microscopy, $\times 4000$)

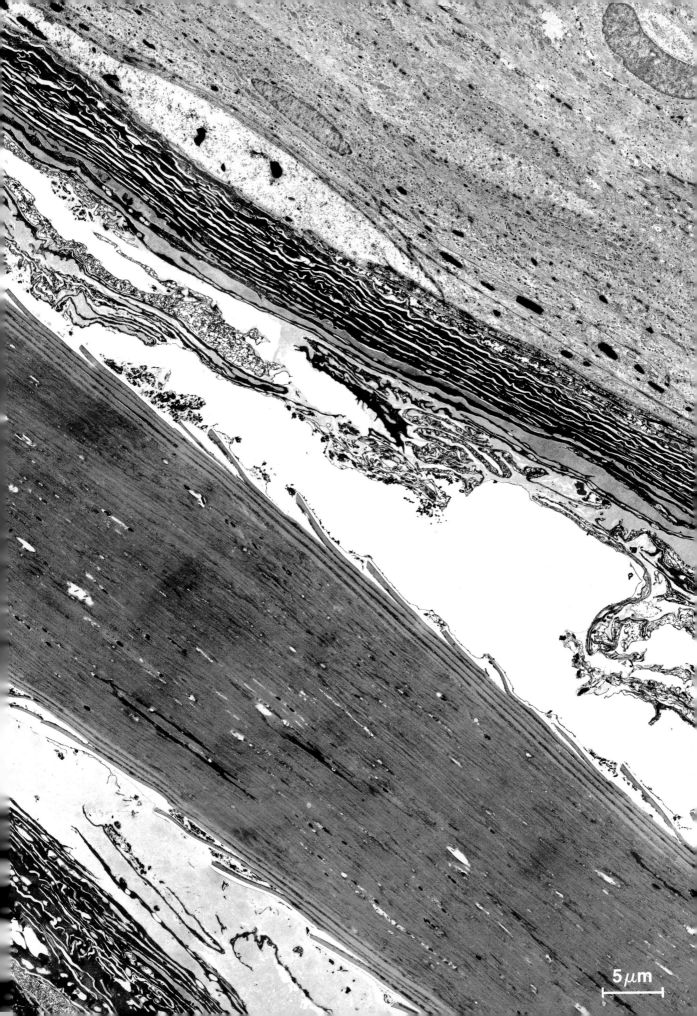

5 μm

Sampling of Follicles
by the Cyanoacrylate Technique

Cyanoacrylate, also known as crazy glue, is a quick-setting polymer which rips off the outermost layers of the stratum corneum, to which are attached vellus hairs and the horny casts within the upper regions of sebaceous follicles. This technique, sometimes referred to as the follicular biopsy, offers a splendid way to collect the contents of sebaceous follicles for a variety of studies, including: (1) density and size of microcomedones, and casts, quantifiable by image analysis; (2) presence and abundance of *Demodex folliculorum* mites; (3) follicular density of *Pityrosporum ovale* and *Propionibacterium acnes*; (4) presence of fascicles of hairs (trichostasis spinulosa); and (5) composition of lipids within microcomedones. The specimens shown here are mounted in immersion oil.

Above

The inset shows the outermost sheet of stratum corneum removed on a glass slide. On the forehead of a healthy person, the vellus hairs are single and not encased in horny material

Below

Left Two sebaceous filaments. A hair is sheathed in a semi-firm mass of corneocytes which thins out toward the root. The presence of only one hair per horny cast indicates that there is no real obstruction. This specimen was from the cheek of an acne patient in whom these follicular casts are typically numerous and thick. They indicate a predisposition to the formation of comedones, corresponding to the clinical picture of large pores and oiliness

Right Microcomedo. Here there are two hairs, the tip of one being barely visible. These are encased in a thick, solid mass of corneocytes, which have begun to distend the follicle. Comedones larger than this, that is closed comedones, are too firmly anchored to be removed by this technique

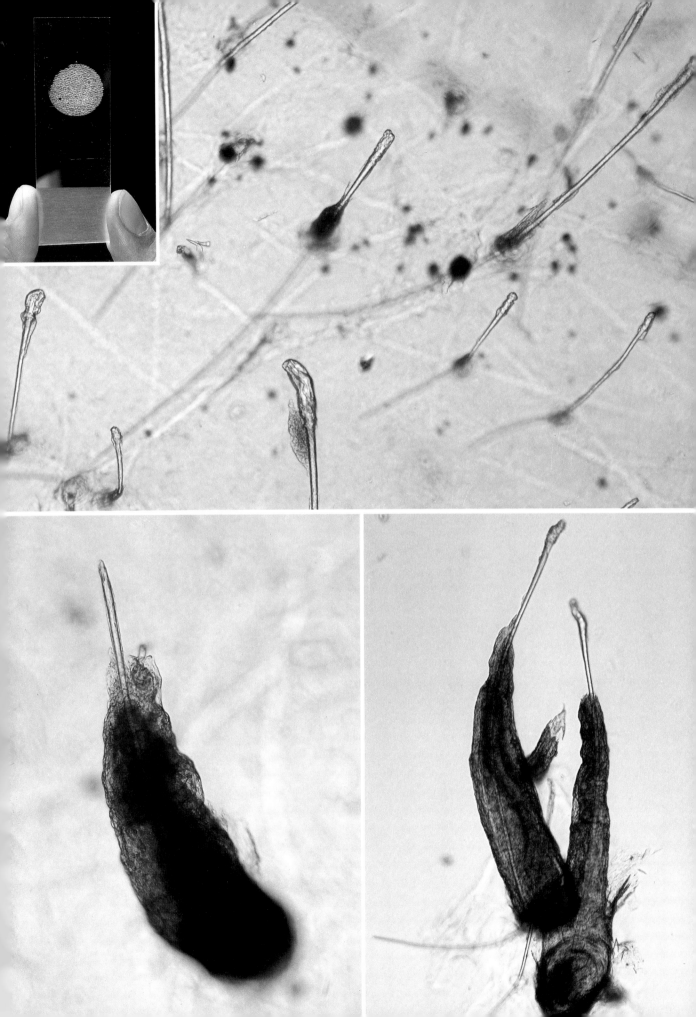

Noninvolved Skin of an Acne Patient:
A Horizontal View

A biopsy of noninvolved skin of the forehead was sectioned horizontally and photographed at the same magnification.

Several points are noteworthy:
- The densely arranged sebaceous and vellus follicles
- The follicular filaments in sebaceous follicles are full of bacteria
- The large sebaceous acini of sebaceous follicles
- The pilary portion associated with each follicle
- The lingering lymphohistiocytic infiltrate

Above

Left   Close to the skin surface, there are many vellus follicles (→) between sebaceous follicles (→). Sebaceous acini are not at this level

Right   Hair papillae and small sebaceous acini (○→) of vellus follicles are present next to spacious infundibula of sebaceous follicles

Below

Left   Level of sebaceous acini of sebaceous follicles. The glands are large and multilobulated (○→). Sebaceous ducts (✱) and cross-sections of hairs (→).

Right   Lower level of sebaceous acini with the pilary portion still mostly outside the glands (→). Perivascular and peribulbar lymphohistiocytic infiltrate is present

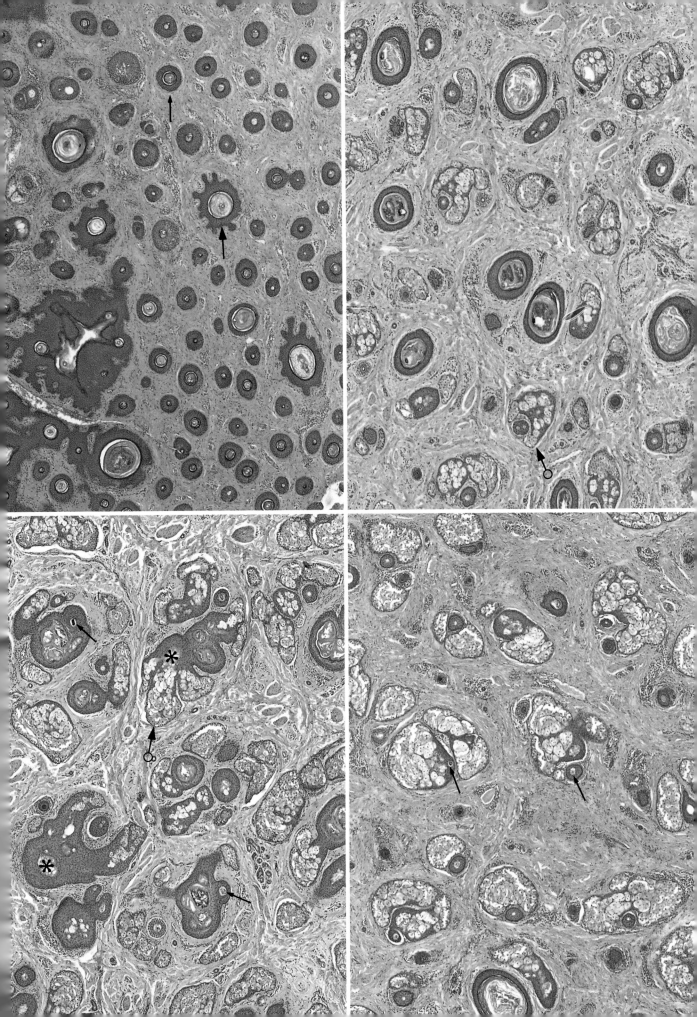

Epidermal Lipids

The lipids synthesized by the epidermis have a composition quite different from sebaceous lipids and serve an entirely different function, principally as a barrier to water loss and the inward diffusion of toxic chemicals.

Epidermal Lipids in Plants and Animals

In most higher terrestrial plants, water is found mainly in the leaves which are covered with a multilayered cuticle rich in lipids. These are usually long-chain, nonpolar hydrocarbons, predominantly *n*-alkanes, but also branched alkanes, wax esters, free fatty acids, and alcohols. Waxes are also deposited on the surface and contribute to the barrier.

In arthropods, the cuticle is similar to that in higher plants. The outermost layer, the epicuticle, is especially rich in lipids and provides the principal barrier. About 80% of the extractable surface lipids are nonpolar hydrocarbons containing *n*-alkanes, wax or alkyl esters, free fatty acids, cholesterol, and free alcohols. There is increasing evidence that the heterogeneous mixture of lipids plays the most important role in barrier function and may be supplemented by proteins and sugars.

Cholesterol should be mentioned particularly because it cannot be synthesized by these insects and therefore must be taken up with their diet. The fact that cholesterol is nevertheless always invariably present indicates that it must have a special function in the arthropod cuticle, e.g., the control of water permeability.

In birds, lipids contribute in two ways to the barrier between the inner sphere of the organism and the environment. Birds spread lipid secretions from the uropygial gland over their feathers, thus preventing water penetration and enabling waterfowl to swim. On the other hand, the avian epidermis actively secretes lipids. These are extruded from membrane-bound droplets within upper epidermal cells into the intercellular spaces of the stratum corneum. Neutral lipids (triacylglycerols, sterol esters, free fatty acids, and hydrocarbons) represent about two-thirds of the total stratum corneum lipids in birds; 25% are sphingolipids (ceramides and glycosphingolipids), and 8% phospholipids. There are many analogies to the mammalian epidermis strongly indicating that this mixture forms the water barrier.

In mammals, lipids constitute approximately 10%–14% of the dry weight of the epidermis. Mainly they consist of fatty acids, cholesterol, and ceramides and lower amounts of phospholipids, cholesterol sulfate, and triglycerides. Their composition varies depending on the cell layer. For example, phospholipids which contain large amounts of unsaturated fatty acids, including linoleic acid and arachidonic acid, predominate in lower cell layers. They are reduced in granular cells and are present in only very small amounts in the stratum corneum. In experiments with rodents it could be shown that linoleic acid, an essential fatty acid, is of great importance for epidermal barrier function. Feeding the rodents with a linoleic acid-free diet resulted in an excessive transepidermal water loss. Unlike birds, mammals possess sebaceous glands, which might be regarded as analogous to the uropygial gland. Nevertheless, the sebaceous lipids do not play a significant role in barrier function.

Epidermal Lipids in Humans

The stratum corneum is a highly differentiated storage and barrier system without which a person would lose about 20 l water transepidermally every day. It also protects the organism from injurious chemical and physical noxae. The lipids of the stratum corneum play a critical role in providing a barrier function and enhancing the water-binding capacity. Human stratum corneum lipids are similar to those of rodents and pigs. All three orders abundantly display sphingolipids, free sterols, and free fatty acids as well as lesser quantities of phospholipids, cholesterol sulfate, triglycerides, and sterol and wax esters. The *n*-alkanes which are present are probably of exogenous origin. In humans, long-chain fatty acids (C_{24} and greater) are exclusively contained in sphingolipids.

Intercellular lipids are synthesized in the Golgi apparatus of the prickle cells of the stratum spinosum and stored in keratinosomes, the so-called lamellar or Odland bodies. In the uppermost layer of the stratum granulosum, these organelles fuse with the cell membrane and secrete their lipid-containing, fine-lamellar material into the intercellular spaces. There, they are reorganized into broad multilamellar layers 4–6 nm in thickness. The secretion of keratinosomal lipids into the intercorneocyte space of the stratum

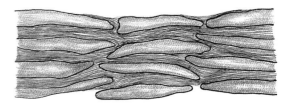

The brick and mortar model

corneum results in a compartimentization into lipid-poor, hydrophilic corneocytes and a hydrophobic matrix rich in neutral lipids.

The stratum corneum is currently considered to be a two compartment system consisting of corneocytes (*bricks*) and intercellular lipids (*mortar*). The stratum corneum lipids are well-ordered throughout the bulk of the membrane, except near the surface. The amount of intercellular lipid per layer decreases with increasing distance from the surface. Corneocytes near the surface have widened intercellular spaces rich in lipids, while deeper down the intercellular spaces are much smaller. Compared to the deeper layers, the outer few layers appear less cohesive, and their intercellular lipids looser and more disrupted. These layers next to the surface finally comprise the desquamating zone.

Qualitative and quantitative changes in the composition of epidermal lipids occur during differentiation. In the basal layers phospholipids, which are necessary for the formation of the cellular membrane, are present in abundance, while during keratinization neutral lipids and sphingolipids increase. These are important for the assembly and stabilization of the lamellar sheets of the stratum corneum.

Increasing amounts of sphingolipids appear as the cells mature, with about 7% in the basal cell layers and 26% in the outer stratum corneum. These compounds, which in the human organism are otherwise only found in the central

27

Structural formulas of major epidermal lipids

Glycerine phosphatides

Phosphatidylcholine

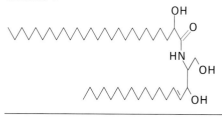

Ceramides

Ceramide 1

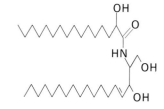

Ceramide 2

Ceramide 3

Ceramide 4

Ceramide 5

Ceramide 6I

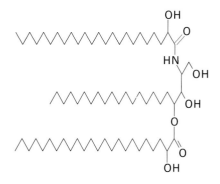

Ceramide 6II

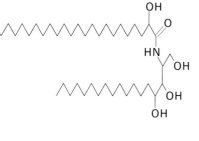

Terpenoids and Sterols

Squalene

Cholesterol

HO

Cholesterol sulfate

O—S—O
O
O

Cholesterol ester

O
C—O

Free fatty acids

Oleic acid

O
C—OH

Linoleic acid

O
C—OH

Triglycerides

Tripalmitylglycerine

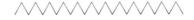

O
H₂C—O—C

O
C—O—CH

O
H₂C—O—C

N-Alkenes

N-Pentacosane

nervous system, consist of sphingomyelin, glucosylceramides, and ceramides. The ceramides increase proportionally in stratum corneum, while glucosylceramides decrease. Ceramides are most important for barrier function and the water-binding capacity of the stratum corneum.

Six structurally different ceramide fractions have been identified so far in human stratum corneum. They consist of the aminoalcohols sphingosine or phytosphingosine that are bound to an amide-linked α-hydroxy fatty acid or nonhydroxy fatty acid, which are mainly saturated and branchless.

The ceramide 1 has a rather unusual structure compared with the other ceramides. It consists of a sphingosine base with an amide-linked long-chain ω-hydroxy fatty acid and an ester-linked nonhydroxy fatty acid, frequently linoleic acid, a twofold unsaturated essential fatty acid.

Because of their long hydrophobic hydrocarbon chains ceramides are presumably capable of forming intercellular lipid membranes, which account for the water permeability barrier of the stratum corneum. It appears that the ceramide 1 molecules serve as rivets for these lipid lamellar sheets, indicating therefore that ceramide 1 holds a key position in barrier function.

In the human epidermis, sterols are largely present as free cholesterol and to a much smaller proportion as cholesterol sulfate which also contributes to the integration of the lamellar lipid sheets of the stratum corneum. The continuous hydrolysis of cholesterol sulfate to cholesterol by the enzyme steroid sulfatase in the lower layers of the stratum corneum seems to be crucial for the destabilization of the lipid sheets and thus for the desquamation of corneocytes.

A malfunction of this mechanism is represented by an inherited disorder, the X-chromosomal recessive ichthyosis. A genetically induced decrease in the enzyme steroid sulfatase causes the concentration of cholesterol sulfate in the epidermis to increase and leads to the manifestation of a retention hyperkeratosis. The special function of the other epidermal lipids has not yet been definitely established.

Bommannan D, Potts RO, Guy RH (1990) Examination of stratum corneum barrier function in vivo by infrared spectroscopy. J Invest Dermatol 95:403–408

Bortz JT, Wertz PW, Downing DT (1989) The origin of alkanes found in human skin surface lipids. J Invest Dermatol 93:723–727

Elias PM (1983) Epidermal lipids, barrier function, and desquamation. J Invest Dermatol 80:44s–49s

Elias PM, Grayson S, Lampe MA, Williams ML, Brown BE (1983) The intercorneocyte space. In: Marks R, Plewig G (eds) Stratum corneum. Springer, Berlin Heidelberg New York, pp 53–67

Elias PM, Menon GK, Grayson S, Brown BE, Rehfeld SJ (1987) Avian sebokeratocytes and mammal lipokeratinocytes: structural, lipid biochemical, and functional considerations. Am J Anat 180:161–177

Freinkel RK (1987) Lipids of the epidermis. In: Fitzpatrick TB, Eisen AZ, Wolff K, Freedberg IM, Austen KF (eds) Dermatology in general medicine, 3rd edn. McGraw-Hill, New York, pp 191–194

Gray GM, White RJ (1978) Glycosphingolipids and ceramides in human and pig epidermis. J Invest Dermatol 70:336–341

Grubauer G, Feingold KR, Elias PM (1987) Relationship of epidermal lipogenesis to cutaneous barrier function. J Lipid Res 28:746–752

Hadley NF (1989) Lipid water barriers in biological systems. Progr Lipid Res 28:1–33

Lampe MA, Burlingame AL, Whitney JA, Williams ML, Brown BE, Roitman E, Elias PM (1983) Human stratum corneum lipids: characterization and regional variations. J Lipid Res 24:120–130

Lampe MA, Williams ML, Elias PM (1983) Human epidermal lipids: characterization and modulations during differentiation. J Lipid Res 24:131–140

Long SA, Wertz PW, Strauss JS, Downing DT (1985) Human stratum corneum polar lipids and desquamation. Arch Dermatol Res 277:284–287

Melnik B (1989) Epidermal lipids and the biochemistry of keratinization. In: Traupe H (ed) The ichthyoses. Springer, Berlin Heidelberg New York, pp 15–42

Proksch E (1990) Die Epidermis als metabolisch aktives Gewebe: Regelung der Lipidsynthese durch die Barrierefunktion. Z Hautkr 65:296–300

Proksch E (1992) Regulation der epidermalen Permeabilitätsbarriere durch Lipide und durch Hyperproliferation. Hautarzt 43:331–338

Schürer NY, Plewig G, Elias PM (1991) Stratum corneum lipid function. Dermatologica 183:77–94

Wertz PW (1992) Epidermal lipids. Semin Dermatol 11:106–113

Wertz PW, Cho ES, Downing DT (1983) Effect of essential fatty acid deficiency on the epidermal sphingolipids of the rat. Biochem Biophys Acta 753:350–355

Wertz PW, Miethke MC, Long SA, Strauss JS, Downing DT (1985) The composition of the ceramides from human stratum corneum and from comedones. J Invest Dermatol 84:410–412

Sebaceous Glands

Introduction

The pathogenesis of acne vulgaris cannot be understood without knowledge of the physiology of sebaceous glands. Nearly all acne patients suffer from seborrhea, excessive sebum production, although not all people with seborrhoea have acne. Acne does not occur when sebum output is low. The efficacy of sebosuppressive drugs such as isotretinoin, antiandrogens, and estrogens provides indirect evidence of the essential pathogenetic role of sebum. A familiar slogan says "sebum fuels the acne flame", which is true, if not exactly scientific.

Anatomy of Sebaceous Glands

With the exception of in the palms and the soles, sebaceous glands are found everywhere in human skin. Their number varies greatly in different body sites. For example, there are more than 800 sebaceous glands per square centimeter on the face and scalp, but less than 50 per square centimeter on the extremities.

The volume of these glands also varies considerably by region. They are largest on the head. In general, the greater the distance from the head, the smaller the glands become. However, their basic structure is the same everywhere. They vary from a single lobule to a complex multilobular structure which delivers sebum into a follicular canal via one or more excretory ducts. The sebaceous glands are surrounded by a capsule consisting of highly vascularized connective tissue from which small trabecules extend, subdividing each lobule into acini. With the exception of the specialized Meibomian glands human sebaceous glands are not innervated and function independently of nerve supply.

Based on the associated hair follicle, three types of sebaceous glands can be distinguished. The smallest ones are associated with fine vellus hairs; larger ones are components of the pilosebaceous units which hold the long, coarse terminal hairs, e.g., of the scalp; and finally, there are huge sebaceous follicles, exclusively found in humans. The products of the giant multilobulated glands of the latter flow into a deep, wide canal to which a tiny, trivial hair unit is attached. These sebaceous gland follicles are particularly abundant in the face, ear canal, V-shaped parts of the chest and back, and on the sides of the upper arms. They are the stage on which the drama of acne is performed. Other mammals lack sebaceous follicles and hence never develop acne.

Histologically sebaceous glands consist of two cell types, sebocytes and the cells of the excretory duct. Sebocytes synthesize sebum, a complex mixture mainly of lipids and small quantities of keratin and cell debris. Secretion of these products is holocrine, i.e., occurs by death of the matured swollen cells full of lipid droplets. Cell reproduction takes place in the basal layer, which is located at the circumference of the sebaceous acini, just above the basement membrane. These cells are small, flat, or cuboidal and mostly undifferentiated, although close inspection, e.g., with the electron microscope, reveals tiny lipid droplets, indicating the start of lipid synthesis. Differentiation progresses from the periphery towards the center. During this process sebocytes increase greatly in size and become round. The volume of a mature cell may be 100–150 times larger than that of the basal cell from which it is derived. Active synthesis of lipids results in great expansion of sebocytes. In contrast to the subcutaneous adipose tissue where the lipids confluate within the adipocyte, mature sebocytes still contain individual lipid vacuoles, sometimes more than 50, separated by fine cytoplasmic strands. The cytoplasm also contains a well-developed Golgi apparatus and rough endoplasmic reticulum. Sebocytes, like the keratinocytes of the epidermis, can also synthesize sparse tonofilaments. These disappear during maturation. At the end of the differentiation process, the different organelles, including the nucleus, are degraded and disappear. Finally the cell ruptures, and the sebum is released.

The cells of the sebaceous ducts show histologic features of both sebocytes and keratinocytes. They contain lipid droplets which are significantly smaller than those of mature sebocytes, but they also possess ultrastructural markers of keratinization, e.g., keratinosomes, keratohyalin, and tonofilaments. They produce a thin horny layer composed of fragile, loose corneocytes which rapidly shed into the lumen. The capability of forming corneocytes becomes especially evident during comedogenesis. Corneocytes stick together to form compact, horny impactions containing gaps through which sebum flows.

Benfenati A, Brillanti F (1939) Sulla distribuzione delle ghiandole sebacee nella cute del corpo umano. Arch Ital Derm Sifilogr Venereol 15:33–42

Downing DT, Stewart ME, Strauss JS (1987) Biology of sebaceous glands. In: Fitzpatrick TB, Eisen AZ, Wolff K, Freedberg IM, Austen KF (eds) Dermatology in general medicine. McGraw-Hill, New York, pp 185–190

Jenkinson M, McEwan D, Elder HY, Montgomery I, Moss VA (1985) Comparative studies of the ultrastructure of the sebaceous gland. Tissue Cell 17:683–698

Sawaya ME (1992) Purification of androgen receptors in human sebocytes and hair. J Invest Dermatol 98:92 S–96 S

Strauss JS, Downing DT, Ebling FJ (1983) Sebaceous glands. In: Goldsmith LA (ed) Biochemistry and physiology of the skin. Oxford University Press, New York, pp 569–595

Tosti A (1974) A comparison of the histodynamics of sebaceous glands and epidermis in man: A microanatomic and morphometric study. J Invest Dermatol 62:147–152

Wheatley VR (1986) The sebaceous glands. In: Jarrett A (ed) The physiology and pathophysiology of the skin, vol 9. Academic Press, London, pp 2723–2761

Physiology of Sebaceous Glands

Cell Cycle of Human Sebaceous Glands

Detailed knowledge of cell kinetics of sebocytes is necessary to evaluate the effectiveness of drugs and other treatment modalities in acne. Very important in this context are: firstly, the duration of the mitotic cycle; secondly, the time between cell division in the basal cell layer and the rupture of the mature sebocytes (the so-called cell transition time); and thirdly, the time between sebum production and its appearance on the skin surface.

The duration of a complete mitosis cycle (G_1, S, G_2, M phase) of sebocytes of the rat, for example, is about 28 h. In human sebocytes, the duration of the mitotic cycle is probably not very different.

To determine the cell transition time, radiolabeled precursors have been injected intradermally and biopsies taken at different times. Besides ^{3}H thymidine, ^{3}H glycine, ^{3}H histidine, and ^{14}C acetate were used in these autoradiographic investigations. However, results from different research groups diverge greatly. We found a significant decrease in radioactivity in sebaceous glands of average size 7 days after injection of radiolabeled amino acids. After 14 days, only trace amounts were demonstrable, whereas after 20–25 days no radioactivity could be detected. The transition time of about 3 weeks, as calculated from these data, was disputed by Downing and co-workers, who pointed out that the last trace amounts of radioactivity might be derived from cells that had undergone one or several divisions after labeling. They used ^{14}C acetate and calculated the total transition time to be about 2 weeks.

So far only rough estimations concerning the time between rupture of sebocytes and the appearance of sebum at the skin surface are possible, especially as the excretory ducts of sebaceous follicles may differ considerably in length and diameter. This interval has been calculated to be 14 h for sebaceous glands of average size.

Our present knowledge of the physiology of sebaceous glands elucidates that swift changes of the amount or the composition of sebum due to exogenous or endogenous factors can be largely excluded.

Downing DT, Strauss JS, Ramasastry P, Abel M, Lees CW, Pochi PE (1975) Measurement of the time between synthesis and surface excretion of sebacous lipids in sheep and man. J Invest Dermatol 64:215–219

Downing DT, Strauss JS (1982) On the mechanism of sebaceous secretion. Arch Dermatol Res 272:343–349

Epstein EH, Epstein WL (1966) New cell formation in human sebaceous glands. J Invest Dermatol 46:453–458

Plewig G, Christophers E, Braun-Falco O (1971) Proliferative cells in the human sebaceous gland. Labelling index and regional variations. Acta Derm Venereol (Stockh) 51:413–422

Plewig G, Christophers E, Braun-Falco O (1971) Cell transition in human sebaceous glands. Acta Derm Venereol (Stockh) 51:423–428

Plewig G, Christophers E (1974) Renewal rate of human sebaceous glands. Acta Derm Venereol (Stockh) 54:177–182

Wheatley VR (1986) The sebaceous glands. In: Jarrett A (ed) The physiology and pathophysiology of the skin, vol 9. Academic Press, London, pp 2763–2796

Methods of Measuring Sebum Secretion

The quantity and composition of surface lipids differ from that of lipids in intact sebocytes because of contamination by epidermal lipids. Furthermore, sebum itself undergoes many metabolic processes. In spite of this, skin surface lipids are used as an indicator of sebaceous gland activity.

Both Strauss and Pochi and Cunliffe and Shuster described a gravimetric method for determining sebum production using cigarette paper. The paper is fixed to the skin for 3 h, after which the lipids are extracted and weighed. A variant of this is to use an absorbent gel containing 15% bentonite clay, a mineral formed by the decomposition of volcanic ash, and 0.2% carboxymethylcellulose. Sebutape, a lipid-absorbent film containing innumerable microcavities, allows the study of sebum excretion at the level of the follicular unit. It yields a punctate pattern of individual droplets which seep into the cavities. Based on their number, size, and distribution, computer image analysis permits the assessment of the activity of individual sebaceous follicles. Some investigators extract skin surface lipids by applying solvents directly onto the skin. One great disadvantage of these methods is that the composition of lipids depends greatly on the test procedure, and especially on the chemical used for extraction.

Many more methods have been developed to make the quantitative measurement of skin surface lipids easier and faster. Schaefer and Kuhn-Bussius, for example, described a photometric technique based on the fact that lipids become translucent on frosted glass. The Lipometre is based on this principle. The glass plate is pressed onto the skin surface for a short time. This method lacks high sensitivity, but is convenient for screening.

One important aspect that is often neglected is that considerable amounts of preformed sebum already exist in the excretory ducts of the sebaceous glands. Thus, above all, one does not measure sebum *production* but sebum *excretion*. Only after delipidation for at least 14 h using cigarette paper or bentonite clay is the reservoir in the sebaceous glands apparently exhausted and only then can the lipids on the skin surface be used to draw conclusions on sebum production.

Cunliffe WJ, Shuster S (1969) The rate of sebum excretion in man. Br J Dermatol 81:697–704

Cunliffe WJ, Kearney JN, Simpson NB (1980) A modified photometric technique for measuring sebum excretion rate. J Invest Dermatol 75:394–398

Downing DT, Strauss JS (1982) On the mechanism of sebaceous secretion. Arch Dermatol Res 272:343–349

Greene RS, Downing DT, Pochi PE, Strauss JS (1970) Anatomical variation in the amount and composition of human skin surface lipid. J Invest Dermatol 54:240–247

Harris HH, Downing DT, Stewart ME, Strauss JS (1983) Sustainable rates of sebum secretion in acne patients and matched normal control subjects. J Am Acad Dermatol 8:200–203

Lookingbill DP, Cunliffe WJ (1986) A direct gravimetric technique for measuring sebum excretion rate. Br J Dermatol 114:75–81

Piérard GE, Kligman AM (1989) An update of the Sebutape® technique. In: Marks R, Plewig G (eds) Acne and related disorders. Dunitz, London, pp 111–112

Saint-Leger D, Berrebi C, Duboz C, Agache P (1979) The lipometre: an easy tool for rapid quantitation of skin surface lipids (SSL) in man. Arch Dermatol Res 265:79–89

Schaefer H, Kuhn-Bussius H (1970) Methodik zur quantitativen Bestimmung der menschlichen Talgsekretion. Arch Klin Exp Dermatol 238:429–435

Stewart ME, Downing DT (1985) Measurement of sebum secretion rates in young children. J Invest Dermatol 84:59–61

Strauss JS, Pochi PE (1961) The quantitative gravimetric determination of sebum production. J Invest Dermatol 36:293–298

The Role of Lipids in the Pathogenesis of Acne

Retention hyperkeratosis of the acroinfundibulum of sebaceous follicles is a primary event in the pathogenesis of acne vulgaris. During comedogenesis, the follicular epithelium becomes hyperplastic and a horny impaction is formed. There are two hypotheses regarding the role played by lipids in comedo formation. Downing and co-workers postulated a *linoleic acid deficiency of the follicular epithelium*. This concept is based upon the finding that the concentration of linoleic acid and acylceramides in the sebum of acne patients is lower than in healthy individuals. In addition, ceramide 1 from comedones contains only one-seventh of the linoleate amount of ceramide 1 from normal stratum corneum. These findings indicate that sebum reduces the concentration of linoleic acid of the epidermal acylceramides. In addition, the linoleic acid concentration of sebum shows an inverse relationship to increasing sebum secretion during puberty. This concept is fascinating, but we think that it overestimates the role of linoleic acid. Although this essential fatty acid is an important constituent of ceramide 1, other structural lipids may also be involved in the pathogenesis of acne.

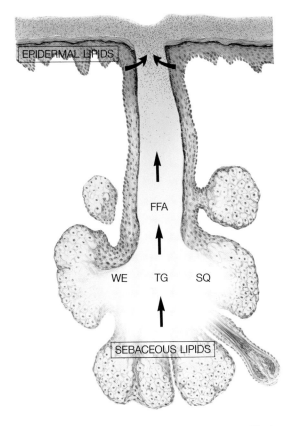

Dilution of the epidermal lipids of the follicular epithelium by sebaceous lipids.

FFA free fatty acids, *WE* wax esters, *TG* triglycerides, *SQ* squalene

Not only ceramides but also other epidermal lipids such as free sterols are reduced in acne comedones. This may lead to an imbalance of free cholesterol and cholesterol sulfate and thus to increased corneocyte adhesion in the acroinfundibulum causing follicular retention hyperkeratosis. Melnik and co-workers were able to show that treatment with isotretinoin, a potent inhibitor of lipogenesis in sebaceous glands, is followed by an increase in lipids of epidermal origin, especially free sterols and ceramides, accompanied by a sharp decrease in lipids of sebaceous origin in initial comedones. They formulated the modified concept of the *follicular deficiency of epidermal lipids in acne.*

Downing DT, Stewart ME, Wertz PW, Strauss JS (1986) Essential fatty acids and acne. J Am Acad Dermatol 14:221–225

Melnik BC (1990) Biochemie und Pathobiochemie des epidermalen Lipidstoffwechsels. Experimentelle Untersuchungen epidermaler Lipide bei Störungen der epidermalen Keratinisierung und Barrierefunktion. Thieme, Stuttgart

Melnik B, Kinner T, Plewig G (1988) Influence of oral isotretinoin treatment on the composition of comedonal lipids. Implications for comedogenesis in acne vulgaris. Arch Dermatol Res 280:97–102

Nicolaides N, Ansari MNA, Fu HC, Lindsay DG (1970) Lipid composition of comedones compared with that of human skin surface in acne patients. J Invest Dermatol 54:487–495

Perisho K, Wertz PW, Madison KC, Stewart ME, Downing DT (1988) Fatty acids of acylceramides from comedones and from the skin surface of acne patients and control subjects. J Invest Dermatol 90:350–353

Stewart ME (1992) Sebaceous gland lipids. Semin Dermatol 11:100–105

Stewart ME, Benoit AM, Downing DT, Strauss JS (1984) Suppression of sebum secretion with 13-*cis*-retinoic acid: effect on individual skin surface lipids and implications for their anatomic origin. J Invest Dermatol 82:74–78

Stewart ME, Grahek MO, Cambier LS, Wertz PW, Downing DT (1986) Dilutional effect of increased sebaceous gland activity on the proportion of linoleic acid in sebaceous wax esters and in epidermal acylceramides. J Invest Dermatol 87:733–736

Wheatley VR (1986) The chemistry of sebum. In: Jarrett A (ed) The physiology and pathophysiology of the skin. vol 9, The sebaceous glands. Chap. 90. Academic Press, London, pp 2829–2872

Concept of the follicular deficiency of epidermal lipids in acne

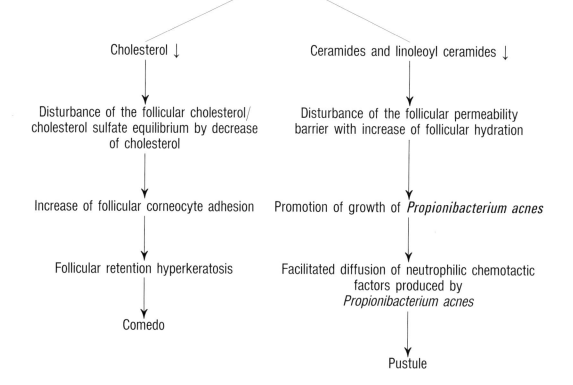

Androgenic stimulation

Increased production of androgens, increased susceptibility
of the sebaceous follicles with genetic predisposition

Increased sebum production

Triglycerides, free fatty acids, squalenes, wax esters

Dilution of the epidermal lipids of the follicular epithelium

Cholesterol ↓

Disturbance of the follicular cholesterol/
cholesterol sulfate equilibrium by decrease
of cholesterol

Increase of follicular corneocyte adhesion

Follicular retention hyperkeratosis

Comedo

Ceramides and linoleoyl ceramides ↓

Disturbance of the follicular permeability
barrier with increase of follicular hydration

Promotion of growth of *Propionibacterium acnes*

Facilitated diffusion of neutrophilic chemotactic
factors produced by
Propionibacterium acnes

Pustule

Factors Influencing Sebum Production

Endocrinologic Influences

Endocrine factors play an important role in the control of the secretory activity of sebaceous glands, and there is evidence that both proliferation and lipogenic activity of sebocytes are influenced by hormones.

Androgens

The skin, like the male genitalia and the prostate gland, is a major site of androgen metabolism and a primary target for the effects of androgens. Under the influence of androgens, mitotic activity, intracellular lipid synthesis, and the thickness of the epidermis increases, and hair growth, and pigmentation are influenced. Sebaceous glands are stimulated by both systemic and topical application of androgens as shown by the sebotropic effect of topical dehydroepiandrosterone (DHEA).

Sebum production is a sensitive indicator of androgenic activity. Sebaceous glands are formed between the 13th and 15th week of fetal life. Their products contribute significantly to the vernix caseosa. Secretion is high immediately after birth, triggered by maternal androgens, and for 3–5 months thereafter, but declines to a very low level throughout childhood.

More than 20 years ago Wotiz and co-workers showed that human skin can metabolize testosterone. The enzyme catalyzing the conversion of testosterone to its more potent metabolite 5α-dihydrotestosterone (DHT) is 5α-reductase which is abundant in sebaceous glands. DHT is the active androgen at tissue level and considered responsible for the stimulation of sebaceous glands. A cytoplasmic receptor for this hormone has been demonstrated in human skin.

According to the current view a complex is formed between DHT and this receptor and is then transferred to the nucleus where it promotes gene expression as a direct response to hormone stimuli, and thus initiates the biochemical reactions leading to the manifestation of the androgenic stimulation.

Androgen receptor levels are similar in men and women with acne as well as in acne lesions and lesion free skin. Neither in acne nor in idiopathic hirsutism does a correlation exist between androgen receptors and androgen serum levels.

In healthy men, about 75% of plasma DHT is derived from the peripheral conversion of testosterone. In women, androstenedione appears to be the major prehormone, as conversion from testosterone accounts only for less than 20% of circulating DHT. It has been shown that the conversion of testosterone to DHT was up to 30 times greater in acne-bearing skin than in normal skin from the corresponding area, with skin from men being more active than that from women. The highest conversion rates were observed in facial skin affected by acne. Plasma levels of testosterone are normal in most acne patients, and thus are not relevant for diagnosis and monitoring therapy.

Estrogens

Estrogens do not significantly affect the proliferation of the sebaceous glands. They may act either by suppressing the secretion of pituitary gonadotrophins and hence the production of androgens, or by enhancing the binding of testosterone to testosterone-binding globulin. Significant differences exist with regard to the number of estrogen receptors between normal and acne-bearing skin in both sexes, being present in almost all female acne patients and in about 80% of male acne patients; however, estrogen receptors could not be demonstrated in normal skin.

Administered systemically, estrogens bring about a reduction in the size and secretion of sebaceous glands in both sexes. This effect, however, can only be achieved with doses exceeding the physiological requirement. Thus it is unlikely that estrogens play a physiological role in the regulation of sebaceous gland activity. Topical application of ethinyl estradiol to the forehead of normal men in rather high concentrations (at least 1%) markedly reduces sebaceous gland secretion. As it causes signs of feminization, this therapy is not suitable for men.

Progesterone

Controversy exists regarding the effects of progesterone on the sebaceous glands. From studies with rats it can be concluded that the response to progesterone is sex-related, as it stimulated sebum secretion only in female and castrated male rats. In normal male rats, this hormone shut down sebum secretion, probably by competitive inhibition of 5α-reductase thus preventing the formation of DHT- from testosterone. In humans, progesterone in physiological amounts has obviously no effect on the activity of sebaceous glands as shown by intramuscular injection of this hormone in women. Administration of synthetic progestins, however, can lead to significant androgenic effects like virilization of newborns after administration of gestagens to their mothers.

Pituitary Hormones

The anterior pituitary gland plays an important role in the control of sebaceous glands. Hypophysectomized rats have a greatly reduced sebum secretion rate, even lower than in castrated animals. Patients with hypopituitarism of different origin, e.g., tumors, hypophysectomy, Sheehan's syndrome, or infections, also have low sebum secretion levels. This can be at least partially reversed by the administration of testosterone, corticosteroids, and thyroxin, since the release of these hormones is under pituitary control.

The pituitary, which is subservient to the hypothalamus, is a central organ for hormonal regulation. Among the hormones secreted by this gland are growth hormone (GH), adrenocorticotrophic hormone (ACTH), prolactin, the gonadotrophins follicle-stimulating hormone (FSH) and luteinizing hormone (LH), as well as thyroid stimulating hormone (TSH), melanocyte stimulating hormone (α-MSH), and β-lipotrophin (β-LPH).

Animal experiments with hypophysectomized rats showed that GH was able to increase sebum secretion, acting synergistically with testosterone. It also stimulates human sebaceous glands, which may explain the increased sebum excretion in patients with acromegaly, supported by the reduced sebum levels in isolated growth hormone deficiency. Recently, GH receptor/binding protein has been localized in epidermis and epidermal appendages, especially also in indifferent and differentiating cells of sebaceous glands in both rats and humans. ACTH exerts its sebotropic effect probably through the stimulation of adrenal androgens. Experiments with hypophysectomized-castrated rats showed that ACTH was able to restore sebum secretion to the level of castrated animals. Simultaneous administration of ACTH and testosterone did not result in a synergistic action.

So far, no certain effect of prolactin on

the sebaceous gland has been established in humans. It has been suggested that the increasing sebum excretion rate associated with advancing pregnancy was due to an increased production of prolactin. Deficiency of gonadotrophins reduces sebaceous gland activity in both sexes. The effect of these hormones is an indirect one.

TSH acts by way of its target gland, since its stimulatory effect on sebum secretion is abolished after thyroidectomy in rats. In humans, the thyroid bears no obvious relationship to sebum secretion, and the low sebum excretion rate in hypothyroidism is attributable to a general reduction in metabolism.

In rodents, α-MSH stimulates the activity of sebaceous glands. A similar action in humans has not been definitely established so far, although a sebotropic action of this hormone in pregnancy has been proposed as an alternative to prolactin.

β-LPH, which had a sebotropic effect in hypophysectomized-ovarectomized rats, is now considered a precursor of β-endorphins and has obviously no independent physiological function.

The existence of a directly acting sebotropic hormone has been discussed for a long time. Some observations imply that, e.g., the finding that L-dopa decreases seborrhea in patients with parkinsonism but not in normal subjects is evidence in favor of inhibition of an unknown pituitary sebotropic hormone. It remains an open issue whether one of the above-mentioned hormones is responsible for this effect.

Adrenocortical Hormones

Three main classes of hormones are produced by the adrenal cortex, glucocorticosteroids, mineralocorticosteroids, and adrenal androgens. The latter have been discussed in detail elsewhere (p. 39). Secretion of glucocorticosteroids and adrenal androgens is controlled by the ACTH. Low levels of cortisol lead to enhanced ACTH-secretion, and increasing levels of cortisol inhibit the release of this hormone. This negative feedback mechanism fails in stress situations, leading to an increase in both ACTH and cortisol.

Unlike adrenal androgens, corticosteroids have obviously no direct effect on the sebaceous glands. In castrated but not in normal men, sebum secretion was suppressed by prednisone. In contrast, substitution with cortisone and hydrocortisone led to a significant increase in sebum production in a patient with Addison's disease. In animal experiments, corticosteroids enhance the effect of testosterone on androgen-susceptible target organs like the prostate. Similar effects could not be substantiated for humans yet.

Bickers DR (1983) Drug, carcinogen, and steroid hormone metabolism in the skin. In: Goldsmith LA (ed) Biochemistry and physiology of the skin, chap 52. Oxford University Press, New York, pp 1689–1186

Bläuer M, Vaalasti A, Pauli SL, Ylikomi T, Joensuu T, Tuohimaa P (1991) Location of androgen receptor in human skin. J Invest Dermatol 97:264–268

Burton JL, Cartlidge M, Cartlidge NEF, Shuster S (1973) Sebum excretion in parkinsonism. Br J Dermatol 88:263–266

Cunliffe WJ (1989) Acne. Dunitz, London, pp 153–162

Drucker WD, Blumberg AM, Gandy HM, David RR, Verde AL (1972) Biological activity of dehydroepiandrosterone sulfate. J Clin Endocrinol Metabol 35:48–54

Goolamali SK, Burton JL, Shuster S (1973) Sebum excretion in hypopituitarism. Br J Dermatol 89:21–24

Levell MJ, Cawood ML, Burke B, Cunliffe WJ (1989) Acne is not associated with abnormal plasma androgens. Br J Dermatol 120:649–654

Lobie PE, Breipohl W, Lincoln DT, García-Aragón J, Waters MJ (1990) Localization of the growth hormone receptor-binding protein in skin. J Endocrinol 126:467–472

Pochi PE, Strauss JS (1974) Endocrinologic control of the development and activity of the human sebaceous gland. J Invest Dermatol 62:191–201

Orentreich N, Matias JR (1988) Local stimulation of sebaceous gland activity by the topical application of dehydroepiandrosterone. J Soc Cosmet Chem 39:291–303

Sawaya ME (1992) Purification of Androgen Receptors in Human Sebocytes and Hair. J Invest Dermatol 98:92 S–96 S

Schmidt JB, Spona J, Huber J (1986) Androgen receptor in hirsutism and acne. Gynecol Obstet Invest 22:206–211

Shuster S, Thody AJ (1975) The control and measurement of sebum secretion. J Invest Dermatol 64:172–190

Shuster S, Hinks WM, Thody AJ (1977) Effect of sex and age at gonadectomy on the sebaceous response to progesterone. J Endocrinol 73:67–70

Strauss JS, Kligman AM (1961) The effect of progesterone and progesterone-like compounds on the human sebaceous gland. J Invest Dermatol 36:309–319

Takayasu S, Watimoto H, Itami S, Sano S (1980) Activity of testosterone 5α reductase in various tissues of human skin. J Invest Dermatol 74:187–191

Thody AJ, Shuster S (1989) Control and function of sebaceous glands. Physiol Rev 69:383–416

Villares JCB, Carlini EA (1989) Sebum secretion in idiopathic Parkinson's disease: effect of anticholinergic and dopaminergic drugs. Acta Neurol Scand 80:57–63

Watts NB, Kefer JH (1989) Practical endocrinology. 4th edn. Lea and Febinger, Philadelphia

Welshons WV, Lieberman ME, Gorski J (1984) Nuclear localization of unoccupied oestrogen receptors. Nature 307:747–749

Wheatley VR (1986) Hormonal regulation of sebaceous gland activity. In: Jarrett A (ed) The physiology and pathophysiology of the skin, vol 9, chap. 89. Academic Press, London, pp 2797–2827

Wotiz HH, Mescon H, Doppel H, Lemon HM (1956) The in vitro metabolism of testosterone by human skin J Invest Dermatol 26:113–120

Nonendocrine Control of Sebaceous Function

Innervation. Sebum secretion is not under neural control. A network of fine cholinesterase positive nerve fibers surrounds the hair follicle but does not reach into the gland. Atropine and acetylcholine have no effect on the activity of the sebaceous gland. In contrast, innervation of some specialized sebaceous glands, e.g., the Meibomian gland of the eyelid or the scent marking glands of some rodents, has been demonstrated. These are exceptions. Damage of nerves from trauma, tumors, or infections can cause a localized seborrhea in the affected area. Excessive oiliness, and sometimes even comedones may be seen after denervation of facial peripheral branches. This is obviously an indirect effect, perhaps mediated by interference with the blood supply.

Effect of Sweating. Sweating and sebum secretion are independent functions. It is only the appearance of oiliness which is increased by sweating. This is a merely visual effect and not attributable to an increased sebum secretion. Sweating makes the skin look greasier than it actually is, causing difficulties in assessing the actual degree of oiliness.

Effect of Temperature. Changes in skin temperature influence the sebum excretion rate by about 10% per degree Celsius. However, as these changes occur within 90 min, the effect is mainly on preformed sebum in the follicular reservoir. Sebum secretion seems to follow a circadian rhythm, being highest during the first hours of sleep, and to increase in the summer months. This might be due to higher skin temperature making sebum less viscous.

UV-Irradiation. Ultraviolet radiation increases the size of sebaceous glands in animals and probably also in man.

Diet. Except for total caloric deprivation which leads to a 40% decrease in sebum secretion, diet has no influence on sebaceous activity. Excessive ingestion of animal and vegetable oils and fats does not increase sebum production, and circulating lipids have no effect on sebocytes. In contrast to common belief even chocolate has no adverse effect.

Genetic Factors. Familial occurrence of acne vulgaris, acne conglobata, and acne inversa indicates a genetic predisposition. This could be partially explained by a genetic control of sebum production.
The possibility of a genetic component involved in the control of sebaceous glands is substantiated by the fact that seborrheic parents normally generate seborrheic children. This is also supported by studies with identical twins who showed similar sebum excretion rates, while nonidentical twins varied significantly in this respect. Investigation of the composition of sebum-derived wax esters in twins suggests that at least the proportion of iso-even fatty acids may be under genetic control.

Age-Related Changes in Sebum Production and Sebum Excretion. Activity of sebaceous glands is age-related, and characteristic patterns of sebum excretion are present in different age groups. In newborns sebum production is comparable to that of young adults. Differences in sebum secretion exist between boys and girls only during the first weeks of life. Afterwards similar sebum secretion rates are found in both sexes, decreasing constantly from the second month onward to the end of the first year of life. This indicates that the androgenic stimulus for sebum secretion has been active before birth. The main candidate is DHEA, the levels of which are 10–15 times elevated at birth in both sexes compared to other androgens.

Sebum excretion markedly increases at puberty with its highest levels in acne patients. In adulthood it gradually decreases, in women especially after menopause. Very old individuals have similar levels of skin surface lipids as well as a comparable composition of fatty acids to newborns.

Agache P, Blanc D, Barrand C, Laurent R (1980) Sebum levels during the first year of life. Br J Dermatol 103:643–649

Archibald A, Shuster S (1973) A non-endocrine control of sebum secretion. Arch Dermatol Forsch 246:175–180

Burton JL, Cunliffe WJ, Saunders IG, Shuster S (1971) The effect of facial nerve paresis on sebum secretion. Br J Dermatol 84:135–138

Cunliffe WJ (1989) Acne. Dunitz, London, pp 140–152

Cunliffe WJ, Burton JL, Shuster S (1970) The effect of local temperature variations on the sebum excretion rate. Br J Dermatol 83:650–654

Fulton JE, Plewig G, Kligman AM (1970) Effect of chocolate on acne vulgaris. JAMA 210:2071–2074

Jacobsen E, Billings JK, Frantz RA, Kinney CK, Stewart ME, Downing DT (1985) Age-related changes in sebaceous wax ester secretion rates in men and women. J Invest Dermatol 85:483–485

Lesnik RH, Kligman LH, Kligman AM (1992) Agents that cause enlargement of sebaceous glands in hairless mice. II. Ultraviolet radiation. Arch Dermatol 284:106–108

Nazzaro-Porro M, Passi S, Boniforti L, Belsito F (1979) Effects of aging on fatty acids in skin surface lipids. J Invest Dermatol 73:112–117

Piérard-Franchimont C, Piérard GE, Kligman AM (1990) Seasonal modulation of sebum excretion. Dermatologica 181:21–22

Stewart ME, McDonnell MW, Downing DT (1986) Possible genetic control of the proportions of branched chain fatty acids in human sebaceous wax esters. J Invest Dermatol 86:706–708

Strauss JS, Downing DT, Stewart ME (1985) Sebum secretion rates in relation to age. J Appl Cosmetol 3:257–266

Thody AJ, Shuster S (1989) Control and function of sebaceous glands. Physiol Rev 69:383–416

Walton S, Wyatt EH, Cunliffe WJ (1988) Genetic control of sebum excretion and acne – a twin study. Br J Dermatol 118:393–396

Wheatley VR (1986) In: Jarrett A (ed) The physiology and pathophysiology of the skin, vol 9. Academic Press, London, pp 2724–2726; 2788–2792

Williams M, Cunliffe WJ, Williamson B, Forster RA, Cotterill JA, Edwards JC (1973) The effect of local temperature changes on sebum excretion rate and forehead surface lipids composition. Br J Dermatol 88:257–262

Wüthrich B, Much T (1977) Akne vulgaris: Ergebnis einer Nahrungsmittel-Allergen-Testung und einer kontrollierten Eliminations-Diät. Aktuel Dermatol 3:177–183

Effects of Drugs

Retinoids. 13-*cis* retinoic acid (isotretinoin) causes a marked decrease in sebum production and a drastic shrinkage of the glands to up to 90% of the level before treatment. The decrease in sebum production is dose-dependent and starts within the first two weeks of treatment. After 3 months, e.g., a reduction of 30% with 0.1 mg, 40% with 0.5 mg, and 90% with 1.0 mg isotretinoin per kilogram body weight per day can be achieved.

This is accompanied by changes in the composition of the surface lipids. The fractions of wax esters and squalene, which are of sebaceous origin, decrease significantly, whereas cholesterol increases. This reflects the pattern in childhood before androgens stimulate the sebaceous glands. What is left on the surface is mainly the contribution from epidermal lipids.

The parent compound retinol can modestly reduce sebum production but only after toxic doses are given, in the order of magnitude of 500 000 IU daily. It is noteworthy that etretinate has practically no effect on the sebaceous glands.

Antiandrogens. The term antiandrogens is applied to drugs which act either by blocking the enzyme 5α-reductase that converts testosterone to DHT or by competing with androgens for receptor-binding sites. Most experience exists with cyproterone acetate, which is often administered together with ethinyl estradiol as used for oral contraception. Cyproterone acetate reduces oiliness by 25%–35% from the second or third cycle. The addition of ethinyl estradiol leads to a further reduction of sebum production. Other antiandrogens are chlormadinone acetate, spironolactone, and cimetidine.

The aldosterone antagonist spironolactone acts by competing with steroids for their receptors on the tubulus cells thus preventing the binding of the steroid. This leads to a reduction of sebum production. Spironolactone needs special mention as it is an alternative to cyproterone acetate in those countries where this drug is not available. It should be kept in mind, however, that all these drugs are effective only after systemic administration. Topically they do not exert their beneficial effects on sebum production. For more details see the chapter on antiandrogens and aldosterone antagonists.

Estrogens. As described elsewhere (p. 39), estrogens reduce sebaceous gland activity and secretion. These hormones are only suitable for women because of the negative effects in men.

Anticholesterol Drugs. Attempts have been made to suppress lipid synthesis using drugs that have been designed to lower cholesterol blood levels. One such drug is the prostaglandin inhibitor eicosa 5,8,11,14-tetraynoic acid. It has been demonstrated that oral administration substantially suppresses sebum secretion. However, serious side-effects after long-term usage rule out clinical applications. The drug is ineffective topically. Other anticholesterol drugs such as clofibrate and nicotinates have not been able to reduce sebum production.

Antibiotics. Neither systemic nor topical antibiotics are capable of reducing the sebum secretion rate. Additional information is provided in later chapters (p. 611).

Topical Drugs. In contrast to common belief, the so-called antiacne topicals do not affect sebum production. Suppression does not occur with sulfur, salicylic acid, resorchinol, tretinoin, naphthol, and azelaic acid. Although the latter is a potent inhibitor of 5α-reductase in human skin under in vitro conditions, sebaceous gland activity remains unaltered using a 20% cream.

Benzoyl peroxide failed to decrease sebum production in acne. In contrast, the topical application of benzoyl peroxide raised the sebum excretion rate in acne patients. We have demonstrated a similar enhancement in hairless mice.

Cunliffe WJ (1987) Evolution of a strategy for the treatment of acne. J Am Acad Dermatol 16:591–599

Cunliffe WJ, Cotterill JA, Williamson B (1972) The effect of clindamycin in acne – a clinical and laboratory investigation. Br J Dermatol 87:37–41

Cunliffe WJ, Holland KT (1989) Clinical and laboratory studies on treatment with 20% azelaic acid cream for acne. Acta Derm Venereol [Suppl 143] (Stockh) 69:31–34

Cunliffe WJ, Stainton C, Forster RA (1983) Topical benzoyl peroxide increases sebum secretion rate in patients with acne. Br J Dermatol 109:577–579

Fanta D (1990) Cyproterone acetate in acne. J Dermatol Treat 1 [Suppl 3]:19–22

Goldstein JA, Pochi PE (1981) Failure of benzoyl peroxide to decrease sebaceous gland secretion in acne. Dermatologica 162:287–291

Hellgren L, Vincent J (1978) Erythromycin stearate in acne vulgaris: its effect on the skin surface lipids and on the activity of purified pancreatic lipase. Dermatologica 156:105–110

Küster W, Rödder-Wehrmann O, Plewig G (1991) Acne inversa: Pathogenese und Genetik. Hautarzt 42:2–4

Lesnik RH, Kligman LH, Kligman AM (1992a) Agents that cause enlargement of sebaceous glands in hairless mice. I. Topical substances. Arch Dermatol 284:100–105

Leyden JJ (1988) Retinoids and acne. J Am Acad Dermatol 19:164–168

Mayer-Da-Silva A, Gollnick H, Detmar M, Gassmüller J, Parry A, Müller R, Orfanos CE (1989) Effects of azelaic acid on sebaceous gland, sebum excretion rate and keratinization pattern in human skin. Acta Derm Venereol [Suppl 143] (Stockh) 69:20–30

Melnik B, Kinner T, Plewig G (1988) Influence of oral isotretinoin treatment on the composition of comedonal lipids: implications for comedogenesis in acne vulgaris. Arch Dermatol Res 280:97–102

Mills OH Jr, Kligman AM (1983) Drugs that are ineffective in the treatment of acne vulgaris. Br J Dermatol 108:371–374

Pochi PE (1983) Hormonal therapy of acne. Dermatol Clin 1:377–384

Shaw JC (1991) Spironolactone in dermatologic therapy. J Am Acad Dermatol 24:236–243

Stamatiadis D, Bulteau-Portois MC, Mowszowicz I (1988) Inhibition of 5α-reductase activity in human skin by zinc and azelaic acid. Br J Dermatol 119:627–632

Stewart ME, Benoit AM, Downing DT, Strauss JS (1984) Suppression of sebum secretion with 13-*cis*-retinoic acid: effect on individual skin surface lipids and implications for their anatomic origin. J Invest Dermatol 82:74–78

Windhager K, Plewig G (1977) Wirkung von Schälmitteln (Resorchin, kristalliner Schwefel, Salicylsäure) auf Meerschweinchenepidermis. Arch Dermatol Res 259:187–198

Large Sebaceous Glands in Acne Patients

These biopsies were obtained from the cheeks of two 17-year-old men, one with smooth skin and no acne, the other with severe inflammatory acne. The tissue was cut horizontally and photographed at the same magnification.

Above   Normal skin. Sebaceous lobules rest around their pilary portion

Below   Acne skin. The huge sebaceous gland is at least four times as voluminous in the acne patient than in the normal subject. The pilary portion is above. Acne patients produce more sebum than nonaffected persons. The more sebum is produced, the severer the acne tends to run. Sebaceous gland are particularly large in patients with acne conglobata

Cotterill JA, Cunliffe WJ, Williamson B (1971) Severity of acne and sebum excretion rate. Br J Dermatol 85:93–94

Plewig G (1974) Acne vulgaris: proliferative cells in sebaceous glands. Br J Dermatol 90:623–630

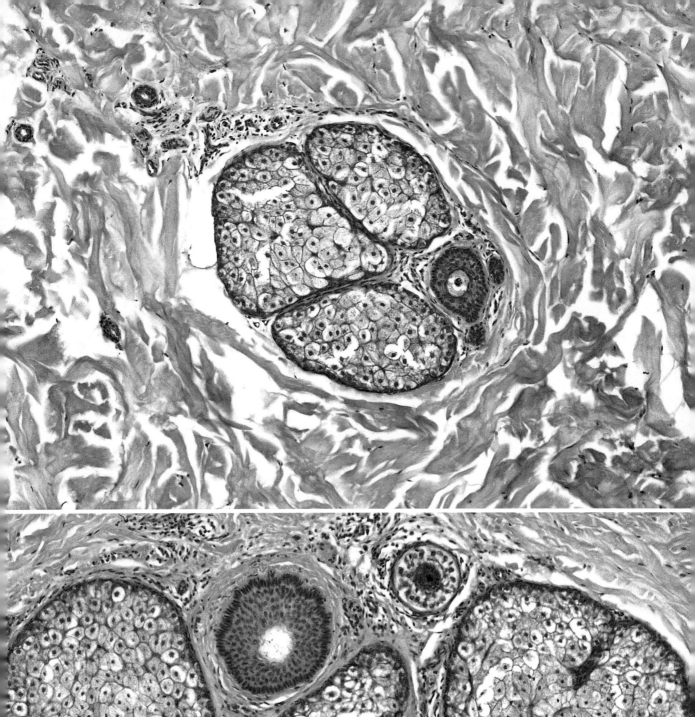
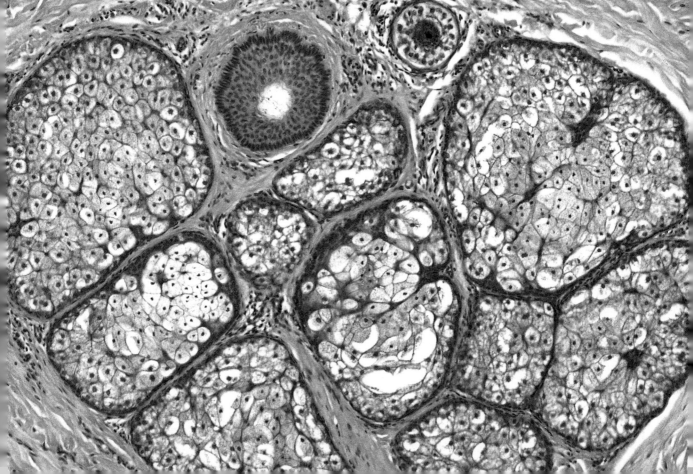

The Sebaceous Filament

Above   Squeezed-out sebaceous filaments. These waxy worms were forced out of the sebaceous follicles of the forehead by strongly pinching the skin between the blades of a hemostat. This was an adult black with oily skin who had had acne in the past. It is much easier to express filaments from the ala nasi of persons with oily skin and large pores. The filament is a cylindrical tube of keratinized cells, actually stratum corneum, enclosing a cheesy mass of sebaceous lipids that are densely colonized by *Propionibacterium acnes.* Sebaceous filaments do not evolve into comedones

Below   Ultrastructure of the sebaceous filament. This view of the central portion reveals a mixture of bacteria and dehiscing corneocytes. The latter are very irregular in size and shape and more like those in ordinary sebaceous follicles than in normal stratum corneum. Many corneocytes seem empty, possibly artifactual. Others contain lipid droplets. Some are swollen and broken, indicating vast imperfections. The bacteria and horny cells are suspended in a matrix of sebum. (Electron microscopy, × 16 600)

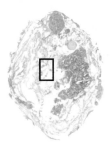

Below: Courtesy of Professor Helmut H. Wolff, Lübeck, FRG

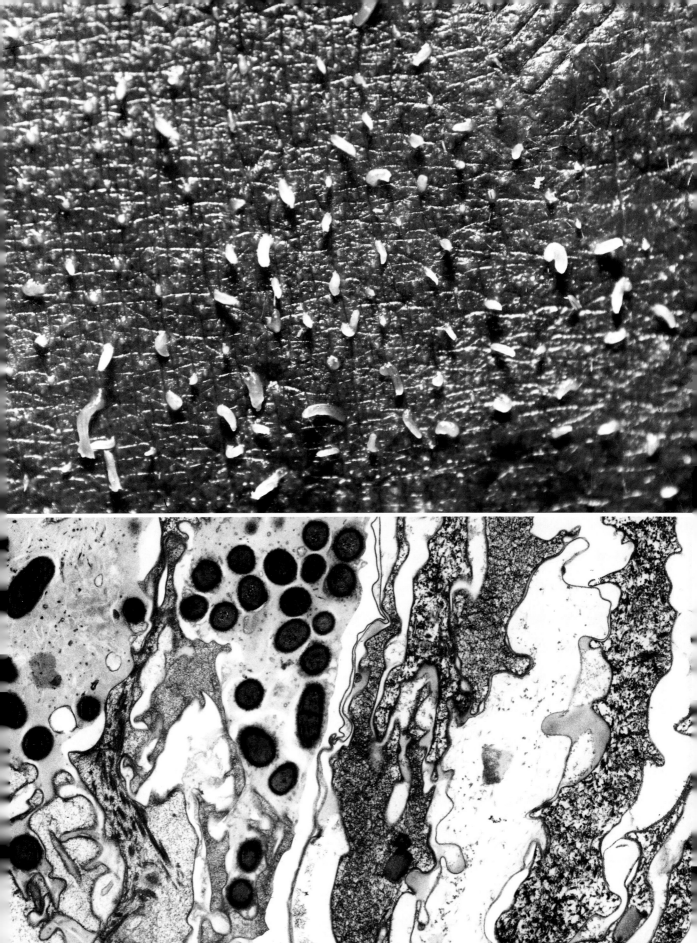

Comparative Ultrastructure of the Acroinfundibulum and the Infrainfundibulum

Above   The acroinfundibulum. The keratinizing epithelium is on the left with prominent keratohyalin granules. Rows of dense corneocytes on the right are compacted into a horny layer. This corresponds to the interfollicular portion of the epidermis. The acroinfundibulum is an extension of the epidermis into the terminal segment of a sebaceous follicle. (Electron microscopy, × 28000)

Below   The infrainfundibulum. This epithelium also keratinizes, but the corneocytes have different characteristics. The keratohyalin granules (*left*) are small and sparse. Adjacent to this diminutive granular layer are three to four rows of poorly formed, jumbled, thin, irregular corneocytes which show signs of disintegration. The amorphous material on the right is sebum. (Electron microscopy, × 28000)

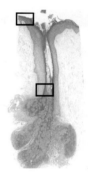

Below: Courtesy of Professor Helmut H. Wolff, Lübeck, FRG

Knutson DD (1974) Ultrastructural observations in acne vulgaris: the normal sebaceous follicle and acne lesion. J Invest Dermatol 62:288–307

Plewig G, Nikolowski J, Wolff HH (1983) Follicular keratinization. In: Marks R, Plewig G (eds) Stratum corneum. Springer, Berlin Heidelberg New York, pp 227–236

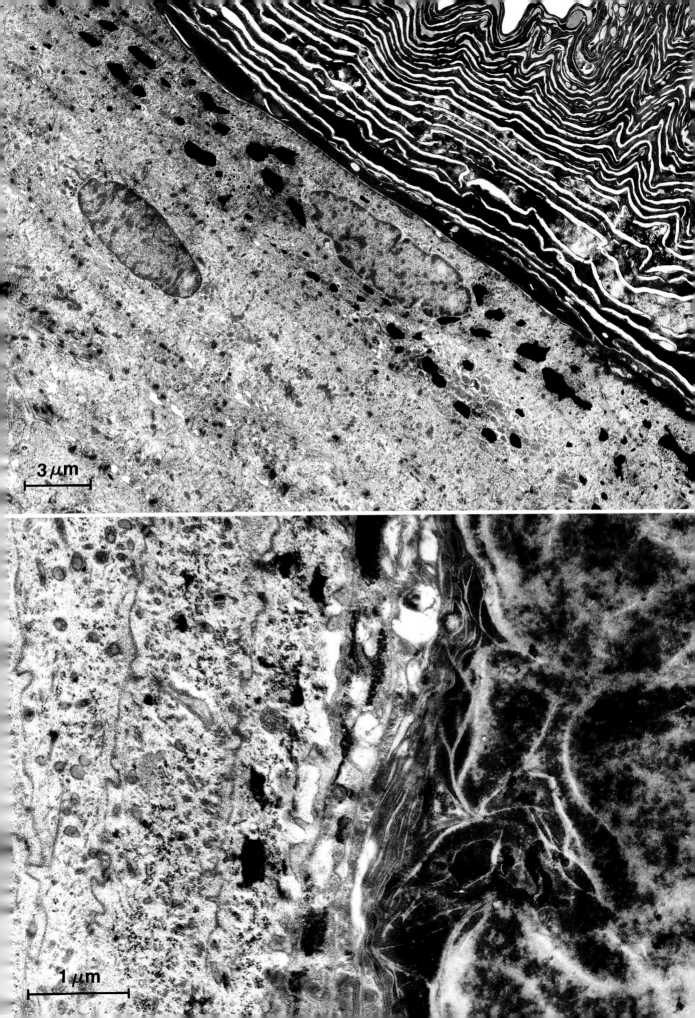

The Appearances of Sebum

Above Comedo stained for lipid. The framework of a comedo is soaked with sebum. This frozen section was stained with oil-red-O. The lipid is found extracellularly in clefts between the corneocytes and in the channels which conduct it to the surface. Lipid droplets within the corneocytes can only bee seen by electron microscopy

Below

Left Lipid-laden cells (sebocytes). Electron microscopic view of mature lipid cells of the sebaceous glands shortly before their rupture. (Electron microscopy, × 6900)

Right Human sebum. Sebum is a yellowish, oily liquid at skin temperature. This was collected by ether extraction from the scalp

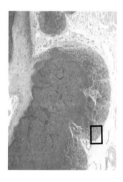

Courtesy of Kenneth J. McGinley, Philadelphia, USA

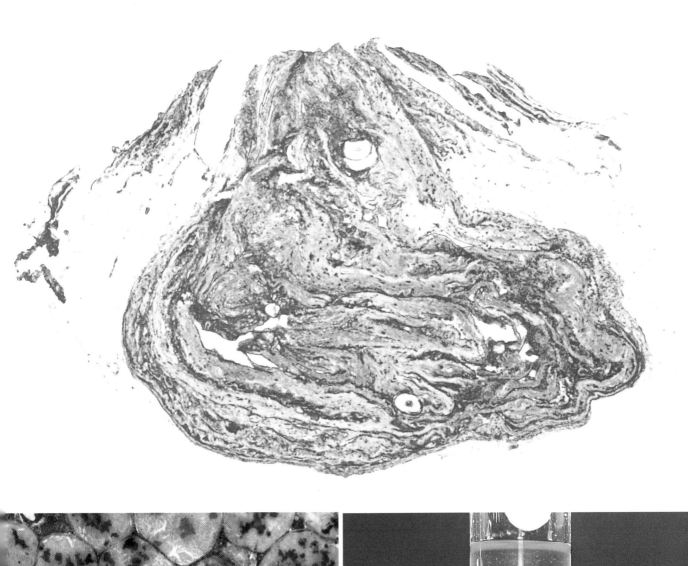
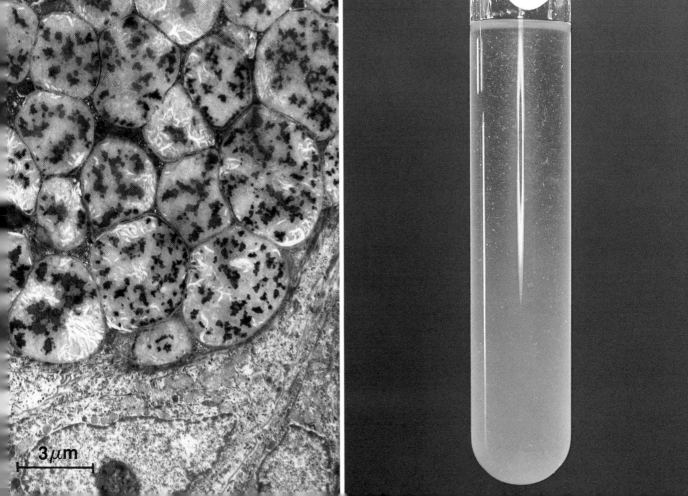

Cell Proliferation of Sebaceous Glands

Autoradiographic techniques give insight into the kinetics of sebaceous glands. In this panel the labeling index after 45 min and the direction and speed of sebocyte migration are shown. Tritiated thymidine, counterstained with hematoxilin.

Above   Labeling index

Left   A sebaceous follicle from the back. About 5% of the epidermal and 8% of the follicular basalar cells are labeled. Sebocytes in juxtaposition to the basement membrane are also labeled. 45 min

Right   Sebaceous follicle from the face. The lowermost part of the infundibulum, sebaceous ducts, and three sebaceous lobules are shown. Labeled cells are seen in each of these structures. 45 min. *Square*: Part of a sebaceous duct; a similar section is shown below left

Below   Cell migration

Left   This is a sebaceous duct corresponding to the square in the upper right figure. Labeled cells have moved from the basal cell layer towards the sebaceous duct lumen (to the left) with considerable speed within 7 days

Right   Sebaceous acinus. Within 17 days, labeled sebocytes have moved far into the center of the lobule with no silver grains left in the basal cell layer. In summary, sebocytes are a quite active cell population with speedy movement

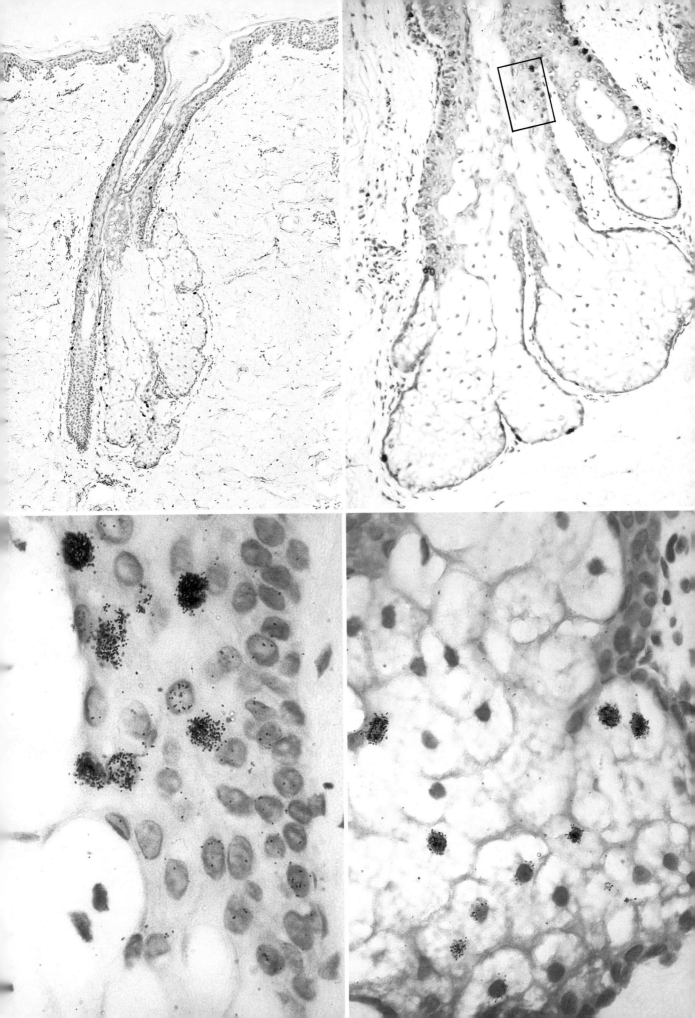

Sebaceous Glands Are Very Active Skin Appendages

Radiolabeling techniques disclose some of the metabolic activities of sebaceous acini.

Above   The same huge sebaceous glands of a sebaceous follicle are photographed with different techniques: *Left* with standard light microscopy, *right* with darkfield microscopy. Tritiated thymidine, 45 min after incorporation, and visualized by autoradiographic techniques, labels the lipid producing sebocytes (fine, dark appearing silver grains) which shine up bright under darkfield illumination

Below   Tritiated thymidine, 5 days after initial incorporation. This sebaceous lobule is viewed with darkfield technique. The basal cell layer appears brownish. The next three to five layers of sebocytes have cleared the tracer, which is slowly moving with the outward movement of sebocytes towards the sebaceous duct

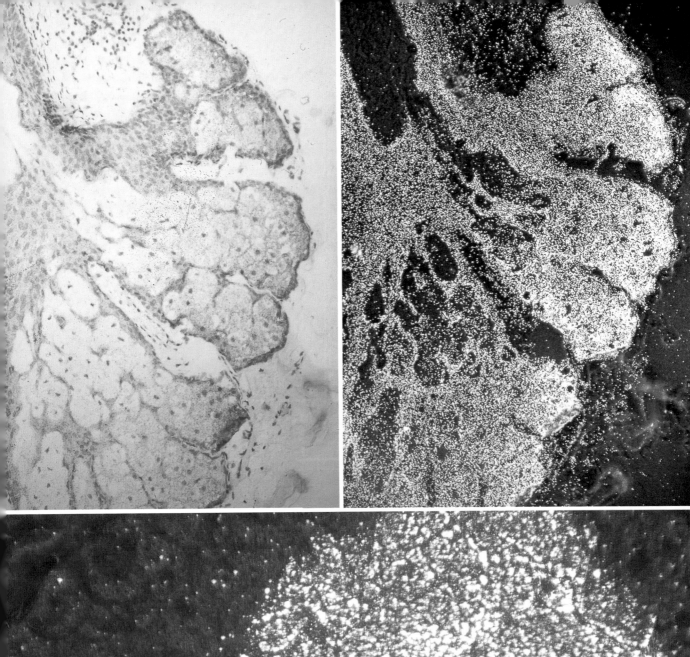
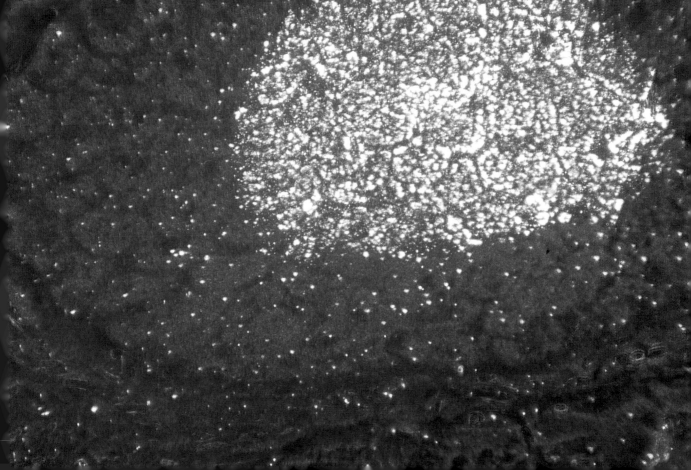

Microorganisms

For a long while acne was considered a bacterial infection; scholars quarreled whether aerobes or anaerobes were the infectious agents. The lesions shared features with pyodermas, namely, redness, tenderness, and, above all, suppuration. Injection of cultured organisms even produced pustules. In addition antibiotics were beneficial. Nonetheless, the question "do bacteria cause acne?" has given way to the more subtle one "do bacteria play any role in acne?"

Only three groups need to be considered:
- *Propionibacterium acnes*
- Cocci, mainly *Staphylococcus epidermidis*
- Lipophilic yeasts of the genus *Pityrosporum*

These organisms are always present in comedones. The failure to demonstrate each of them in all cases reflects technical error. The same organisms occur on the normal face and are hence part of the resident microflora. The fact that an organism is a regular and harmless inhabitant does not exclude a pathogenic role. Many healthy persons carry unnoticed virulent staphylococci and streptococci in their nose and throat; infections only result after host resistance changes.

Formerly, the nonvirulent aerobic resident cocci of the skin were all called *Staphylococcus albus*. Modern taxonomy recognizes two genera of the family Micrococcaceae, namely *Staphylococcus* and *Micrococcus*, each with several species. A classification widely used until the late 1970s was that of Baird-Parker, which has been replaced by that of Kloos and coworkers. The latter classification is based on more reliable biochemical, physiological, and morphological phenotypic characteristics. Unfortunately, there is no direct relationship between both systems.

Practically all of these cocci can occur in the face; the dominant one is *Staphylococcus epidermidis*, a coagulase-negative bacterium. By sampling successive thin slices of comedones, it can be shown that the great bulk of *Staphylococcus epidermidis* is situated near the surface. It is far outnumbered by facultative anaerobes which live monopolistically in the deeper portions. Because of their location, one rarely sees cocci in histologic sections of ruptured comedones. Cocci can be recovered from pustules only when the horny kernel is sampled along with the pus. Interestingly, their numbers are not reduced by antibiotics as they quickly become resistant. This is mediated by plasmids.

Yeasts and cocci produce lipases in vitro and so are able to hydrolize glycerides to fatty acids. The aerobes chiefly colonize the orifices of sebaceous follicles and are not situated in the deeper infrainfundibulum, where only the microaerophilic *Propionibacterium acnes* can survive. There is no evidence that they are comedogenic; nor can they cause the rupture of comedones. They are bystanders only.

Morphologically two types of *Pityrosporum* can be distinguished in sebaceous follicles and comedones: *Pityrosporum ovale*, by far the most common, and *Pityrosporum orbiculare*. Recent investigations indicate that these are merely morphological variants of the same organism. It has not been possible to establish an etiologic role for yeasts in acne. Their presence or absence is immaterial. Rare pustular acneiform eruptions of the trunk caused by oral tetracyclines is not a result of excessive growth of this yeast, although this is a common belief. Experimental inoculation of human skin does not evoke pustules.

We are thus left with *Propionibacterium acnes*. There can be little doubt of its pathogenic role, although some important questions remain to be answered. First of all, *Propionibacterium acnes* is microaerophilic, growing best under strictly anaerobic conditions. This commits it to an intrafollicular existence. It also utilizes sebum as a nutrient and is accordingly most abundant in the sebum-rich regions where the density of deep follicles is greatest. The highest counts obtained by scrubbing the surface are recovered from the face and the scalp, where they are 10–100 times greater than on the upper back. This can be very misleading, however, because the follicles on the back are comparatively far apart. One can understand that scrubbing the surface will not provide a true count of the organisms within the follicles. This holds especially for sebaceous follicles with their deep, wide canals. A sebaceous follicle on the back doubtlessly can support as many *Propionibacterium acnes* as one in the face. Some are packed with *Propionibacterium acnes*, others seem empty. The quantity can only be accurately ascertained when the contents are extruded in one piece as in follicular filaments or in comedones. The important information is the density per follicle, not the quantity per square centimeter. This can be studied with quantitative bacteriologic techniques like microdissection, and by sampling follicular casts extracted by the cyanoacrylate follicular biopsy technique.

The number of *Propionibacteria* usually exceeds, that of aerobes in open and closed comedones. They are more numerous in closed comedones than in open ones, reflecting lower oxygen tension. Since open comedones are drier, they also contain fewer aerobes on a weight basis. The high density of organisms in closed comedones may correlate with the greater tendency to rupture.

Corynebacterium acnes was the term previously applied to these anaerobes. Those from the face have been divided into two groups, type I and type II, on the basis of morphology, phage susceptibility, biochemical reactions, and immunologic specifity. Type I and type II *Corynebacterium acnes* are now called *Propionibacterium acnes* and *Propionibacterium granulosum*, respectively. Fortunately, typing can be done with almost complete reliability by simply looking at the colonies.

Propionibacterium avidum (type III) occurs in nonacne areas such as the axilla. It is rarely isolated from the face and its pathogenicity is problematic. It has been suggested that *Propionibacterium granulosum* may be more prevalent in individuals with the severer forms of acne. This is of more interest because *Propionibacterium granulosum* shows high in vitro activities. It is more proteolytic, more antigenic, and tends to produce a more pronounced reaction when injected intradermally. However, it frequently cannot be isolated in severe acne which brings into question the relevance of in vitro findings. This is a generalized role in biology. *Propionibacterium acnes* has a higher prevalence and is more numerous than *Propionibacterium granulosum*, whether obtained from acne patients or not. *Propionibacterium acnes* can be isolated from practically all subjects. Usually, only one species is recovered from one follicle, but mixtures do occur. *Propionibacterium acnes* is certainly not a pathogen in the usual sense, and in rare cases it has been incriminated in systemic infections such as endocarditis in compromised patients. There are no convincing reports of its capability to cause infections in skin or other organs. Because it is a normal resident organism, it is often recovered in samples submitted for bacteriologic work-up. Consequently, a number of diseases of unknown cause, for example, acne necrotica, have been erroneously attributed to this organism. Attempts to demonstrate that *Propionibacterium acnes* can multiply within human skin have failed completely. We found that:

● It took more than a billion organisms injected intradermally to evoke a pustule.
● The same response could be secured with heat-killed organisms.
● Suspensions of comedones produced persistent papules with the histologic characteristics of foreign body granulomas whether or not the suspension was heat-treated to kill *Propionibacterium acnes*. When these induced lesions were excised (*Propionibacterium acnes* or comedones), there was more than 90% killing in a few hours, with no survivors after 24 h.

Sampling inflammatory lesions has been instructive. The bacteria are transported passively into the tissue when comedones rupture. *Propionibacterium acnes* can be demonstrated histologically in the extruded horny core, but not free in the inflammatory tissue. Recovery by culture is low, even in fresh lesions; the latter are frequently sterile. Larger inflammatory lesions such as nodules typically contain very few organisms. Not only is *Propionibacterium acnes* quickly mopped up by neutrophils, but the oxygen tension of the inflammatory environment is unfavorable for its survival. All these observations are consistent with the view that *Propionibacterium acnes* acts only indirectly in pathogenesis, namely by inciting comedones and by producing substances which lead to their rupture.

As regards the formation of the comedo, *Propionibacterium acnes* produces a lipase which releases free fatty acids from triglycerides. Lipolysis is virtually complete wherever the organism is very numerous as in follicular filaments or comedones. Free fatty acids are considerably more comedogenic than the triglycerides from which they are derived. Lipoidal extracts of the organisms themselves are strongly comedogenic in comedo assays. The commencement of the comedo is always preceded by a huge massing of *Propionibacterium acnes* in the canal. The only exception to this is the formation of the first comedones in prepubertal children. Its important role in causing rupture of comedones has been deduced from the following observations.

1. The cysts of steatocystoma multiplex are sterile. They also possess sebaceous glands and hence contain sebum. When injected with *Propionibacterium acnes*, the organism will proliferate, the cyst wall degenerates, and the dumping of its contents into the dermis incites an inflammatory lesion, typical of acne. This does not happen when cocci are injected.
2. Comedones induced in humans by topical application of coal tar, which contains phenolic substances with antibacterial properties, do not undergo inflammatory breakdown; they harbor very few *Propionibacterium acnes*.
3. Sebum-induced comedones in the rabbit ear canal are never colonized by *Propionibacterium acnes* and attempts to implant the organism fail. These bacteria-free comedones never become inflamed.

4. *Propionibacterium acnes* within comedones produce toxic substances which can attack the follicular epithelium and incite rupture, e.g., the lipolysis of glycerides leads to high concentrations of free fatty acids. Additionally, the organism produces a number of enzymes which attack the follicular epithelium and lead to extrusion of comedonal contents. These include protease, lipase, lecithinase, hyaluronate lyase, neuramidase, phosphatase, phospholipase, proteinase, and RNase: quite a cocktail of active materials. More will be discovered that are proinflammatory: histamine and interleukins are already under investigation.

An interesting theory centers around the importance of the follicular environment. Differences in the microenvironment between involved and noninvolved follicles may influence the production of biologically active compounds. After all, only a small proportion of the total sebaceous follicles become involved at any one time. In support of this concept it has been found that low-chain-length fatty acids, especially propionic acid, a major end product of *Propionibacterium acnes* metabolism, possesses cytotoxic activity in different test systems. The production of propionate was enhanced when glucose was added as an energy source. There is an analogy here with periodontal disease, in which plaque-forming microorganisms also secrete low molecular weight fatty acids which attack the tissues.

Another finding which points to the critical role of the follicular microenvironment is the extreme dryness of the skin induced by oral isotretinoin. The counts of aerobes and anaerobes fall sharply. Sebum production markedly decreases before this happens. The low density of *Propionibacterium acnes* persists for several months after the end of treatment, despite the return of sebum levels to normal. Isotretinoin-induced dryness leads to the virtual elimination of *Propionibacterium acnes* and gram-negative bacteria. At the same time colonization by *Staphylococcus aureus* may be enhanced, first in the nasal antrum. *Propionibacterium acnes* also produces porphyrins. These can be easily visualized under Wood's light examination of culture plates or localized at the orifices of large sebaceous follicles, as on the nose. The role of porphyrins in the evolution of comedones or the initiation of inflammatory acne lesions is uncertain. It has been proposed that porphyrins accelerate squalene oxidation. Squalene is a highly effective oxygen-trapping compound which could lower the oxygen tension within sebaceous follicles, thus favoring colonization of *Propionibacterium acnes*. This might help to account for the variability of involvement from follicle to follicle.

Propionibacterium acnes synthesizes antigens which can induce circulating antibodies. Immediate wheals to intradermally injected antigens are more common and intense in acne patients than in matched controls. The titer of circulating antibodies is higher in acne patients, but this problem reflects repeated extrusion of *Propionibacterium acnes* into the dermis via the rupture of comedones. Intradermal injection of *Propionibacterium acnes* extracts also provokes an inflammatory reaction suggestive of cell-mediated delayed allergy. However, the histopathologic picture is not consistent with delayed-type allergy and the responses are similar in patients and controls. Thus, while immune processes may be initiated these are probably secondary events. The therapeutic efficacy of antibiotics and of isotretinoin is compelling proof of the central role of *Propionibacterium acnes*. The disease is always moderated by those drugs which cause a sharp reduction in the *Propionibacterium acnes* population or in the proportion of free fatty acids in the surface lipids. Finally, there is a striking difference in the evolution of *Propionibacterium acnes* colonization of subjects with and without acne. At puberty, the quantity of *Propionibacterium acnes* on the face and cheek goes up sharply in acne patients, remaining rather constant throughout adult life. In nonacne subjects, however, *Propionibacterium acnes* counts stay relatively low till early adulthood. After about 20–25 years of age, the population is the same in both groups. Interestingly, there is no correlation between the density of *Propionibacterium acnes* and the severity of the disease. This may be misleading since solely the surface organisms are being recovered by the scrubbing method. Besides, *Propionibacterium acnes* does not survive in inflammatory lesions.

Akamatsu H, Nishijima S, Takahashi M, Ushijima T, Asada Y (1991) Effects of subliminal inhibitory concentrations of erythromycin, tetracycline, clindamycin, and minocycline on the neutrophil chemotactic factor production in Propionibacterium acnes biotypes 1–5. J Dermatol 18:247–251

Allaker RP, Greenman J, Osborne RH, Gowers JI (1985) Cytotoxic activity of Propionibacterium acnes and other skin organisms. Br J Dermatol 113:229–235

Baird-Parker AC (1974) The basis for the present classification of staphylococci and micrococci. Ann NY Acad Sci 236:7–14

Bibel DJ, Aly R, Maibach HI, Leyden JJ, Shinefield HR, Akers WA, Burnett JW (1976) Nomenclature of staphylococci and micrococci. Arch Dermatol 112:1614–1615

Cove JH, Holland KT, Cunliffe WJ (1983) Effects of oxygen concentration on biomass production, maximum specific growth rate and extracellular enzyme production by three species of cutaneous propionibacteria grown in continuous culture. J Gen Microbiol 129:3327–3334

De Young LM, Young JM, Ballaron SJ, Spires DA, Puhvel SM (1984) Intradermal injection of Propionibacterium acnes: a model of inflammation relevant to acne. J Invest Dermatol 83:394–398

Hoeffler U, Ko HL, Pulverer G (1976) Antimicrobial susceptibicity of Propionibacterium acnes and related microbial species. Antimicrob Agent Chemother 10:387–394

Holland KT (1989) Microbiology of acne. In: Cunliffe WJ Acne. Dunitz, London, pp 178–210

Kloos WE, Schleifer KH (1975) Isolation and characterization of staphylococci from human skin. II. Description of four new species, Staphylococcus warneri, Staphylococcus capitis, Staphylococcus hominis, and Staphylococcus simulans. Int J Syst Bacteriol 25:62–79

Lavker RM, Leyden JJ, McGinley KJ (1981) The relationship between bacteria and the abnormal follicular keratinization in acne vulgaris. J Invest Dermatol 77:325–330

Leyden JJ, McGinley KJ, Foglia AN (1986) Qualitative and quantitative changes in cutaneous bacteria associated with systemic isotretinoin therapy for acne conglobata. J Invest Dermatol 86:390–393

McGinley KJ, Webster GF, Ruggieri MR, Leyden JJ (1978) Regional variations of cutaneous propionibacteria. Correlation of Propionibacterium acnes population with sebaceous secretion. J Clin Microbiol 12:672–675

Metze D, Kersten A, Jurecka W, Gebhart W (1991) Immunoglobulins coat microorganisms of skin surface: a comparative immunohistochemical and ultrastructural study of cutaneous and oral microbial symbionts. J Invest Dermatol 96:439–445

Nordstrom KM, Labows JN, McGinley KJ, Leyden JJ (1986) Characterization of wax esters, triglycerides and free fatty acids of follicular casts. J Invest Dermatol 86:700–705

Puhvel SM, Amirian DA (1979) Bacterial flora of comedones. Br J Dermatol 101:543–548

Puhvel SM, Sakamoto M (1977) An in vivo evaluation of the inflammatory effect of purified comedonal components in human skin. J Invest Dermatol 69:401–406

Singer RE, Buckner BA (1981) Butyrate and propionate: important components of toxic dental plaque extracts. Infect Immun 32:458–463

Webster GF, Cummins CS (1978) Use of bacteriophage typing to distinguish Propionibacterium acne types I and II. J Clin Microbiol 7:84–90

The Microflora of Acne

Three organisms are constantly found on the face: *Propionibacterium acnes*, *Staphylococcus eidermidis*, and yeasts of the genus *Pityrosporum*.

These panels compare the light-microscopic (*left*) and the electron-microscopic (*right*) appearances of these organisms in tissue at the same magnification.

Above *Pityrosporum*. These budding years congregate in bead-like patterns at the tip of the comedo and also in the acroinfundibulum of normal follicles. Note the very thick wall. *Left*, semithin section, periodic acid – Schiff, ×960; *right*, electron microscopy, ×3200

Middle *Staphylococcus epidermidis*. These bacteria prefer superficial locations in the acroinfundibulum and at the tips of comedones. They are recognized by their round shape. *Left*, semithin section, methylene blue, ×960; *right*, electron microscopy, ×25000

Below *Propionibacterium acnes*. This microaerophilic diphtheroid almost exclusively occupies the deeper portions of the sebaceous follicles and comedones. The bacterium varies a good deal in size and shape, sometimes even showing coccoid forms. *Left*, semithin section, methylene blue, ×960; *right*, electron microscopy, ×64000

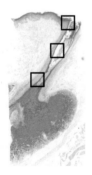

Below: Courtesy of Professor Helmut H. Wolff, M.D., Lübeck, FRG

Wolff HH, Plewig G (1976) Ultrastruktur der Mikroflora in Follikeln und Komedonen. Hautarzt 27:432–440

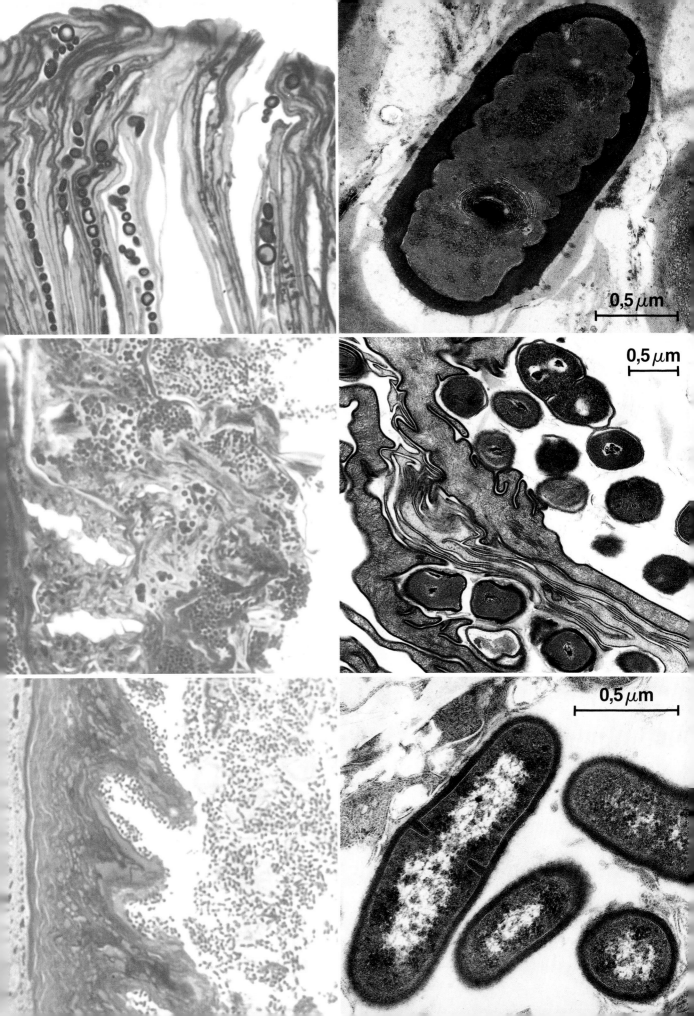

Follicular and Comedonal Flora

The deep anaerobic or semianaerobic recessus of follicular structures is an El Dorado for bacteria, richly nourished by the constant flow of sebum.

Above

Left   A normal sebaceous follicle of a person with no acne. The follicular filament is saturated with solid colonies of bacteria, most of which are *Propionibacterium acnes* and *Staphylococcus epidermidis.* Sebaceous glands provide nutrition (Gram stain)

Right   An old open comedo has multiple spacious cavernas (✱) in its inner structure, providing space and ambient living conditions for *Propionibacterium acnes.* Between the lamellae of corneocytes at the tip numerous *Pityrosporum ovale* yeasts (→) enjoy undisturbed growth. They have nothing to do with the acne process. The pilary portion is to the lower left (periodic acid – Schiff stain)

Below

Left   Horizontal section through a biopsy from the cheek of a person with moderate acne on the back Multiple large sebaceous follicles and their adjacent sebaceous acini are seen. The blue stain signals bacterial colonization. Thus every follicle is colonized (Gram stain)

Right   Higher magnification of two follicular canals of sebaceous follicles. The follicular filament is a cast of corneocytes, with multiple channels in the center which are full of bacteria. Each channel is the draining system of a sebaceous duct below. *Propionibacterium acnes* loves this nutrient broth. The hairs (→) enter the follicular canal at this level (Gram stain)

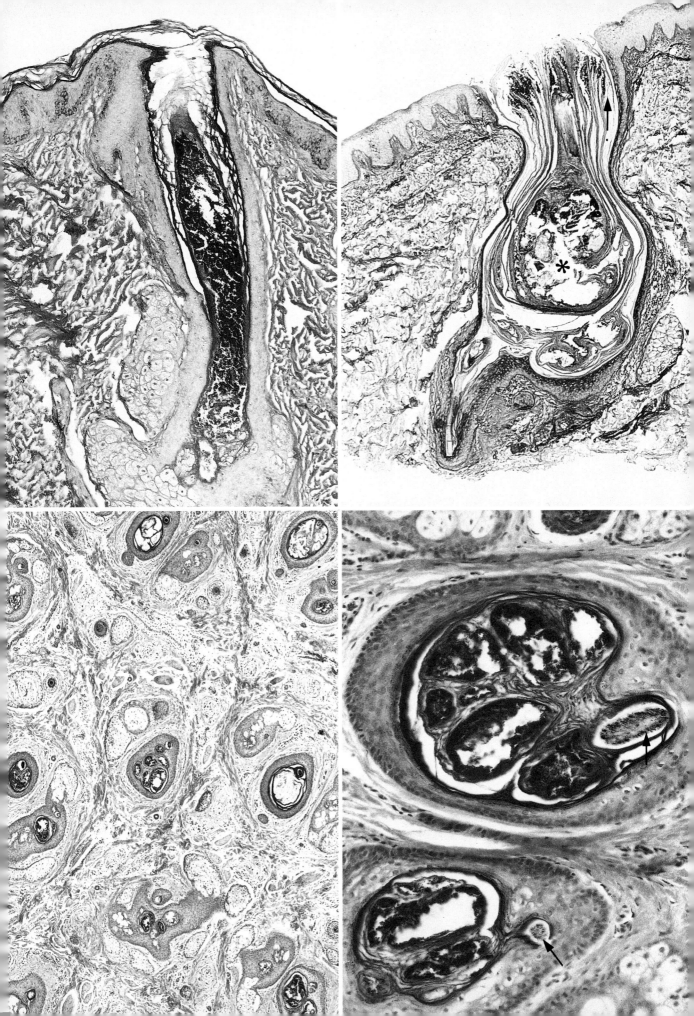

Internal Structures of Old Open Comedones

Comedones removed with comedo extractors were cut horizontally. Despite their compact external appearance large open comedones are often full of holes like Swiss cheese.

Above   In very large, aged comedones there are rows of chambers, all exiting into a single giant cavity. Finger-like projections of corneocytes divide the gallery. These chambers are full of *Propionibacterium acnes*, most of which fell out during histologic preparation

Below   The individual cavernas are sealed by concentric layers of tightly adherent corneocytes. Masses of *Propionibacterium acnes* are trapped, floating in a sea of sebum. The cavernas communicate at other levels of the comedo, while they meander to the comedonal core

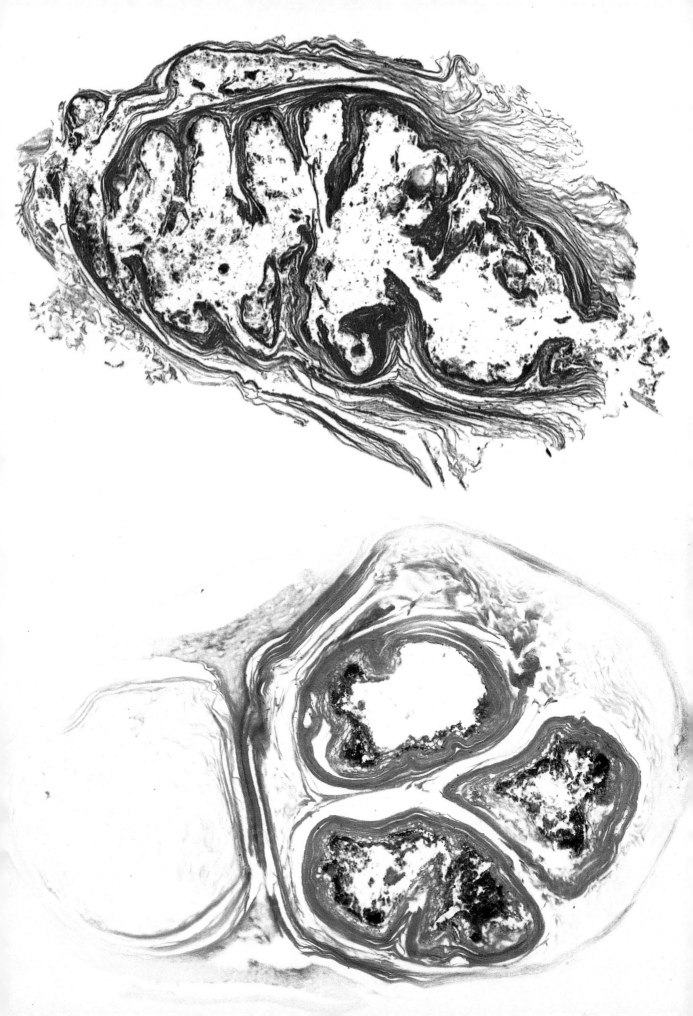

Follicular Fluorescence

Propionibacterium acnes produces porphyrins which fluoresce under Wood's light. The characteristic orange-red fluorescence can thus be visualized in follicles which harbor a dense population of these microorganisms. Sebum itself fluoresces slightly yellow.

Above

Left Fluorescent follicles are most easily observed on the nose. The cheesy "worms" that can be pressed out of the alae nasi fluoresce brilliantly and contain millions of *Propionibacteria*. The percentage of brightly fluorescing follicles varies greatly from person to person. Fluorescence is a rough but useful indicator of the quantity of *Propionibacterium acnes*. Persons who show bright fluorescence over their forehead and cheeks invariably have high numbers of these microaerophilic microorganisms. As a rule acne patients show an intense and widespread fluorescence compared to nonacne subjects. After antibiotic or antimicrobial treatment, fluorescence diminishes greatly owing to suppression of *Propionibacterium acnes*. This can be used to evaluate the efficacy of antibiotics in acne treatment

Right Fluorescent colonies of *Propionibacterium acnes* on agar. Only the surface colonies fluoresce brightly

Below Skin surface biopsy obtained with the cyanoacrylate technique, viewed with fluorescent light. The follicular filaments containing one hair are easily seen. *Inset*, higher magnification of one follicular filament. Not only sebum, but also horny material shows a yellow fluorescence

Below: Courtesy of Gerhard Sauermann, M.D., and Udo Hoppe, M.D., Beiersdorf AG, Hamburg, FRG

Cornelius CE, Ludwig GD (1967) Red fluorescence of comedones: production of porphyrins by Corynebacterium acnes. J Invest Dermatol 49:368–370

Formanek I, Fanta D, Poitscheck CH, Turner J (1977) Porphyrinproduktion des Propionibacterium acnes. Arch Dermatol Res 259:169–176

Hoppe U, Sauermann G (1990) Moderne kosmetische Wirkstoffe und der Nachweis ihrer Funktion. Z Hautkr 65:123–131

Martin RJ, Kahn G, Gooding JW, Brown G (1973) Cutaneous porphyrin fluorescence as an indicator of antibiotic absorption and effectiveness. Cutis 12:758–764

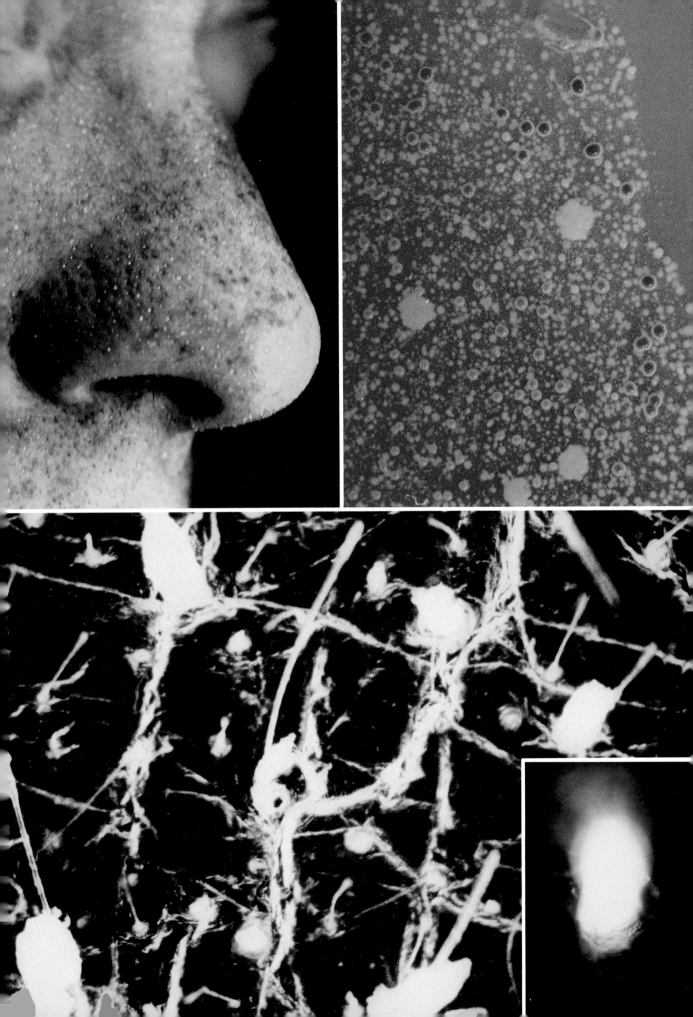

The Dynamics of Inflammatory Acne: Immunologic Factors

The gram-positive microaerophilic diphtheroid *Propionibacterium acnes* is the dominant organism in sebaceous follicles. It grows in dense colonies within the lacunae of follicular filaments, microcomedones, and both closed and open comedones. *Propionibacterium acnes* depends for nutrition on the triglyceride fraction of sebum. It is absent in animals, and the density is low to absent in prepubertal children. It is the glycerol moiety of sebaceous triglycerides which the bacteria need for nutrition; they get access to it by their extracellular lipase. The split-off (deesterified) free fatty acids remain in the sebum. Their concentrations are directly related to the density of the bacterial population, and it is believed, not without controversies, that these play a key role in creating inflammatory lesions. Two types of inflammatory responses may be recognized. The commonest is a frank rupture of the comedonal epithelium. The comedo contains corneocytes, hairs, sebum, bacteria, and a mixture of cellular debris, and these are dumped into the dermis provoking a foreign body reaction. The other is a rather silent affair with no evidence of epithelial discontinuity and is discovered histologically. Masses of neutrophils congregate within the intact comedo, hugging the epithelial wall which may be spongiotic. This suggests the leakage of diffusable substances from the comedonal kernel. This is a kind of brush war which may be followed by frank rupture. In this silent early phase, immunoglobulins, e.g., IgG and complement, e.g., C_3 can be detected in the blood vessels surrounding the comedo as well as in the clinically uninvolved skin of acne patients. The chemoattractant has been partially characterized. It may be extracted from comedones into aqueous solutions, and it is heat stable, dialyzable, and does not require complement for activity. The molecular weight is around 2000. Its small size would explain its ability to diffuse from intact follicles or comedones into the dermis, thus attracting neutrophils. Once neutrophils are present, further inflammatory steps ensure. Neutrophils possess a number of enzymes which can digest the follicular epithelium as well as collagen. Complement is deposited in the dermis. *Propionibacterium acnes* is a potent activator of both the classical and alternative pathway of complement. There is evidence that the classical pathway is mediated by anti-*Propionibacterium acnes* antibodies, whereas the alternative pathway is mediated by carbohydrates derived from cell walls of the bacteria. The activation of complement is proportional to the levels of *Propionibacterium acnes* in comedones. The next step following classical or alternative complement activation is the generation of C_5-derived neutrophil chemoattractants, completing the vicious circle of inflammation.

The reversal, the resolution of inflammation, is only poorly understood. One important finding ist that *Propionibacterium acnes* is very resistant to degradation by neutrophils or monocytes which have ingested the organism. In an in vitro study, less than 10% of the *Propionibacterium acnes* mass was degraded within 24 h. More than 1 week is necessary to reduce the *Propionibacterium acnes* mass by half, and about 3 weeks to reduce it by 90%. This parallels the clinical observation of persistent papules or small nodules in acne patients for several weeks, in contrast to the situation in staphylococcal folliculitis, which resolves in a few days. Another feature that may contribute to persistence is the fact that *Propionibacterium acnes*, once phagocytized, remains viable for days despite antimicrobial treatment. The organism dies quickly when free in the tissue.

In contrast to the probable role of circulating antibodies and complement activation, the pathogenesis of acne is problematic and controversial. Macrophages and lymphocytes are routinely found in persistent inflammatory lesions. These can release a great many cytokines which can aggravate inflammation, including activation of T-cell subsets.

Allaker RP, Greenman J, Osborne RH (1987) The production of inflammatory compounds by Propionibacterium acnes and other skin organisms. Br J Dermatol 117:175–183

Ingham E, Gowland G, Ward RM, Holland KT, Cunliffe WJ (1987) Antibodies to P. acnes and P. acnes exocellular enzymes in the normal population at various ages and in patients with acne vulgaris. Br J Dermatol 116:805–812

Lee WL, Shalita AR, Sunthralingam K, Fiberig SM (1982) Neutrophil chemotaxis to Propionibacterium acnes lipase and its inhibition. Infect Immun 35:71–78

Leeming JP, Ingham E, Cunliffe WJ (1988) The microbial content and complement C3 cleaving capacity of comedones in acne vulgaris. Acta Derm Venereol (Stockh) 68:468–473

Puhvel SM, Sakamoto M (1977) A re-evaluation of fatty acid as inflammatory agents in acne. J Invest Dermatol 68:93–99

Puhvel SM, Sakamoto M (1977) An in vivo evaluation of the inflammatory effect of purified comedonal components in human skin. J Invest Dermatol 69:401–406

Puhvel SM, Sakamoto M (1980) Cytotaxin production by comedonal bacteria. Propionibacterium acnes, Propionibacterium granulosum and Staphylococcus epidermidis. J Invest Dermatol 74:36–39

Webster GF (1990) Inflammatory acne. Int J Dermatol 29:313–317

Webster GF, Indrisano JP, Leyden JJ (1985) Antibody titers to Propionibacterium acnes cell wall carbohydrate in nodulocystic acne patients. J Invest Dermatol 84:496–500

Webster GF, McArthur WP (1982) Activation of components of the alternative pathway of complement by Propionibacterium acnes cell wall carbohydrate. J Invest Dermatol 79:137–140

The Evolution of the Comedo

The comedo is the initial, primary lesion of acne. It is an impaction of horn within sebaceous follicles. Comedones develop through the following stages.

Primary Comedones

The *microcomedo* is an early distention of the follicle by corneocytes. Its existence can only be verified in histologic sections.

The *closed comedo or whitehead* is the first visible lesion, a whitish firm nodule resembling a milium, generally 1–2 mm in diameter. The pore is tiny and generally cannot be seen with the naked eye.

The dilatation of the orifice by a protruding mass of darkly pigmented horny material marks the onset of the *open comedo or blackhead*. It may attain a diameter of 5 mm, sometimes even more.

Secondary Comedones

The rupture and re-encapsulation of comedones creates secondary comedones. The same comedo may experience focal blow-ups many times. Secondary comedones can usually be differentiated because they have irregular shapes, are generally larger than the primary ones, and show histologic signs of a prior inflammatory episode. Three types of secondary comedones are sufficiently specialized to warrant specific designations.

The *cyst* is a large, skin-colored, rubbery nodule, resembling a trichilemmal cyst (synonyms are *atheroma* or *wen*). 5–20 mm in diameter, occurring mainly on the back and sometimes the cheeks of individuals with ongoing or past acne conglobata. Puncture releases a cheesy, crumbly material consisting of corneocytes, hairs, bacteria, and sebum.

The *fistulated (polyporous) comedo* looks like a cluster of two or more blackheads, occurring mainly on the back in acne conglobata. These are interconnected and share common openings. Fistulated comedones can also be viewed as a peculiar type of scar.

A late sequel, probably starting with a primary comedo, then engulfing other follicles, comedones, papules and abscesses results in a *draining sinus*.

The latter two will be dealt with in a later chapter (p. 88).

The Life History of the Comedo

Above

Left   Normal sebaceous follicle. A normal sebaceous follicle with its extravagant glands, miniscule hair (telogen stage) and cavernous canal

Middle Early microcomedo. The canal has begun to distend with coherent layers of corneocytes. Inside these are bacteria-filled channels (stained blue), reaching well into the sebaceous ducts. The hair is an anagen

Right   Late microcomedo. The epithelium is hyperplastic. A horny impaction has dilated the follicle. This is still too small to be visible with the naked eye. The sebaceous ducts are also hyperkeratotic. Regressing of the sebaceous acini has started. Gram-positive rods (*Propionibacterium acnes*) have densely colonized the central channels

Below

Left   Mature closed comedo. The pore is microscopic. Horny squamae are densely packed into concentric lamellae, though whorling has jumbled the pattern. The channels are larger and more irregular than in microcomedones. They contain solid masses of *Propionibacterium acnes*. The glands are small. The pilary portion is intact, with several hairs being trapped in the horny mass

Right   Open comedo. There are now numerous bacteria-filled spaces which belie the solid appearance of the comedo. The sebaceous glands are very small, but never absent. The pilary portion is normal and continues to shed hairs into the comedo. Here and there are cross-sectional cuts of trapped vellus hairs. Yeasts (*Pityrosporum ovale*) are congregated at the tip. A comedo is a melange of corneocytes, bacteria, yeasts, hairs and sebaceous lipids

All drawings are of the same magnification

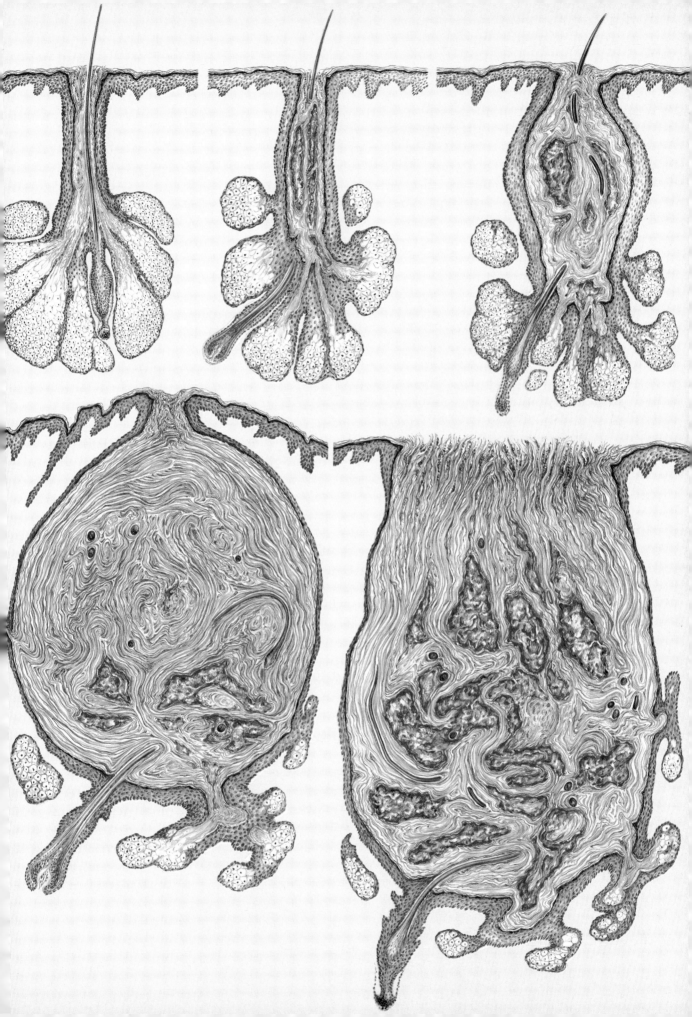

The Dynamics of Primary Comedo Formation

Two tactics have been of inestimable value for observing the anatomical changes of the evolving disease: these are biopsying and serial sectioning the apparently uninvolved areas of acne-bearing skin. Without the latter the earliest changes cannot be seen and without serial sections one can obtain only glimpses, not a full picture. One section of the same specimen may almost look normal while elsewhere there may be startling alterations. Asymmetry is quite characteristic of acne lesions.

A peculiar change in the pattern of keratinization of the infrainfundibulum marks the onset of comedo formation. A granular layer appears, sturdier corneocytes are produced and, most important of all, these begin to stick together to form a coherent kernel made up of well-defined horny lamellae.

The microcomedo originates from follicles harboring sebaceous filaments; these might be regarded as precomedones. However, it is very important to appreciate that sebaceous filaments do not inevitably evolve into comedones. In fact they usually do not since they are common in adults with oily skin who no longer have acne. Moreover, sebaceous filaments are common on the nose where comedones are rare. They are simply a stage through which the sebaceous follicles pass on their way to comedo formation. The filament has an outer envelop of compacted corneocytes, literally a thick horny layer, encasing a softish amalgam of sebum, sloughed empty sebocytes, undifferentiated cells from sebaceous acini, and flimsy corneocytes from sebaceous ducts or the lower portion of the infrainfundibulum. A paramount finding is masses of *Propionibacterium acnes* within the core of the filament. These play a crucial role in the formation of the comedo. The lumen is congested but not obstructed. Sebum issues through the orifice.

The transformation of a sebaceous filament into a microcomedo is a continous process with no sharp definition. The key change, however, is decreased dehiscence of corneocytes. They stick together tightly like bricks and form a solid compact mass which steadily expands. The intercellular cement must change in some way so as to act as a nondegradable glue. Probably there are qualitative and quantitative alterations of the intercellular lipids, in particular the ceramides. Perhaps lytic enzymes are no longer secreted into the intercellular spaces to weaken the cement. In any case the cells become permanently tied together. Speculation concerning these events now centers around the keratinosomes or membrane coating granules. These are lysosome-like structures which extrude their lipid-rich contents into the intercellular spaces. These lipids are essential for the barrier function of the stratum corneum and also apparently regulate desquamation in some unknown fashion. Membrane-coating granules are numerous in the normal infrainfundibulum, but have been reported to decrease when comedones form, suggesting that shedding of corneocytes becomes limited in their relative absence. This is a disputed subject. Another explanation for the tight cohesion of corneocytes is that the desmosomes which bind epidermal cells together fail to desintegrate as keratinocytes reach the horny layer. Their persistence in the horny layer would prevent desquamation.

Another component of importance for the cell-to-cell-adhesion not only in the living epidermis but also in the stratum corneum (or comedones) are desmosomes. Corneosomes are modified desmosomes in the stratum corneum. Corneosome breakdown and corneocyte shedding are closely related. In any case, the failure of corneocytes to slough normally produces a hyperkeratosis of the retention type. There is also an increased production of corneocytes. The upper follicular epithelium becomes hyperproliferative. Both processes, increased production and increased retention of corneocytes, contribute to the distension of the infundibulum by the horny impaction. It should be emphasized that this hyperkeratosis is not simply a result of irritation. Toxic substances characteristically produce loose horny layers which fall apart rapidly in contrast to comedogenic agents with cause cohesion. For example propionic acid is very irritating and noncomedogenic, while oleic acid is comedogenic and only mildly irritating.

It is the better part of wisdom not to offer any mechanistic explanation for comedo formation. We do not know how this happens or why among the thousands of sebaceous follicles only a few evolve into comedones at any time. To this very day, the customary belief of how a comedo forms is a fanciful misconception. It is always said that it begins with an obstruction of the orifice. The orifice becomes blocked and a bag of sebum results; this might be called the plug or cork version.

Nothing like this happens; indeed quite the opposite. The acroinfundibulum or pore region does not participate at all. If the acroinfundibulum became hyperkeratotic, the orifice would dilate from the very start; the first visible lesion would be an open not a closed comedo. This never happens in acne vulgaris. However, it can be brought about artificially when a potent comedogenic agent such as coal tar is applied. In this case the acroinfundibulum becomes immediately involved in retention hyperkeratosis. The horny mass distends and protrudes through the pore. The first visible lesion is then an open not a closed comedo in contrast to acne vulgaris. In acne vulgaris, only the infrainfundibulum participates in comedo formation. Hence the follicle swells below and the orifice does not dilate. Instead of a cork at the outlet, the whole follicular canal becomes filled with compact corneocytes. Acne would be an easier disease to treat if the cork conception were true. Advertisements promoting the sale of abrasives and peeling agents are often based on uncapping this supposedly superficial plug.

Closed comedones ordinarily do not grow beyond a size of about 2 mm. They take approximately 5 months to reach this degree of maturity. The larger ones sometimes contain two hairs, rarely more, which is evidence of their youth. Closed comedones (microcomedones in their start-up stage) suffer one of two fates: either they rupture and incite an inflammatory lesion or they gradually enlarge into open comedones. Autoradiographic studies show that the production of corneocytes does not slow down as the comedo enlarges; hence, if it does not explode, continued accumulation of corneocytes will force the orifice to dilate. The tip of the horny mass will then be exposed, giving birth to the open comedo. At first, the pigmented tip may be not more than 1 mm wide. As the orifice dilates, the core of protruding horn gets thicker and may eventually reach a size of 5 mm or more. The open comedo has a very long career, being a rather stable structure. Unlike the closed comedo, horny material continuously moves through the orifice in a glacier-like fashion and is eroded away. Semi-liquid substances such as sebum can escape to the surface. Drainage of sebum and products excreted by masses of *Propionibacterium acnes*, is almost completely obstructed in the closed comedo; hence its tendency to rupture. It has been dubbed the time bomb of acne.

As the open comedo enlarges, the pilary portion continues to produce and shed hairs. These are of course retained and become curled and tangled within the horny matrix. Medium sized blackheads generally contain six to eight hairs. An aged comedo may contain as many as fifteen hairs. Allowing 80 days for a complete anagen–telogen hair cycle, the longevity of such a comedo would be over 3 years. During that time the horny mass would of course have been replaced or turned over many times. Throughout the life of a comedo, the shrunken sebaceous lobules continue to secrete sebum which streams to the surface through tor-

tuous, bacteria-filled central channels. In aged blackheads, the channels tend to fuse and become large cavities containing dense communities of *Propionibacterium acnes*. It is likely that bacterial enzymes, mainly proteases, contribute to the widening and merging of the channels. The fact that products of these bacteria can lyse horny material can be shown in a very simple way; clear zones form around colonies of *Propionibacterium acnes* growing on agar plates seeded with keratinized scales.

Chapman SJ, Walsh A (1990) Desmosomes, corneosomes and desquamation. An ultrastructure study of adult pig epidermis. Arch Dermatol Res 282:304–310

Lavker RM, Leyden JJ, McGinley KJ (1981) The relationship between bacteria and the abnormal follicular keratinization in acne vulgaris. J Invest Dermatol 77:325–330

Leyden JJ, Kligman AM (1972) Hairs in acne comedones. Arch Dermatol 106:851–853

Plewig G, Fulton JE, Kligman AM (1971) Cellular dynamics of comedo formation in acne vulgaris. Arch Dermatol Forsch 242:12–29

Plewig G, Wolff HH (1976) Follikel-Filament. Arch Dermatol Forsch 255:9–21

Wolff HH, Plewig G (1976) Ultrastruktur der Mikroflora in Follikeln und Komedonen. Hautarzt 27:432–440

Channels in Sebaceous Filaments and Comedones

Sebaceous filaments and comedones often exhibit peculiar cavernas filled with masses of bacteria. Not only provide they space for bacterial colonization but also act as sewage canals to drain sebum from the sebaceous ducts to the skin surface.

Above

Left   A microcomedo with one cavity. A transitional stage from follicular filament to a microcomedo. The only one cavity drains the single large sebaceous lobule below. The passage through the sebaceous duct (✱) is not in this particular cut

Right   A microcomedo with one cavity. In this lesion the direct communication with the sebaceous duct is tangentially cut (✱). Like in many other specimen, considerable parts of the bacterial colonies get lost during sectioning. Empty spaces are artifacts

Below

Left   Every sebaceous acinus has one sewage canal system. This large sebaceous follicle is drenched by three channels, each one directly associated with a sebaceous duct (✱)

Right   More than half of the space of this sebaceous filament is occupied by a chamber, densely stuffed with bacteria. Deep down mostly *Propionibacterium acnes* colonizes, mixed with *Staphylococcus epidermidis*. The toxic material from bacteria is perfectly sealed off from the follicular infundibulum. No inflammation is present

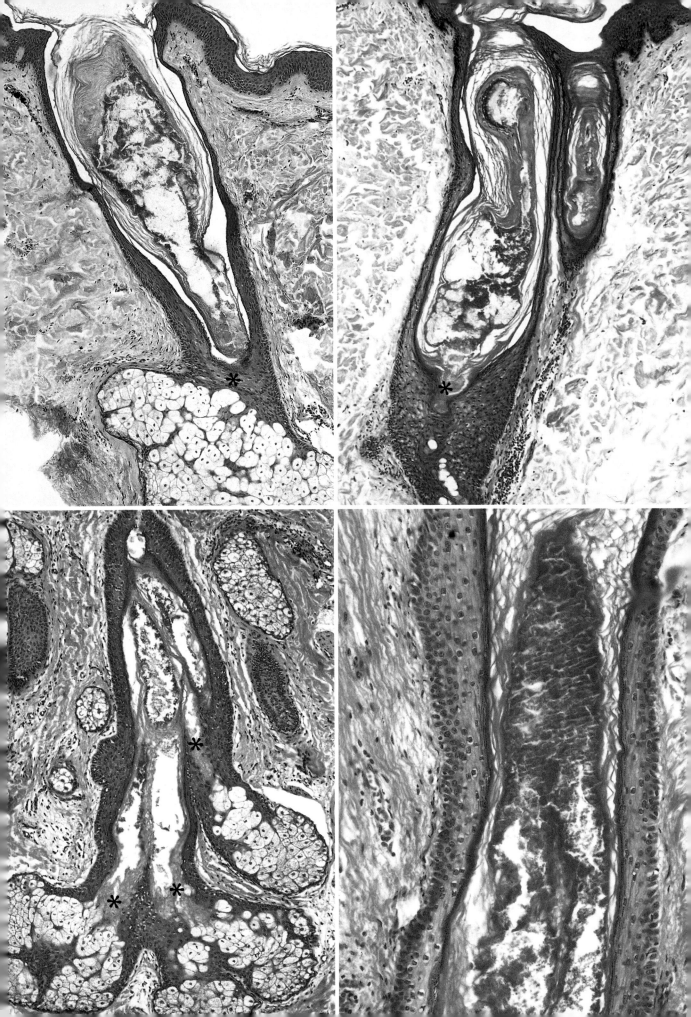

Patterns of Keratinization in Sebaceous Filaments and Microcomedones: A Horizontal View

The waxy worms that can be squeezed out from spacious sebaceous follicles are either normal impactions in large follicles, or the intermediate stage to microcomedones. In this plate the architecture of a microcomedo in oil acne is compared with the one of a sebaceous filament in normal skin from an acne patient.

Above   Oil acne. Oil acne is the result of inadequate exposure to comedogenic compounds of various industrial oils and greases, including cutting fluids. A clinical example is shown on p. 365

Left   A microcomedo. Densely packed corneocytes, about 30, form a cylinder around the horizontally cut hair with very little sebaceous matter and debris between the hair and the concentric layers of corneocytes. Bacteria are notably absent, characteristic of oil acne. (Electron microscopy, × 10500)

Right   The follicular epithelium (acroinfundibulum) immediately adjacent to the epidermis is to the right with keratohyalin granules. It produces dense and coherent corneocytes, indistinguishable from interfollicular epidermis. The toxic material responsible for oil acne inhibits bacterial growth. (Electron microscopy, × 15000)

Below   Sebaceous filament. Sebaceous filaments (synonymous with follicular filaments or follicular casts) are numerous and well developed in oily skin of patients with acne.

Left   The hair is to the left. Loose cellular debris, swollen corneocytes, lipid droplets, and bacteria form a soft, pasty material. (Electron microscopy, × 8900)

Right   The periphery of the filament consists of roughly 15 layers of corneocytes, five of which are shown here. They are swollen and show a few lipid inclusions. Many bacteria are embedded in an amalgam of sebaceous matter. (Electron microscopy, × 11600)

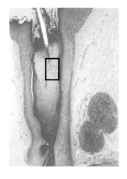 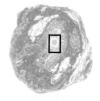

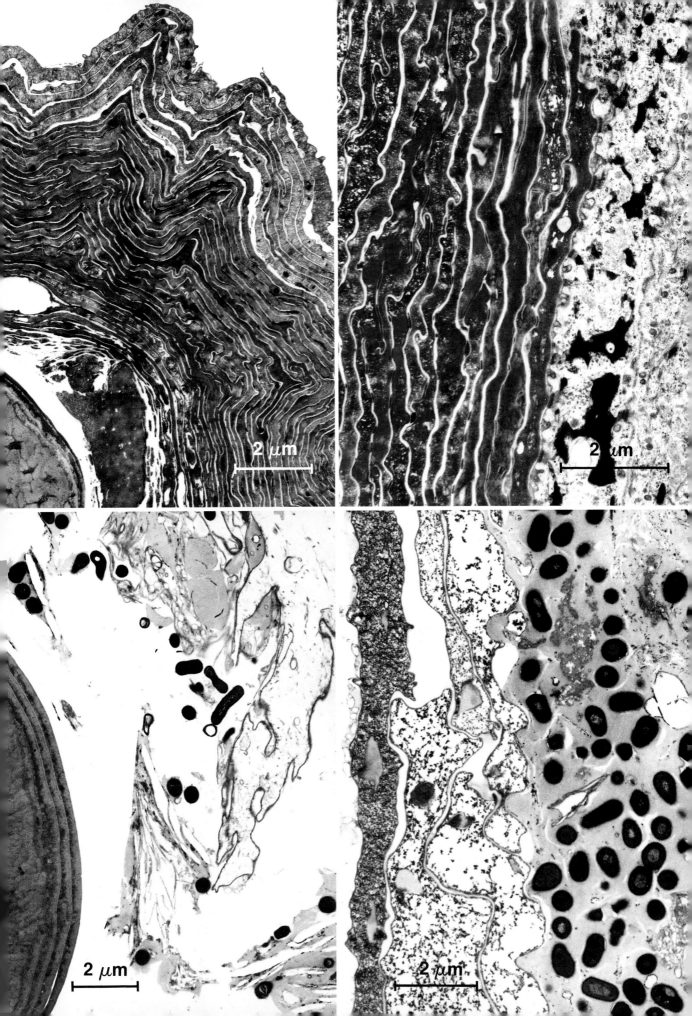

The Dynamics of Secondary Comedo Formation

Rupture, abscess formation and re-encapsulation is the key sequence which underlies the creation of secondary comedones. These can only arise when rupture is partial, and generally not from nodules. Substantial segments of comedonal epithelium must survive the inflammatory storm. Because focal rupture and re-encapsulation may happen once or many times, secondary comedones cannot be placed in such neat categories as primary ones; they are exceedingly variable in size and shape. Some of them may look like closed or open comedones. Secondary comedones can be identified with certainty only by histologic examination.

Diagnosis is made by finding evidence of an earlier inflammatory event. If this was recent, there will be hyperplasia of the epithelium and a chronic inflammatory reaction. Later, there may be only a scattering of lymphocytes. The connective tissue presents the ultimate clue, a scar consisting of fine, parallel bundles of collagen. The fibers are arranged in loose laminae, often in concentric patterns. Within the scarred tissue, all elastic fibers have been destroyed. An elastic stain, therefore, is helpful to delineate the extent of scarring.

After repeated episodes of rupture and re-encapsulation the internal structure of the comedo becomes altered. The horn is not so dense, the lamellae are looser and not in such neat concentric patterns. The bacteria are more sparse; the habitat seems less hospitable for *Pro-pionibacterium acnes*. Three varieties of secondary comedones are clinically distinctive.

The Cyst

True cysts have an epithelial lining. The opening is not very evident in most of them; others have a clearly visible punctum. Cysts are almost always part of the scenery of acne conglobata. Their chief territory is the back, from the shoulders straight down to the hips, and to a lesser extent the face, neck, nape, and ear lobes.

Acne cysts are smooth, dome-shaped, elevated, freely movable, skin-colored, round to ovoid structures. They are usually 7–15 mm large, but may attain great sizes, as much as 2–5 cm in diameter. Large cysts are old lesions and can be up to 5–10 years of age. There is some confusion regarding nomenclature. Torpid nodules and abscesses, typical of acne conglobata, are practically always called cysts. They are, however, not cysts and lack epithelial lining.

Cysts will release a cheesy to waxy material (corneocytes with bacteria, debris from previous inflammatory episodes) when nicked. Deep puncture with a scalpel will yield more of this content. Discharge can also occur spontaneously. The contents often have an offending odor like foul, rotten material. Hairs are typically few or may even be absent in large, old cysts. In the latter case, the pilary unit and sebaceous glands have been destroyed by successive inflammatory episodes. Cysts are like time bombs: one never knows when they will rupture. Rupture may be limited to a small segment of the epithelium with swift re-encapsulation, or it can be a total explosion. Large, very painful abscesses can develop within a few days. The overlying and neighboring skin and subcutis is edematous, red, very tender, and painful when the patient leans against a chair or lies on his back, for example. It is a common mistake to diagnose a boil (furuncle). Cultures are generally sterile with no evidence of *Staphylococcus aureus* infection.

Histopathology. One finds an epithelial-lined cystic cavity with an apical opening, mostly small in size, and sometimes serial sections are required for visualization. The epithelium keratinizes to form corneocytes, which are associated with a well-developed stratum granulosum. Sebaceous acini are absent. Occasionally small buds of undifferentiated sebaceous glands cling to the cyst epithelium. The pilary portion is almost always destroyed so that few or no hairs lie within the cavity. Pericystic fibrosis is always present.

Treatment. Cysts never disappear spontaneously. There are only two fates: rupture with abscess formation leaving a bad scar, or surgical removal of the cyst wall. Of course, surgery is preferable, and the results gratifying. Surgical interventions are underused in acne.

The Fistulated Polyporous Comedo

Like the cyst, the polyporous comedo is a typical feature of acne conglobata; again it predominates on the back. Usually there are several lesions; indeed it is not rare to encounter patients whose back is studded with hundreds of these communicating comedones. Fistulated comedones have always fairly wide openings, with pigmented tips protruding through the pore. Their formation takes place over years, after a complete series of ruptures and encapsulations.

Histopathology. A localized rupture occurs which by encapsulation becomes a lateral diverticulum lined by keratinizing epithelium. By subsequent ruptures, the diverticulum extends in length and finally breaks into a nearby follicle which also becomes or may have been the site of a comedo. Groups of two or more follicles become linked up in this fashion. When there are two openings the term double comedo is used. One could likewise refer to a triple comedo.

Fistulated comedones evolve through inflammatory stages from ordinary comedones, and therefore have to be classified as secondary comedones. They could also be placed into the category of scars, in which they are embedded. The scar tracks and tunnels are stuffed with a comedo-like paste of corneocytes. Fistulated comedones are dealt with again in a later chapter (p. 172).

The Draining Sinus

A somewhat similar series of events leads to the formation of another dreadful lesion: the draining sinus. This is nothing but a monstrous, long, and particularly deep-seated fistulated sinus tract which empties to the surface. It most often occurs in acne conglobata patients; rarely is it seen in patients with rosacea. In contrast to fistulated comedones it prevails on the face: cheeks, saddle of nose, chin, and neck. There may be one or two tracts, rarely more. Inflammation is much more extensive than with the fistulated comedo. Like a volcano it erupts at unforeseeable intervals. Of course, there is progessive scarring as in fistulated comedones.

Plewig G (1974) Follicular keratinization. J Invest Dermatol 62:308–315

Watson JB (1959) Monoporous and polyporous acne. Arch Dermatol 80:167–170

Comedogenesis

All stages of primary comedogenesis can be studied in this panel.

Above

Left   A large sebaceous follicle with a follicular filament full of bacterial cavernas is on the left. A microcomedo is on to the right. The keratinization of the sebaceous duct is typically for rapidly growing comedones

Right   A closed comedo is to the left, with a tight opening and dedifferentiating sebaceous lobules. A large sebaceous follicle with debris but no appreciable keratinization in its three sebaceous ducts is to the right

Below

Left   A closed comedo with hardly anything left of its sebaceous lobules. The pilary portion is intact

Right   An open comedo, densely stuffed with corneocytes. The sebaceous acini are but a small bud, the pilary unit still functioning

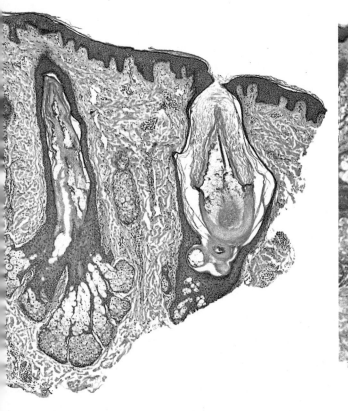
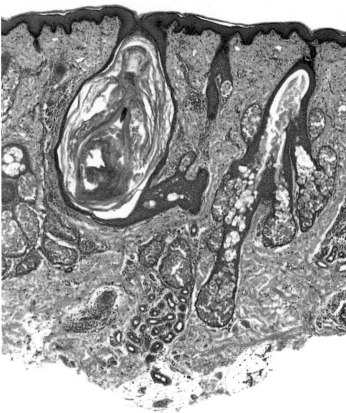
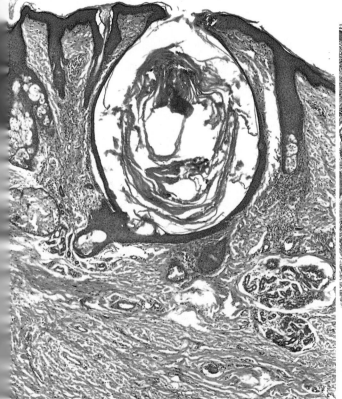
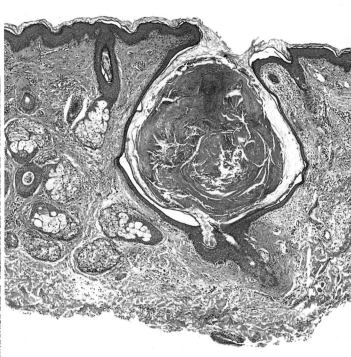

Sebaceous Ducts Keratinize
and Become Part of the Comedo

With slow enlargement of open and closed comedones, the sebaceous glands gradually disappear. The formerly large sebaceous acini become small buds with only a few sebocytes. The sebaceous ducts are integrated into the comedonal epithelium.

Above The sebaceous ducts are the most vulnerable section of follicles and comedones. Often small foci of inflammation are found here. The sebaceous duct is distended by parakeratotic and orthokeratotic debris

Below This open comedo has only small sebaceous glands (*left*) in its base compared with the large sebaceous acini of a sebaceous follicle (*right*). The sebaceous ducts keratinize like the rest of the comedonal epithelium. The more the comedo becomes inflated by its growing kernel, the more sebaceous ducts are integrated into the comedo wall

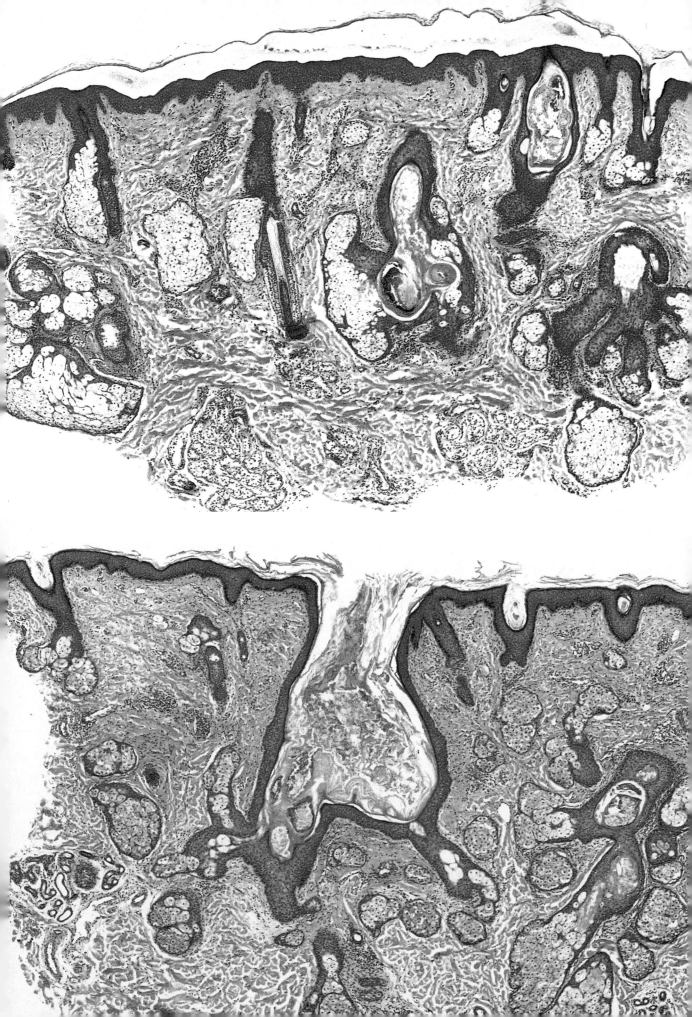

Closed Comedones

Above Macrophotography of acne-bearing skin reveals many closed comedones, some of them in an intermediate stage to open comedones. The central pore is tightly constricted like a pouch

Below The histopathologic counterpart reveals a microcomedo to the left, a fully developed closed comedo in the center, and an oblique cut through a micro-comedo to the far right. No inflammation disturbs the scene

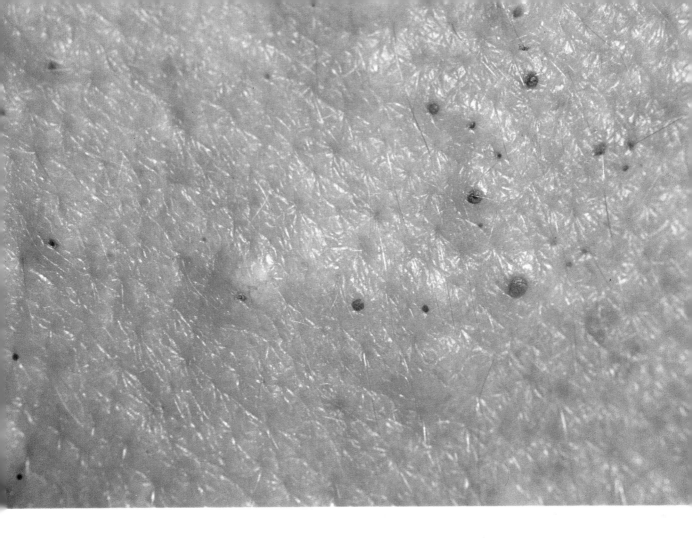

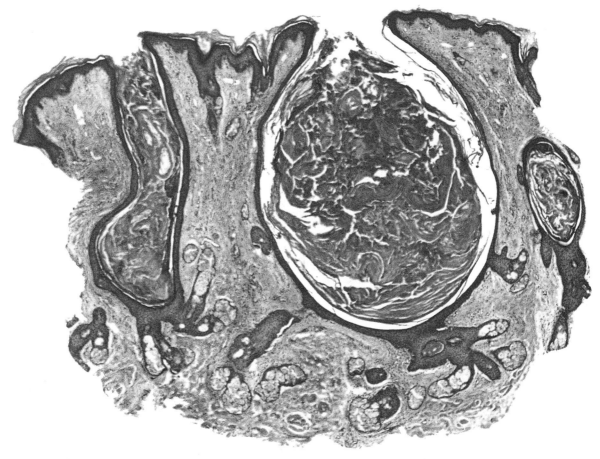

Gross and Microscopic Anatomy
of Open Comedones

In some patients open comedones silently sit in the skin, do not become inflamed, and reach old age, often remaining for years. The comedonal opening is more or less patent, exposing the pigmented apical portion, which makes the lesion look ugly.

Above

Left   Modern macrophotography opens a new dimension of viewing skin surface structures and follicular disorders. The comedo is wide open, with only a veil-like stretch of epidermis locking it firmly into its cavity

Right   An open comedo of this stature has reached old age. One can assume there have been 1–2 years of maturation. The opening reveals a compacted pigmented core; the cystic cavity is much broader, almost 5 mm across. The comedo bulges at the skin surface, a characteristic typical of old lesions

Below

Left   Histopathology of an open comedo with no signs of inflammation. The wall is stretched out, but bears no signs of leaks or inflammatory pockets. The sebaceous acini are still quite large, revealing that the lesion is not extremely old. The sebum exits through sebaceous ducts, one of which is seen in this section. The sebum then flows in channels through the comedo. This is the favorite location for bacterial chambers

Right   An old, compacted, open comedo, also not inflamed. Several cuts through hairs are visible (brownish ovoid structures). The sebaceous glands dedifferentiate

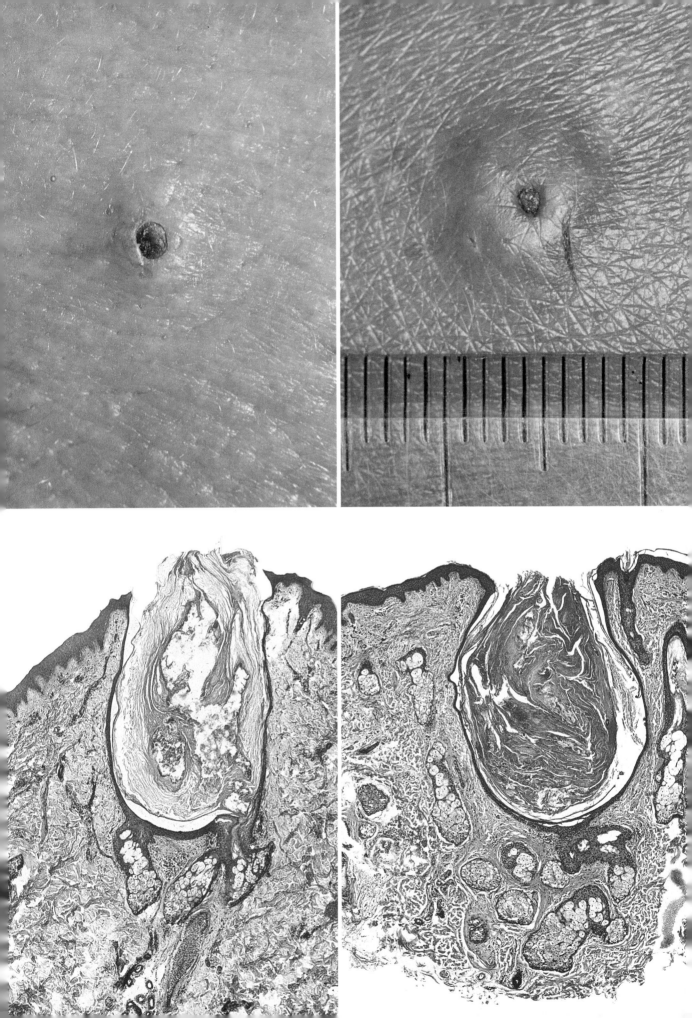

The Majestic Comedo

This is a whole biopsy which has been cleared with methyl salicylate to allow a three-dimensional view of the shape and contents of an open comedo. Coiled-up hairs of different diameters and lengths are trapped in the horny impaction. The tip of one has wondrously managed to extrude through the orifice. Major rupture of a comedo with displacement of hairs, horn, and lipids into the dermis provokes persistent indurated papules and nodules. Large, open comedones are end-stage lesions which rarely rupture.

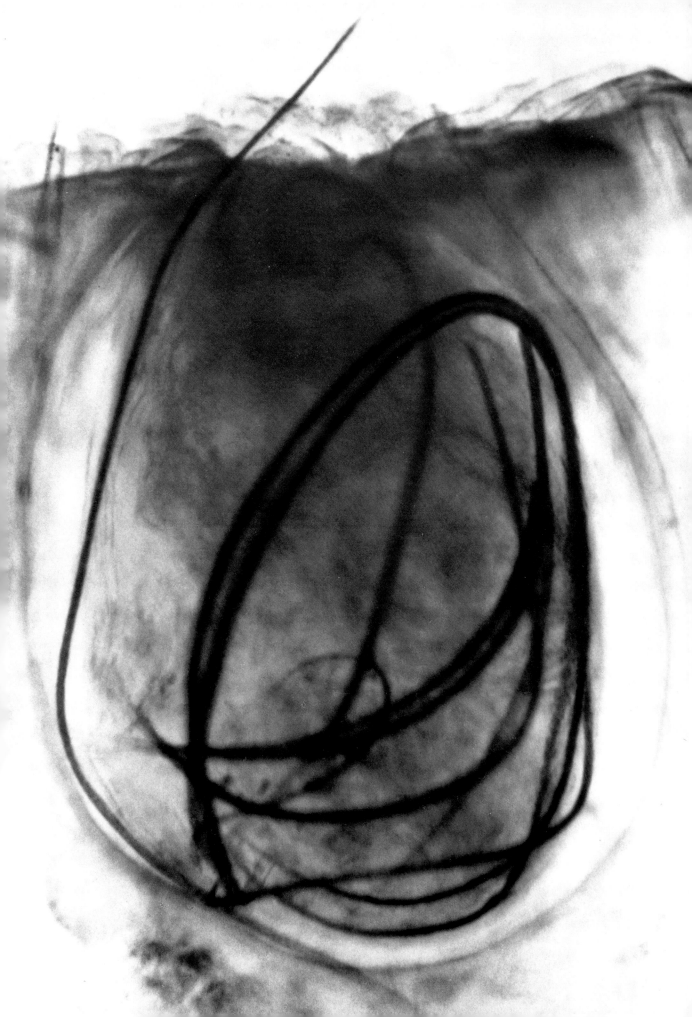

Corneocytes: The Bricks of Comedones

The bricks of the horny framework of comedones are corneocytes. Those from the interfollicular epidermis form the stratum corneum of the skin, those from the follicular infundibula of sebaceous follicles the comedones. The intercorneocyte material is the mortar, cementing the bricks properly together. This brick-and-mortar model is now being employed to explain epidermal barrier functions. Cellular adhesion is also provided by desmosomes. The morphology of corneocytes is quite distinct. In this plate epidermal and comedonal corneocytes are compared.

Above

Epidermal corneocytes. Mostly they are of regular, often even symmetrical shape. Hexagonal and pentagonal patterns prevail. The cells have no nuclei and overlap at the edges. The size of corneocytes differs because of regional variations and the effects of age. The surface area of epidermal corneocytes on the chest of adults is about 1000 μm^2. The cells increase in size, e.g., from about 900 μm^2 in the newborn to about 1150 μm^2 in the octogenarian.

Left   Monolayer of corneocytes from the shoulder

Right   A single corneocyte from a darkly pigmented patient shows a central cluster of melanin granules

Below

Comedonal corneocytes. The bricks from follicular filaments or comedonal kernels are of other quality than their epidermal counterparts. Variable size and shape with convex and concave borders, and thin translucent fragile cells prevail. There are often nuclei or nuclear remnants. Above all they are much larger than those from the epidermis, between 50–70 μm in diameter

Left   A single corneocyte from a comedo. It contains numerous lipid-like droplets

Right   Individual corneocytes from a closed comedo. Irregular configurations, large size, nuclear, and nucleolar remnants are typical features

Hölzle E, Plewig G, Ledolter A (1986) Corneocyte exfoliative cytology: a model to study normal and diseased stratum corneum. In: Marks R, Plewig G (eds) Skin models. Models to study function and disease of skin. Springer, Berlin, pp 183–193

Plewig G (1970) Zellmorphologie im Exprimat von Nasenflügel-Follikeln und Comedonen. Arch Klin Exp Dermatol 237:703–716

Plewig G (1970) Regional differences of cell sizes in the human stratum corneum. Part II. Effects of sex and age. J Invest Dermatol 54:19–23

Plewig G, Marples RR (1970) Regional differences of cell sizes in the human stratum corneum. Part I. J Invest Dermatol 54:13–18

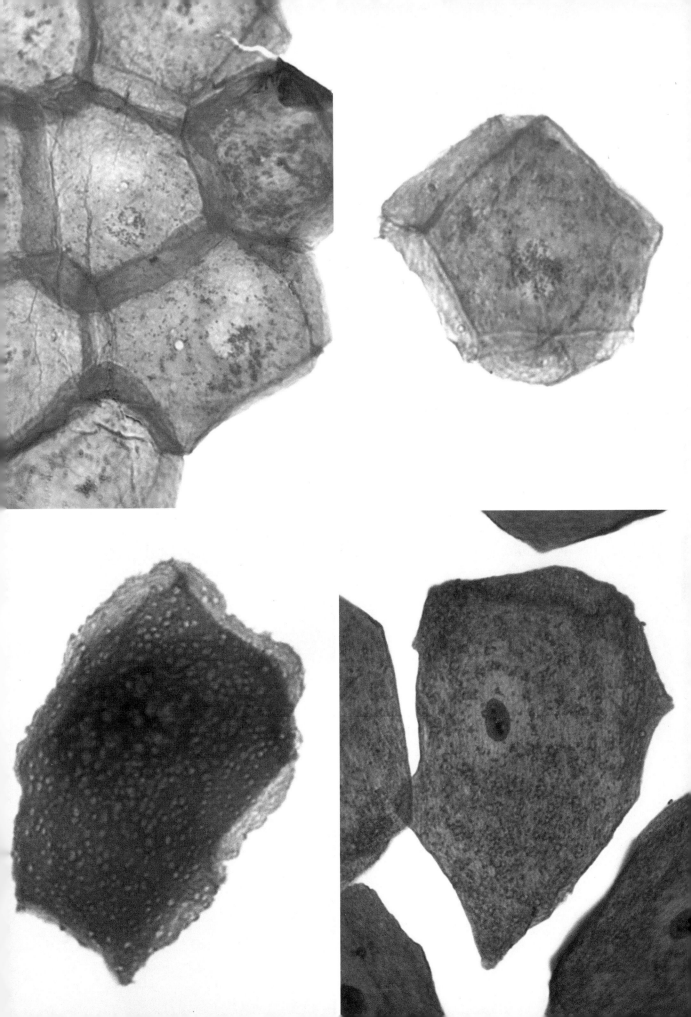

Ultrastructural Tableau of the Horny Framework of a Comedo

Horny cells comprise the hard skeleton of the comedo. Processing of tissue for electron microscopy eliminates the artifacts of cracks and fissures between horny lamellae that one always sees in specimens prepared for light microscopy. Note the tight packing of cells and absence of empty spaces between them. The narrow interspaces are filled with a cement substance which is responsible for cohesiveness. A portion of an epithelial cell with dark keratohyalin granules is at the lower right. (Electron microscopy, × 22 000).

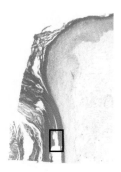

Courtesy of Professor H.H. Wolff, Lübeck, FRG

1 μm

Differences Between Corneocytes of Epidermis and Comedones

The complex structure of the stratum corneum has only recently come to light. Special staining methods and electron microscopy are required to show details which are hidden in routine light microscopy. Even so, artifacts are abundant.

Above   Stratum corneum of normal epidermis. The granular layer at the bottom contains prominent keratohyalin granules. The corneocytes are densely packed with fibrous protein, compacted into a stratum corneum about 15 cell layers thick. The spaces between the corneocytes are rich in lipids and sugars. This mixture is thought to keep the cells together, providing a barrier to inward diffusion of external substances as well as outward diffusion of water. Also evident are electron-dense disks (desmosomes, sometimes called cementosomes or corneosomes in the stratum corneum), which provide strong cell-to-cell attachments. The brick (corneocytes) and mortar model can be appreciated from this electron microscopic picture, × 22000

Below   Comedonal corneocytes. There are tightly compacted, densely filled corneocytes with variably sized lipid droplets, reflecting rapid turnover. The empty spaces are artifacts. They contain bilaminar membranes made up of various lipid classes. (Electron microscopy, × 18000)

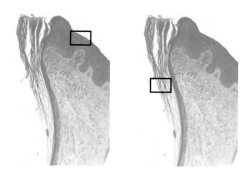

Below: Courtesy of Professor Helmut H. Wolff, Lübeck, FRG

Knutson DD (1974) Ultrastructural observations in acne vulgaris: the normal sebaceous follicle and acne lesions. J Invest Dermatol 62:288–307

Plewig G, Nikolowski J, Wolff HH (1983) Follicular keratinization. In: Marks R, Plewig G (eds) Stratum corneum. Springer, Berlin Heidelberg New York, pp 227–236

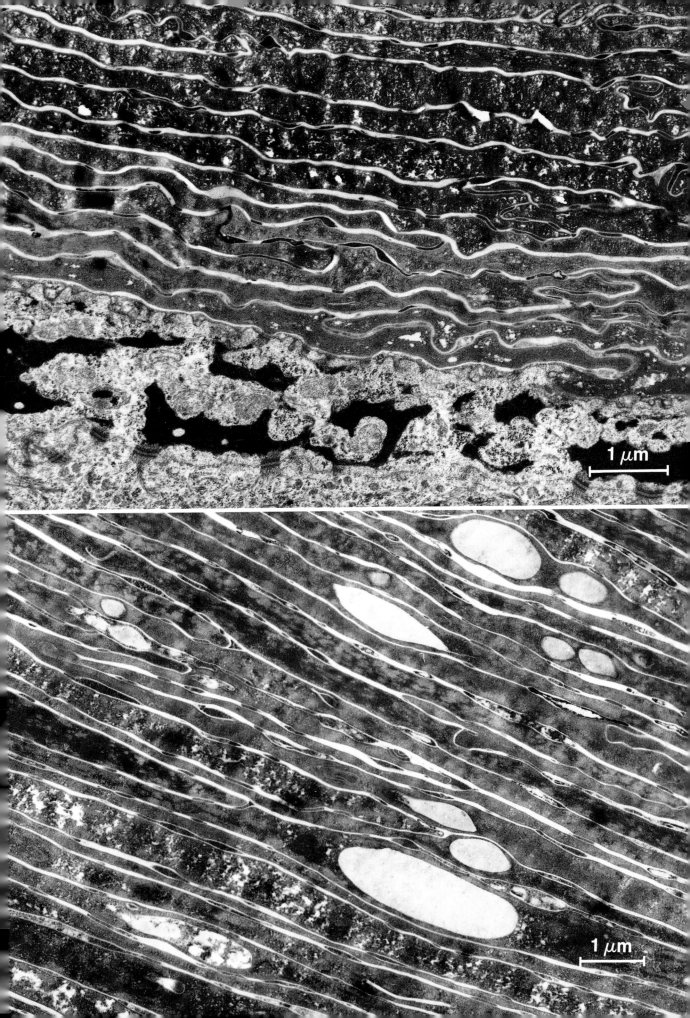

Ultrastructure of Intercorneocyte Epidermal Lipids

High-resolution electron microscopy together with careful fixation permits the viewing of a new dimension: the ultrastructure of the mortar which holds together the bricks (corneocytes) of human stratum corneum or comedones. The membrane structure in the middle and outer parts of the stratum corneum consists of more than 20 lipid layers. The electron-lucent (hydrophobic) and electron-dense (hydrophilic) layers are of comparable thickness. In some areas there are electron-lucent lamellae with interrupted appearance and continuous lucent bands of a certain regularity. These were previously shown in mouse skin, and are shown here for the first time in human skin.

Above   Volar side of forearm, middle part of stratum corneum. The primary fixative was acrolein vapor, the secondary fixative 0.5% ruthenium tetroxide with 0.25% potassium ferrocyanide. Embedding in Spurr's resin. (Electron microscopy, × 190000)

Below   Volar side of forearm, upper part of stratum corneum. (Electron microscopy, × 270000)

Below: Courtesy of Privatdozentin Manigé Fartasch, Erlangen, FRG

Fartasch M, Bassukas ID, Diepgen TL (1992) Hornschicht-Strukturen als Träger der normalen und veränderten Barrierefunktion: Strukturelle Atopiemerkmale der Hornschicht. In: Klaschka F (Hrsg) Empfindliche Haut. Diesbach, Berlin, pp 1–11

Hou SYE, Mitra AK, White SH, Menon GK, Ghadially R, Elias PM (1991) Membrane structures in normal and essential fatty acid-deficient stratum corneum: characterization by ruthenium tetroxide staining and x-ray diffraction. J Invest Dermatol 96:215–223

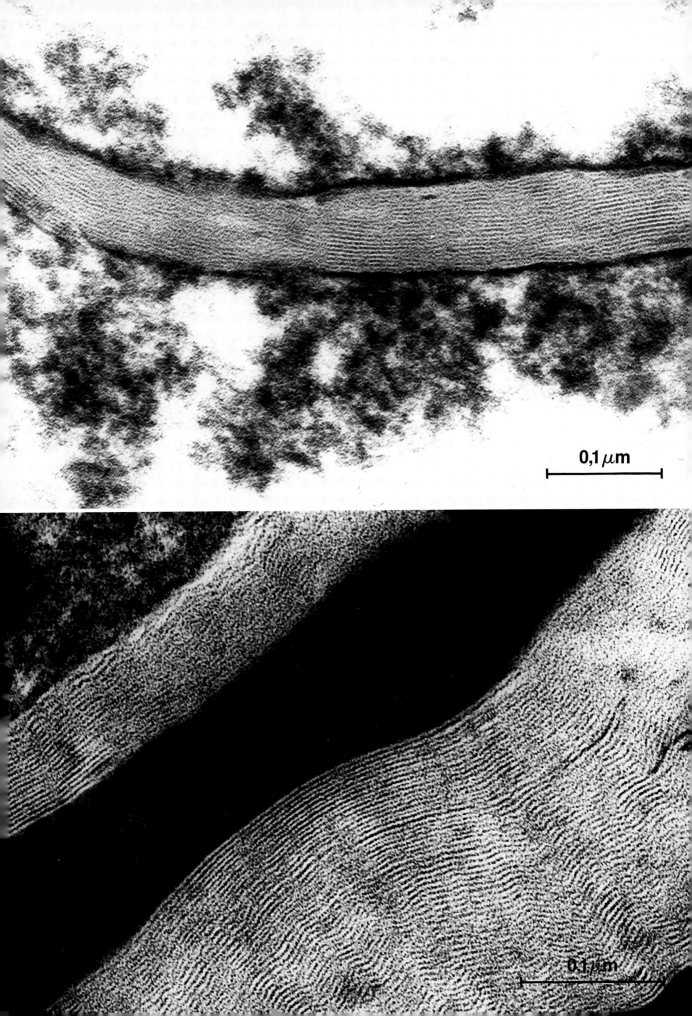

0,1 μm

0,1 μm

Inside a Comedo

The core of a comedo is a skeleton of tightly packed corneocytes. In the horny layer of the epidermis, they are stratified and stacked; in a comedo, both stacking and disarray concur.

Above   Swirled corneocytes. The cells seem to push each other into meandering patterns. (Electron microscopy, × 10000)

Below   In the central chambers of the comedonal kernel, detached corneocytes swim in an amalgam of sebum and debris. (Electron microscopy, × 21800)

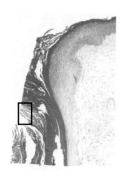

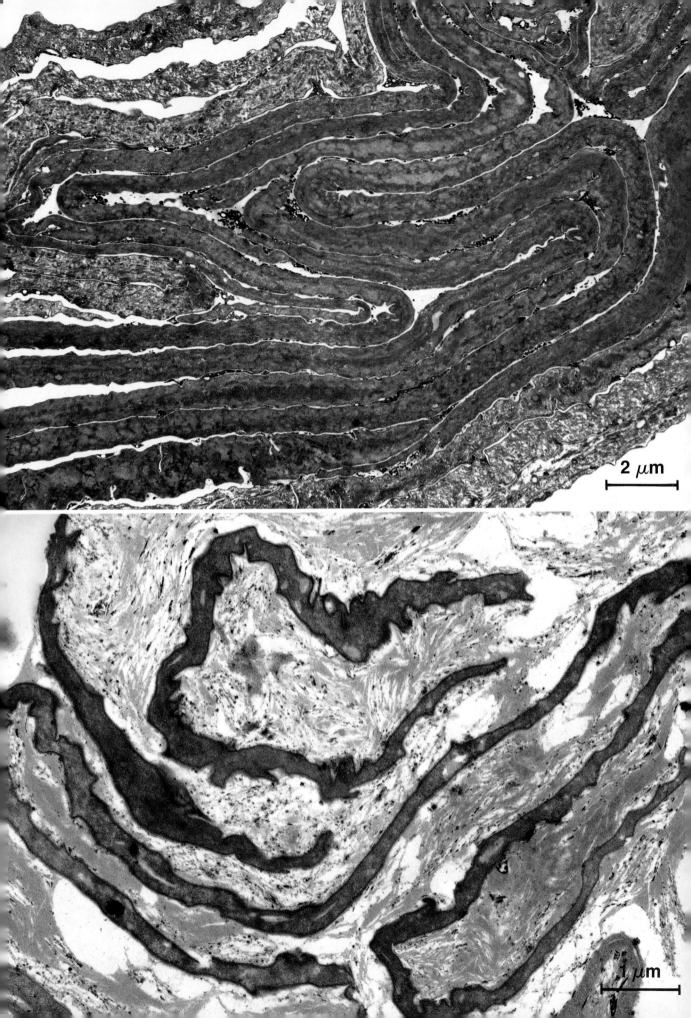

2 μm

1 μm

The Fast Turnover of Comedonal Epithelia

It was only with the advent of radioactive labeling that the proliferative activity of sebaceous glands and follicular epithelia was discovered. Tritiated histidine was used as a tracer.

Above Segment of a comedo 45 min after labeling. The entire viable epithelium is studded with silver grains, being particularly dense over the stratum granulosum, a histidine-rich zone sui generis. There is no labeling at all of the comedonal core; but some over fibroblasts in the dermis. (Hematoxilin, light microscopy)

Middle Tritiated histidine was injected 1 week prior to the biopsy. The silver grains have been transported in corneocytes produced within the past 7 days. The leading front is sharp. The comedonal epithelium (brownish structure) is almost free of the tracer. (Darkfield microscopy)

Below Tritiated histidine was twice injected, 18 and 10 days prior to the biopsy. Two perfectly symmetrical bands of silver grains show the direction and speed of newly produced corneocytes. The comedonal epithelium is at the bottom. (Darkfield microscopy)

Plewig G, Fulton JE, Kligman AM (1971) Cellular dynamics of comedo formation in acne vulgaris. Arch Dermatol Forsch 242:12–29

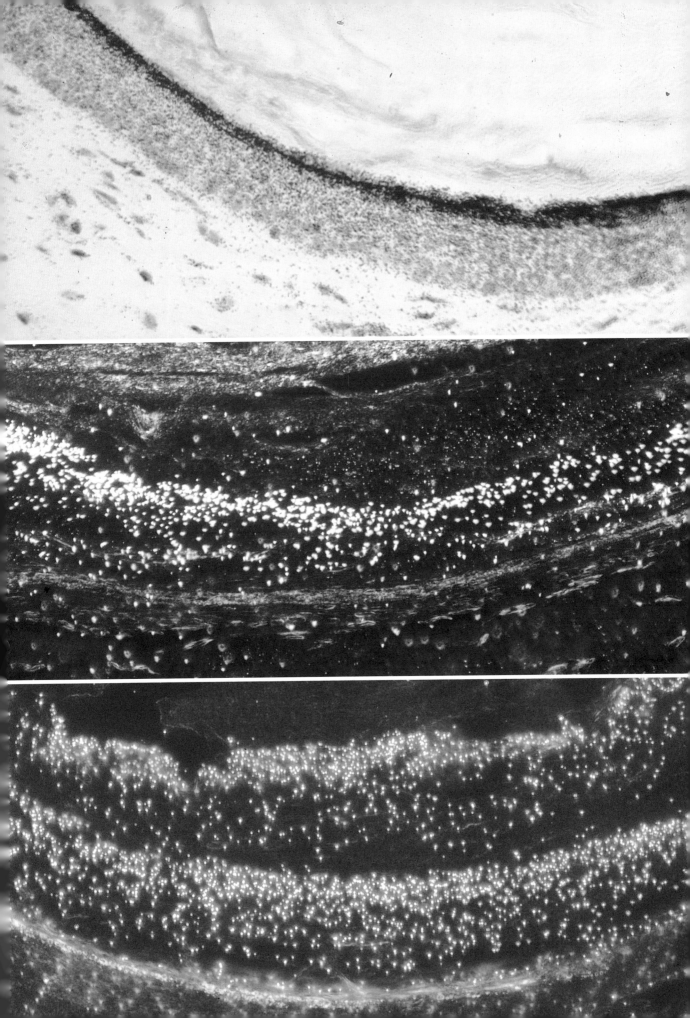

Hairs in Comedones

The wispy, puny hairs that are trapped in comedones are easily overlooked. They are of no clinical significance except when an explosion extrudes them into the dermis.

Above   Cross-section of an extracted comedo. The corneocytes are arranged in concentric lamellae. A number of hairs are cut in cross-section

Below   An immersion-oil squash mount of an open comedo. The corneocyte matrix becomes transparent and allows visualization of individual hairs which can be teased out and counted. The latter are tangled and coiled

Leyden JJ, Kligman AM (1972) Hairs in acne comedones. Arch Dermatol 106:851–853

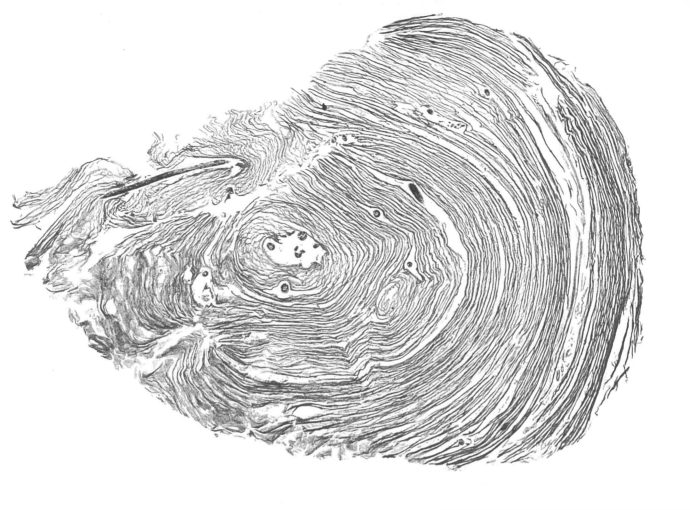
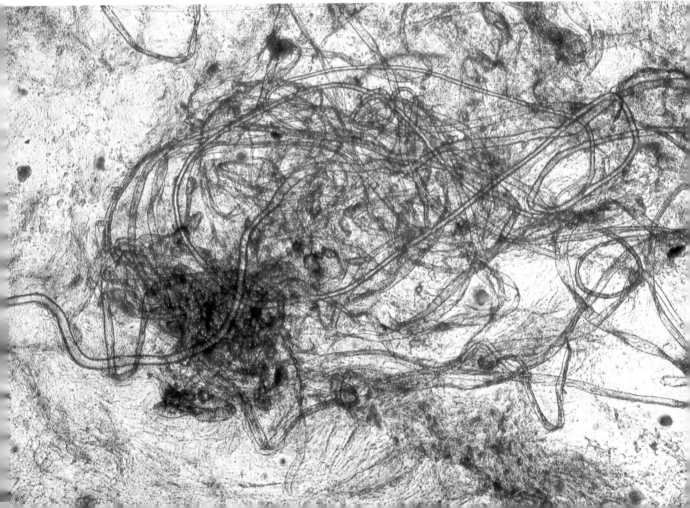

Pigment in Comedones

Pigment in comedones, seen macroscopically in open but only microscopically in closed ones, is melanin and not dirt.

Above

Left In this darkly pigmented subject, not only melanocytes but also the basal keratinocytes of the acroinfundibulum and interfollicular epidermis are packed with melanin. The lower part of the infundibulum does not contain melanin-synthesizing cells. (Silver stain)

Right All four comedones lifted up with a comedo extractor display a melaninpigmented cap, and a whitish nonpigmented lower portion and tail. (Unstained)

Below Melanin-synthesizing cells are confined to the acroinfundibulum and the interfollicular epidermis. The closed comedo on the *right* bears no pigment. The pigmented hair trapped in the comedo is cut twice tangentially. (Silver stain)

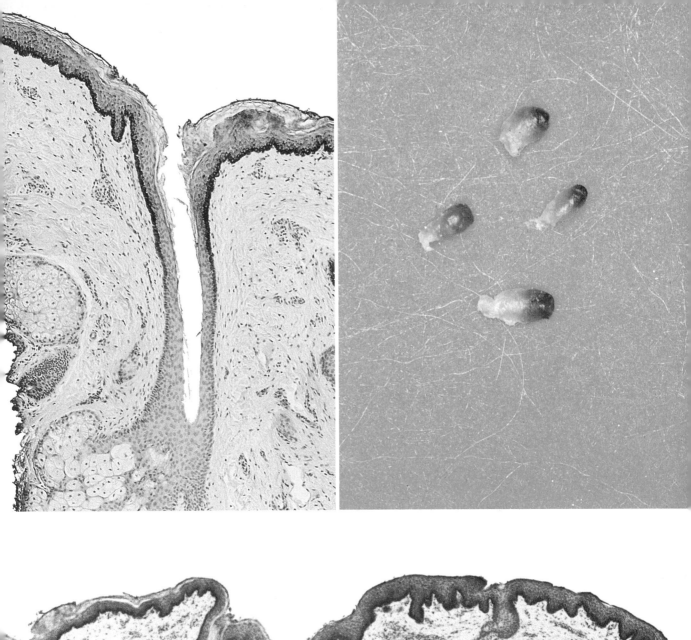
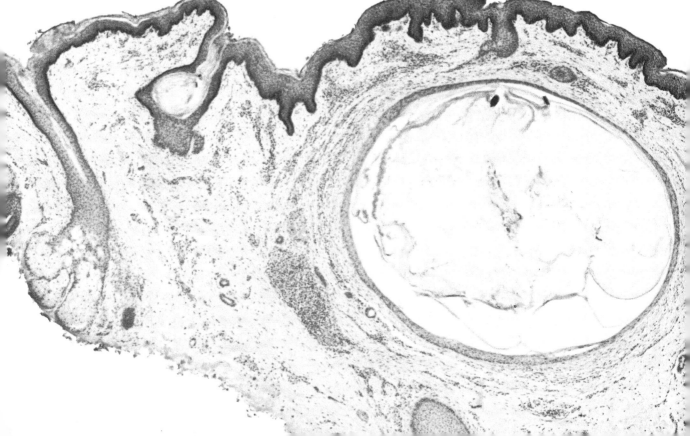

Pigment in Comedones Is Melanin

The black cap seen to varying degrees in open but not closed comedones is neither dirt, nor oxidized lipid matter, but melanin. Melanin is produced in the apical portion of the comedonal epithelium and then transferred into the corneocytes. Giant melanosomes, large packages of clumped melanin, ride with the corneocytes. Hundreds of condensed corneocytes provide enough pigment to produce a deep brown–black color.

Above   Tip of an open comedo with many giant melanosomes within corneocytes. (Electron microscopy, × 35000)

Below   For comparison corneocytes from a benign pigmented skin lesion (lentigo senilis) is shown. Likewise giant melanosomes ride upwards with the corneocytes. (Electron microscopy, × 32000)

Below: Courtesy of Privatdozent Wilhelm Stolz, Munich, FRG

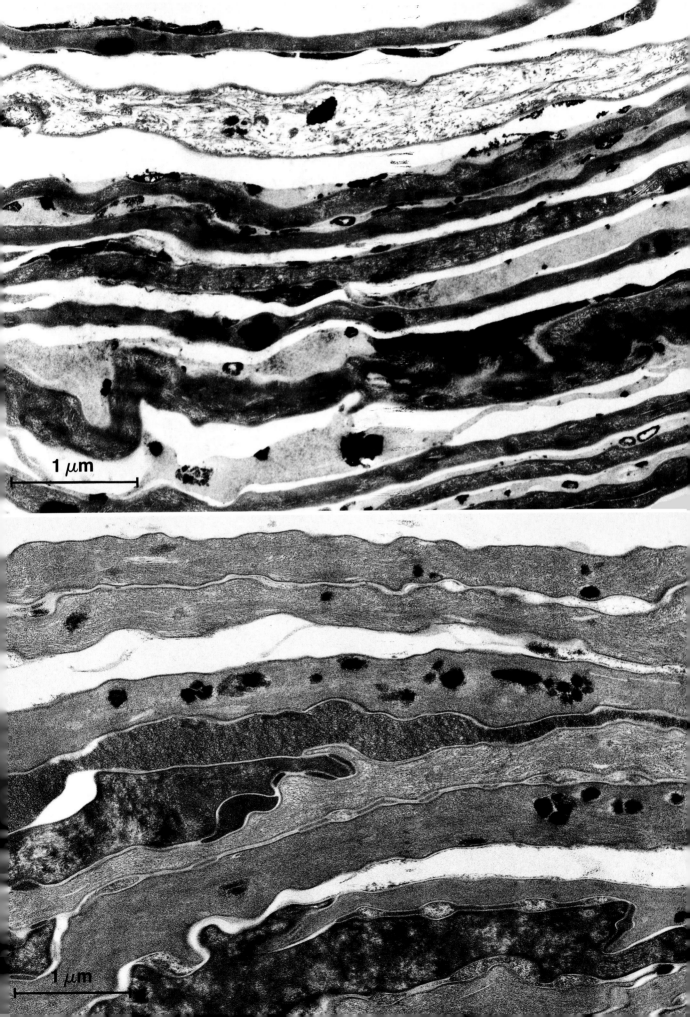

The Multiple Faces of Comedones

Comedones have variegate faces; no two look alike. Yet there is always something present that is specific to the key histopathologic features.

Above

Left   A well-matured comedo which was never blasted by inflammatory episodes. This can be said because it is symmetrical and whirled patterns of the comedonal core and pericomedonal fibrosis are absent. The sebaceous glands have all regressed. The pilary unit is intact, with one hair shed into the comedo. A few lymphocytes linger around at the site where the sebaceous acini once resided

Right   The opening of this comedo is spatulate. The core consists of densely packed corneocytes, with only a few bacteria in between. The large sebaceous lobule below still connects with the comedo, as could be judged from serial sections

Below

Left   The slight asymmetry, the pericomedonal fibrosis, remnants of parakeratotic corneocytes mixed with debris from granulocytes and lymphocytes (*right upper* portion), and multiple cross-sections through hairs all indicate that this comedo is old, and has undergone several although not lethal inflammatory episodes, from which it recovered. It is bizarre that two sebaceous acini are still releasing sebum into the comedo

Right   A very mature open comedo. Its belly is hollow like an old tree. Multiple cystic cavernas make up a good portion of the kernel; they are all densely filled with bacteria. Most of them are *Propionibacterium acnes*. The comedo seems to graciously lift itself up. This is an artifact from the pressure when the anesthetic was injected

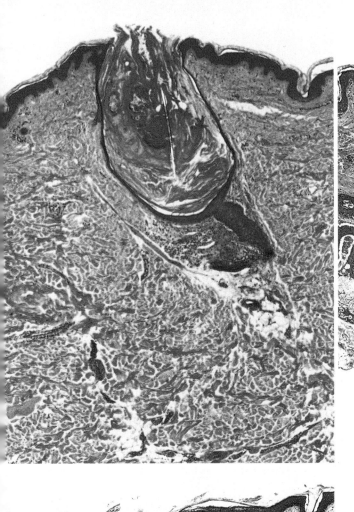
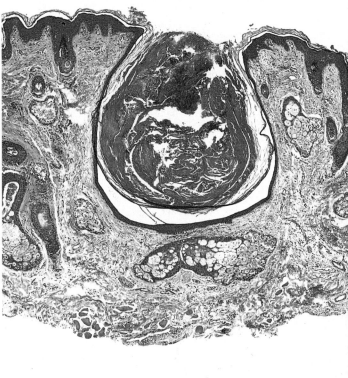
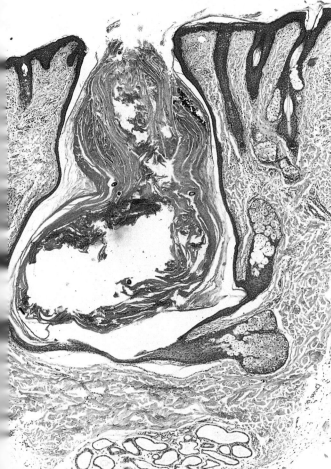
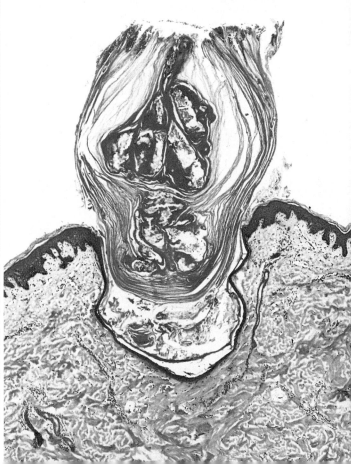

The Evolution of Comedones

Above   A beautiful closed comedo (*right*). Its pore is tight, the epithelium stretched out and thin, the sebaceous gland atrophic, and the comedonal kernel tightly packed. It was never inflamed. For comparison a normal sebaceous follicle can be seen on the *left*

Below   This is also a closed comedo, but more specifically a macrocomedo or epithelial cyst. Its pore is tight, though artificially distended for histotechnical reasons. The epithelium is extremely thin. No sebaceous glands can be detected, even in step-section. The pilary portion has been destroyed. Perilesional fibrosis indicates earlier inflammatory phases. If left alone, these lesions can become very old and persist for years or decades

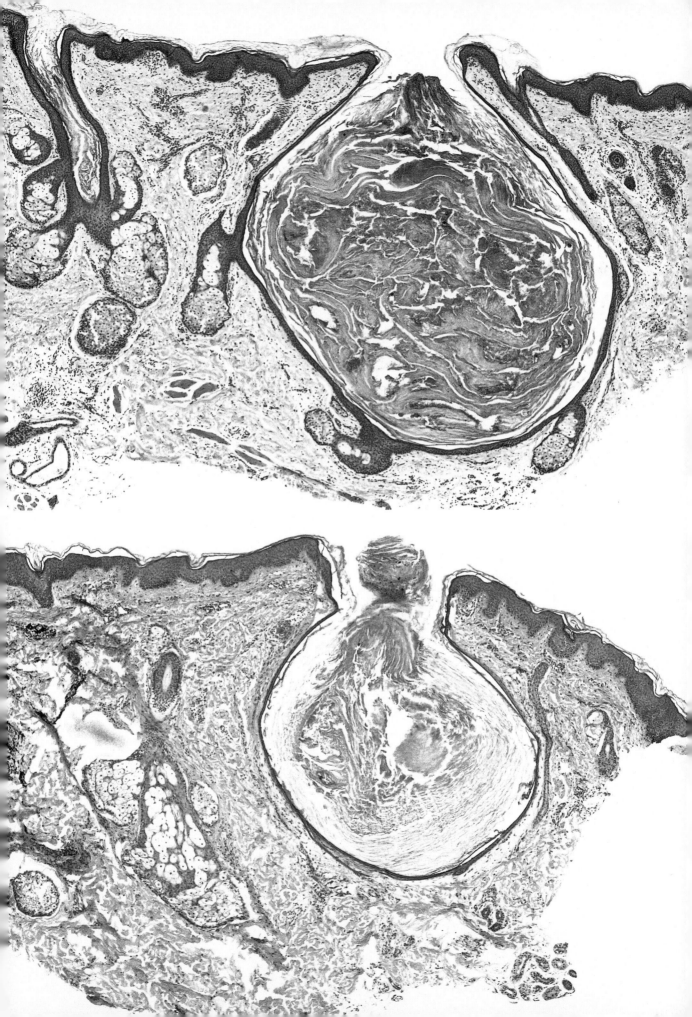

The Dynamics of Inflammation

It is a popular conception that free fatty acids formed within sebaceous follicles are irritants which attack the follicular epithelium, thus causing breaks in the lining. Presumably sebum then flows out and provokes an inflammatory reaction. Theoretically a pustule could spring up in this way from a normal sebaceous follicle. However, with rare exceptions pustules originate mainly from preexisting comedones, whether these are visible or not. There is no doubt that sebum is a toxic material. Intradermal injection of a dilute suspension provokes within 24 h a tender, intensely red papule, lasting for many days. However, there is no proof that the normal follicular epithelium is leaky because of the toxicity of sebum. Spongiotic changes of the follicular epithelium are quite uncommon in our experience.

Comedones are generally not clinically evident when one looks at pustules or papules. The reason for this is that comedones frequently burst before becoming large enough to be visible. Besides, the inflammatory reaction itself tends to mask the underlying comedo. Expressing the contents of pustules often enables one to tease out the horny kernel. The most conclusive demonstration is by histologic evaluation. We have done this hundreds of times. A comedo, often very small or sometimes also of much larger size, is invariable present. The tendency for closed comedones to blow up has led to the expression "time bombs" of acne. This sobriquet is well earned. The toxic materials produced within them cannot get out easily through the microscopic pore. By contrast, open comedones are relatively inert. When they do occasionally rupture, their large size and pigmentation makes it easy to discover them within the infiltrate. Inflammatory lesions arising from open comedones tend to be rather limited; the reaction is usually not strong enough to discharge the comedones.

The more a comedo matures, the less likely it is to rupture. Mature old comedones have very small sebaceous glands left, which provide only minuscule amounts of fuel for explosion. This is why one often sees patients whose lesions are mainly comedones with but a scattering of pustules. Blackheads are stable end stages. On the other hand, comedones are typically rare in patients with numerous inflammatory lesions. As a rule, there is an inverse relationship between the visibility of comedones and the prominence of inflammatory lesions. In acne conglobata, for example, primary comedones are not conspicuous. These patients have such fragile microcomedones that early collapse is almost inevitable once horny distention is under way. In patients with many papulopustules, rupture usually occurs at the microcomedo stage. Of course some patients have both comedones and papulopustules; in these, some follicles get past the "time bomb" stage.

The follicular population is heterogeneous. Why some follicles are more susceptible than others is a mystery. Microcomedones are not visible, thus manual extraction is not feasible for prophylaxis. The removal of visible closed comedones is helpful in moderating papulopustular acne. The extraction of open comedones is cosmetically satisfying but does not alter the course of the disease. As always there are exceptions.

Application of cyanoacrylate to remove early follicular impactions is possible, but not as a routine procedure. The inflammatory lesions that make up the characteristic repertoire of acne vulgaris are papules, pustules, papulopustules, and nodules, all ending in scars, visible or not. Pressure is not an important factor in the rupture of comedones. Various other cystic lesions such as steatocystoma multiplex and trichilemmal cysts which reach much larger size would rupture even more readily. The latter usually have very thin walls, but they stay intact.

The earliest event in the development of an inflammatory lesion can only be discovered by chance. This requires taking random biopsies of apparently uninvolved skin in patients with numerous inflammatory lesions. This is of course a hit-and-miss technique; sometimes the histologic findings are normal. Occasionally, however, one catches the earliest change. This consists of the accumulation of a few neutrophils hard up against the outside of the follicular epithelium. At this stage the lining seems intact, although perhaps leukotrienes and other proinflammatory peptides may have leaked out at that focus. Subsequently, the neutrophils invade the epithelium and induce spongiotic changes. The epithelial cells swell and detach from each other. Leukocytes soon begin to pool on the inner side of the epithelium within the comedo. The epithelium at that site then degenerates. This is the event specified by the term "rupture". The contents of the follicle leak out and masses of neutrophils are called forth, extending well beyond the rupture. An intrafollicular and perifollicular abscess is thus formed. The massive pooling of granulocytes inside and outside the comedo is archetypical of acne vulgaris. The segment of epithelium which undergoes necrosis is of variable length. It may be so tiny as to never surface clinically. Minor border incidents of this kind are fairly common in biopsies of comedones which did not show any trace of inflammation clinically. These tiny breaks heal swiftly and would remain entirely undetected except for histologic observations. Old open comedones frequently show traces of these little "brush fires," with variable degrees of fibrosis.

The capacity of the epithelium to restore continuity after a break is very impressive. We have pushed sterile needles completely through closed and open comedones expecting to incite a pustule. With two and even three such perforations the comedo usually remained serene. Histologically, these artificial breaks healed within several days. A small nest of neutrophils collected outside the perforation; the epithelial edges quickly linked up.

We envision that toxic substances, particularly products produced by *Propionibacterium acnes*, accumulate in the comedo. These attach a weak point in the epithelial lining, permitting diffusion into the dermis. Neutrophils rush to the scene and destroy the epithelium completely, forming an intrafollicular abscess. Components of the comedo now pour into the surrounding tissue and initiate a perifollicular abscess.

Dahl MGC, McGibbon DH (1979) Complement C_3 and immunoglobulin in inflammatory acne vulgaris. Br J Dermatol 101:633–640

Lee WL, Shalita AR, Suntharalingam K, Fikrig SM (1982) Neutrophil chemotaxis by Propionibacterium acnes lipase and its inhibition. Infect Immun 35:71–78

Puhvel SM, Sakamoto M (1977) A re-evaluation of fatty acids as inflammatory agents in acne. J Invest Dermatol 68:93–99

Puhvel SM, Sakamoto M (1977) An in vivo evaluation of the inflammatory effect of purified comedonal components in human skin. J Invest Dermatol 69:401–406

Puhvel SM, Sakamoto M (1978) The chemoattractant properties of comedonal components. J Invest Dermatol 71:324–329

Puhvel SM, Sakamoto M (1980) Cytotaxin production by comedonal bacteria (Propioniobacterium acnes, Propionibacterium granulosum and Staphylococcus epidermidis). J Invest Dermatol 74:36–39

Scott DG, Cunliffe WJ, Gowland G (1979) Activation of complement – a mechanism for the inflammation in acne. Br J Dermatol 101:315–320

Webster GF (1990) Inflammatory acne. Int J. Dermatol 29:313–317

Inflammatory Lesions and Sequels

The Pustule

Pustules frequently start as solid lesions (papules) which soon liquefy. These are hybrids for which the term papulopustule is more exact, although not favored. The pustule represents a partial breakdown of the comedo. A variable segment of the epithelial lining survives and will reconstitute itself. Blow-outs close to the epidermis are less serious than deeper ones in the dermis and create smaller, more elevated lesions. Usually, the roof of the pustule bursts, allowing pus to escape. The battered remnants of the comedo are then discharged. Healing occurs in a very characteristic way that does not differ from normal wound repair. The severed ends of the follicular epithelium, literally immersed in a pool of pus, begin to thicken and soon send out irregular, hyperplastic sheets of undifferentiated epithelial cells. This migrating epithelium cleaves its way through the tissue around the periphery of the abscess, searching for viable dermis on which to implant. The epithelial ends link up and a continuous lining is re-established. The abscess thus becomes re-encapsulated. Hyperplasia gradually diminishes, and redifferentiation into a keratinizing epithelium occurs.

What happens to the comedonal core? Fortunately, it is usually not extruded into the dermis; enough epithelium remains to keep it in place. If extruded, however, granulocytes partially liquefy and disperse the horny matrix. Hydrolytic enzymes of the granulocytes, especially proteases, attack corneocytes and break them down. This is described later in more detail (p. 122).

Small pustules may resorb without retaining horny fragments. Following re-encapsulation the polymorphous neutrophils slowly disappear. About 10 days after rupture, lymphocytes and histiocytes become prominent. A loose cell-rich connective tissue surrounds the re-formed epithelium. The presence of concentrically arranged fine collagen fibers with many fibroblasts always indicates an earlier rupture. Inflammatory cells remain on the spot for an extraordinarily long time, at least several weeks after clinical healing. Eventually, nothing is left but a histologic scar. By tattooing the vicinity of pustules and then taking biopsies at various times after their clinical disappearance, much can be learned about their fate. This field, however, needs more investigation. Two outcomes have been observed, excluding serious scarring:

1. The epithelium may resume the production of coherent corneocytes; the comedo then continues its growth after a brief inflammatory interlude. Thus the secondary comedo is born. Re-encapsulation inevitably results in a variable enlargement of the lesions. Depending on the place and extent of rupture the outline of the secondary comedo will be variably irregular. The appearance may be that of simple pushing outwards, a tubular diverticu-

lum, a ballooning, or other odd shapes. The same comedo may rupture repeatedly. Large cystic lesions can arise from this.

2. The sebaceous follicle may be reconstituted usually with some distortion in architecture. The sebaceous glands reform, but are peculiarly shaped. The epithelium reverts to the production of loose horny material. The comedo's life is terminated. This is probably the more usual outcome. As a rule pustules heal without much visible scarring though one can often find the site with a magnifying glass.

The Papule

The collapse of the comedo gives rise to the deep-seated, long-lasting papule. The papule may be considered as a small nodule. The destruction of the epithelial lining is complete in most cases. The comedonal core is often not discharged to the surface and remains within the tissue as a foreign body. The horny core floats in a huge sea of inflammatory cells. In the ensuing inflammation, fragments of horn become sequestered in the dermis. Hairs, too, are dumped out. The skin has no effective means to rapidly remove lipid, horny detritus, and hair fragments; hence, the devastating quality of the papule. Tissue enzymes are not suited for this type of mop-up.

A foreign-body granuloma is provoked within a week or so and then takes many weeks and months to resolve. The violent inflammatory response extends widely in all directions. The neutrophilic flood may lap against neighboring sebaceous follicles and down into the subcutaneous fat as well. It may break into nearby follicles or comedones. Further out, it still seeps along vascular channels encircling the secretory coil of eccrine sweat glands. Here and there one finds thickened irregular remnants of the follicular epithelium struggling vainly to link up with other epithelial islands. These are all necrotic and heavily infiltrated with granulocytes. Nuggets of horny material are sometimes scattered far away from the destroyed follicle. Fragments of vellus hairs litter the scene, sometimes swallowed by foreign-body giant cells. Trichogranulomas are particularly persistent pestilential sequels. Later the infiltrate consists of a mixture of granulocytes, lymphocytes, histiocytes, and Langhans' foreign-body giant cells. Eventually, granulation tissue forms with many new vessels and fibroblasts. Histologic evidence of inflammatory activity persists long after the lesion has become clinically quiescent, usually for months. Scarring is inevitable, macroscopically as well as microscopically.

The Nodule

The nodule represents the total disintegration of a comedo with far-flung consequences. Two or more adjacent comedones often break down and fuse to create these monstrous lesions (giant papules). While the papule is a relatively localized explosion, the nodule is a volcanic eruption which destroys a large surrounding territory. A huge abscess engulfs neighboring follicles or comedones and destroys these too. The dissolution of adjacent pilosebaceous units propagates the inflammatory reaction. Hemorrhage and pools of serum are always part of this violent reaction. The abscess dissects well down into the subcutaneous tissue; panniculitis is always prominent. Every living structure within a radius of 10–30 mm is destroyed – sweat glands, vellus follicles, sebaceous follicles, nerves, and vessels. Fragments of hairs and comedonal kernels float like flotsam in the necrotic tissue. Foreign-body giant cells are numerous. Acute inflammation slowly gives way to a chronic one with many mononuclear cells and histiocytes. Histologic activity lasts for many months. Granulation tissue finally forms and scarring is, of course, massive.

The Draining Sinus

The draining sinus is a truly malevolent hybrid lesion, and features the combination of nodules and scars at the same time. It develops in the face, especially in the nasolabial folds, cheeks, and the neck. It is a huge tender lesion which periodically drains and crusts. In this case remnants of follicular epithelium somehow manage to survive. These dissect through the necrotic tissue and create tunnels of hyperplastic epithelium. They form a complicated, bizarre labyrinth of galleries which connect with the surfaces at various places. The epithelium is constantly breaking down so that the sinus tracts are not completely lined with epithelium. The lesion thus propagates itself, often extending linearly to form huge inflammatory ridges several centimeters long. The tunnels lie in a matrix of chronic granulation tissue composed of a variable mixture of neutrophils, lymphocytes, histiocytes, and foreign-body giant cells. The epithelium lining of the tunnels is very restless and sends out buds, ribbons, and tongues to form bizarre patterns which often suggest hamartomatous growths. Here and there, ruptures occur and epithelium immediately encapsulates the new areas of necrosis. Sebaceous lobules and pilary units persist for a variable period, but are destroyed with time. There is a constant tug of war between athe process of rupture and repair. The draining sinus is entirely analogous to the pilonidal cyst of the coccygeal area. It may grow relentlessly for years, intermittently calming down only to start draining again. Spontaneous healing does not occur.

Treatment is a real challenge and very difficult. It is done conservatively with aspiration of the hemorrhagic contents and injection of a corticosteroid crystal suspension, with tightly fitting compression badages worn afterwards for several days. Oral antibiotics are nearly always ineffective. Isotretinoin provides only temporarily and inconsistent relief, though it seems to be the treatment of choice. Sometimes only surgical excision of the entire labyrinth provides a final cure.

Profiles of Inflammation

A wide variety of inflammatory lesions arise from the rupture of comedones.

Above The closed comedo. The closed comedo is the first visible lesion in acne, sometimes called a time bomb. There are masses of *Propionibacterium acnes* in the central channels. Products of this invariable incite rupture. A normal sebaceous follicle is shown on the left. Two vellus follicles and one eccrine sweat gland are on the right

Middle

Left The pustule. Disintegration of the upper epithelial lining has created an intrafollicular abscess with a perifollicular inflammatory reaction. The basal portion of the comedo is intact. Healing will occur by re-encapsulation; while a scar will form, it will generally not be clinically apparent, except for some minor distortion of the orifice

Right The papule. Here the comedo has totally collapsed and the epithelial lining has been destroyed completely. Neutrophils have spread far into the tissue and even into the subcutaneous fat. The lesion persists for several weeks and will heal slowly, leaving a depressed scar

Below The nodule. The comedo has been shattered. Remnants of horn and hairs have been extruded into the tissue. The acute neutrophilic phase will give way to a chronic foreign body granuloma, remaining in place for weeks or even months. An ugly permanent scar is certain. A vellus follicle is to the left, a sebaceous follicle with incipient inflammation to the right. If the nodule links up the sebaceous follicle, a fistulated comedo is created

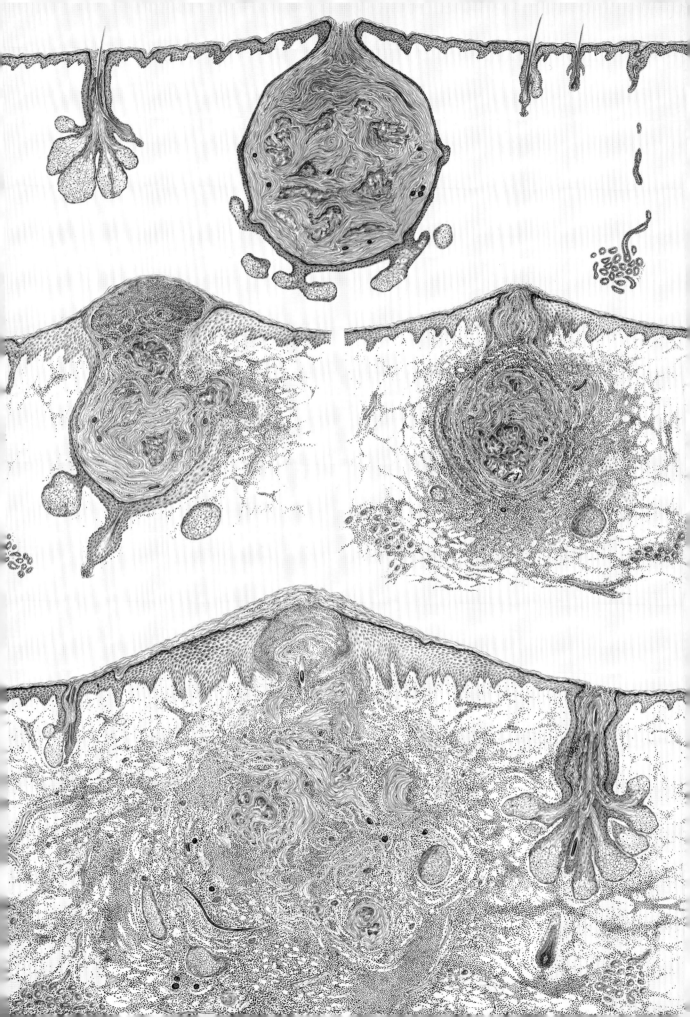

Dynamics of Inflammatory Acne in Men

Above

Left   Irrespective of grading systems, anyone can easily understand that this is bad acne. Face, neck, and shoulders bear papules, nodules, even hemorrhagic ones. Many closed comedones on the maxilla complete the varied spectrum of lesion

Right   A much milder course of acne, but troublesome. This patient has had this acne for years. It is now mostly inflammatory. The facial pores are wide, the skin oily, and fine scars are already present. The dusky red hue on his nose may be a very early sign of a rosacea diathesis, a disease which may follow acne

Below

Left   These many superficial and deep papules and nodules are aggressive and violent. Some persist for many weeks. Seborrhea is a typical cofeature. This is not the picture of gram-negative folliculitis, and no gram-negative organisms could be cultured despite several attempts

Right   Severe, destructive, necrotizing acne, almost acne conglobata on forehead, saddle of nose, temples, jawline, lateral sides of neck and shoulders. Extensive and intensive scarring is inevitable

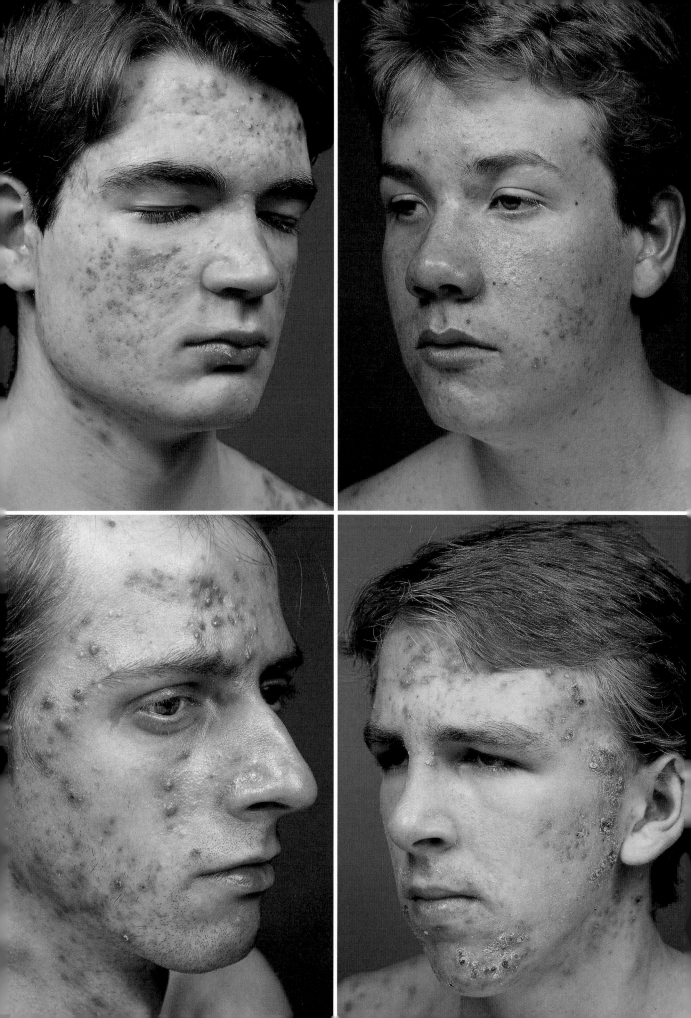

Folliculitis Versus Fragile Follicles

Folliculitis, mostly of the impetigo type (impetigo Bockhart) is a pyoderma, and could be misinterpreted as an acne pustule, which is by definition not a pyoderma.

Above   Staphylococcal folliculitis

Left   This lesion is a typical bacterial infection of a sebaceous follicle. *Staphylococcus aureus* is retrieved in great numbers from such lesions. The entire follicular canal is filled with granulocytes; there is no comedonal kernel

Right   Another example of bacterial folliculitis, with minimal accumulation of corneocytes swimming as an eosinophilic flotsam in a sea of pus. The sebaceous glands, as in the lesion to the left, are intact

Below   Fragile follicles. Some acne patients, particularly those with acne conglobata and acne fulminans, have very fragile follicles. They rupture at an early phase before a substantial comedo can be built up

Left   Fragile follicles from a patient with acne conglobata. The follicle has ruptured to the upper right. The comedonal kernel has been partly lost during sectioning, but loose corneocyte debris is still present. The pilary portion is to the left

Right   Fragile follicle from a patient with acne fulminans. The canal is filled with granulocytes and debris, with a microcomedo close to the sebaceous ducts. Both lesions in this lower panel harbor *Propionibacterium acnes* and *Staphyloccus epidermidis*, but no pyogenic organisms

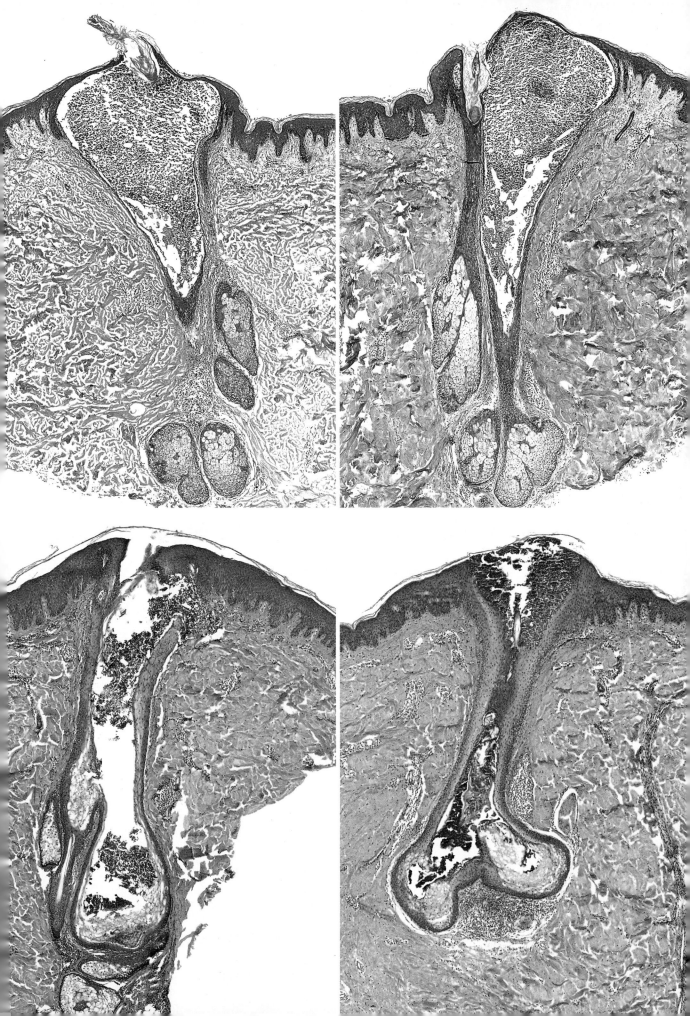

Variegate Histopathology
of Pustules and Papulopustules

Open but much more often closed comedones undergo focal areas of inflammation. Depending on its site and degree variable pustular elements are the result.

Above

Left   The quite old open comedo, with a dense central core, multiple bacterial cavities, a thin comedonal epithelium, and almost completely regressed sebaceous acini has become inflamed. Pockets of granulocytes are dissecting along the entire comedonal epithelium, with a major collection of pus subcorneally. It is expected that this comedo will survive to become a secondary comedo

Right   Deep papulopustule. The comedonal kernel is in the center. The entire comedonal epithelium has been destroyed. The inflammatory infiltrate extends far beyond the original lesion. Healing will be slow with a bad scar without reconstitution of a follicle

Below

Left   This aged open comedo ruptured in its bottom portion. The comedonal epithelium has been reconstituted. Pericomedonal inflammation attacks the sebaceous acini and pilary unit. It is assumed that they will survive

Right   An old closed comedo has been shattered at various points along the epithelial lining and is now a papulopustule. The pilary unit together with the sebaceous acini are destroyed; a cyst is born

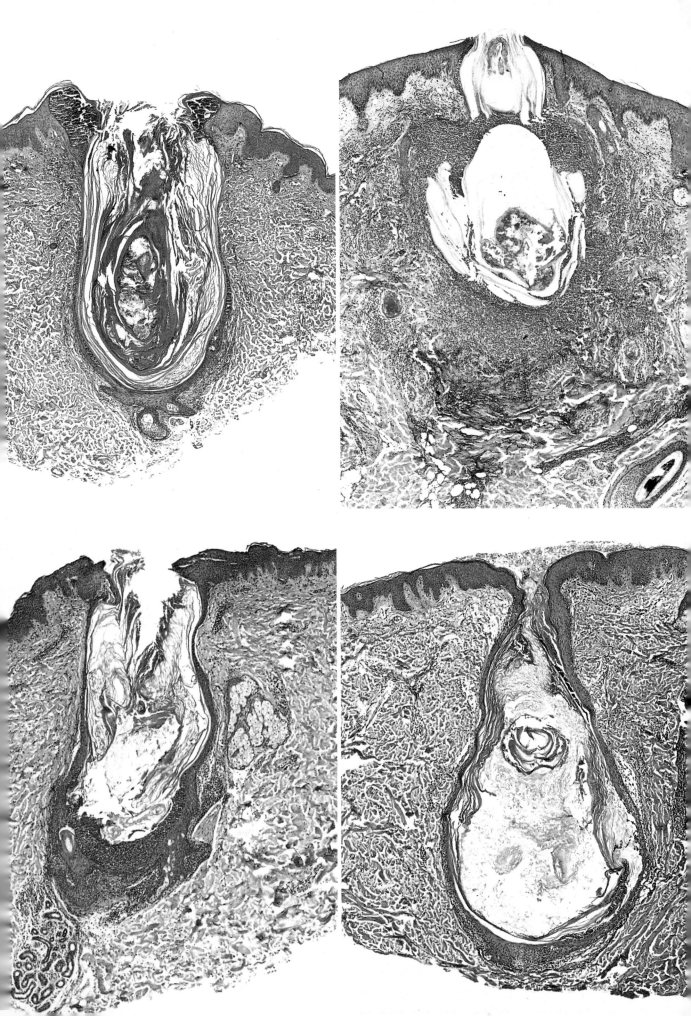

The Hateful Pustule

Pustules are very conspicuous lesions and therefore hated by all acne patients.

Above   A large succulent pustule. Acne pustules arise from comedones; the latter are usually invisible. Here, the brownish comedonal core floats on a yellow sea of pus, surrounded by erythema

Below   The histologic counterpart. This is an abscess with a horny kernel. Only a short segment of the comedonal epithelium to the right is still intact, too small to re-encapsulate the entire inflammatory lesion

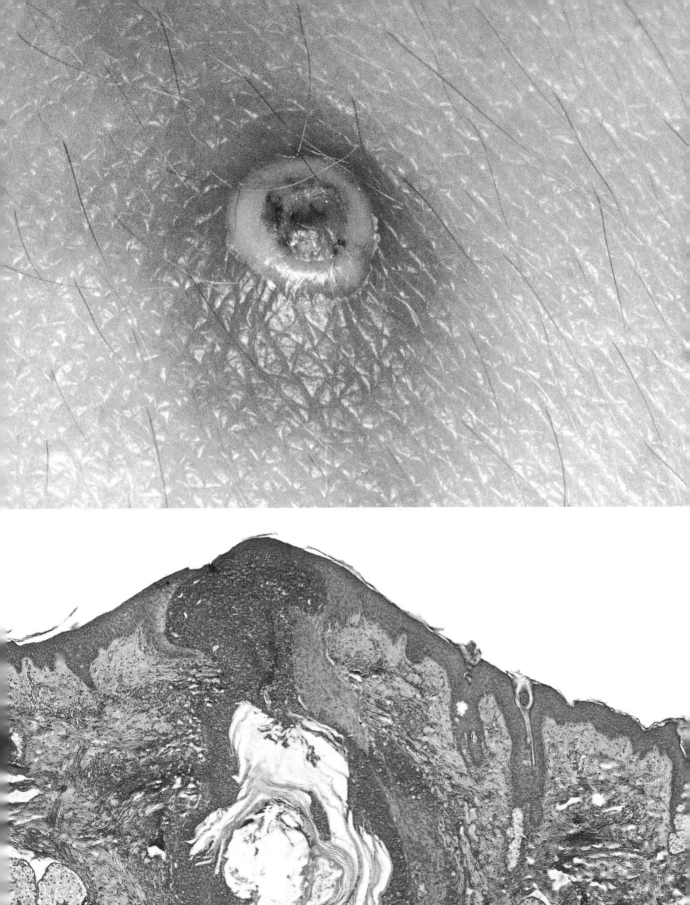

Draining Sinus: A Nasty Lesion

Above   An illustrative example of a draining sinus that runs for more than 5 cm from the nose to the corner of the mouth. It is still inflamed and tender, with stretches of atrophic scarring

Below   Histopathology of a similar lesion explains why a draining sinus cannot come to rest. The tunnel is completely epithelialized, opens at multiple sites into the epidermis, and is chronically inflamed

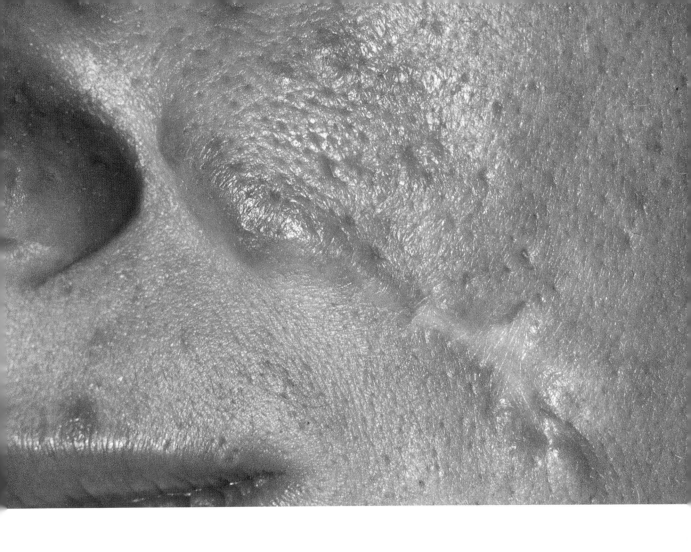

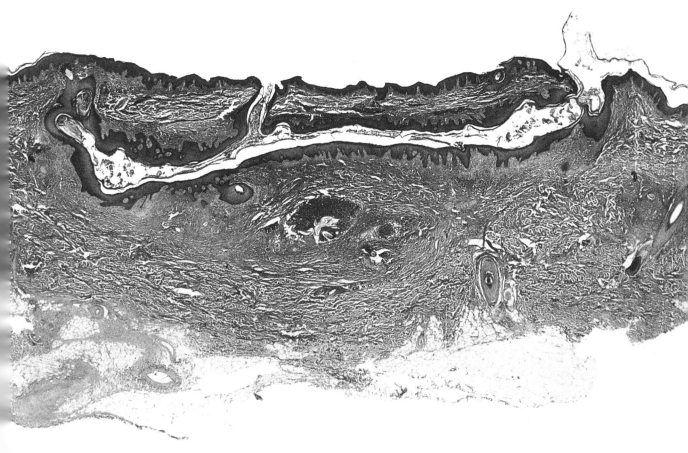

The Old Open Comedo

Histologic view of a large, long-standing open comedo. Old blackheads often show little "brush-fires" of inflammation along their borders. Sometimes the epithelial lining is very thin or absent. Pericomedonal fibrosis reveals that rupture and repair have occurred many times. The inflammatory reaction is limited because the really toxic soluble contents of the comedo are bottled up in the central chambers. The periphery of this comedo constitutes a dense capsule of corneocytes which is an effective barrier. The blue-staining amorphous material in the large multi-loculated central cavities is a dense population of *Propionibacterium acnes*, luxuriating in a sea of sebum. Fortunately mature open comedones rarely rupture and thus do not spill their toxic contents into the dermis, an event that would, of course, wreak havoc. The horny capsule mainly seals off the internal contents, although not completely, as seen from the pericomedonal neutrophilic infiltrate.

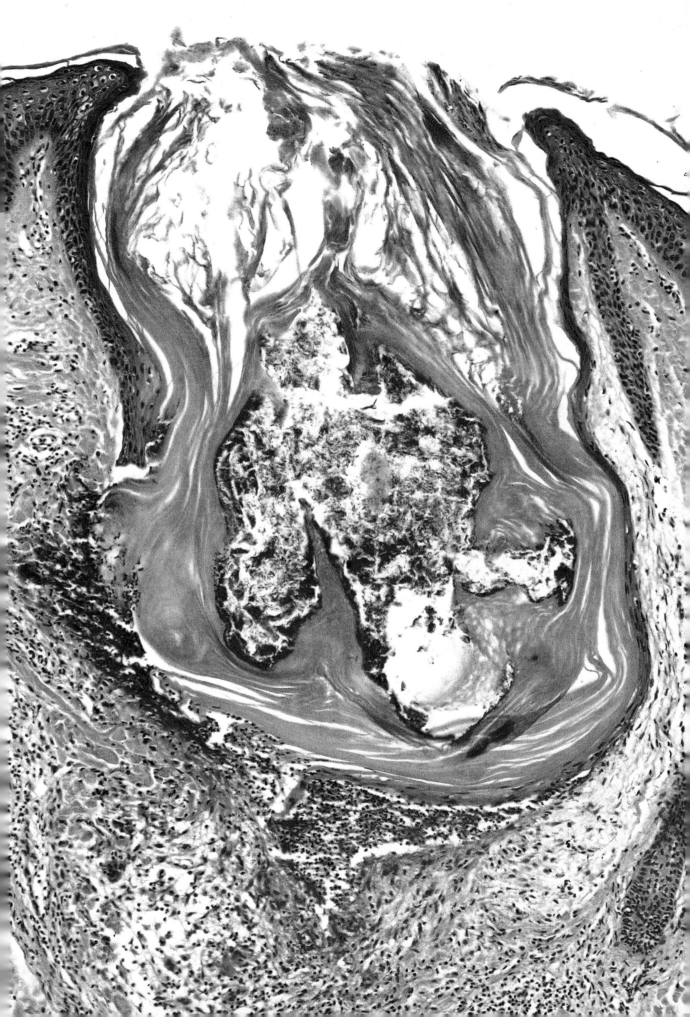

Early or Late Rupture of Comedones

Above

Left   A microcomedo, just on its way to becoming a closed comedo, has ruptured. The biopsy is from a patient with acne conglobata. The still small comedonal core is layered between inflammatory cells and the severed, acanthotic comedonal epithelium. It is a poor sign that the abscess has dissected deep down into the dermis. There is much more inflammation than was suspected clinically

Right   In contrast to the figure on the left, this is an old open comedo with a wide pore. Parts of the comedo are bacteria-filled chambers. The comedonal epithelium is extremely thin, almost absent on the right side. The pilary portion but not the sebaceous acini, are intact. Pericomedonal edema and fibrosis signal multiple earlier inflammatory episodes from which the comedo survived

Below   A quite symmetrical closed comedo has ruptured, for the first time, on its upper right side. The inflammation is mainly localized in the apical portion, classifying it clinically into a pustule. Healing will be fast, with almost no scarring. For comparison a normal sebaceous follicle with sebaceous acini, a pilary unit, and one hair in the follicular canal is seen on the left

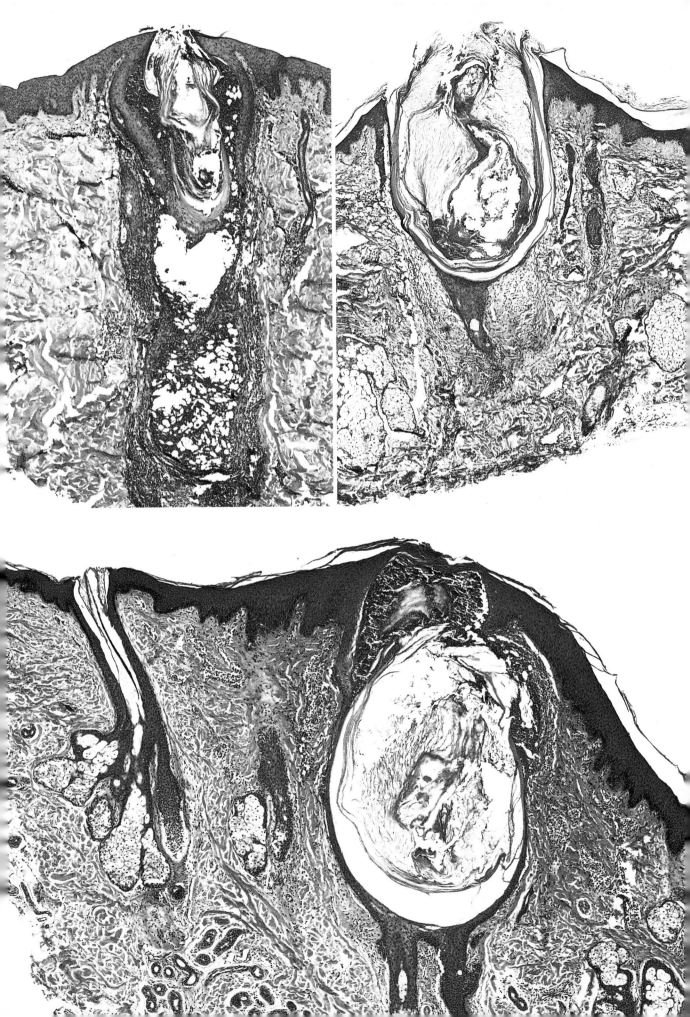

Deep-Seated Papules

Papules are histologically hybrids: papulopustules. Superficially located lesions often drain to the skin surface and leave less trouble behind than deep-seated ones.

Above   A comedo has ruptured at its lower pole. One third of its bottom lining has been destroyed; the comedonal contents exploded far into the surrounding skin. This lesion will persist for many weeks or months before all of this inflammatory disaster has been cleared away. Scarring is inevitable

Below

Left   The entire comedonal epithelium has been dissolved. The comedonal contents are exposed to the vasculature and connective tissue, inciting a heavy proinflammatory response. A bystanding sebaceous follicle to the left has been attacked already

Right   Higher magnification reveals the comedonal kernel with bacterial chambers. The bacteriology of papulopustules can only be studied if this comedonal kernel is secured. Scarring is inevitable and substantial once this acne lesion has calmed down. Healing will take months

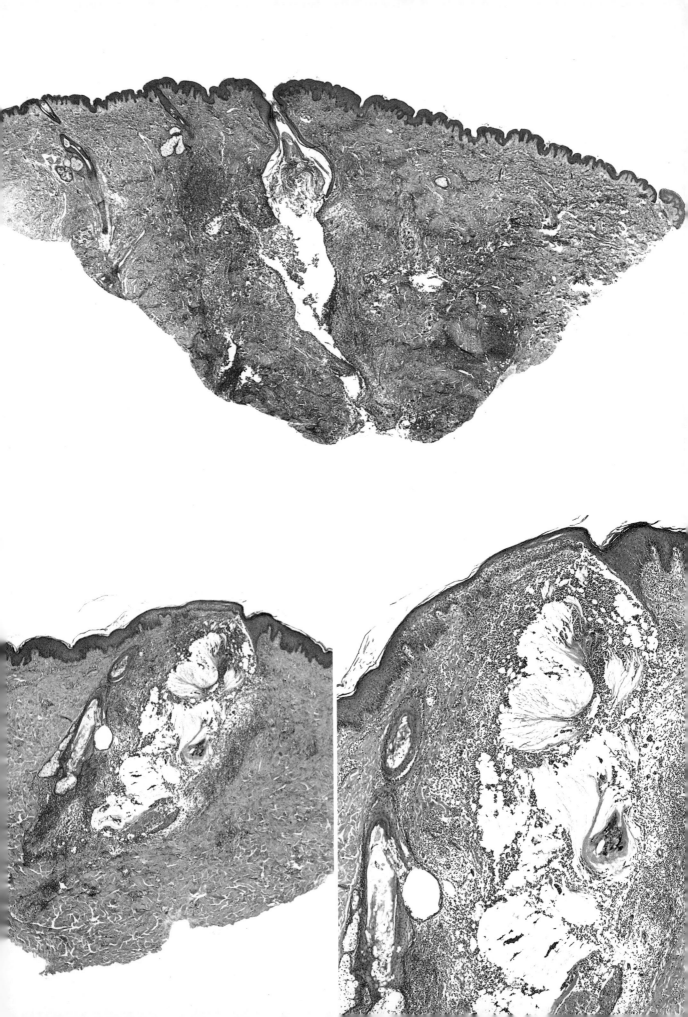

Regenerative Capacity of Comedones

Comedones take various assaults quite well, overcome mechanical and inflammatory attacks, and keep on minding their own business. Experimental injury was performed by 18-gauge sterile injection needles.

Above   An open comedo was pierced with the needle, and the site biopsied several minutes later. The needle had lacerated the comedonal epithelium, which partly retracts. Two fairly wide breaches expose toxic comedonal contents to the vasculature and cellular components of corium. There is no inflammatory response yet

Below   The same experiment was performed with this open comedo, but the biopsy was obtained 7 days later. One can study the wound healing of the comedo. This all went very swiftly. The epithelial dehiscences have been corrected by migration of sprouts and reconnection of the comedonal wall. The parakeratotic corneocytes, mixed with inflammatory cells, have been tightly sealed off. The comedo wall is acanthotic; the pericomedonal hemorrhage and fibrosis reveals the recent inflammatory episode. This is now a secondary comedo

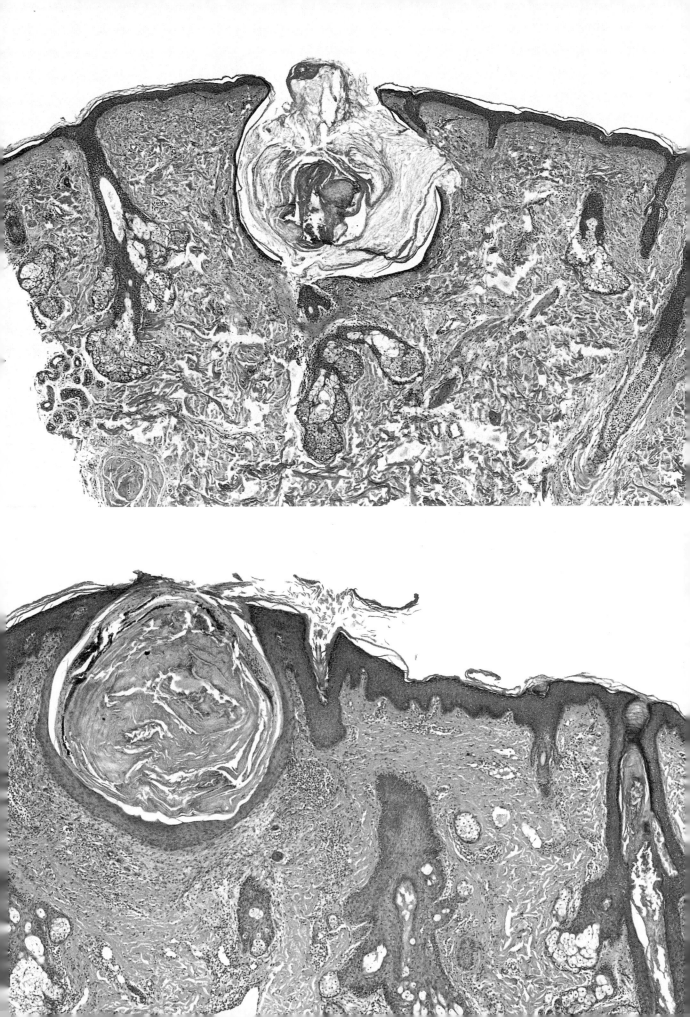

Hemorrhagic Nodules

Some patients with acne conglobata and acne fulminans react at the peak of the stormy disease with frank bleeding into the skin. Intact hemorrhagic nodules and dome-shaped elevations form, or the skin ulcerates early on, leaving wide-open bloody craters. Biopsies are only rarely taken from this severely afflicted patients; this one is from the upper back.

Above   Two dome-shaped hemorrhagic nodules on top of an atrophic scar. Multiple other scars are seen in this patient with acne fulminans

Below   Biopsy from a similar lesion. A hemorrhagic abscess occupies the middle and lower dermis. Gelatinous material is in the center, dissecting in all directions. The dermis is totally necrotic. The debris is surrounded by a dense infiltrate. The contents of such hemorrhagic skin necrosis are sterile

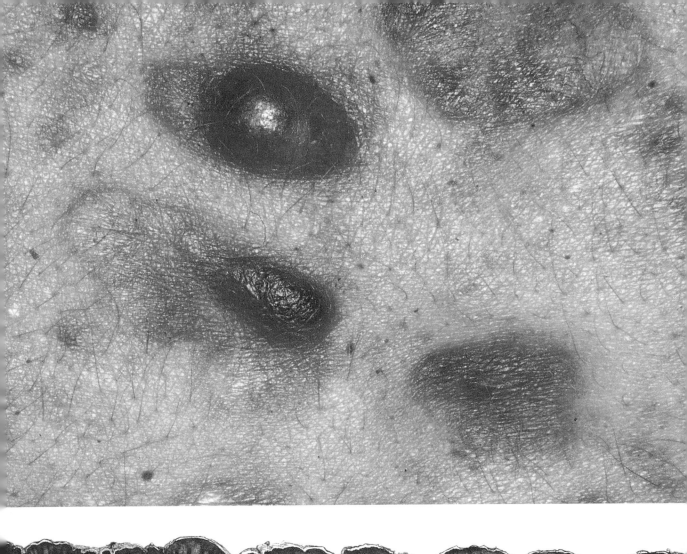
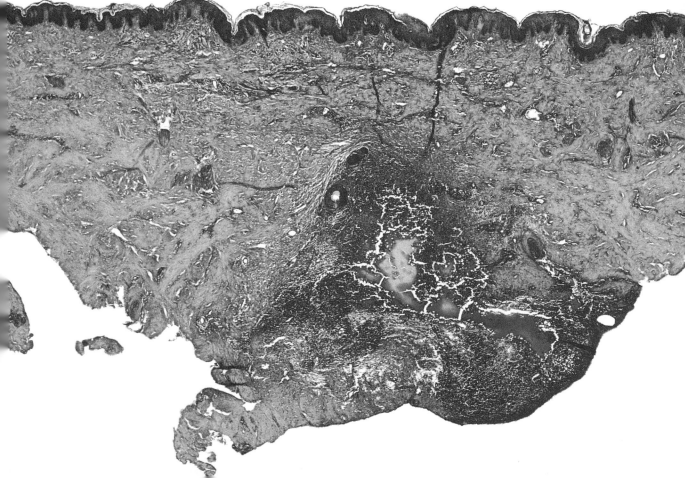

Nodules

Patients with severe acne can develop nodules of fantastic size and at the most unusual locations.

Above

Left   One predilection site is the ear lobes. The nodules persist for a long while and can re-erupt intermittently. They cause discomfort and pain. Aspiration yields a reddish or brownish viscous fluid. Unfortunately refilling occurs within a few days. Sometimes intralesional injection of triamcinolone acetonide crystal suspension is helpful. Otherwise nodules have to be excised, if possible, once they have come to a temporary rest

Right   The bridge of the nose is another choice location for hemorrhagic nodules. Sometimes nodules turn into draining sinuses

Below

Left   The extensive tissue destruction can be seen in this lower-power view. The abscess extends below the lateral and lower margin of this photograph. The remnant of the comedonal kernel is in the center. No comedonal epithelium has survived

Right   The ruptured comedo and parts of its epithelium are still alive. The abscess spreads far in all directions

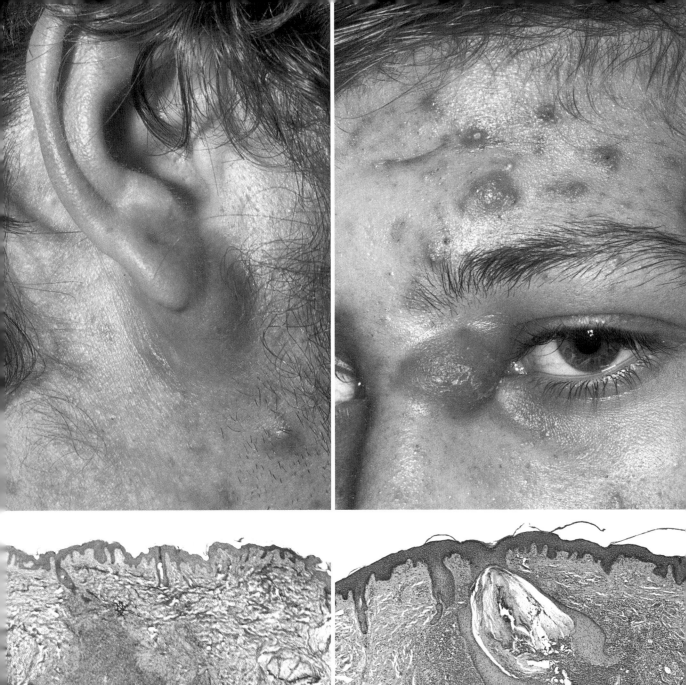
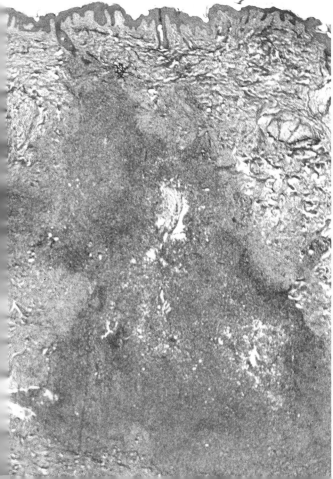
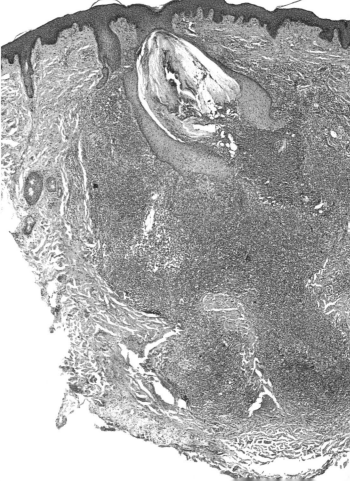

Explosion of Closed Comedones

A complete rupture blew up this closed comedo, dispersing some of its contents into the corium. This is clinically equivalent to a deep persistent papule or nodule.

Above   The comedonal core is in place. The comedonal epithelium has ruptured to the left and right, is now acanthotic, and tries to reconnect. Pericomedonal inflammation is far-flung

Below   Close-up of the breach shown in the upper photograph. Tangential cuts through three hairs, which are now lying outside the comedo. A foreign-body reaction will persist for many weeks or months before this alien material has been completely resorbed

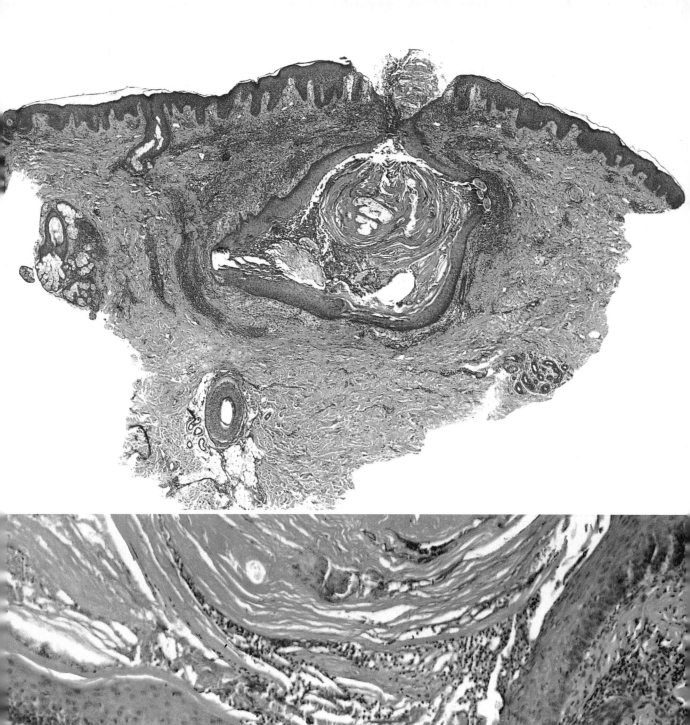
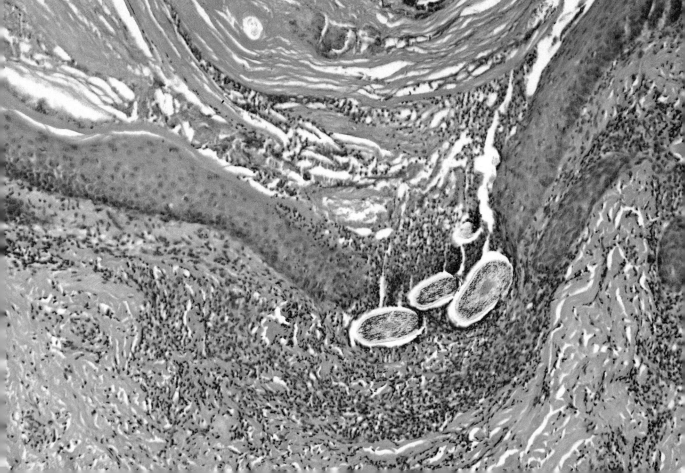

Secondary Comedones

Secondary comedones are always postinflammatory stages of open or closed comedones. Their fate is variable. Some remain in the same category of open or closed comedones, others develop into cysts, and even others into fistulated comedones. The worst outcome would be a draining sinus. Two of these possibilities are presented here.

Above A fistulated comedo. A large comedo has sustained a bad blow-up; miraculously it survived. The comedo is sandwiched between inflammatory debris. The comedo wall is acanthotic and sends out tongues of epithelium. The widespread and heavy chronic infiltrate with many multinucleated giant cells show that the clean-up job is still to be done. An innocent neighboring sebaceous follicle to the right has become involved in the abscess, and is now permanently linked with its aggressor; thus a fistulated complex is formed. If more than two follicles or comedones are linked up, there is always the danger of a draining sinus ensuing

Below A cyst. The comedo has also escaped total destruction by the previous inflammatory episode. Its wall is sealed again, locking up the comedo core and debris. However, none of the sebaceous glands nor the pilary unit survived. Only a miniscule bud of epithelium (⟶) remains to show where the sebaceous acinus once prospered. The area surrounding of the cyst is still chronically inflamed

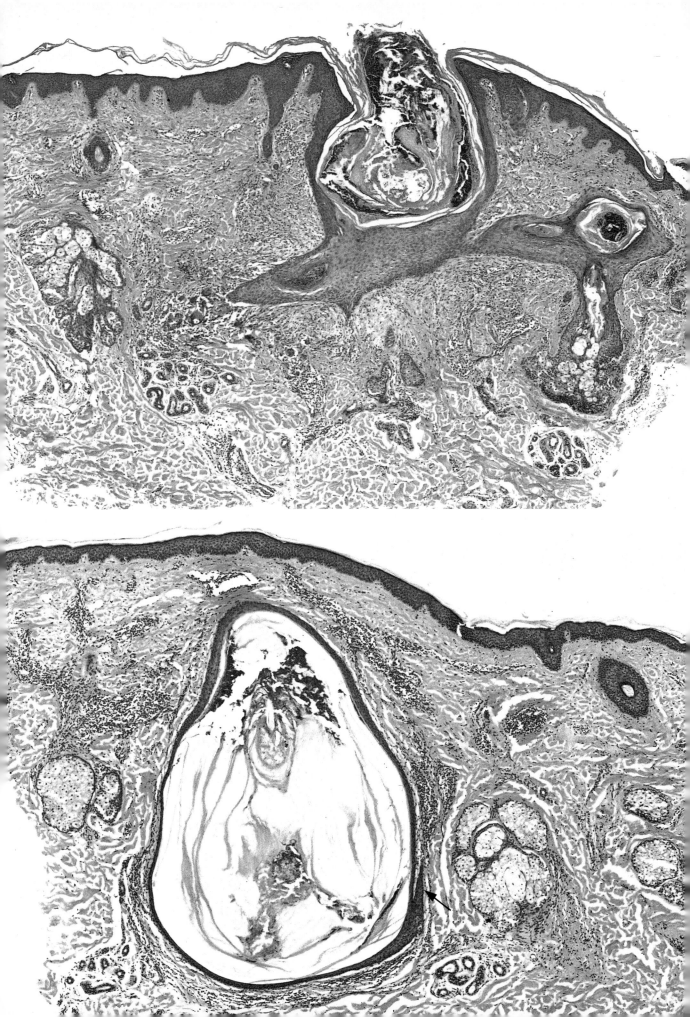

Pustules and Their Sequels

Above   In this instance an invasion of the follicle by neutrophils has floated the comedo out of the follicle in a sea of pus. The follicle will reform because the epithelium is still intact. Scarring will be minimal and can be diagnosed only histologically by perifollicular fibrosis

Below   This was a deep-seated pustule which ruptured several weeks ago. The pustule unfortunately, did not empty towards the skin surface but into the deeper dermis, where it caused a widespread inflammatory response. The comedonal epithelium has reformed, thus creating a secondary comedo. The irregular shape, acanthosis, and loose corneocytes are indicative for a secondary comedo

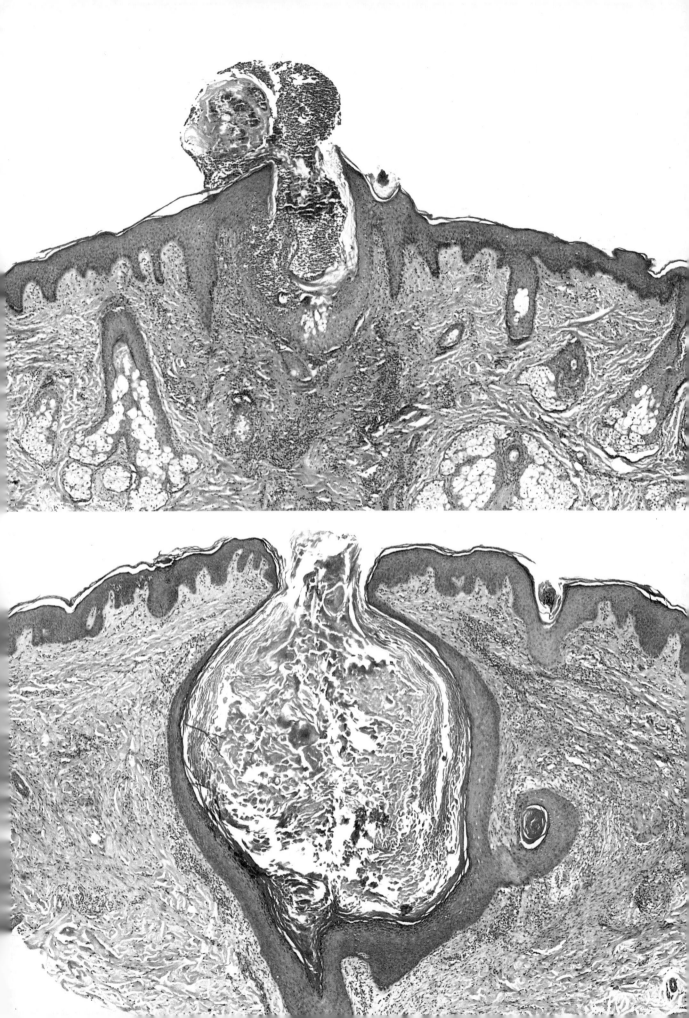

Secondary Comedones

It is fairly easy to come to a correct classification of secondary comedones:

- Asymmetrical shape
- Acanthosis mixed with atrophy of the comedo wall
- Pericomedonal fibrosis
- Variable portions of sebaceous acini: atrophy or total destruction of glands
- The pilary portion is mostly destroyed

Above

Left   A secondary comedo with loose corneocytes, irregular wall, and pericomedonal fibrosis

Right   This secondary comedo survived from a bad inflammatory reaction. The scar to its sides and bottom is extensive. Sebaceous acini and the hair unit were destroyed

Below

Left   A secondary comedo on its way to a cyst. If the secondary comedo survives long enough, it often gets bigger and bigger and thus turns into an epidermal cyst

Right   A good example of a secondary comedo with asymmetry, loss of the pilary unit, pericomedonal fibrosis, and a regressing sebaceous gland on its base

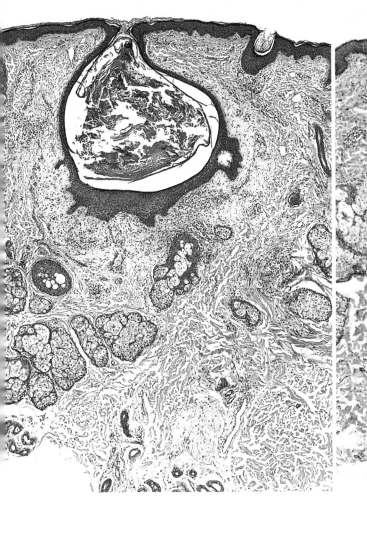
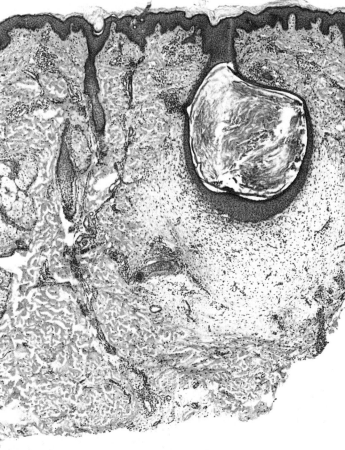
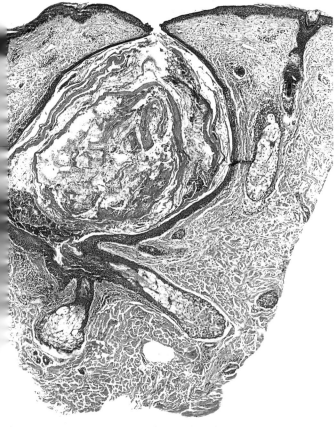
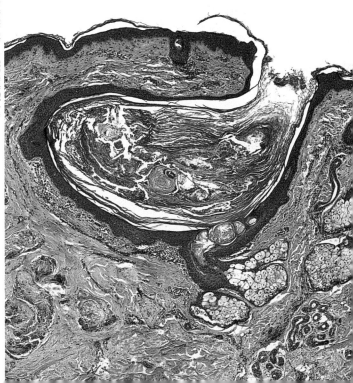

Fistulated (Polyporous) Comedones: A Clinical View

Fistulated comedones can be classified as secondary comedones or, eventually, as scars. They have a complicated history and take a long time to develop. They are rare on the face, but common on the back, and they are late and permanent sequelae of acne conglobata.

Above This adult man seems to have many giant blackheads. On closer inspection, one notes that the comedones are distributed in clusters. Indeed, each comedo is a member of a complex system of interconnected horn-filled galleries. Other stigmata of acne conglobata are also present: atrophic and hypertrophic scars and invariably a few hot spots where the disease refuses to die, even after decades

Below A probe inserted in any opening can be made to issue from any of the others in the complex. A part of the horny plug has been pushed out. These comedones are really specialized scars filled with corneocytes. The pigment is melanin. The gaping and irregular outlines are telltale signs of scarring

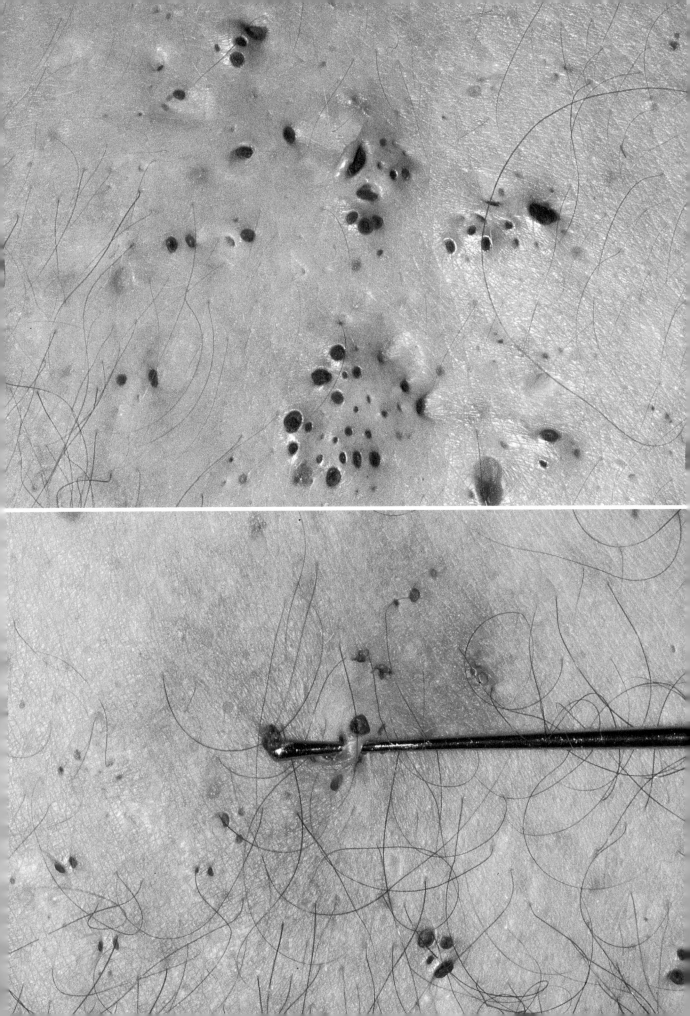

Late Events of Inflammation

Biopsying acne skin several weeks or months after the acute inflammatory phase discloses peculiar leftovers.

Above   Several weeks previously this was the site of a papulopustule. The location was carefully identified and biopsied 10 weeks later. Clinically it was just a fairly fresh, slightly red scar. Histopathology showed more than was anticipated. Remnants of the comedo are present as foreign material, and a whole string of multinucleated giant cells slowly digests the debris and corneocytes. Chronic, lymphocytic perivascular, and diffuse infiltrates as well as ectatic venules remain as a sign of the ongoing inflammation. The follicle remains even after the comedo has long been eradicated

Below   More than 12 weeks previously, a deep-seated tender papule developed, persisted, and at the time of biopsy inflamed skin was still seen. Deep in the dermis, spectacular inflammatory elements are present. Quite a large portion of the comedo, though devoid of its epithelium, drifts around. Two segments of epithelium (✻) float in a sea of pus. The lymphocytic infiltrate reaches far beyond the bundaries of this section

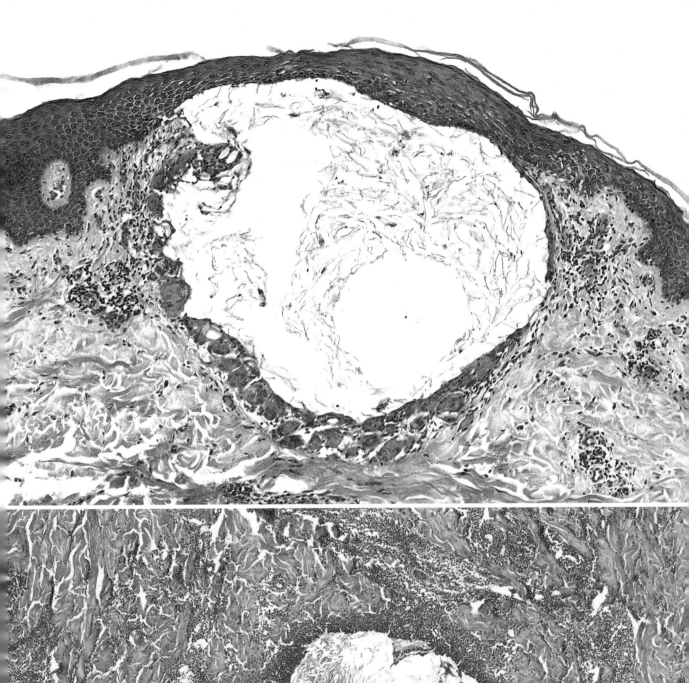
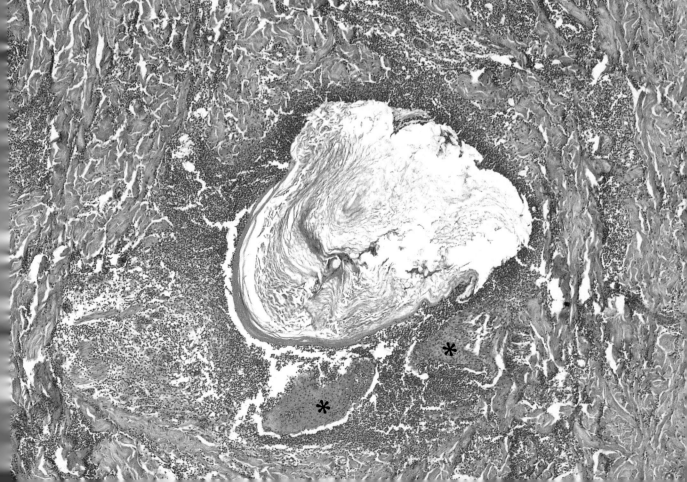

Spontaneous Healing of Pustules and Papulopustules

Pustules usually heal quickly, at least clinically. Histopathologically, though, long-standing inflammation and variable scarring are inevitable.

Above

Left   A facial pustule spontaneously discharged 8 days prior to the biopsy. The follicular structure is intact with a small comedonal kernel. A parakeratotic mound is still present, and there is dense perifollicular lymphohistiocytic infiltrate

Right   A week earlier this papulopustule fell out. The follicular epithelium is acanthotic. The surrounding tissue is still inflamed. The tattoo to the right identifies the correct area under investigation

Below

Left   Twenty-two days before this site was biopsied, a facial pustule dried up. The follicular epithelium was badly damaged and is now bizarre in shape with acanthotic and atrophic stretches. Fibrosis and scarring is eminent. The facial pore is distended, thus leaving a visible scar

Right   Fifteen days prior to the biopsy a pustule was present. Histologically a scar extends between two neighboring follicles. The skin surface is almost smooth, thus leaving no visible problem for the patient

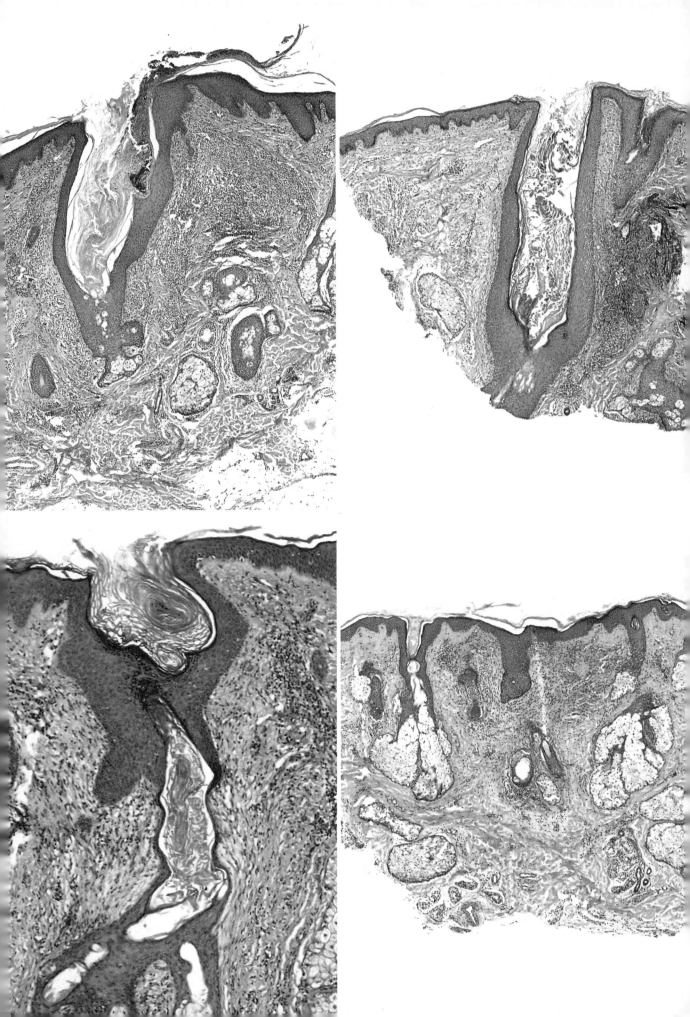

Cysts

The term cystic acne is somewhat of a misnomer. Cysts are primary epithelial-lined cavities. The cysts in acne are a result of repeated ruptures and re-encapsulations, best defined as large secondary comedones.

Above Cysts can be found everywhere in the territory of acne, mostly on the trunk. However, the face is not spared. This black man has one cyst behind the ear (*left*) and many on the cheeks (*right*). Puncture reveals a cheesy, horny material. The epithelial sac can be delivered by a small curette, a permanent end to the cyst

Below Cysts are soft and fluctuant. They have a widespread distribution in this man, occurring on his face, chest, shoulders, and back. They slowly enlarge over time, some attaining gigantic size. At that stage the epithelial wall becomes quite thin and can easily rupture by trauma. Ruptured cysts leave abscesses in their wake. Patients are well advised to have their cysts shelled out to prevent rupture and subsequent inflammatory nodules

Left Multiple cysts on temple, cheek, chin, and chest

Right This white man in his late fifties has had acne all his life, which is not unusual for acne conglobata. He also has many scars and secondary open comedones

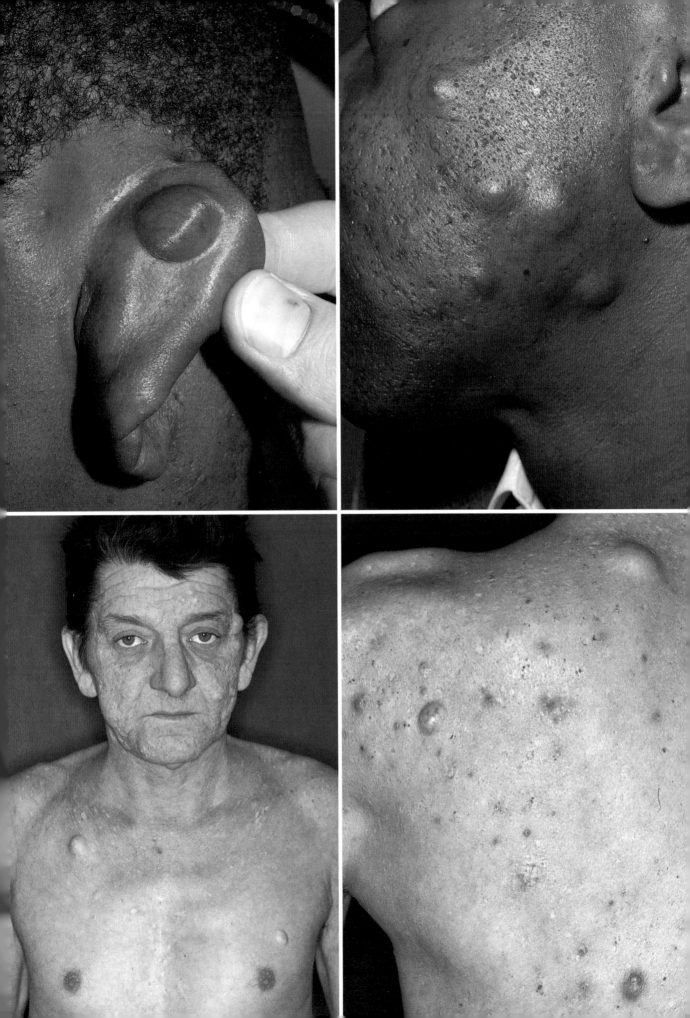

Acne Cysts

The repertoire of acne is vast, and some of the actors are strange characters, among them are cysts.

Above

Left   The cyst is a late lesion of acne conglobata, but not a burned-out inflammatory lesion. It is a soft, seemingly lifeless, flesh-colored, round mass which, on close inspection, sometimes shows a central dimple. In fact it is a huge secondary comedo formed by repeated rupture and re-encapsulation

Right   After puncture or with pressure alone, one can force out a string of whitish, curdy horny material. To prevent re-formation one must also deliver the epithelial sac, or excise it completely

Below

Left   A single cyst shelled out by blunt dissection

Right   Histology shows a huge epithelium-lined sac containing loose horny matter. There are no hairs, the pilary unit having been destroyed long ago. Though a pore was not visible clinically, there is a tiny orifice. A localized inflammatory reaction goes on at the bottom of the lesion like a brush fire

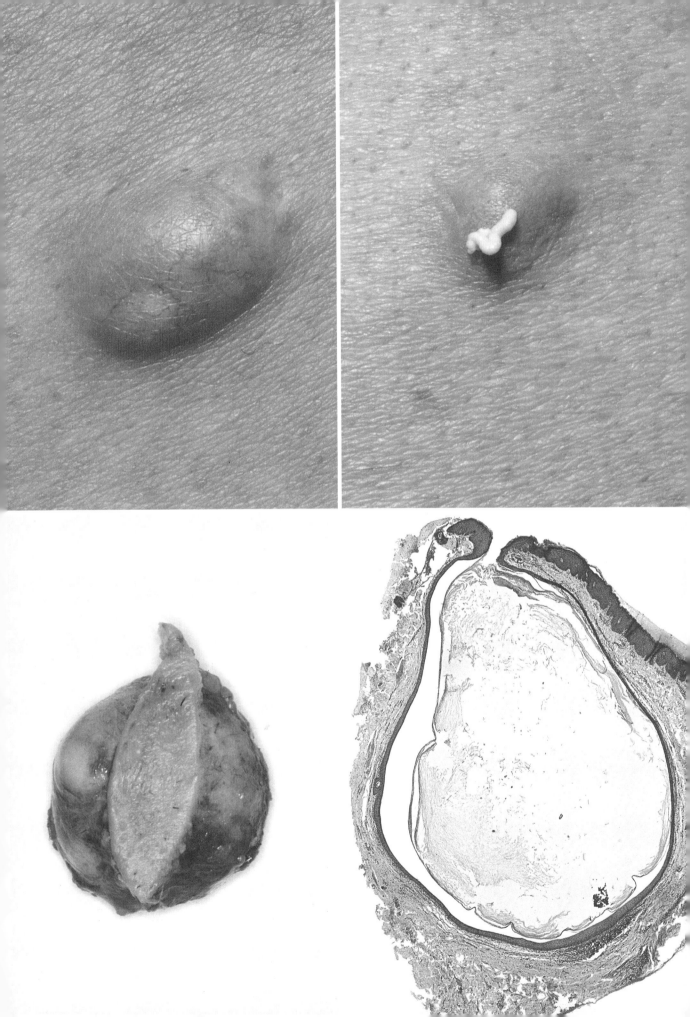

The Scope of Scars

Next to comedones scars are the hallmark of acne. Permanent scarring is the most dreaded outcome of this disease. Scarring can be the natural consequence of inflammatory lesions, or the result of self-manipulation. The latter is too often overlooked. Both types may coincide. In this chapter only spontaneous scars will be discussed. A separate chapter is devoted to self-inflicted scars (p. 356). The spectrum of scars extends from invisible to severely mutilating.

Pitted, Crateriform, and Ice Pick Scars

Typical examples of the variety of acne scars are represented by pitted, crateriform, and ice pick scars. Exclusively confined to the face, they are variably shaped crater-like depressions, pits, and ice pick scars (reminiscent of steepsided pits in a glacier from an ice pick). Pitted scars may become confluent to form broad retiform extremely ugly scars. The rim of the scar can be steep or shallow. This makes real difference to the bearer. Steep rims throw shadows and cause the scars to be conspicuous. Bevelled rims allow light to flood the base, without shadows. These scars are less noticeable.

Histopathology. The picture is variable, but one always finds horn-filled canals, lined by an irregularly thickened epithelium budding off into ribbons. Signs of foreign-body granulomas are present with mixtures of inflammatory cells. There are variable inflammatory changes, inevitably accompanied by a surrounding fibrosis. In short, scars are extremely pleomorphic depending on their stage and the severity of the preceding inflammatory lesion.

Trough Scars

Usually one or a few shallow soft depressions develop that are limited entirely to the face.

Atrophic Scars

Small flat scars can occur on the face. Much larger ones, several centimeters in size, may develop on the upper parts of the back over the shoulder blades. Atrophic scars are the insignia of acne conglobata. Fresh ones are pink to red, older ones alabaster-white to yellowish. Some of them are cigarette-paper thin, wrinkled, and transparent. As the collagen bed is extremely thin and atrophic, the blood vessels are visible through the thin overlying tissue. All skin adnexa are completely wiped out by the fibrotic process. Looking at the surface under magnification, one cannot see a single opening of remnants of follicles, nor for that matter sweat glands.

Histopathology. Quite distinctive is the extremely flattened-out thin epidermis, void of rete ridges. Whithin the dermis there are numerous ectatic lymph and venous vessels with fine, horizontally arranged collagen bundles, numerous fibroblasts, and irregular foci of lymphohystiocytic cells. Remnants of arrector pili muscles, nerves, clusters of debris, giant cells, calcification, or even bone formation are variably present. No appendageal structures remain.

Hypertrophic Scars

These are also called fibrotic nodules. They are preceded by deep inflammatory nodules of acne conglobata, commonest on the back, shoulder, or over the sternum. The lesions are large, often 1–2 cm wide, dome-shaped, and elevated 5–10 mm above the surface. First there are fiery-red, later becoming porcelain yellowish-white. These are very hard and lumpy. The surface is shiny, without follicular openings. With time these lesions flatten, a process that may take years. Itching is frequently reported.

Histopathology. A low-power view is useful for diagnosis. The scar is composed exclusively of dense collagen bundles of varying size and in complete disarray. Most of the collagen is stratified horizontally. The skin appendages have all been destroyed. Elastic fibers are absent or sparse. Vessels are scarce. This is the picture of extreme fibrosis.

Perifollicular Papular Scars

Perifollicular papular scars are elevated, firm, hard growths that are prevalent on the back, rarer on the chest, and absent on the face. The scars are round to oval, white, and slightly elevated lesions. Several terms are used to describe them: papular acne scars, perifollicular elastolysis, postacne anetoderma-like scars, and papular elastorrhexis. The latter has been mistaken for a connective tissue nevus. They resemble closed comedones, hence the name closed comedo-like scar. We prefer the term perifollicular papular scars. These are best seen when the skin is pinched together between the fingers. They are frequently mistaken for closed comedones. Puncturing the apex with a pointed scalpel differentiates comedones. Nothing comes out.

Histopathology. The extent of the scar is best visualized by staining elastic fibers. The perifollicular papular scar is larger than it appears clinically. The elastic fibers are completely destroyed. The surrounding elastic fibers mark the borders of the scar. Generally, the appendages have been destroyed, though sometimes a hair-bearing unit survives with a fine hair protruding, hence the name perifollicular papular scar. Fibrosis is evidenced by dense bundles of collagen with straggly vessels.

Calcified Scars

One of the late sequelae of severe inflammatory acne is calcification. Even bone formation (osteoma) may occur. These scars are not diagnosed clinically. Sites of predilection are the face, especially the cheeks and chin, followed by the upper back. X-rays show many opacities, often an accidental finding. Sometimes calcified nodules can be suspected in a badly scarred face, when densities hard as stone are felt by palpation.

Histopathology. Small or large calcified nodules are dispersed throughout the corium. Multinuclear giant cells often bear calcified deposits. Osteoma cutis is described elsewhere (p. 535).

Keloids

Keloids are a terrible form of scars which occur more often in blacks than in whites. Sites of predilection are the sternum, breasts, lateral sites of upper arms, shoulders, back of neck, and the V-shaped area of the back. Keloids do not arise spontaneously, but start with trauma, often minor. In acne they follow inflammatory lesions which may simply be papulopustules, but more often are inflammatory nodules in acne conglobata. Keloids are often mistaken for hypertrophic scars. The two are not interchangeable, as many seem to think. True keloids extend far beyond the original zone of inflammation. They are thick, raised, lobulated fibrotic plaques, with a great tendency to recur after removal. They do not flatten with time. Elevated hard scars in white persons are almost always hypertrophic scars. The color is deep red to brownish, with a shiny surface. After many years they become skin-colored. No fine texture, wrinkles, or pores are visible. Itching, sometimes associated with pain, is very common. Keloids never regress spontaneously even after decades, as may happen with hypertrophic scars.

Histopathology. Nothing very specific can be seen histopathologically, except for densely packed, whorled, mostly horizontally arranged collagen bundles. In between are ectatic blood vessels and sparse lymphohistiocytic infiltrates. Elastic tissue is completely absent, as in all scars. Any search for adnexal structures will be in vain. Histopathologists all too commonly fail to appreciate that keloids can be distinguished from hypertrophic scars. The fibrous tissue in the former are arranged in nodules with circumferential bands of collagen delimiting each nodules. This architecture is absent in hypertrophic scars where the collagen is in disarray.

Fistulated Comedones (Polyporous Comedones)

Fistulated comedones are described elsewhere (p. 88). They are sequelae to acne conglobata, mainly located on the back and achieve their final form over many years of inflammatory activity. Quite often, dozens or even hundreds of clusters of comedo-like lesions are spread over the upper trunk. Each cluster is a system of interconnected horn-filled galleries. Between 2 and 20 openings may show on the surface of these complex units. A blunt probe inserted into one opening may issue from others nearby, indicating that one is dealing with a labyrinth of epithelium-lined channels. A comedo-like kernel can be pushed out; its surface is often dark black. The pigment is melanin.

There is a smoldering low-grade inflammation, causing tender abscesses to form, off and on. The bacteriology is that of the normal skin flora. Dumping of foreign material into the dermis, e.g., corneocytes, trapped hairs, and epithelial remnants accounts for abscesses and foreign-body granulomas. Other stigmata of acne conglobata with atrophic and hypertrophic scars are often in close proximity. Fistulated comedones never heal spontaneously and stay with the bearer for the rest of his life.

Incision with fine scissors unroofs each gallery (marsupialization). The horny impactions fall out and do not reform. The opened lesions are allowed to heal by secondary intention. To clean up hundreds of fistulated comedones is a herculean task, although rewarding. Elimination of the rancid odor is in itself very gratifying to patients.

Histopathology. Tunneled galleries, interconnected with each other, with a variable number of gully-like openings, are lined with keratinizing epithelium. Sebaceous lobules are usually destroyed, though occasionally a bizarrely shaped acinus is connected with the labyrinth. The tunnels are stuffed with densely packed corneocytes. Inflammatory pockets, small or large, are part of the spectrum. Melanin is produced around the openings, so that the horny material becomes black.

The Draining Sinus

This is the most grotesque and disturbing lesion of the acne repertoire. Typically these inflammatory tunnels are located in the face, notably the nasolabial folds, cheeks, bridge of the nose, chin, and sides of the neck. Suppurative material drains to the surface more or less continually. These are sausage-like thickenings which are linear, often several centimeters long. They are tender, smelly, and offensive with their periodic foul discharges.

Histopathology. Multiple openings on the skin surface connect a set of galleries traversing through the middle and deep corium. The tunnels are lined with a restless epithelium forming odd patterns with innumerable sprouts and ribbons. The appearance varies with each cut. Trapped in the tunnels are loose corneocytes, parakeratotic debris, all kinds of inflammatory cells, and sometimes curled-up hairs. The perilesional collagen is fibrotic. One finds pockets of inflammation with a variable mixture of lymphohistiocytes and granulocytes, sometimes calcification.

Actively smoldering draining sinuses can be treated by intralesional injection of corticosteroids, notably triamcinolone (p. 160). Unfortunately flare-ups are common. Final cure can only be achieved by surgery; the entire gallery has to be excised, resulting of course in a linear scar. Plastic surgeons can sometimes do wonders in excising and repairing draining sinuses.

Ahn ST, Monafo WW, Mustoe TA (1991) Topical silicone gel for the prevention and treatment of hypertrophic scar. Arch Surg 126:499–504

McGregor AJ (1971) Calcification in scars of healed acne vulgaris. Oral Surg 32:829–830

Millikan L, Banks K, Purkait B, Chungi V (1991) A 5-year safety and efficacy evaluation with Fibrel in the correction of cutaneous scars following one or two treatments. J Dermatol Surg Oncol 17:223–229

Plewig G (1974) Follicular keratinization. J Invest Dermatol 62:308–315

Quinn KJ (1987) Silicone gel in scar treatment. Burns 13 (Suppl):33–40

Quinn KJ, Evans JH, Courtney JM, Gaylor JDS (1985) Non-pressure treatment of hypertrophic scars. Burns 12:102–105

Varadi DP, Saqueton AC (1970) Perifollicular elastolysis. Br J Dermatol 83:143–150

Watson JB (1959) Monoporous and polyporous acne. Arch Dermatol 80:167–170

Wilson BB, Dent CH, Cooper PH (1990) Papular acne scars. A common cutaneous finding. Arch Dermatol 126:797–800

Acne: Mild in Expression But Still Scarring

All four men portrayed here have relatively mild acne. The disease smolders for years, leaving a variety of shallow or ice pick-like scars.

Above

Left   Slightly depressed scars on cheeks and temples with still smoldering inflammatory papules and pustules are late signs of acne. A dermabrasion could improve this patient's condition

Right   Multiple flat scars from the hairline to the neck have left their mark on this man's face

Below

Left   The boy is 17 years old and seriously attacked by his aggressive acne: many closed comedones which readily rupture, deep-seated papules, and confluent nodules. Some of the ensuing scars are deep and ice pick-like. A course of isotretinoin was prescribed which completely eliminated comedones and inflammatory lesions. Surgical techniques to improve scars are the next step

Right   Burned-out acne with many shallow scars. A variety of surgical techniques including punch elevation grafts and dermabrasion would be helpful

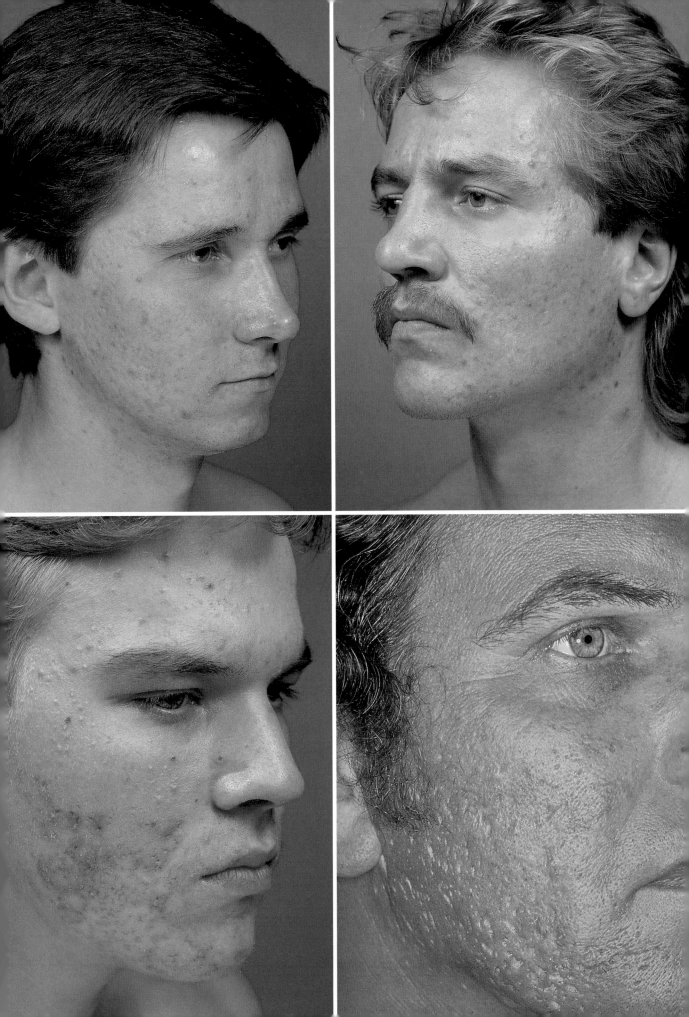

Acne Scars Can Be Improved by One Means or Another

One of the questions most often asked by acne patients is: Can my scars be removed or improved? Various techniques are available, including dermabrasion, punch elevation, punch replacement, and collagen and silicone injections, to name but a few.

Above

Left   The shallow depressions are the most common scars. These are highly amenable to dermabrasion. Ongoing inflammatory lesions are not a contraindication, although we prefer to treat them first

Right   Multiple, small, shallow scars respond well to dermabrasion and chemical peels

Below

Left   Numerous deeper scars call for expert evaluation. Soft tissue augmentation with collagen is an option. Replacement punch biopsies from postauricular skin is another

Right   These deep, canyon-like scars can be compared to ice picks hammered into a glacier, hence the term ice pick scars. The steep sides throw shadows which make the pits more noticeable. Bevelling off the rims by dermabrasion reduces their visibility

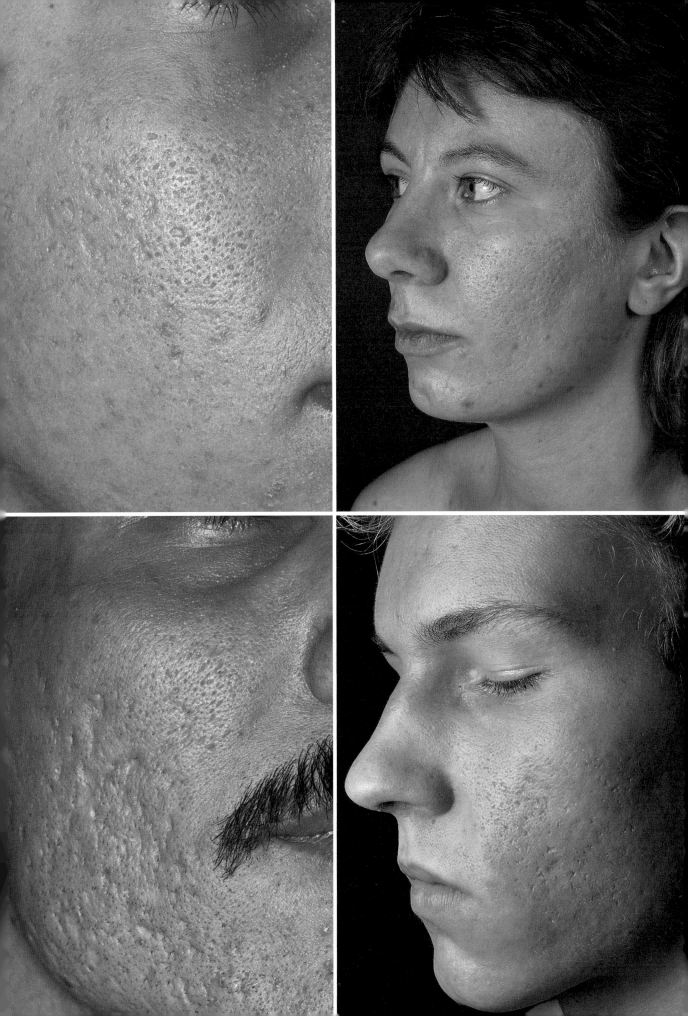

Variety of Scars

A man well in his adulthood has gone through serious attacks of acne more than 30 years ago. It is easily perceived where he fought the disease. The photographic portraits on this page documents more than a legend.

The entire face and neck are scarred, even his nose. The facial pores are wide, and the skin oily, despite the destruction of many sebaceous glands during the active phase of the disease. Ingrown beard hairs pose an additional problem.

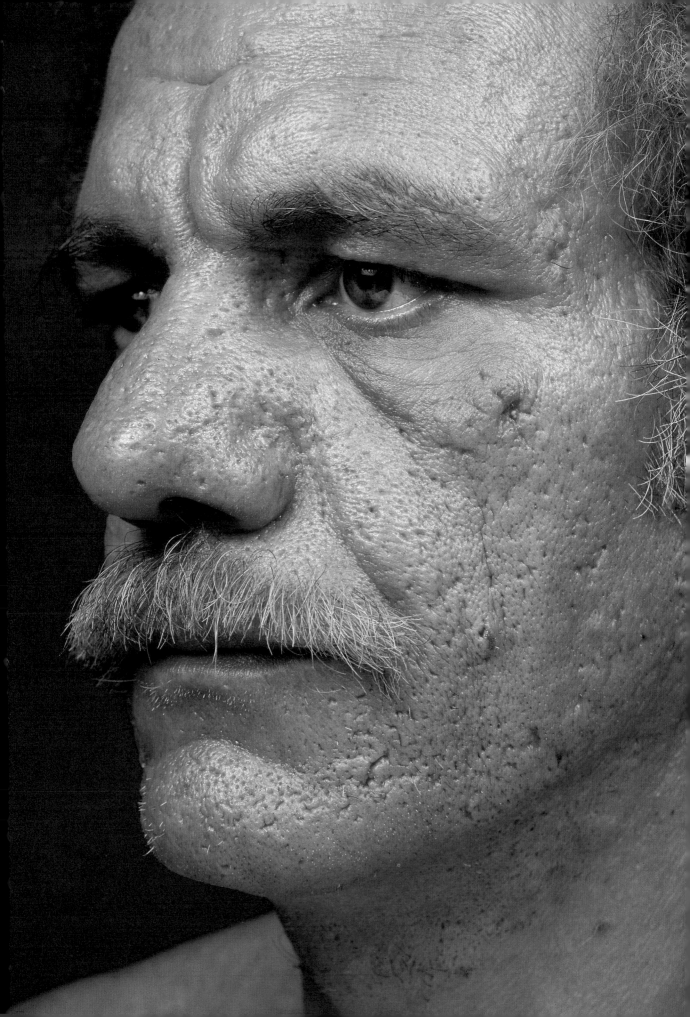

Scars

These biopsies came from scarred facial skin.

Above   Shallow scar. Clinically this is only a slightly depressed scar, which throws no shadows due to its gentle slopes. Beneath the epidermis, however, a remarkable scar is identified. It extends beyond the right and bottom margin of this figure. The collagen is dense and rich in blood vessels, which are surrounded by lymphocytes. The adnexa have been wiped out

Below   A trough-like scar. Clinically this is a cumbersome scar. Its sides are steep, allowing for light-and-shadow phenomena. Histopathologically, however, it is a fairly punched-out limited defect. One sebaceous acinus is connected with its base, as are sprouts of epithelium, possibly remnants of sebaceous acini. The collagen beneath is horizontally arranged with little inflammation

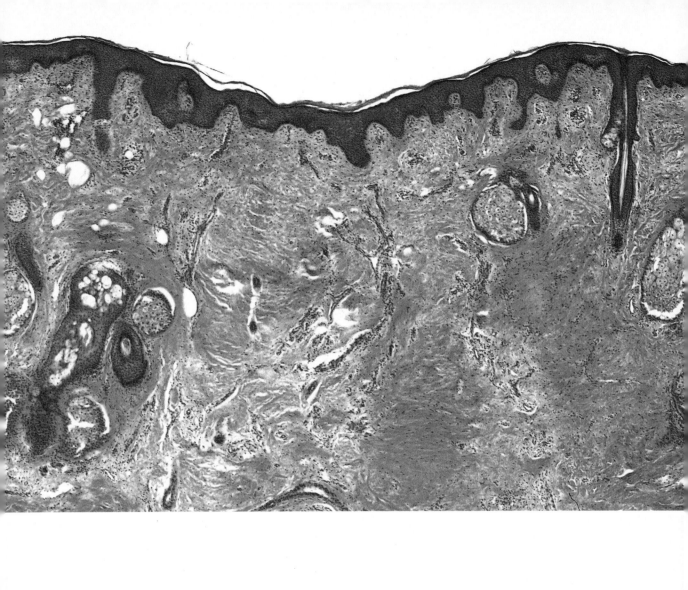
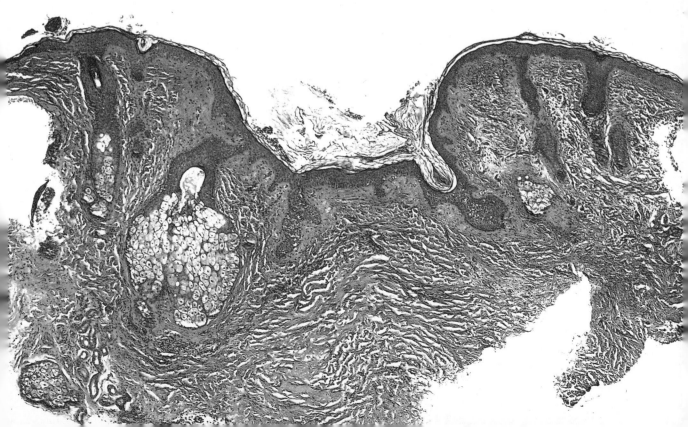

Histopathology of Shallow Scars

Above   Clinically, this was a shallow scar on the cheek of an acne patient. Histologically, the scar is easily identified. Surprising are its depth and the dense chronic inflammation extending beyond the margins of the section

Below   The special stain for elastic tissue reveals that the scar is void of elastic fibers. All adnexa have been destroyed. (Van Kossa stain)

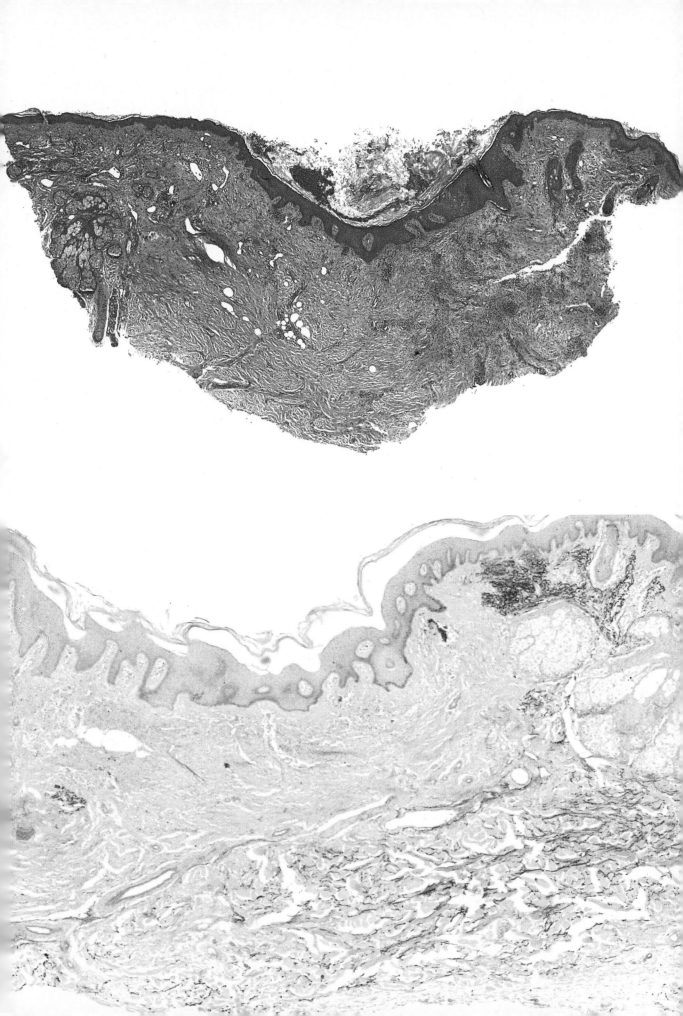

Variegate Expression of Acne in Women

All these women are out of their teens and are disfigured by acne.

Above

Left   Widespread acne scars on cheeks, chin, and forehead following a course of more than 10 years of severe inflammatory acne. She was not a picker; all scars followed papules and nodules. This calls for scar correction

Right   Two types of scars bother this woman. Multiple, fine pit-like scars, which are not so prominent, and two monstrous draining sinuses on her left cheek and mandible. Draining sinuses are the worst of all acne lesions, and almost incurable. The upper one is 8 cm long, broad, has half a dozen openings, and drains periodically. The upper and the lower sinus could eventually merge

Below

Left   Acne conglobata in a very seborrheic woman. On close inspection there are many more acne lesions: closed comedones, papules, pustules, and postinflammatory hyperpigmentation. Vigorous treatment is indicated before she becomes indefinitely scarred

Right   Stubborn acne, predominantly with papules and pustules encroaching on the hairline. Appropriate treatment should ban the further stigmas of this disease

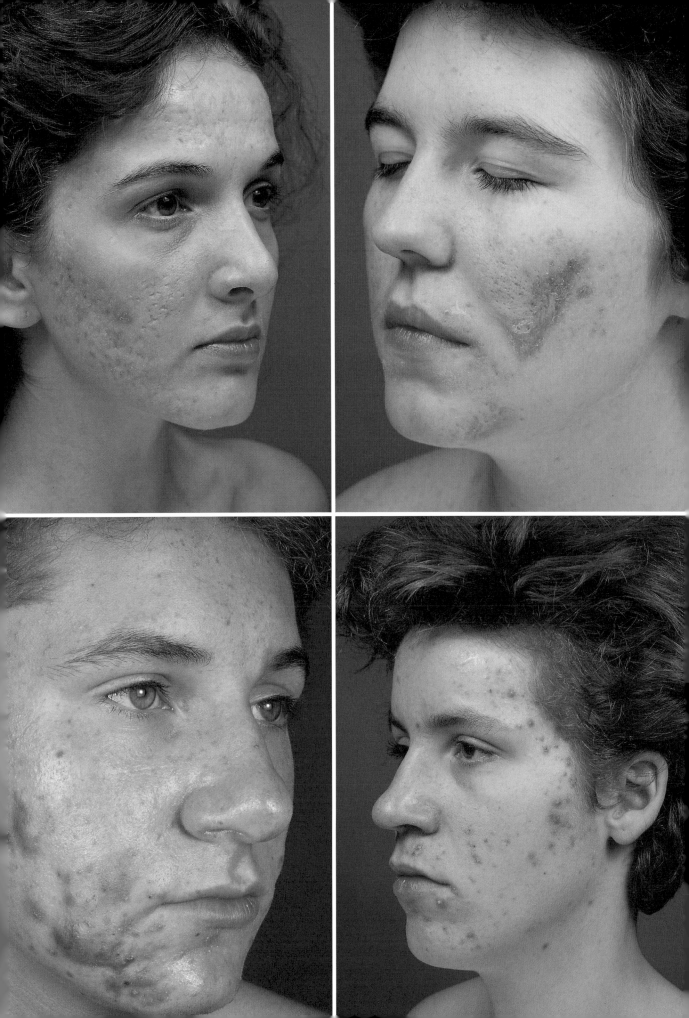

Portrait of Scars

A man well into his adulthood has suffered serious attacks of acne which marked his face. The inflammatory storm has passed. Left over permanently are deep criss-cross and icepick-like scars, even on the nose and neck. The facial pores are wide, and the skin oily, despite the destruction of many sebaceous glands during the active phase of the disease. The man wears a beard to conceal these dreadful marks. Ingrown beard hairs emerge from several scars.

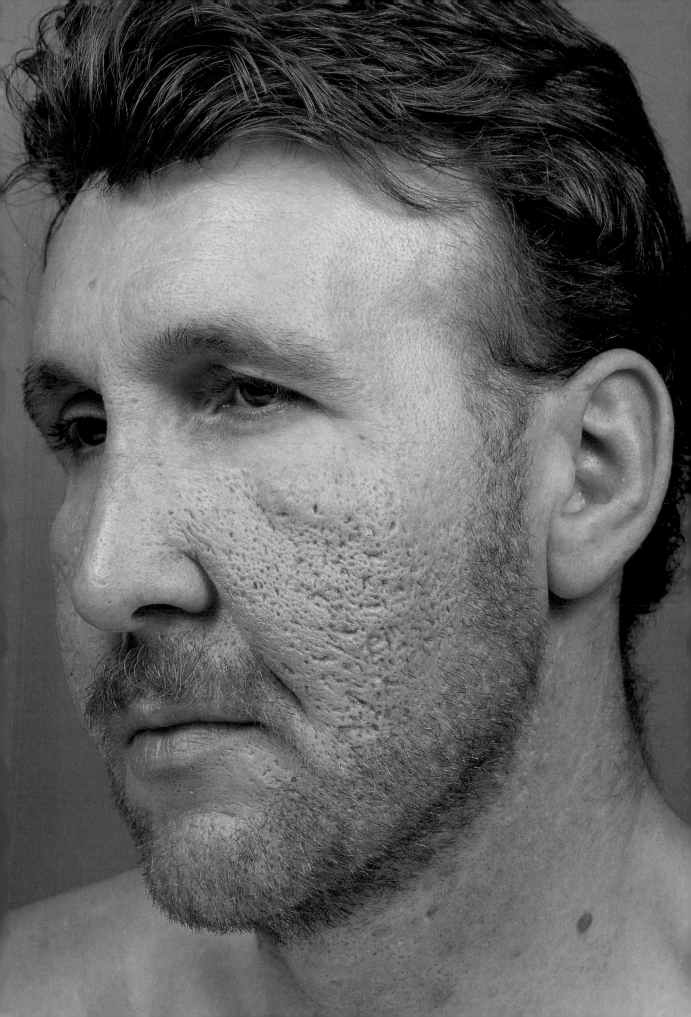

Pustules and Scars

Most pustules and papulopustules in acne patients will leave a scar, histologically and clinically.

Above   A localized papulopustule with trapped remnants of the comedo kernel. The pus will be discharged pretty soon. The lower portion of the comedonal epithelium will stay intact and could leave a scar as depicted below

Below   A pit in the skin with steep sides and loosely arranged corneocytes. This cannot be concealed by camouflage. The histopathology reveals the extent and disaster of such scars. The base of the scar connects with strands of epithelium traversing through the skin. The dermis is scarred with horizontally arranged fine fibrils, many fibroblasts, lymphocytes and histiocytes

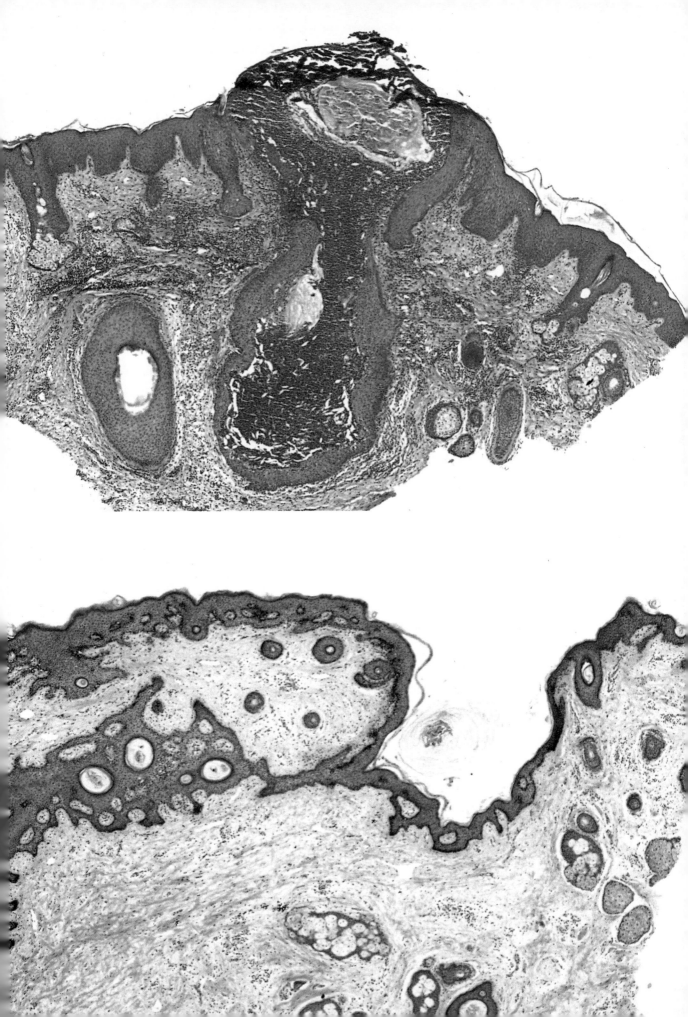

The Spectrum of Scars

Scars are multifaceted permanent records of tissue destruction.

Above   The face of this acne patient bore many crateriform deep scars. The biopsy, though cut somewhat oblique, tells of the dimension and configuration of the scar. Wide segments of the cheek were destroyed. Epithelium with bizarre sprouts has finally closed the defect, leaving an irreparable steep tunneled crater forever, unless it is excised. One lonely sebaceous acinus not associated with a hair unit any more has survived the previous abscess. Scars are always chronically inflamed

Below

Left   An ice pick-like scar from the cheek was surgically removed and cut horizontally. Irregular diverticula with bizarre epithelial projections are embedded in dense fibrotic collagen. This scar is too steep to be improved by dermabrasion. Punch replacement or excision with primary closure would be proper maneuvers

Right   A special form of scar is burned-out fistulated comedones. These scars occur almost esclusively on the back. The epithelium is thin, and no sebaceous glands or hair follicles are left. A comedo-like compacted core of corneocytes with pigmented tips fills this scar. The only meaningful therapeutic measure is to dissect the small epithelial bridge above, thus liberating the horny kernel

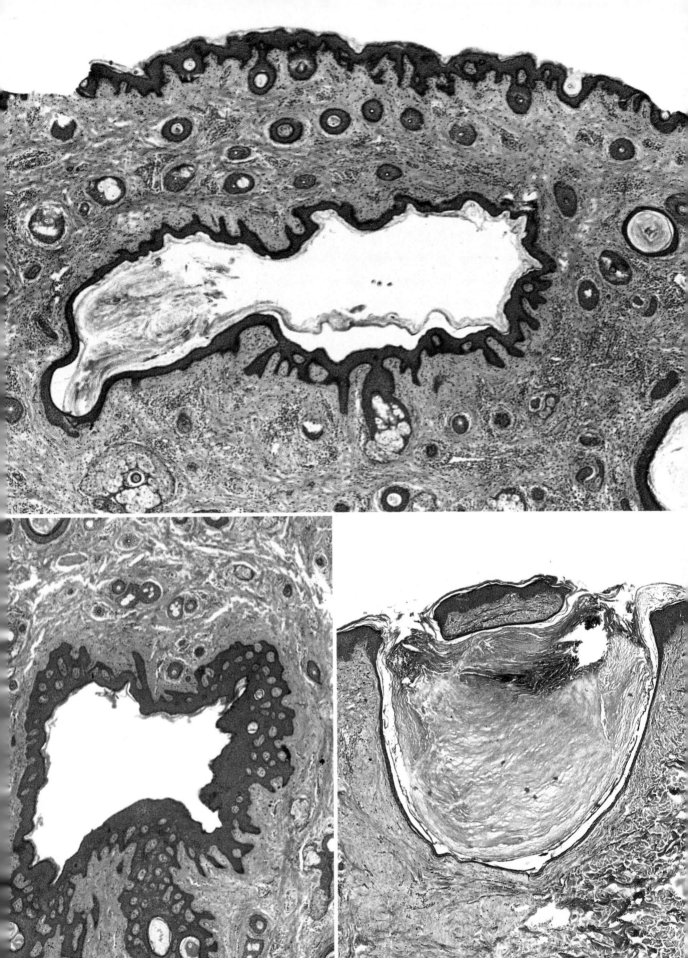

Atrophic Scars

Above   Huge irregular scars are eloquent evidence of the tendency of acne conglo-bata to engulf large areas of skin. Through fusion of lesions, only islands of normal skin remain. Most of the scarring on the back of this 16-year-old boy is of the flat, cigarette paper-like, atrophic kind. The destruction has not come to an end yet, as there are still hemorrhagic crusts covering necrotic tissue (far left)

Below   The normal tissue is to the left of the arrows (⟶). The scar has an atrophic epidermis with loss of rete ridges. The skin appendages have been destroyed. Numerous ectatic vessels, a chronic lymphohistiocytic infiltrate, a few multi-nucleated giant cells, fibroplasia and interstitial edema characterize the scar

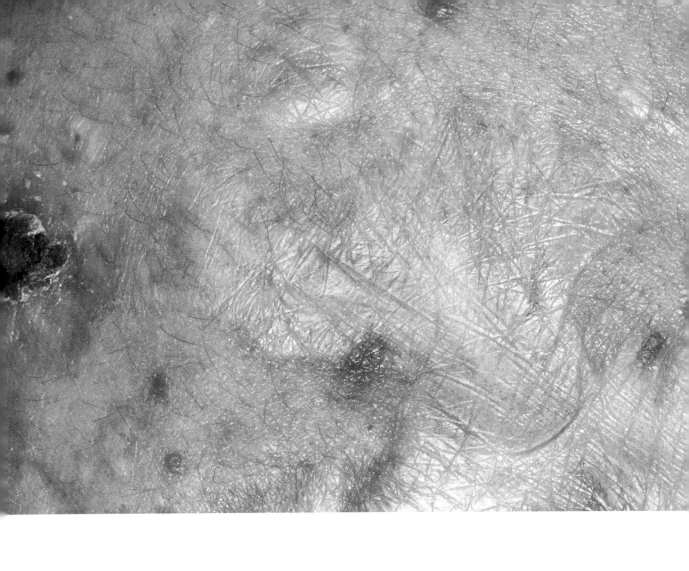
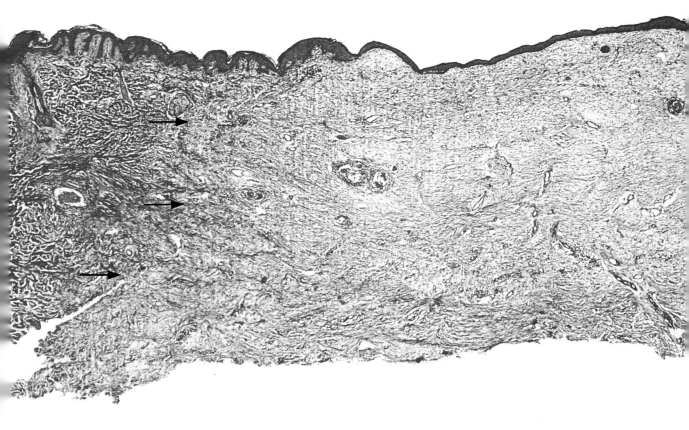

The Hypertrophic Fibrotic Nodule or Plaque

Above   This irregular, massive, hard, lumpy growth is a sequela of inflammatory nodules in acne conglobata. Fibrotic nodules are commonest on the back, shoulders, or upper arms. With time they slowly flatten. The process can be accelerated by injecting corticosteroids intralesionally

Below   This is a low-power view of a fibrotic nodule. Collagen bundles are in disarray and of variable size. Numerous characteristic thin-walled, dilated vessels are evident. The skin appendages have all been destroyed. The scar extends further down than shown by this photograph

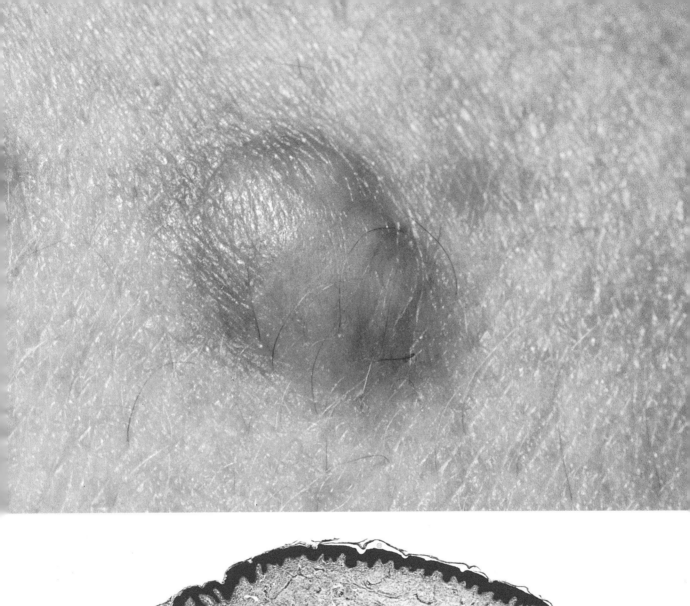
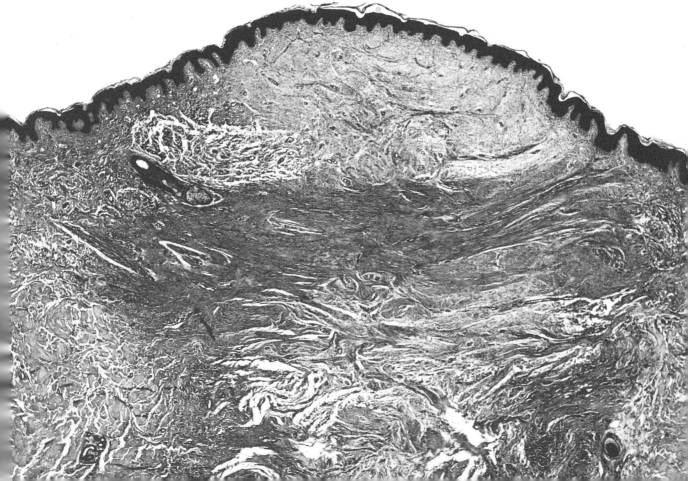

The chest (*above*) and upper back (*below*) of this man with long-standing, severe acne are covered with hundreds of small, white, dome-shaped papules, associated with inflammatory acne lesions. They are all scars and commonly mistaken for closed comedones. One can also call these closed comedo-like scars. They almost never occur on the face. While these scars may flatten a little after many years, no effective treatment is available. The scars are sequelae of prior inflammatory lesions. This man also displays larger hypertrophic scars scattered among inflammatory lesions.

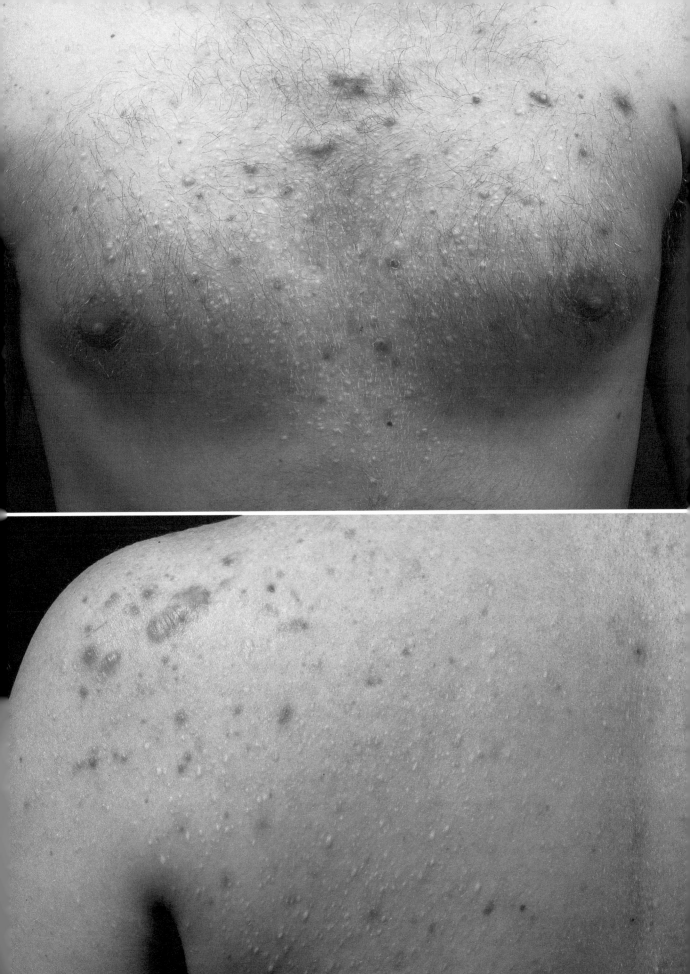

The Scope of Scars

A fantastic variety of scars occur in the wake of inflammatory acne. Besides comedones, scars are the hallmark of the disease.

Above Multiple criss-cross, pitted, and crateriform scars distort the face of this unfortunate man. The neck is similarly afflicted. Another late sequela of acne is the huge horn-filled cyst on the left side of the neck

Below Often these noninflammatory whitish, dome-shaped elevations, strictly follicular in distribution, are mistaken as closed comedones. In fact they are small hard hypertrophic scars. The decisive finding is the failure to express horny material when the lesion is punctured or squeezed with a comedo extractor. Why they form in some people is a mystery. These comedo-like scars are more frequent on the back than on the chest and rarely occur in the face. Note that inflammatory lesions are also present

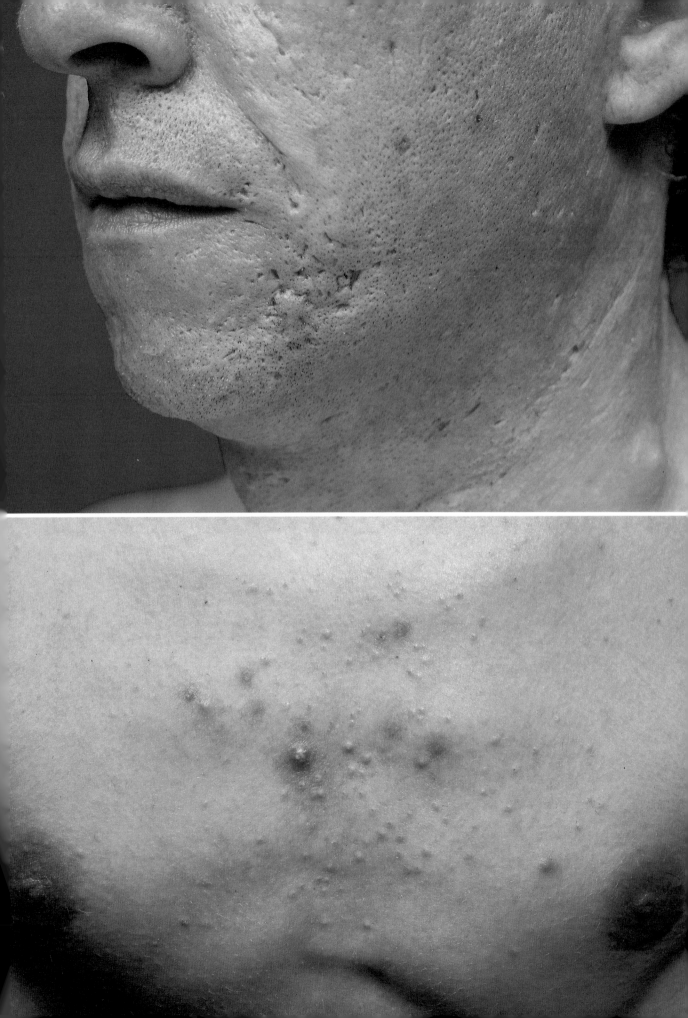

Perifollicular Papular Scars
(Closed Comedo-like Scars)

These small, elevated, hard growths prevail on the skin of back and chest. In contrast, atrophic, depressed scars are more likely to be found on the face. For better visualization of the lesions, one should compress the skin between two fingers.

Above

Left   These round, white, elevated lesions are often mistaken for closed comedones. In most of them a centrally or excentrically located fine hair reveals the follicular origin

Right   The photograph reveals that a pilary unit is in the center, though tortured from previous inflammation, hence the name perifollicular papular scar. The scar extends far beyond the right, left, and lower margins of this picture with twisted collagen bundles, ectatic blood vessels, and a chronic lymphohistiocytic infiltrate

Below   The comedo-like scar is larger than it appears clinically. Its true extent can be determined by staining for elastic fibers. The latter are generally destroyed and do not regenerate. The original elastic fibers are found only beyond the boundaries of the scar (→). The collagen bundles are rather coarse, densely packed, and eosinophilic. There are many dilated vessels of variable size in a disorderly arrangement typical for scars. The appendages have been destroyed

Wilson BB, Dent CH, Cooper PH (1990) Papular acne scars. A common cutaneous finding. Arch Dermatol 126:797–800

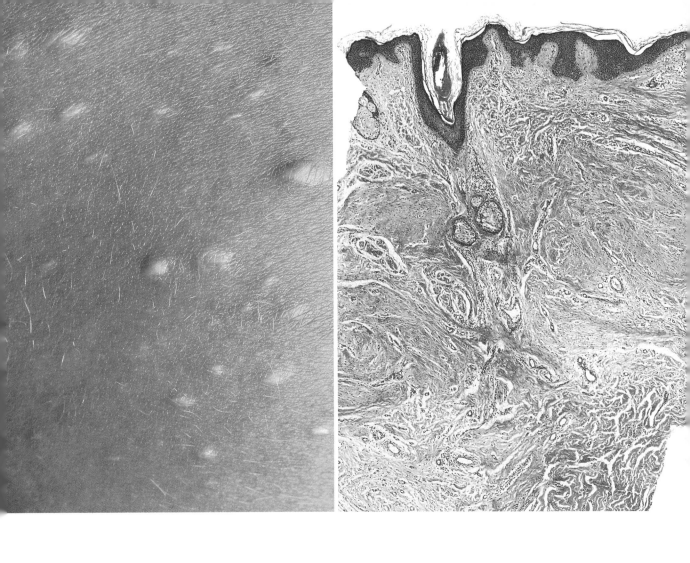

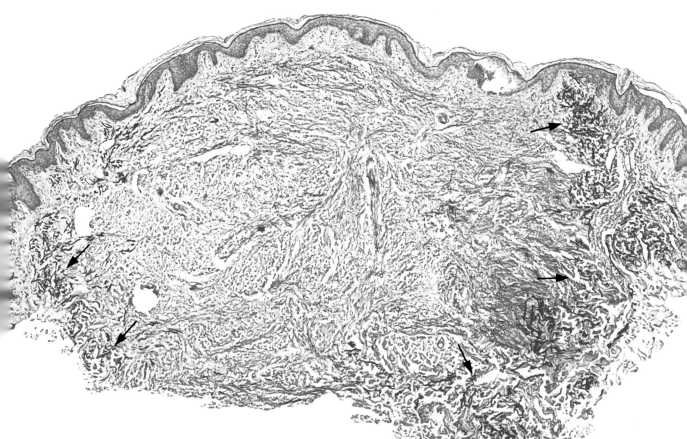

Keloidal Scars Versus Keloids

The spectrum of acne scars includes unusual forms. In Blacks, true keloids may occur; they are fortunately uncommon and virtually never develop in the face. In Caucasians inflammatory lesions may be followed by thick, elevated, lobulated, fibrotic plaques which resemble true keloids. They are, however, hypertrophic scars and are less likely to recur when excised. Laser treatment also seems to work in some patients. Sites of predilection are the V-shaped area of chest and back, particularly over the sternum, the breasts, the lateral aspects of the upper arms, and the shoulders.

Above   In this 18-year-old girl, the keloidal scars and keloids are limited to the areas of previous acne: chest, upper arms, and shoulders

Below

Left   Scattered keloidal scars on the upper back and upper arm in a young woman with previous acne

Right   High-power view from the back of a man with previous acne conglobata. Keloidal scars do not appear spontaneously. All scars arise from acne lesions. Repeated rupture and inflammation caused excessive fibrillogenesis by fibroblasts

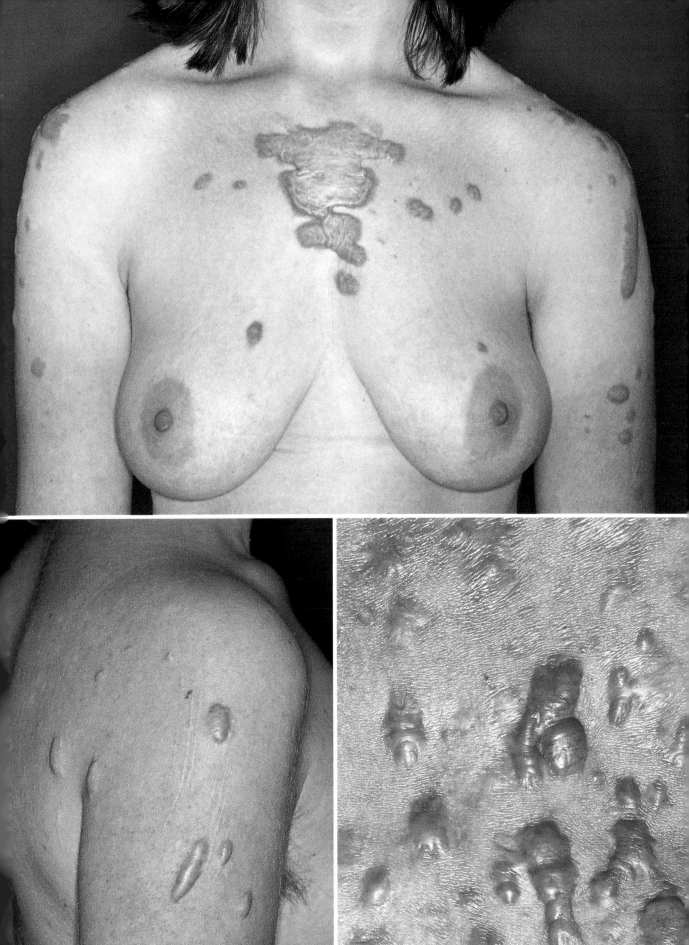

Keloids: The Worst Type of Scar

Keloids are expanding growths of fibrous connective tissue usually secondary to trauma. In this unusual case inflammatory acne lesions stimulated uncontrolled fibroplasia. The man has had acne conglobata. Thick, raised, red, itchy, and painful growths stud this man's back, chest, and shoulders.

Above   Discrete keloidal scars on the chest which could be mistaken for hypertrophic scars

Below   Confluent, huge expanding fibrous plaques on the back establish the unequivocal diagnosis of keloids. Keloids are extremely difficult to treat, unlike hypertrophic scars, and tend not to flatten with time

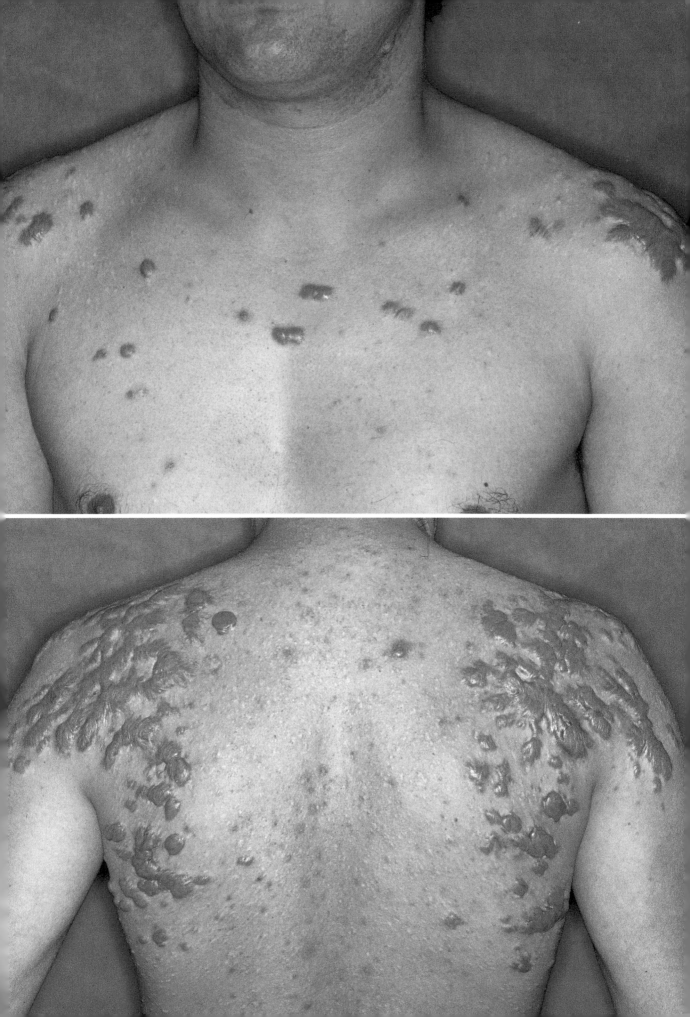

Widespread Scars

Above   The skin of the chest, neck, and upper back is a mess. The V-shaped area of the chest bears multiple, shallow, through-like scars, closed comedo-like scars, and a few papules

Below   The rear side, on closer inspection, is a mess. Open comedones, fistulated comedones retaining heavily pigmented corneocyte impactions, and scattered papules are a burden

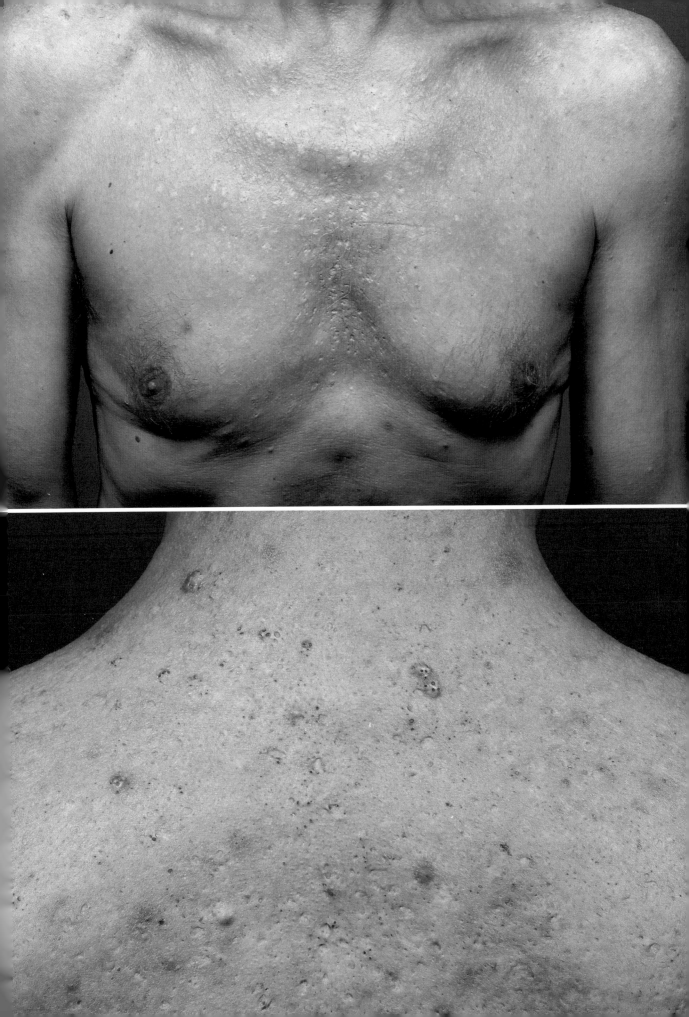

Fistulated Comedones

Fistulated comedones, also called polyporous comedones, have two or more openings. Sometimes there are twenty outlets. The whole structure may be compared to a rabbit hole. Fistulated comedones are actually scars.

Above Much of the skin of the back of this adult man has been mutilated by innumerable inflammatory episodes in the past. The inflammatory battle is over. What is left are hundreds of thick, dark comedonal structures full of dense horn. The black comedo-like impactions are dry, solid masses of corneocytes. These are interconnected complexes with two to more than a dozen openings. The pigment is melanin. The only effective treatment is the dissection of the overlying epithelial bridges, setting free the keratinized debris

Below The way polyporous comedones originate is illustrated here. Two sebaceous follicles have fused via an inflammatory process, leaving a joint horn-filled cavity below with two chimneys above. There is a diffuse inflammatory process with fibrosis surrounding the comedo. The sebaceous acini have been destroyed or are reduced to small undifferentiated epithelial buds, shown at the base. For comparison, there is an intact sebaceous follicle on the left

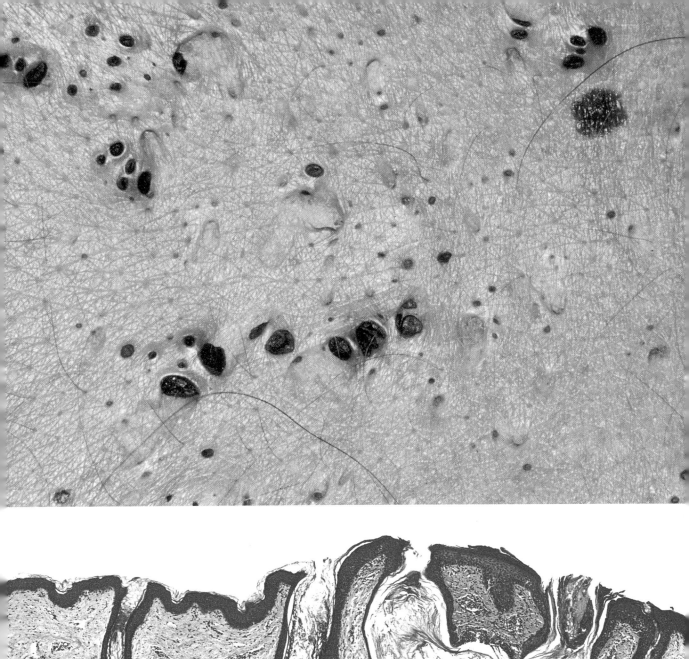
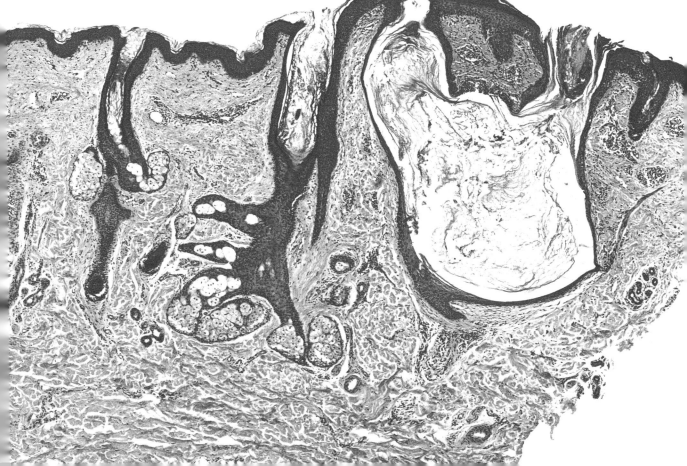

The Draining Sinus Should Not Be Incised

Draining sinuses are too often misdiagnosed, resulting in inappropriate surgical intervention. While draining sinuses and nodules inevitably leave a scar, incisions produce far worse scarring. Intralesional injection of triamcinolone acetonide is the preferred local approach, sometimes combined with orally given isotretinoin.

Above   Bilateral draining sinuses in a 14-year-old girl, an unusual presentation to say the least. Acne lesions on her forehead provided the diagnostic clue. Within the next 4 years she developed severe inflammatory acne on the face and back

Below   Examples of baleful effects of incision and drainage

Left   The draining sinus in a young girl received an incision 2 cm long. The lesion not only refilled but left an ugly scar

Right   Deep incisions (*above*) of a large draining sinus on the cheek of a 16-year-old girl. Unfortunately an unsightly scar (*below*) remained

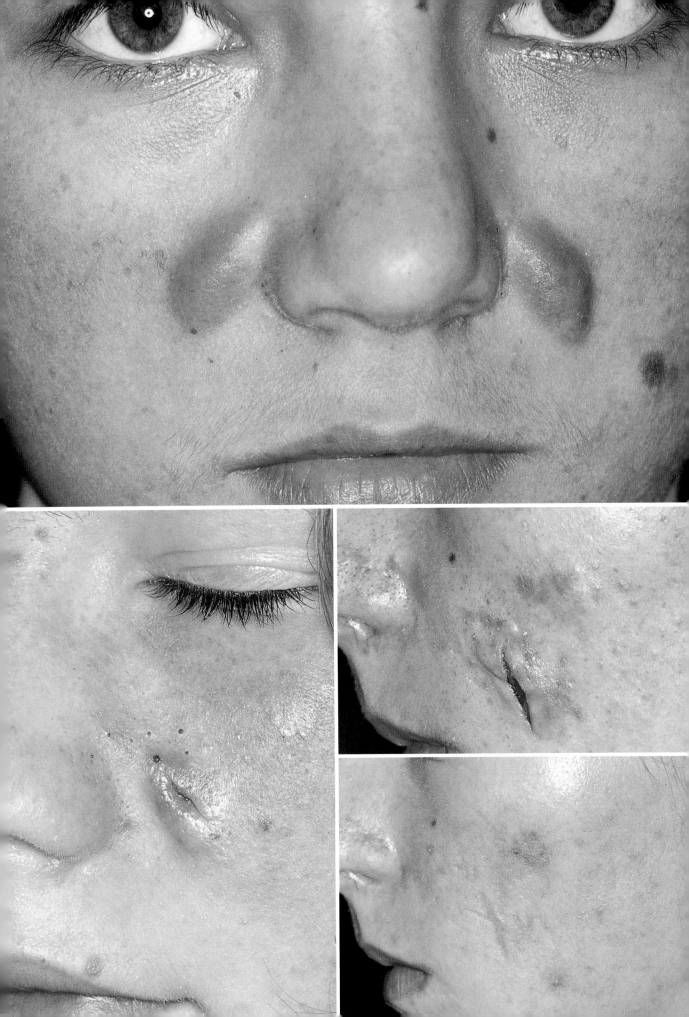

The Misery of Draining Sinuses

Above

Left   The boy not only suffers from acne conglobata but also from draining
          sinuses on the bridge of the nose, the right nasolabial fold, and the chin

Right   A bulging abscess, linear in configuration, is a draining sinus

Below   Acne conglobata has left variable scars on the cheek of this patient. The
          linear scar is a draining sinus, producing discharge from multiple openings
          and re-erupting occasionally like a vulcano

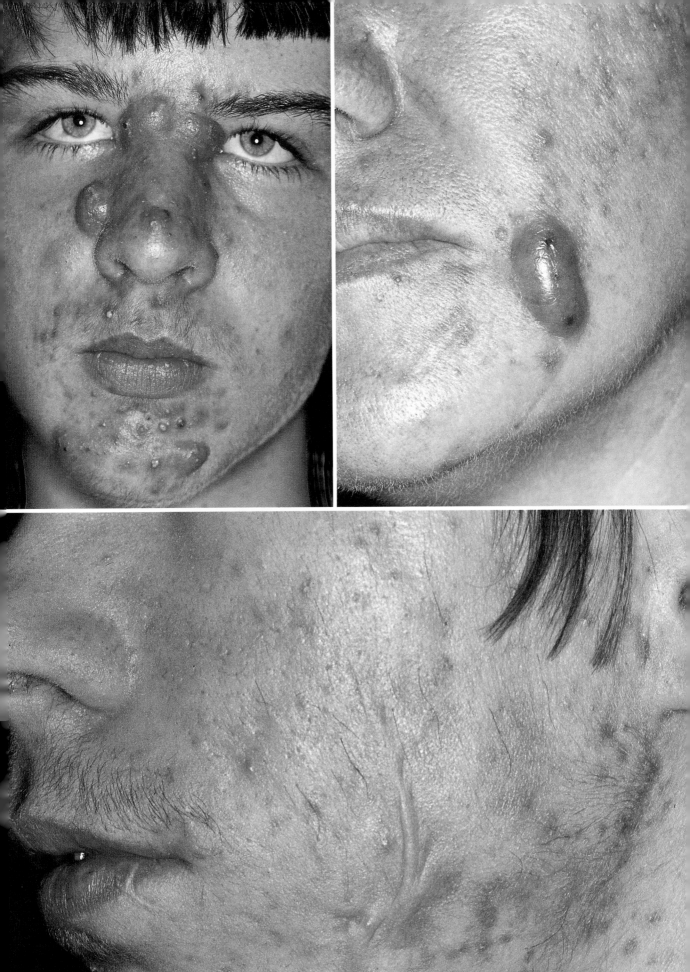

The Draining Sinus

One of the most relentless and horrifying lesions of acne, typical for the face and refractory to most treatments, is the draining sinus. These leave ugly scars and polyporous comedones. Two siblings afflicted with the same lesions are shown here. Draining sinuses are often, but not always, associated with acne conglobata. Both siblings showed acne conglobata on the trunk.

Above

Left   For 6 months a monstrous draining sinus on the cheek of this 17-year-old girl (*a*) was constantly refilling and draining from several openings. Oral tetracyclines had no effect

Right   A vigorous therapeutic attack was designed. This included aspiration (*b*) of about 5 ml of hemorrhagic fluid (*c*) and a pressure bandage for several days. The beneficial result was evident 5 days later (*d*). Oral isotretinoin brought the disease into remission

Below

Left   This huge hemorrhagic lesion appeared on the left cheek of the above patient's 19-year-old brother (*e*). He was also successfully treated with aspiration, compression bandages, and oral isotretinoin. When he was only 13 years old (*f*) he already had two draining sinuses on his right cheek, a portent of troubles to come

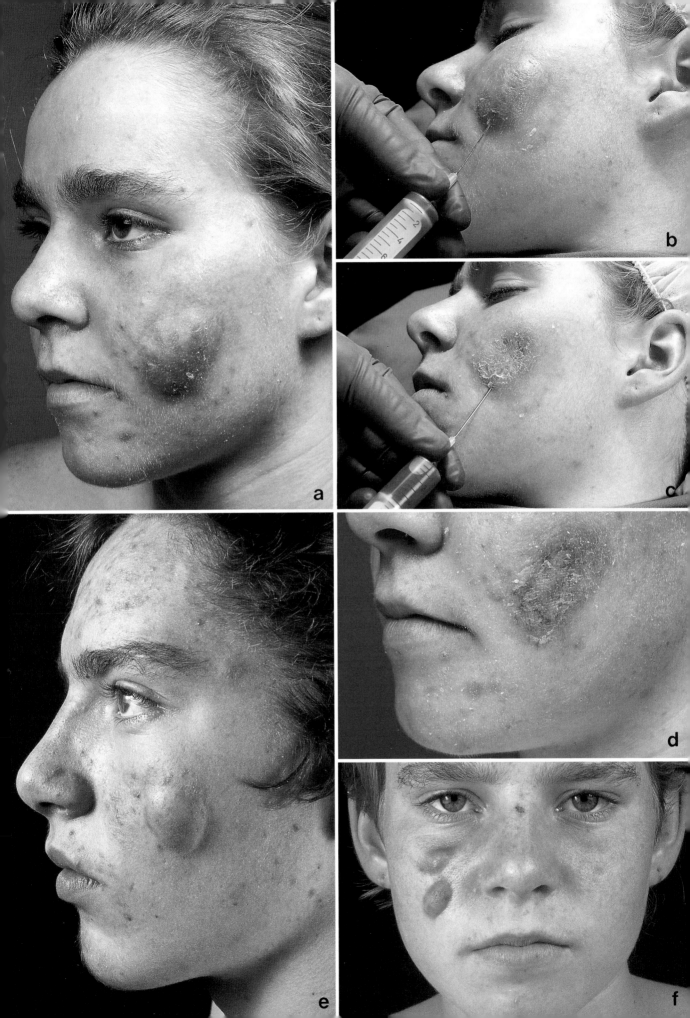

Experimental Reproduction of Sinus Tracts and Fistulated Comedones

The surgical thread placed into the skin provides a model to study the generation of sinus tracts and interconnecting comedones.

Above   Sinus tract. The surgical thread left in place for several days has led to the formation of a horizontal tract, completely epithelialized. Many neighboring follicles are interconnected with remnants of sebaceous acini still present. The tract is filled with inflammatory debris and communicates with the skin surface through multiple follicles, as was shown by serial cuts

Below   Double comedo. Two sections of the thread are in this section. The foreign material has linked up two closed comedones and one sebaceous follicle. Spontaneous rupture, inflammation, and wound healing similarly lead to hooked-up comedones and follicles

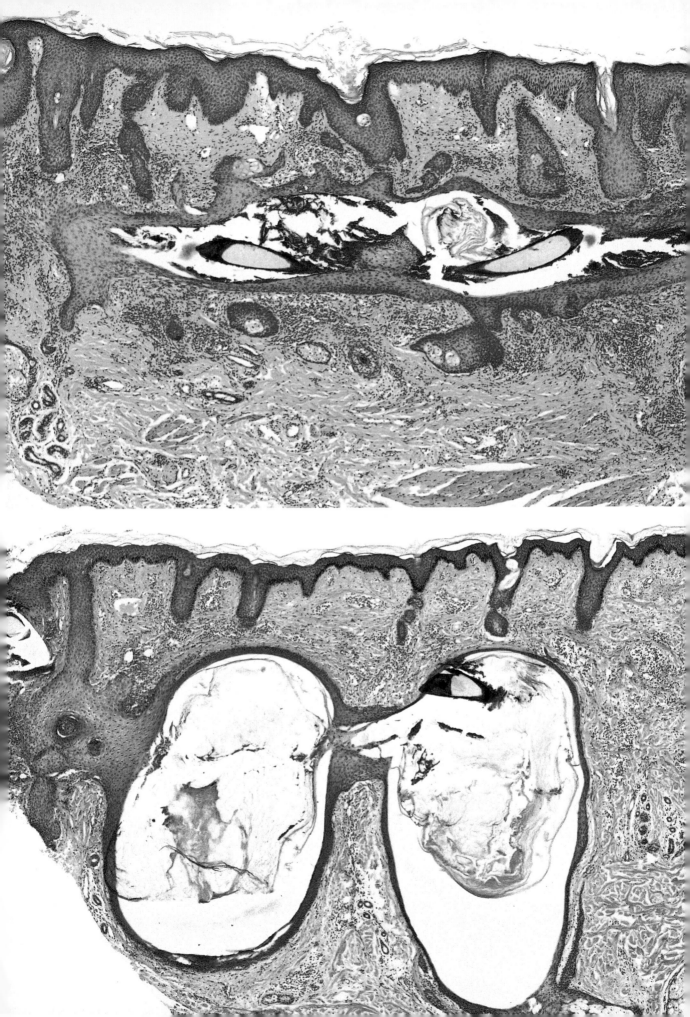

Cinematographic View of Fistulated Scars

Serial sections of scars disclose bizarre patterns not expected clinically. Often scars, like this one from the chin, have surprising extensions. Epithelial-lined, sinus-like tracts traverse the skin. The epithelium is bizarre, pouching out into various directions. Fistulated scars connect multiple follicles. This scar originated from a draining sinus. Most of the inflammation has cooled off, leaving a dense scar deep in the dermis with horizontally arranged collagen bundles and a chronic perivascular inflammation. Stiff beard hairs pinch through the scar, making clean shaving a problem. Acne is still present with comedones as seen in the *bottom* section.

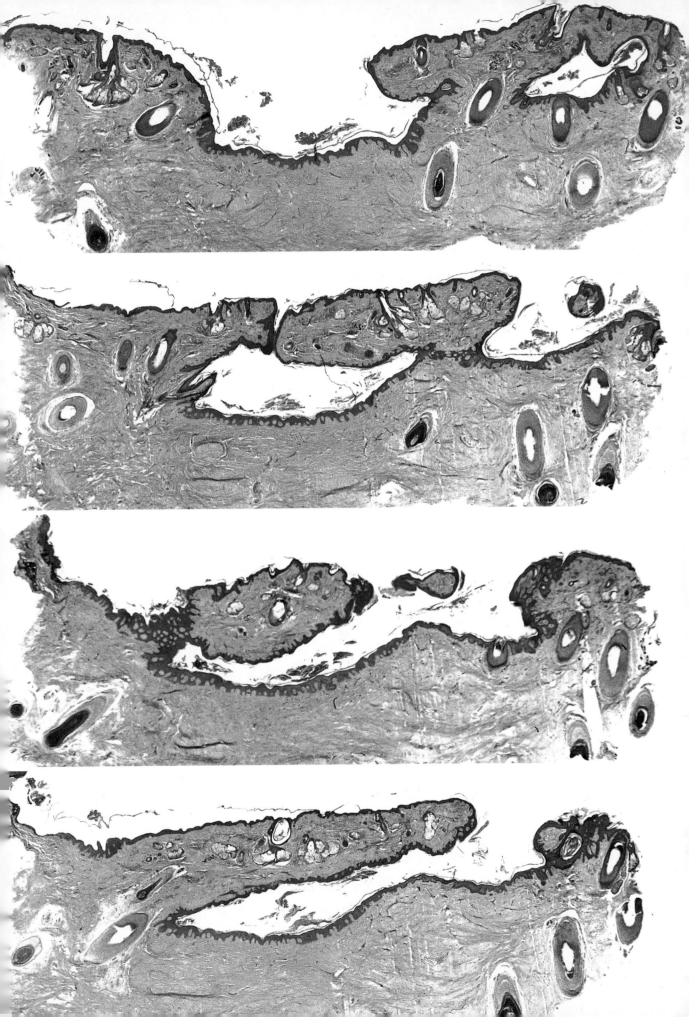

Classification of Acne

Nosology does not rank high among the interests of acne researchers. Yet, the lack of a common international standard for classifying and grading the severity of acne has been a distressing source of confusion and controversy. The result is that epidemiologic data and classifications from different sources cannot be compared because the criteria are different. This adversely affects every field of investigation, for example, surveys concerning the prevalence of acne in different countries. At present we have no information as to whether acne is more prevalent in meat eaters than in vegetarians, in cold or warm climates, in different ethnic groups, etc. What dermatologists may classify as severe acne in Japan might be considered mild by American dermatologists.

Consequences regarding the efficacy of antiacne remedies are egregious. Widely divergent views are held concerning the efficacy of the same drug. Perhaps worse than differences among observers is the problem of inconsistencies by the same observer. In the absence of objective criteria the same physician seeing the same patient at different times is highly susceptible to biased readings.

The extraordinary effectiveness of placebo therapy (vehicle) in many studies doubtlessly stems from the subjective way in which the severity of acne is judged. The most widely used grading systems are quite unsatisfactory, enduring only because of their simplicity. For example, patients are commonly classified as having mild, moderate, or severe acne. This is usually based on the dominant lesions. Comedonal acne, even when the face is densely studded, is generally graded as mild. Papulopustular acne is deemed moderate, while nodules imply severity. But one may ask who is worse off, the patient with hundreds of closed comedones or the patient with three nodules? Therefore we must take into account not only the quality of the lesions but their quantity as well.

We have come to realize that no simple description (mild to severe) or numerical system (grade I to IV) can encompass the appraisal of both quality and quantity. Our empirical approach may be summarized as follows:

The first step is to divide the disease into its three main subtypes with reference to facial acne: *comedonal acne, papulopustular acne*, and *acne conglobata*. The latter is a spectacular disease and can be easily identified. By definition, acne conglobata is never mild. The disease is at the far end of the spectrum of acne and its nosologic position is explicit.

In comedonal acne the lesions are dominantly open and closed comedones. Some inflammatory lesions may be, and frequently are, present, but there are usually no more than five on one side of the face.

The severity of *comedonal acne* is classified as follows, based on the number of lesions on one side of the face:

Grade I	less than 10 comedones
Grade II	10–25 comedones
Grade III	26–50 comedones
Grade IV	more than 50 comedones

The majority of cases falls into grades I and II. In short, comedonal acne is for the most part rather mild. It is chiefly encountered when the disease makes its debut around puberty. What starts as comedonal acne often evolves into more serious disease. Nonetheless, older adolescents sometimes have mainly grade IV comedonal acne. Comedonal acne is usually first apparent on the nose, then on the forehead, descending to the chin over months or even years.

Papulopustular acne is by far the commonest type in midadolescence, or beyond. Actually, it is a mixture of comedones and inflammatory lesions which can be further divided into papules and pustules. Actually, clinical papules are pustules histologically. We routinely combine these under the designation of papulopustules. Assignment to this category is based solely on the prevalence of inflammatory lesions, regardless of the number of comedones:

Grade I	less than 10 papulopustules
Grade II	10–20 papulopustules
Grade III	21–30 papulopustules
Grade IV	more than 30 papulopustules

As a rule the higher grades are associated with fewer comedones. Moreover, there will be more larger, harder, deeper, and persistent papules. In severe inflammatory acne, microcomedones flare up before they mature into clinical comedones, hence the inverse relationship.

Acne conglobata, being so severe, usually does not warrant grading, except for descriptive purposes. It connotes the worst expression of the disease. The importance of proper classification, accompanied by counting lesions, should not be underestimated, especially with regard to therapeutic outcomes. Inflammatory acne is treated differently than the comedonal variety.

Another classification is that by Cunliffe. He uses ten grades. We feel that this is too complex and literally requires training in his clinic. On the other hand, when high resolution, color blow-up photos are available for reference, Cunliffe's system may have merits. Of course, one must always have a complete set of photos which are exactly alike.

The latest classification is based on an international consensus conference. Experts from the USA, Great Britain, and Germany came up with the following consensus (adapted from Report of the Consensus Conference on Acne Classification 1991):

For all practical purposes, acne grading can be best accomplished by the use of a *pattern-diagnosis* system, which includes a global, semiquantitative estimate of lesion density. In severe inflammatory acne, additional descriptions are used, for example, pain, drainage, hemorrhage, ulceration, etc.

The most destructive forms of the disease, e.g., acne conglobata, acne fulminans, and acne inversa, are never mild. These entities are easily recognized and should be designated as very severe.

Acne comprised only of comedones, even when they are present in large numbers or are extensively distributed, can rarely be designated as severe acne.

Inflammatory acne lesions are to be classified as papulopustular and/or nodular. A severity grade based on an approximate lesion count would lead to the designation of mild, moderate, or severe.

This approach is based on the reasonable assumption that global grading in experienced hands is fairly reliable and may facilitate evaluations by eliminating counting, a procedure which is by far more pre-

Severity	Comedones	Papules/pustules	Nodules
Mild	Few to several	Few to several	None
Moderate	Several to many	Several to many	Few to several
Severe	Numerous	Numerous and/or extensive	Many

cise than commonly supposed. The reproducibility of lesion counts is quite poor. Regulating authorities understandably favor counts, no matter how unreliable, for purposes of statistics.

- A strictly quantitative definition of acne severity cannot be established because of the variable expressions of the disease.

- The clinical diagnosis of severe acne should be based on the presence of any of the following characteristics: persistent or recurrent inflammatory nodules, extensive papulopustular disease, ongoing scarring, persistent purulent and/or serosanguineous drainage from lesions, or the presence of sinus tracts.

- Another dimension of severity deserves more attention, namely the psychosocial consequences of the disease. Psychologic disability – depression and anxiety – affects the patient at the workplace and in social and sexual relationships

- Finally, refractory acne which fails to respond adequately to conventional therapies is a class by itself. Such patients should be sent to acne experts who have therapeutic resources not accessible to otherwise welltrained dermatologists, including antiandrogens and anti-inflammatory drugs (corticosteroids, adrenal suppression, hormonal therapy, etc.). There are only few cases of acne that cannot be helped, even if they cannot be completely controlled.

Allen BS, Smith JG Jr (1982) Various parameters for grading acne vulgaris. Arch Dermatol 118:23–25

Cook CH, Centner RL, Michaels SE (1979) An acne grading method using photographic standards. Arch Dermatol 115:571–575

Cunliffe WJ (1989) Acne. Dunitz, London, pp 115–122

Finlay AY (1990) The pathogenesis, disability and management of acne. Indian J Dermatol Venereol Leprol 56:349–353

Motley RJ, Finlay AY (1989) How much disability is caused by acne? Clin Exp Dermatol 14:194–198

Plewig G, Kligman AM (1975) Acne: morphogenesis and treatment. Springer, Berlin Heidelberg New York, pp 162–163

Report of the Consensus Conference on Acne Classification (1991) J Am Acad Dermatol 24:495–500

Samuelson JS (1985) An accurate photographic method for grading acne: initial use in a double-blind clinical comparison of minocycline and tetracycline. J Am Acad Dermatol 12:461–467

Problems of Classification.
Is This Mild or Severe Acne?

This boy has many closed and some open comedones. Many would call this mild (grade I) acne because there are only a few scar-forming inflammatory lesions. However, grading of acne requires evaluation of the quantity as well as the quality of the lesions. When hundreds of closed comedones are present, as in this case, the affliction falls into the serious category (grade IV) and deserves intensive therapy. Closed comedones are often more easily felt than seen. Patients know this very well since they minutely examine every corner of the face. The skin of this boy is worse than it looks to the casual observer.

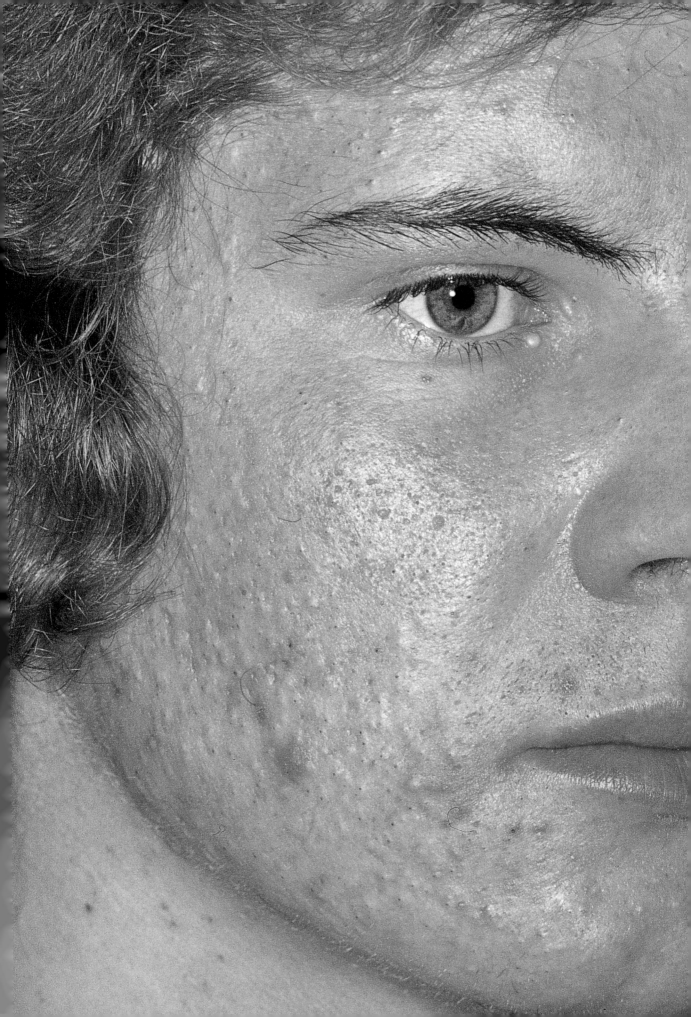

ANIMAL MODELS

Acne does not occur spontaneously in any animal species. Acne is uniquely a human disorder. Still, certain species possess sebaceous-like follicles and are therefore suitable to assess the comedogenicity of chemicals, the comedolytic effects of drugs, and androgen metabolism of sebocytes. We recognize the limitations; yet these models have proved to be valuable both in research and pharmacologic testing.

Syrian Hamster Model

Sebaceous Gland Assays

Sebaceous glands in humans and animals are androgen-sensitive structures. Sebocyte activity depends on androgen stimulation. Without androgens there would be no acne. History informs us of the blemish-free skin of eunuchs. The "miracle" drug isotretinoin nearly completely shuts down sebum production, though not through the classical antiandrogen pathway.

The search for antiandrogens to treat acne systemically or topically has been going on for more than 25 years.

Androgen-sensitive tissues include the prostate gland, testes, and seminal vesicles. It is now appreciated that the Golden Syrian Hamster has two androgen-dependent sebaceous gland regions which are very well suited to hormonal experiments. The presently available antiandrogens cyproterone acetate, megestrol acetate, and spironolactone were effectively screened in this system. It has been a frustration that only orally administered antiandrogens are effective in humans.

Flank Organ

The costovertebral flank organ is a paired nipple-like swelling, 3–5 mm in diameter, containing an aggregation of huge sebaceous glands. Three structures of this organ are androgen dependent: the sebocytes, the pigmented coarse hairs, and dermal melanocytes. Castration of male animals causes shrinkage of the sebaceous glands, regression of hairs, and loss of dermal pigment. Androgens stimulate each of the three components in females. Testosterone, after enzymatic conversion to dihydrotestosterone (DHT), binds to androgen receptors. This DHT–androgen receptor complex then binds to DNA. Thereafter protein synthesis via mRNA is stimulated, as is lipid synthesis. The cDNA for androgen-regulated mRNA in the flank organs has been characterized. Antiandrogenic effects can be assayed by a variety of morphological and biochemical methods. One can measure diameters, weight, histologic cross-sectional areas, as well as use radiolabeling techniques to gain insight into cellular kinetics (labeling index, turnover time, transit time), and protein content. All classical antiandrogens work in this system.

Ears

The dorsal and ventral sides of the pinna are studded with many large sebaceous glands, in shape and organization not unlike sebaceous follicles in humans. They have two to three large sebaceous lobules, draining into a common sebaceous duct and follicular infundibulum, with one small vellus hair unit attached. The follicular canal can retain corneocytes and thus build up comedo-like impactions. Access is via the ventral side.

Dozens of sebaceous follicles are available for histologic, morphometric, autoradiographic, and biochemical analyses. As there is no adipose tissue, the ear lobe has a great advantage over the flank organ.

Bacteria do not colonize these follicles. *Propionibacterium acnes* cannot be implanted. Therefore, bacteria-related phenomena of comedogenesis and inflammatory stages of papulopustules cannot be studied in these animal systems.

Hisaoka H, Ideta R, Seki T, Adachi K (1991) Androgen regulation of a specific gene in hamster flank organs. Arch Dermatol Res 283:269–273

Lucky AW, McGuire J, Nydorf E, Halpert G, Nuck BA (1986) Hair follicle response of the Golden Syrian hamster flank organ to continuous testosterone stimulation using silastic capsules. J Invest Dermatol 86:83–86

Luderschmidt C, Plewig G (1977) Effects of cyto-proterone acetate and carboxylic acid derivatives on the sebaceous glands of the Syrian hamster. Arch Dermatol Res 258:185–191

Luderschmidt C, Bidlingmaier F, Plewig G (1982) Inhibition of sebaceous gland activity by spironolactone in Syrian hamster. J Invest Dermatol 78:253–255

Plewig G, Luderschmidt C (1977) Hamster ear model for sebaceous glands. J Invest Dermatol 68:171–176

Seki T, Ideta R, Shibuya M, Adachi K (1991) Isolation and characterization of cDNA for an androgen-regulated mRNA in the flank organ of hamsters. J Invest Dermatol 96:926–931

Takayasu S, Adachi K (1970) Hormonal control of metabolism in hamster costovertebral glands. J Invest Dermatol 55:13–19

Vermorken AJM, Goos CMAA, Wirtz P (1982) Evaluation of the hamster flank organ test for the screening of anti-androgens. Br J Dermatol 106:99–101

Syrian Hamster Model

This animal species provides the special structures to study hormonal mechanisms.

Above   The flank organ. The overview depicts the entire flank organ, an accumulation of large sebaceous acini, follicular canals, and coarse, pigmented hairs. The flank organ is supported by adipose tissue, below which is a layer of costovertebral musculature.
The flank organ is androgen dependent. Antiandrogens make it shrink to an undifferentiated cell bud; testosterone stimulation in castrated male animals inflate it to the size shown here

Below   Sebaceous follicle of the ear lobe. The ear lobe is studded with hundreds of sebaceous follicles, particularly the ventral side of the pinna. There is close resemblance to sebaceous follicles in the human, with a short infundibular canal, sebaceous ducts, sebaceous acini, and one pilary unit. Bacteria are notably absent in this animal. Like the flank organ these sebaceous acini follow the rules of androgen stimulation and antiandrogen inhibition

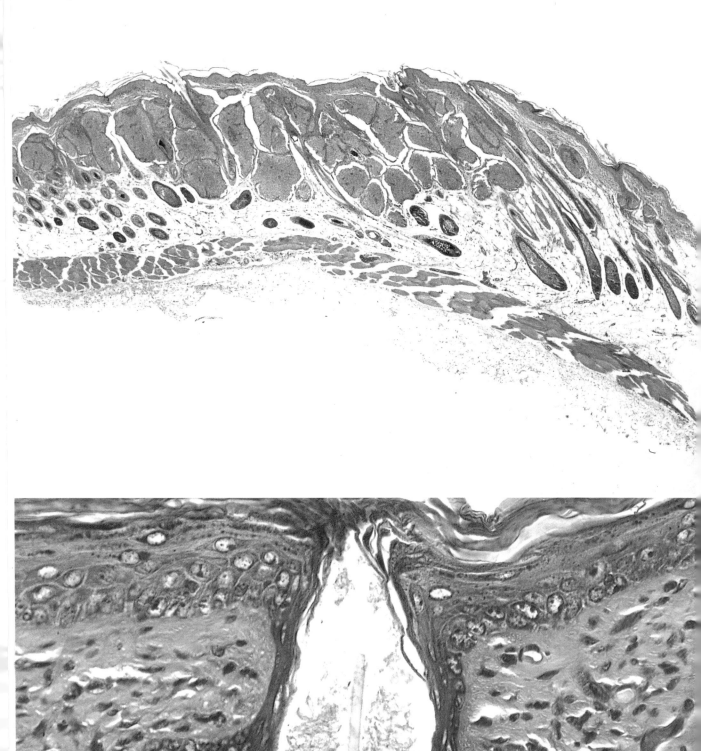

The Rabbit Ear Comedogenicity Assay

The ventral surface just outside the ear canal contains large, numerous follicles with multilobular sebaceous glands. The architecture resembles human sebaceous follicles somewhat. Substances which induce comedones in the rabbit ear are also comedogenic in humans.

Above

Left Horizontal section of a normal follicle with a pilary unit in the center from which sebaceous acini radiate in all directions

Right A whole mount, stained with oil-red-0 to show the distribution of the multilobulated sebaceous glands of six closely spaced follicles

Below Horizontal view of a 4 + comedogenic reaction to coal tar. The follicles are distended by masses of dense coherent corneocytes. Bacteria are notably absent in this model. The coal tar model can be effectively used to assay comedolytic agents

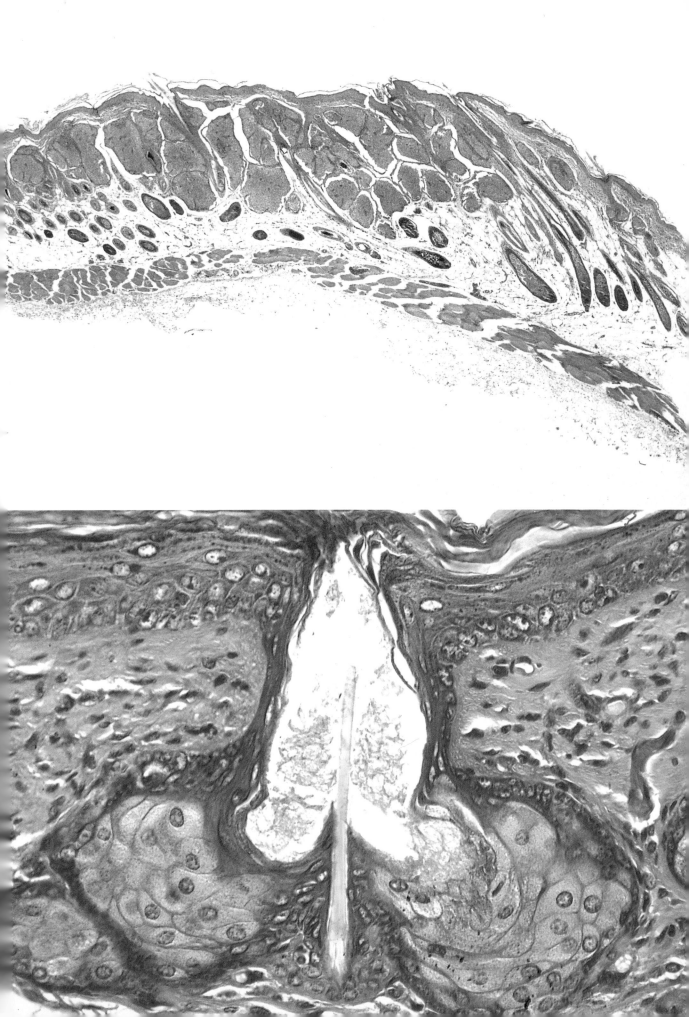

Rabbit Ear Model

The term comedogenic refers to the ability of substances to induce horny impactions, that is, comedones. The rabbit ear has long served as a model for assaying comedogenic materials. However, we now realize that this assay can provide a good deal more information. One must first distinguish between dense (comedonal) and loose (hyperproliferative) horn. This cannot be judged clinically, only histologically. Some substances are predominantly comedogenic, others are mainly irritating, producing loose horn (scales), and are both comedogenic and irritating. These hybrids are not uncommon and are certainly more troublesome. Those may all look alike on the surface, but are vastly different histologically. Because of this we have abandoned gross inspection.

We have elected to use the broader term *acneigenic* instead of *comedogenic*. This encompasses inflammatory responses of which the most relevant is folliculitis, actually histologic pustules. It turns out that some chemicals in cosmetics, toiletries and even drugs mainly provoke inflammatory reactions expressed as pustules and papulopustules, a form of chemical folliculitis with little or no inflammatory components.

Historical Note

The rabbit ear model for assessing the comedogenic potential of topically applied substances is almost half a century old. Adams and co-workers, stimulated by a severe outbreak of occupational acne among workers handling chlorinated chemicals, identified the offending substances. Application to the external ear canal of rabbits induced follicular horny impactions (comedones). Subsequently, Hambrick and Blank applied chlorinated aromatic hydrocarbons to the ear canal and not only demonstrated the formation of comedones in less than one week, but also delineated high-potency comedogenic compounds from medium- or low-strength ones. This model is very sensitive and no credible alternative has been found so far. We have recently standardized the procedure and provided guidelines for interpreting the histologic change. Responsible manufacturers routinely assay their products for comedogenicity (acneigenicity).

Informed consumers search labels on cosmetics to ascertain that the product is noncomedogenic. Unfortunately, controversies have arisen among experimenters who have reported conflicting results on the same materials. Three examples may be given: sodium lauryl sulfate is wrongly said to be comedogenic by some authors, but is only irritant according to our view. D & C red pigments are said to cause comedones, but we judge them to be harmless. Sulfur is rated harmless by some, but found to be rather strongly comedogenic by us. A major source of these controversies is the publications of Fulton; these should be read to understand how disagreements arise. For example, Fulton mainly depends on naked eye examination.

Selection of Animals

Rabbits, like humans, vary considerably with regard to the size of their sebaceous follicles. Animals in which the orifices within the pinna are hard to see with the naked eye must be rejected. Large-pored animals should be preselected by the supplier. Young animals just weaned are unacceptable. The capability to form comedones increases with age. Male rabbits are more reactive than females; they should weigh about 4 kg.

Test Protocol

Within the rabbit ear canal there are numerous, large pilosebaceous units reminiscent of human sebaceous follicles. These have multilobulated sebaceous glands which empty their contents into a wide lumen. One tiny hair is associated with each unit. The epithelial lining of the follicular canal is highly reactive to comedogenic chemicals, much more so than in humans. Within the ear canal the follicles are highest in density, largest, and most reactive. Their size and density declines sharply a few centimeters outside the canal; therefore applications should be placed immediately adjacent to the canal. Insertion of the test material into the canal is not recommended. The applications are "blind" and often the rabbits become agitated. We recommend a glass rod to apply test materials liberally to the concave area directly outside the external ear canal. The amount varies from 125 to 250 mg. Three animals are used per test agent. The compounds are applied once daily, 5 days a week for 3 weeks. This is sufficient, even for weakly comedogenic agents. Longer times do not appreciably

increase the size of comedones. Prolonged application of irritants may result in accommodation, which can underrate irritation. Irritation peaks in about 3 weeks and decreases thereafter. Unlike in humans, the prolonged application of irritants does not lead to secondary comedones in the rabbit. On the contrary, strong irritation induces corneocyte shedding and is antagonistic to comedo formation. Cocoa butter is applied to the opposite ear as a positive control. The response to the control must be at least 1+. If a stronger positive control is desired, 0.1% crude coal tar in USP hydrophilic ointment will consistently yield 2+ to 3+ comedones.

Evaluation

Visual Assessment. Visual assessment is based on dilatation and prominence of the follicular orifices. The test is simple, though too often misleading. Some authors condemn the use of substances which react positively. We do not share this attitude. False-positive reactions are the most common problem because irritating substances often induce follicular swellings which are confused with true comedogenic impactions. The naked eye merely sees prominence and distension of the orifices. Without histology it is impossible to distinguish an inflammatory response from comedogenicity.

Attempts have been made to approve the objectivity of the visual method by making silicon replicas of the surface. Each follicular orifice is measured after being projected on a screen. Nevertheless the same objections hold.

We improved the original technique by using stereomicroscopic inspection of isolated sheets of epidermis. By immersing the tissue in hot water for 1 min the epidermis can be lifted off, carrying with it the material contained in the follicular infundibulum. Global assessment of comedones on a scale of one to three can be made. This technique was upgraded by staining the sheet with oil-red-0 and determining the surface area covered with comedones by image analysis. The problems of false-positive results remain. A negative reading is meaningful, indicating that the test agent is neither comedogenic nor irritating.

Comedones are graded histologically on a zero to three plus scale:

0 Normal loose corneocytes in the infundibulum.

1+ Small accumulations of adherent horn in the infundibulum without distension.

2+ Moderate horny impaction distending the follicle, extending into the sebaceous duct, along with hyperplasia of the sebaceous duct. Corresponds to microcomedones in the human.

3+ Follicle widely distended with dense horn. Marked epithelial hyperplasia, and partial regression of sebaceous glands. Corresponds to open comedones in the human.

Histopathology

The most reliable technique is histopathology. Obtain a 2-cm long elliptical section of tissue excised along the longitudinal axis, as close as possible to the end of the canal. The tissue is split along the cartilage, fixed in formalin, sectioned at 6 μm semiserially, and stained with hematoxylin and eosin. An alternative is to make horizontal cuts parallel to the surface, offering a view of many follicles in the same section. The follicles closest to the canal are the most reactive and are most important for grading.

Comedogenic compounds will always produce acanthosis of the epidermis, along with compact retention hyperkeratosis.

Hyperplasia of the follicular epithelium accompanies comedo formation. The difficulty is that irritants also produce hyperplasia of the epidermis and the follicular epithelium. We merely describe rather than grade inflammatory reactions. Most commonly found is a perifollicular lymphocytic infiltrate. Neutrophils signify strong irritation. Accompanied by a loose aggregate of horny cells we have called these "pseudocomedones." It should be recalled that an agent may be both comedogenic and irritating.

Occupational Versus Cosmetic Acne

The workplace may involve exposure to potent substances which can induce devastating acne. An example is chloracne due to halogenated aromatic hydrocarbons as witnessed in the immediate past in Japan, Taiwan, Spain, and Italy. A few micrograms of these substances will provoke comedones in rabbits and humans. For dioxin, nanogram amounts are sufficient. All these industrial hazards yield strong responses in the rabbit ear.

With cosmetics the situation is very different. The ingredients are never more than moderately reactive in the rabbit ear model. Usually they are quite mild. Histologic examination is required for assessing these weekly positive substances.

Conclusions

● A negative rabbit ear test assures safe use in the human.
● A strong positive test forecasts clinical trouble.
● An unresolved issue, at present, is how to interpret a weakly positive test result. No sensitive assay in the human is

presently available for identifying weak acneigens.

- Histopathologic evaluation of the rabbit ear is a reliable method for assessing the comedogenic or irritating potential of products designed for daily use on the face.

American Academy of Dermatology Invitational Symposium on Comedogenicity (1989) J Am Acad Dermatol 20:272–277

Fulton JE Jr (1989) Comedogenicity and irritancy of commonly used ingredients in skin care products. J Soc Cosmet Chem 40:321–333

Fulton JE Jr, Pay SR, Fulton JE III (1984) Comedogenicity of current therapeutic products, cosmetics, and ingredients in the rabbit ear. J Am Acad Dermatol 10:96–105

Hambrick GW Jr, Blank H (1956) A microanatomical study of the response of the pilosebaceous apparatus of the rabbits ear canal. J Invest Dermatol 26:185–200

Kaidbey KH, Kligman AM (1974) A human model of coal tar acne. Arch Dermatol 109:212–215

Kligman AM (1989) Updating the rabbit ear comedogenic assay. In: Marks R, Plewig G (eds) Acne and related disorders. Dunitz, London, pp 97–106

Kligman AM, Kwong T (1979) An improved rabbit ear model for assessing comedogenic substances. Br J Dermatol 100:699–702

Lanzet M (1986) Comedogenic effects of cosmetic raw materials. Cosmet Toilet 101:63–72

Mezick JA, Thorne EG, Bhatia MC, Shea LM, Capetola RJ, Raritan NJ (1987) The rabbit ear microcomedo prevention assay. A new model to evaluate anti-acne agents. In: Maibach HI, Lowe NJ (eds) Models in dermatology, vol. 3. Karger, Basel, pp 68–73

Mills OH Jr, Kligman AM (1982) A human model for assessing comedogenic substances. Arch Dermatol 118:903–905

Morris WE, Kwan SC (1983) Use of the rabbit ear model in evaluating the comedogenic potential of cosmetics ingredients. J Soc Cosmet Chem 34:215–225

Strauss JS, Goldman PH, Nacht S, Gans EH (1978) A reexamination of the potential comedogenicity of sulfur. Arch Dermatol 114:1340–1342

Tucker SB, Flannigan SA, Dunbar M Jr, Drotman RB (1980) Development of an objective comedogenicity assay. Arch Dermatol 122:660–665

The Rabbit Ear Comedogenicity Assay

The ventral surface just outside the ear canal contains large, numerous follicles with multilobular sebaceous glands. The architecture resembles human sebaceous follicles somewhat. Substances which induce comedones in the rabbit ear are also comedogenic in humans.

Above

Left   Horizontal section of a normal follicle with a pilary unit in the center from which sebaceous acini radiate in all directions

Right   A whole mount, stained with oil-red-0 to show the distribution of the multilobulated sebaceous glands of six closely spaced follicles

Below   Horizontal view of a 4+ comedogenic reaction to coal tar. The follicles are distended by masses of dense coherent corneocytes. Bacteria are notably absent in this model. The coal tar model can be effectively used to assay comedolytic agents

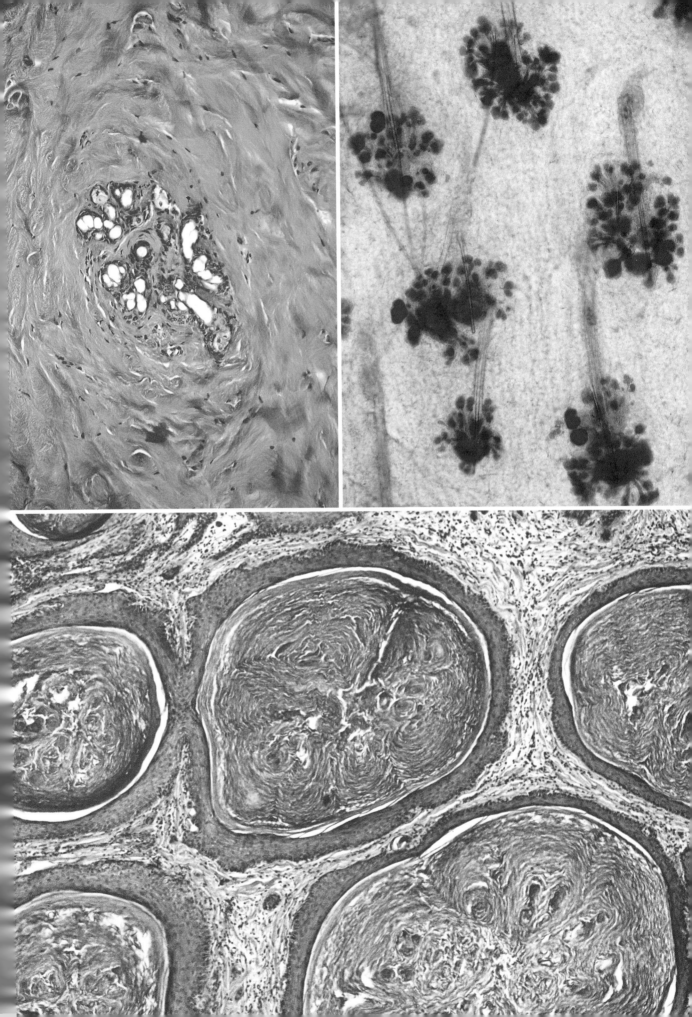

Rhino Mouse Model

Rhinocerous mice which have excessively wrinkled skin were first described in 1856 by Gaskoyne, although a detailed description of these peculiar changes was not given until a century later by Mann.

The rhino mouse (hr^{rh} hr^{rh}) is allelic to the smooth-skinned hairless (hr hr) variety. This is an ugly, repelling animal with its nudity draped into rhinocerous-like folds and ridges. Newborn rhino mice are hairy. With the first telogen phase, a fault in the catagen hair cycle results in permanent hair loss. Remnants of the hair papillae and the external root sheath epithelium separate from the ascending follicle during catagen. This sequestered epithelium forms a keratinous cyst; the pilary canal forms an ampulla-like cavity, an utriculus, which is full of retained corneocytes. The utriculus bears some resemblance histologically to open comedones in humans. These cannot be squeezed out manually, do not contain *Propionibacterium acnes*, and never become inflamed. Actually, the corneocytes are loose and not at all like the hard horny impactions in men. Nonetheless, the comedolytic effect of topicals can be quantitatively assessed. Reduction in size or diameter of the horn-filled utriculus can be estimated histologically or in whole, cleared mounts.

Topical tretinoin rapidly expels corneocytes with shrinkage of the utriculus. Other retinoids, like isotretinoin, etretinate, and motretinide have been shown to be less effective. Oral retinoids have similar comedolytic effects.

Old-fashioned, so-called peeling agents such as resorcinol and sulfur show no comedolytic activity. In fact, elemental sulfur expends the utriculi and is therefore comedogenic. Salicylic acid, as expected, is moderately effective, while the α-hydroxy acids and benzoyl peroxide are inactive.

The rhino mouse can be used to assess drugs which affect epithelial differentiation and comedolysis, like retinoids, or descaling agents like salicylic acid, which promote loss of cohesion between corneocytes.

Ashton RE, Connor MJ, Lowe NJ (1984) Histologic changes in the skin of the rhino mouse induced by retinoids. J Invest Dermatol 82:632–635

Bernerd F, Ortonne JP, Bouclier M, Chatelus A, Hensby C (1991) The rhino mouse model: the effects of topically applied all-*trans* retinoic acid and CD271 on the fine structure of the epidermis and utricle wall of pseudocomedones. Arch Dermatol Res 283:100–107

Gaskoyne JS (1856) On a peculiar variety of Mus musculus. Proc Zool Soc Lond 24:38–40

Kligman LH, Kligman AM (1979) The effect on rhino mouse skin of agents which influence keratinization and exfoliation. J Invest Dermatol 73:354–358

Lowe NJ, Weingarten D (1989) The effects of hyperproliferative agents on the rhino mouse: Variable effects on keratin utricles. In: Marks R, Plewig G (eds) Acne and related disorders. Dunitz, London, pp 165–167

Mann SJ (1971) Hair loss and cyst formation in hairless and rhino mutant mice. Anat Rec 170:485–499

Mezick JA, Bhatia MC, Capetola RJ (1984) Topical and systemic effects of retinoids on horn-filled utriculus size in the rhino mouse. A model to quantify "antikeratinizing" effects of retinoids. J Invest Dermatol 83:110–113

The Rhino Mouse

Horn-filled utriculi of the rhino mouse can be used to study comedolytics.

Above A neat row of utriculi, each one filled with eosinophilic keratinized material. The opening is usually narrow. Small sebaceous glands are connected to the bottom portion. Untreated control

Below Topical application of tretinoin has completely expulsed the utricular retention hyperkeratosis. Only very minute amounts of eosinophilic corneocytes reside in the follicular opening. The sebaceous acini are intact. Developmental failure of the pilary units to connect with the utriculi above accounts for the Swiss-cheese-like cysts; these are not connected with the skin surface

Below: Courtesy of Loraine H. Kligman, PhD, Philadelphia, USA

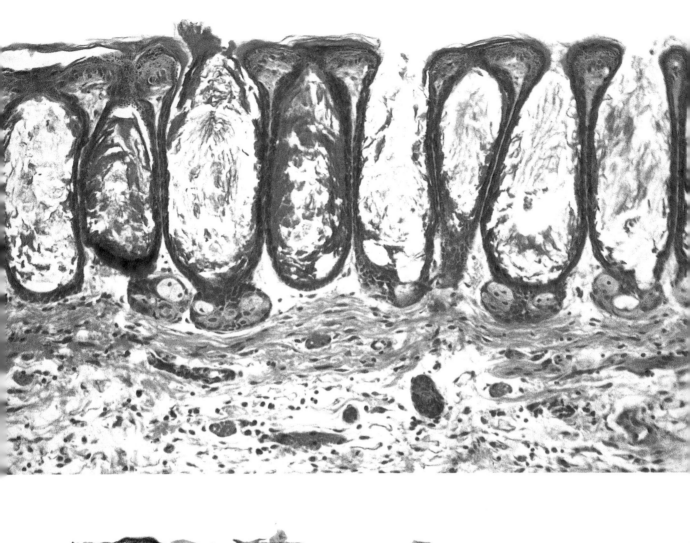

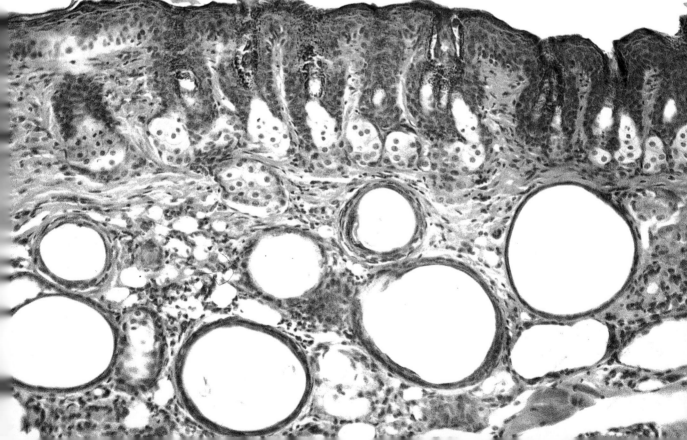

THE ACNES

Acnes

Synopsis of the acnes. The various forms of acne are subdivided like genus and species, e.g., acne venenata, and variations, e.g., pomade acne

Acne neonatorum

Acne infantum

    Acne conglobata infantum

Acne juvenilis

    Acne comedonica
    Acne papulopustulosa
    Acne conglobata
    Acne inversa
    Acne fulminans
    Solid persistent facial edema in acne
    Acne mechanica

Acne adultorum

    Acne on the back in adults
    Acne tropicalis
    Postadolescent acne in women
    Premenstrual acne
    Postmenopausal acne
    Masculinizing syndromes in women
    Polycystic ovary disease
    Androluteoma of pregnancy
    Androgen excess in men
    XYY acne conglobata
    Body building acne
    Doping acne (power athlete acne)
    Testosterone-induced acne fulminans in extremely tall boys

Acne venenata (contact acne)

    Acne cosmetica
    Pomade acne
    Chloracne (skin contactants, inhalants, ingestants)
    Oil, tar, and pitch acne

Comedonal acne due to physical agents

    Solar comedones (Favre-Racouchot's disease)
    Mallorca acne (acne aestivalis)
    Acne due to ionizing radiation: X-ray and cobalt acne

Acne in Infancy

We generally think of acne as a disease which begins in adolescence. Its presentation in infancy is disturbing but not necessarily serious. Several types are recognized.

Acne Neonatorum

Acne neonatorum occurs at birth or shortly thereafter, mostly in boys. Closed comedones, sometimes accompanied by a few open ones, and often a scattering of papulopustules are found on the cheeks and forehead. The eruption is generally mild and usually regresses spontaneously in the next few months. The term acne neonatorum is quite appropriate for this disease of early onset, low level, which is self-abating. It is certainly a good deal more common than the approximately 100 cases reported so far. Pediatricians are familiar with it and regard it casually because of its short duration. The more one looks the more one sees. The incidence may be more than 20% if one includes the presence of only a few comedones. The pathogenetic mechanisms are speculative. Maternal and fetal androgens, especially from the hyperactive adrenals in the neonate, have been incriminated.

It is important to differentiate acne venenata induced by ointments and oils, acne infantum, and acneiform eruptions due to drugs given to the mother during pregnancy (hydantoin, lithium).

Treatment is usually unnecessary; a few comforting words will do. If required, topical tretinoin alone is sufficient. Babies tolerate comedolytic agents quite well. Inflammatory lesions can be treated with low strength benzoyl peroxide (2.5%) or topical erythromycin.

Acne Infantum

Acne infantum, like acne neonatorum, is a true acne variant and not an acneiform eruption. We differentiate this from acne in the newborns. It has a later onset, usually from the third to the sixth month of life, and tends to be more severe. More boys than girls are affected. We are ignorant of its pathogenesis.

The lesions are confined to the face and are generally fairly numerous. Comedones predominate, mainly on the cheeks, and are often dense. Inflammatory lesions are frequent, rarely including cystic nodules, which heal with scars. Papules and pustules come and go.

The disease lasts for many months, even for years. Resistant acne infantum calls for endocrinologic screening (total and free testosterone; dehydroepiandrosterone, DHE, and its sulfate, DHE-S; FSH; LH; etc.). It is hypothesized that this may represent precocious secretion of androgens by the gonads.

Acne infantum has its ups and downs, but fortunately tends to burn itself out in a year or two. Rare cases go right on to adolescence. Acne in both parents sometimes forms the background of acne infantum.

Differential diagnosis includes acne neonatorum (in neonates only) and acne venenata (from comedogenic oils, creams, and lotions applied by parents).

Acne infantum requires decisive treatment and can be a real challenge. A comedolytic agent such as tretinoin (retinoic acid, vitamin A acid) is usually helpful. Topical antibacterials like benzoyl peroxide and erythromycin may be tried as adjuncts to tretinoin. Oral antibiotics, especially erythromycin, may have to be added to bring the process under control. Parents must be informed that treatment, as in adolescent acne, may be prolonged. Intralesional steroids may be tried for deep inflammatory lesions.

Acne Conglobata Infantum

Rarely, acne conglobata may occur in infants. The lesions are confined to the face, which is disfigured by papules, pustules, nodules, and draining sinus tracts. The parents are understandably very much concerned. Depressed scars are a dreaded result and an indication for aggressive treatment. The disease may endure right into puberty and be followed by severe acne conglobata.

Differential diagnosis is limited to pyodermas and panniculitis of various origins. Otherwise the picture is so dramatic that no other form of acne needs to be considered.

Treatment is the same as for severe acne infantum. Topical and systemic modalities may be started at the same time. Tetracyclines must not be used because of danger of damage to the teeth, including yellowish discoloration. In refractory cases oral isotretinoin may be considered for several months. This is followed by topical tretinoin (retinoic acid)

to prevent relapse. Great improvement is the rule. Scars are to be avoided by all means.

Acne Venenata Infantum

Acne venenata infantum is contact acne. (Venenum means poison in Latin.) Topically applied comedogenic substances provoke the lesions. These products are often greasy salves, creams, pomades, and oils, applied by parents and grandparents. Not all greases are acneigenic. Ethnic and cultural peculiarities determine the prevalence of acne venenata infantum in different groups. The condition is common in some Mediterranean countries and also among American Blacks. Within the first 3–4 months of life, but not at birth, dense crops of tiny closed and open comedones spring up on cheeks, nose, forehead, temples, but rarely on the trunk or extremities. Removing the contactagent terminates the problem, but the time to clearing may be surprisingly long.

Differential diagnosis includes acne infantum, or acne venenata from other sources, e.g., topical use of corticosteroids.

Treatment is not always necessary. Mild cases resolve spontaneously. Topical tretinoin is usually effective. Treatment should be kept as simple as possible.

Steroid Acne in Infants

Oral and topical corticosteroids induce steroid acne. Children are unusually susceptible to these agents. Crops of inflammatory papulopustules should arouse suspicion. Treatment entails withdrawal of the steroid. The eruption responds well to tretinoin and/or benzoyl peroxide.

Hippie Acne, Chap-Stick Acne, McDonald's Acne, and Kelp Acne

Odd variants of acne are mostly seen in adolescents, but may also occur in childhood. These are described elsewhere (p. 376).

Chloracne in Children

A more detailed description of chloracne, a horrendous condition, will be given elsewhere (p. 376). In 1976 there was an industrial catastrophe in Seveso, Italy, whereby 2,3,7,8-tetrachlorodibenzo-p-dioxin (TCDD) was released, and approximately 4 kg of this toxin contaminated in the form of a gas cloud several square miles around the factory. Within months some 25 patients developed comedo-like lesions on the face, upper and lower arms, thighs, and lower legs. Children as young as 5 years developed extremely severe chloracne. Two years later about two hundred cases were seen.

Despite the horrible and extensive skin lesions no systemic adverse effects have been reported, in contrast to other TCDD-poisoned victims. Unfortunately massive pox-like scarring, particularly in the face, developed in some children. Gas chromatography mass spectrometry of comedones has failed to demonstrate the presence of dioxins in these lesions.

Similar disasters occurred in Japan in 1968 (Yusho or oil disease), in Taiwan in 1979, where a salad oil contaminated with polychlorobiphenyl was identified, and in Spain in 1987, when contaminated and adulterated olive oil was sold. Everywhere children were among the victims.

Certain dioxins are superpotent acneigens, usually by surface contact, but also by inhalation and ingestion. Children are at risk to ingest toxins of contaminated soil by swallowing dust while playing. Dioxin can also enter the food chain and induce acne in this way.

Chloracne is usually limited to the skin without concomitant internal disease. Dioxins and other potent chloracneigens selectively destroy sebaceous acini and cause the development of compact comedones in an unusually dense and wide distribution over the body.

Chloracne is difficult to manage at any age. Treatment is topically and orally as in severe acne conglobata. Isotretinoin is the drug of choice in severe cases.

Fetal Hydantoin Syndrome

Women who take hydantoin during early pregnancy may give birth to premature babies with the fetal hydantoin syndrome. This is charcterized by growth retardation, peculiar facies, variable limb defects, and dry hair. Neonatal acne may also be a feature of this syndrome. This acneiform eruption is provoked by transplacental drug transfer from the mother to the fetus. It resolves spontaneously within the first months of life.

Androluteoma Syndrome of Pregnancy

A persistent corpus luteum with excessive testosterone production causes severe abnormalities due to an excess of androgen. The mother becomes masculinized with seborrhea, hypertrichosis, deep voice, papulopustular acne, and even acne conglobata. Female fetuses are at risk and can be born with signs of masculinization, including acne.

This tumor is rare, with only 14 cases reported so far. Diagnosis is based on ultrasound identification of the tumor in

Disease	Age	Sex	Cause
Fetal hydantoin syndrome and acne neonatorum	Newborns	m+f	Hydantoin therapy of the mother during pregnancy
Androluteoma syndrome of pregnancy and masculinized female fetuses	Newborns	f	Virilizing luteoma (androluteoma) in pregnancy
Acne neonatorum	Newborns and first weeks of life	m+f	Maternal and infantile androgens?
Acne infantum	>3 months	m+f	Androgens of child?
Acne conglobata infantum	>3 months	m+f	Androgens of child?
Acne venenata	>3 months	m+f	Contact with comedogenic compounds
Variants Steroid acne	>1 year	m+f	Local or systemic corticosteroids
Pomade acne	Babies and infants	m+f	Comedogenic care products

m, male; f, female

the ovary and excess androgenic hormone levels in the peripheral blood. Surgical removal of the androgen-producing corpus luteum during pregnancy is curative.

Ayres S (1926) Infantile acne vulgaris. Arch Dermatol Syph 14:12–13

Caputo R, Monti M, Ermacora E, Carminati G, Gelmetti C, Gianotti R, Gianni E, Puccinelli V (1988) Cutaneous manifestations of tetrachlorodibenzo-p-dioxin in children and adolescents. Follow-up 10 years after the Seveso, Italy, accident. J Am Acad Dermatol 19:812–819

Chew EW, Bingham A, Burrows D (1990) Incidence of acne vulgaris in patients with infantile acne. Clin Exp Dermatol 15:376–377

Duke EMC (1981) Infantile acne associated with transient increases in plasma concentrations of luteinizing hormone, follicle-stimulating hormone, and testosterone. Br Med J 282:1275–1276

Koßmann E (1988) Acne neonatorum und Acne infantum. Hautarzt (Suppl 8) 39:113

Latif R, Laude TA (1982) Steroid acne in a 14-month-old boy. Cutis 29:373–376

Menni S, Brancaleone W (1992) Cosmetic acne in a child. Eur J Dermatol 2:242–243

Nanda A, Kaur S, Bhakoo ON, Kapoor MM, Kanwar AJ (1989) Fetal hydantoin syndrome: a case report. Pediatr Dermatol 6:130–133

Passi S, Nazzaro-Porro M, Boniforti L, Gianotti F (1981) Analysis of lipids and dioxin in chloracne due to tetrachloro-2,3,7,8-p-dibenzodioxin. Br J Dermatol 105:137–143

Stankler L, Campbell AGM (1980) Neonatal acne vulgaris: a possible feature of the fetal hydantoin syndrome. Br J Dermatol 103:453–455

Wagner G, Schmidt KU, Rensing H (1987) Acne conglobata infantum. Aktuel Dermatol 13:306–307

Zander J, Mickan H, Holzmann K, Lohe KJ (1978) Androluteoma syndrome of pregnancy. Am J Obstet Gynecol 130:170–177

Acne Neonatorum

Some babies are born with comedones and inflammatory lesions or develop them soon after birth. Excessive androgens of the newborn, typical for this period, is blamed for the eruptions. Most babies lose their acne spontaneously within a few months.

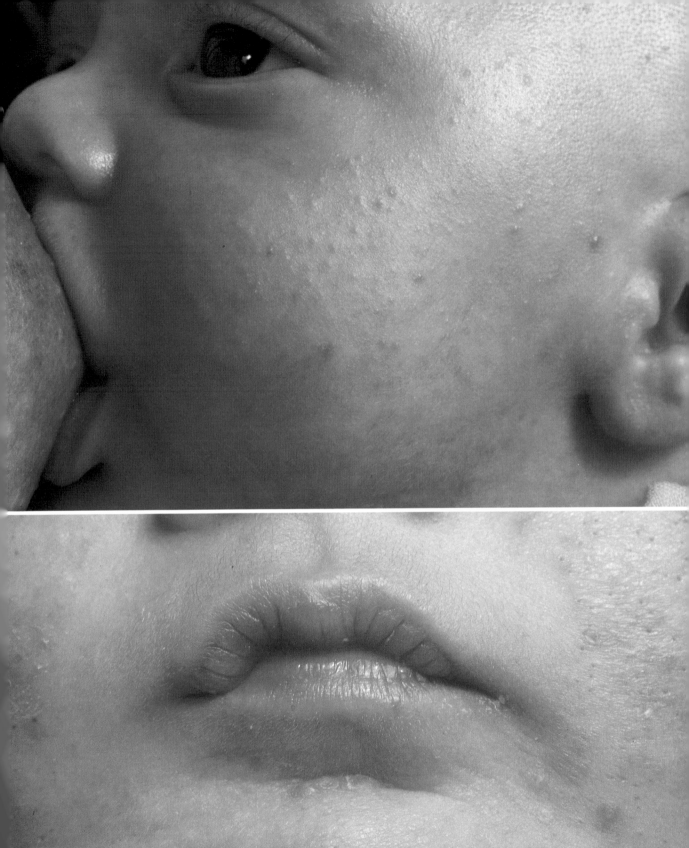

Acne in Infancy

It is not unusual that newborns present some signs of acne in their face. Also in early childhood acne can appear with many variations.

Above

Left   Acne neonatorum. Many papulopustules and small comedones cover the face of this boy. The skin is oily, signifying androgen-stimulated sebaceous gland activity

Right   This could pass as acne neonatorum or acne infantum but is actually acne venenata in a 5-month-old infant. Some mothers have an irresistible urge to grease the skin with exotic salves. In this case an unidentifiable ointment had been applied several times daily. Aggregations of comedones always suggest an exogenous cause. As a rule infants and children, who have immature follicles, are relatively resistant to acne

Below

Left   Acne infantum. Indurated deep papules and nodules persist for many months, with new lesions coming up periodically

Right   Acne conglobata, the most severe form of acne infantum. Understandably the parents of this girl worry about the outcome of this severe inflammatory variant of acne. Scarring is inevitable

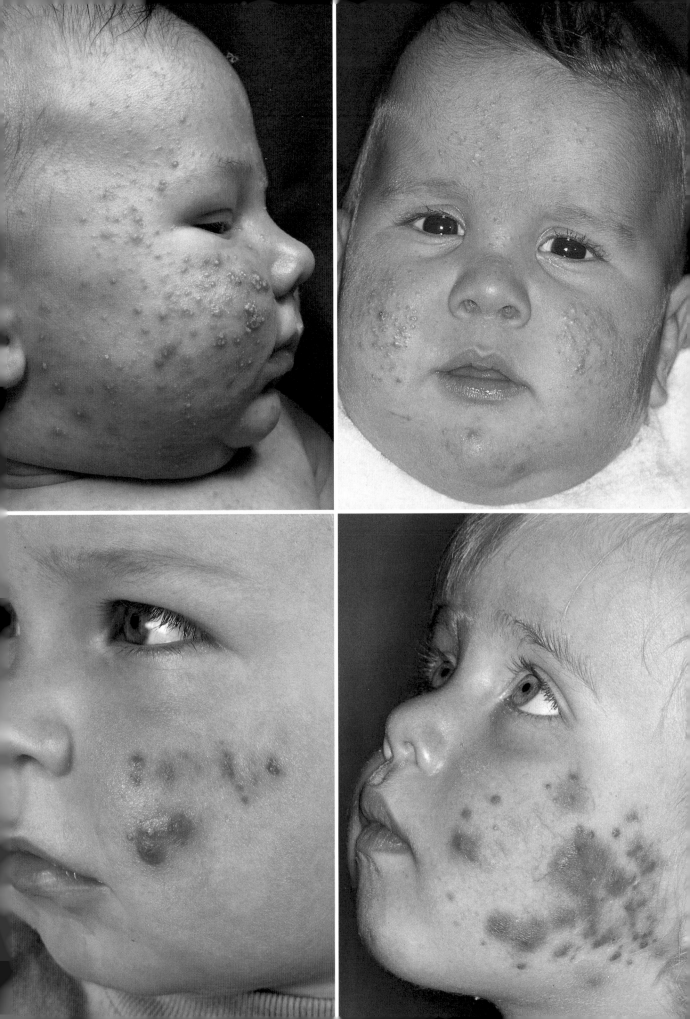

Acne Comedonica (Comedonal Acne)

Acne vulgaris makes its debut with the comedo. This is the undisputed hallmark of the disease. Several features distinguish acne comedonica.

Onset is early, often before the more obvious signs of puberty. Comedones appear earlier in girls than in boys. Onset is related to measures of pubertal age such as secondary sex characteristics, not chronologic age. It is not at all rare for small comedones to emerge on the nose of 8- to 10-year-old girls, years before menarche. Experienced dermatologists have come to believe that early onset acne is a relatively recent phenomenon. In rare cases comedonal acne can begin as acne infantum and goes on straight through to puberty.

Seborrhea preceeds the appearance of comedones. Not only the face but also the scalp becomes oily. These changes may be subtle clinically but have been validated by measurements of sebum excretion such as Sebutape pore patterns. The hair has to be shampooed more frequently than before.

Acne comedonica starts in quite typical areas. Chief locations are the dorsum of the nose and the alae nasi. Acne then encroaches on the forehead and spreads to the cheeks and finally to the chin. The general time pattern is downwards. The trunk is affected much later and often escapes altogether.

Odd locations like behind or on the ear should be examined. It is not uncommon to find multiple black open comedones on the concha along with closed comedones.

These are not likely to be self-reported. Another peculiar site for comedones is the ear lobe. These cyst-like closed comedones can be better palpated than seen. They feel like lead shot, rarely exceeding 2–3 mm in diameter. Next is the mastoid area, where open and closed comedones are hidden in the shadow of the ear.

The first comedones are the closed ones, which later enlarge and become open comedones. Often the nose and forehead are studded with many small whitish closed comedones, giving the skin surface a rough sandpaper-like aspect, easily felt. The further course of the disease shows great individual variations. Some patients never produce more than a few comedones, happily remaining at a benign stage, which has been termed acne minor. Others produce inflammatory lesions along with new comedones. The appearance is polymorphic with comedones, papules, and pustules. In some unfortunate individuals this erupts into a ferocious expression of the disease (acne major).

Those with only comedones and practically no inflammatory lesions belong to the category of acne comedonica. However, severity varies widely in this group. We divide comedonal acne into four grades (p. 221). A patient with many closed comedones, i.e., more than 50 on one side of the face, has severe comedonal acne. A high density of closed comedones bespeaks therapeutic stubbornness. The popular patient term for closed comedones is whiteheads.

Closed comedones, which have no visible opening, are prone to rupture, creating a variety of inflammatory lesions.

Open and closed comedones are not peculiar to acne vulgaris. Comedones can be induced by a number of agents, such as ultraviolet radiation in solar comedones or subsequent to X-rays. Comedogenic substances are widely distributed among cosmetics, toiletries, and even topical drugs. Certain occupations involve a high exposure to potent comedogens (chloracne).

Comedones occur only in humans, except in unusual species like the Mexican hairless dog. However, comedones can be artifically induced in the rabbit ear. This animal is suitable for assays of comedogenic materials.

Not everything that looks like an open comedo is one. Some confusion may occur in depressed scars filled with pigmented corneocytes, dilated facial pores, pilar sheath acanthomas, and the horny impactions of nevus comedonicus.

Debut of Acne

Acne starts earlier in girls than in boys, often by 2–3 years.

Above This girl is only 8 years old. The lesions consist of open and closed comedones, along with small papules and pustules. The nose is often involved, at the start; by contrast nasal lesions are rare. Acne which is this severe early on demands aggressive treatment

Below

Left Acne started 3 years previously on the nose of this 12-year-old girl. Thereafter it extended to the forehead. Inflammatory lesions appeared later on on the cheeks. This sequence of localizations is typical. The chin is the last region to become affected

Right This is a homozygous twin; her sister had exactly the same distribution and severity, bespeaking the importance of heredity. At age 16 intensive seborrhea and densely set comedones, papules, and pustules are present. It is not a good sign when there is a high density of mixed lesions already present in teenagers. Therapy should be vigorous initially

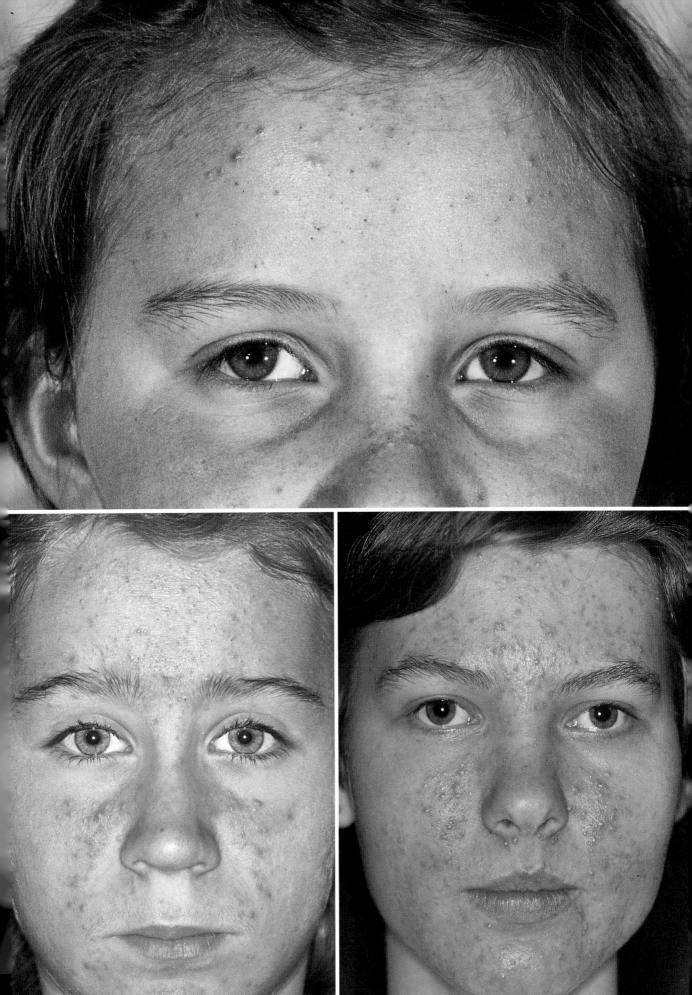

Comedonal Acne in Teenagers

The initial lesions in acne are closed comedones which occur on the nose and forehead and appearing on the cheeks.

Above   Acne may make its debut first on the forehead. The many closed comedones are not very visible, unless the skin is stretched by the fingers. Large pores, accompanied by seborrhea, indicate the probability of more severe disease later on in this young girl. Early aggressive treatment usually prevents inflammatory, scarring lesions

Below   In this girl of the same age, acne also began as dense closed comedones but these have evolved into small inflammatory papules. It is important to use effective comedolytics before they rupture. Patients and parents are typically negligent in starting therapy when the first comedones surface

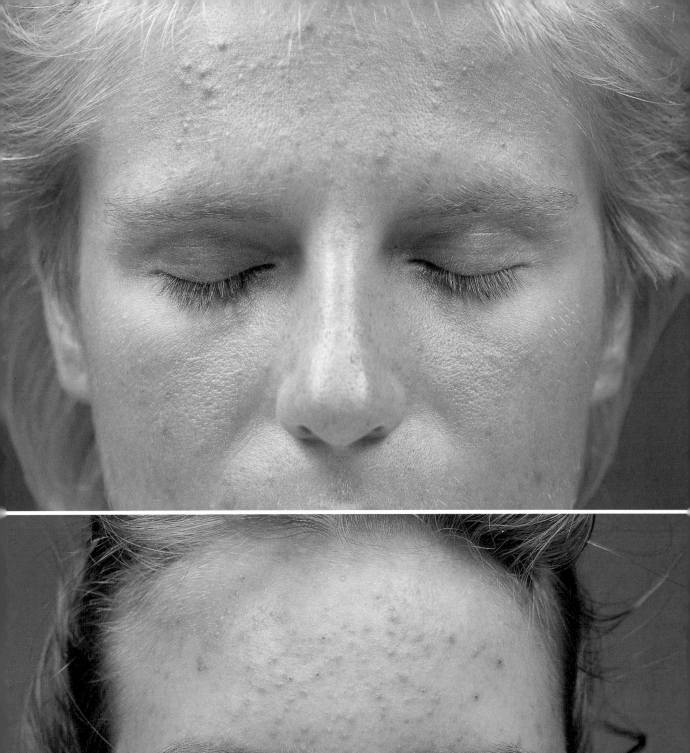

Acne Papulopustulosa (Papulopustular Acne)

Most patients with acne fall into this category. The clinical picture is straight forward and the face is the favorite site of localization.

Papules and pustules are always secondary lesions. The sequence is as follows: a comedo, be it only of microscopic size (the microcomedo), precedes the inflammatory stage. Open and closed comedones are always present to varying degrees, intermingled with papules and pustules. The hybrid term papulopustules is an acceptable clinical designation.

The disease runs an unpredictable course, remaining mild in many patients and progressing to more serious disease in others. Not rarely some patients suffer from this type of inflammatory acne all through puberty, early adulthood, and well into their twenties. Papulopustules may also occur on the neck and trunk. All inflammatory lesions heal with a scar which in most cases, fortunately, is only noticeable in histologic sections. Deeper and larger indurated papulopustules leave clinically evident scars.

We classify papulopustular acne into four stages of severity, in homology to acne comedonica (p. 223).

It is important to recognize that the presence of papules and pustules does not automatically lead to a diagnosis of acne vulgaris. Similar lesions may originate from a variety of causes and are classified under the general title of acneiform eruptions. These are discussed elsewhere.

High-Density Acne Lesions in a 15-Year-Old Girl

Few follicles are spared in this intensive affliction. The full spectrum of lesions are present, e.g., closed comedones, small papules, and pustules. The chest and back were also involved. Extreme seborrhea forms the background for the unusually numerous lesions. Aggressive therapy is indicated to prevent progression to an even more frightening disease. The emotional impact in this girl was understandably disabling.

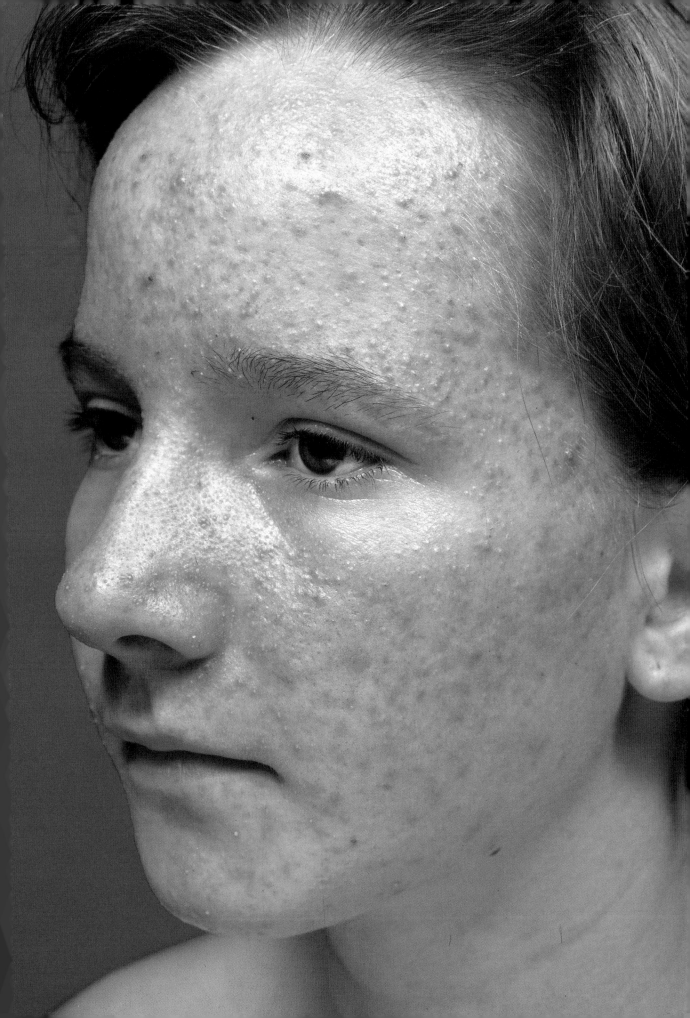

A Portrait of Acne

The face is rich in sebaceous follicles, the target structures of acne. The dynamics of lesion formation can be appreciated from this picture, showing various stages. The primary lesions are closed comedones (whiteheads), which are small inconspicuous whitish elevations, located here near the nasolabial folds and on the forehead. They should not be confused with a few milia on the left lower eyelid. Whiteheads are time bombs of acne and sooner or later rupture to provoke variably sized inflammatory pustules and papules, mainly distributed here on the cheeks and forehead.

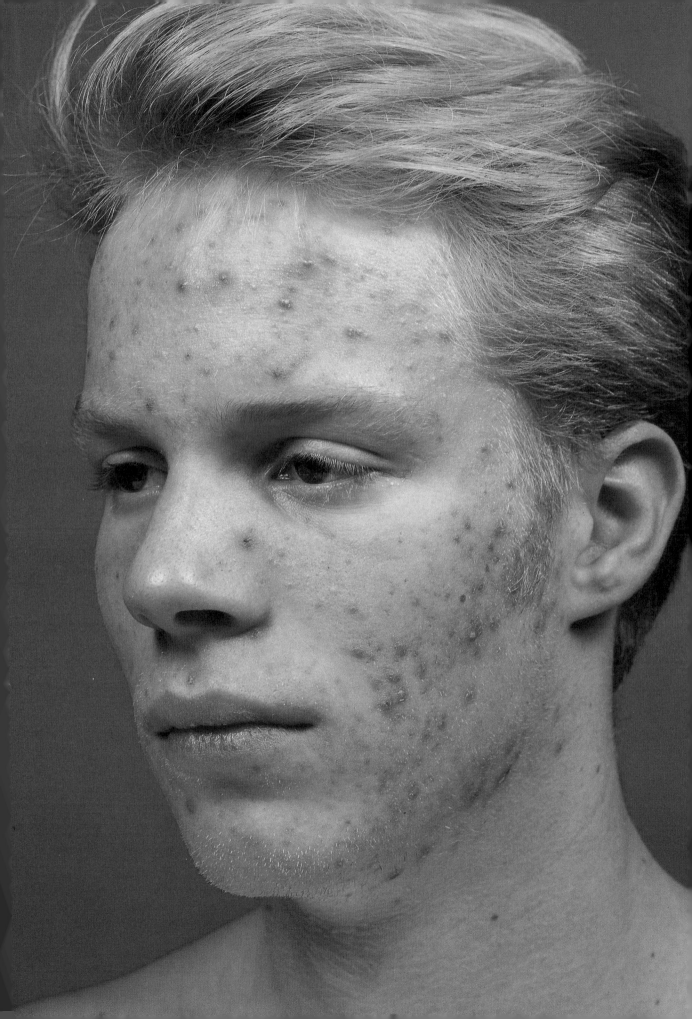

The Spectrum of Acne

Above

Left   Sadness is evident in this picture. The young woman has conglobate acne. Immediate action is required before she becomes scarred physically and mentally. Isotretinoin is indicated, provided all contraindications are ruled out and guidelines are strictly followed

Right   Though not as severe as the picture to the *left*, this is nonetheless troublesome acne. Inflammatory papules and deep persistent nodules are mingled with the initial comedones

Below

Left   Acne conglobata in a 16-year-old adolescent. This is serious acne, programmed to run for years and decades unless appropriately treated. In the middle of the cheek confluent abscesses dissect the skin; a draining sinus can result from this

Right   The complexion is not good in this woman. The face is obviously oily and papules pop up, leaving scars. Excoriations inflicted by her fingers add another facet to the disease. Hormonal treatment, especially with antiandrogens, could be indicated

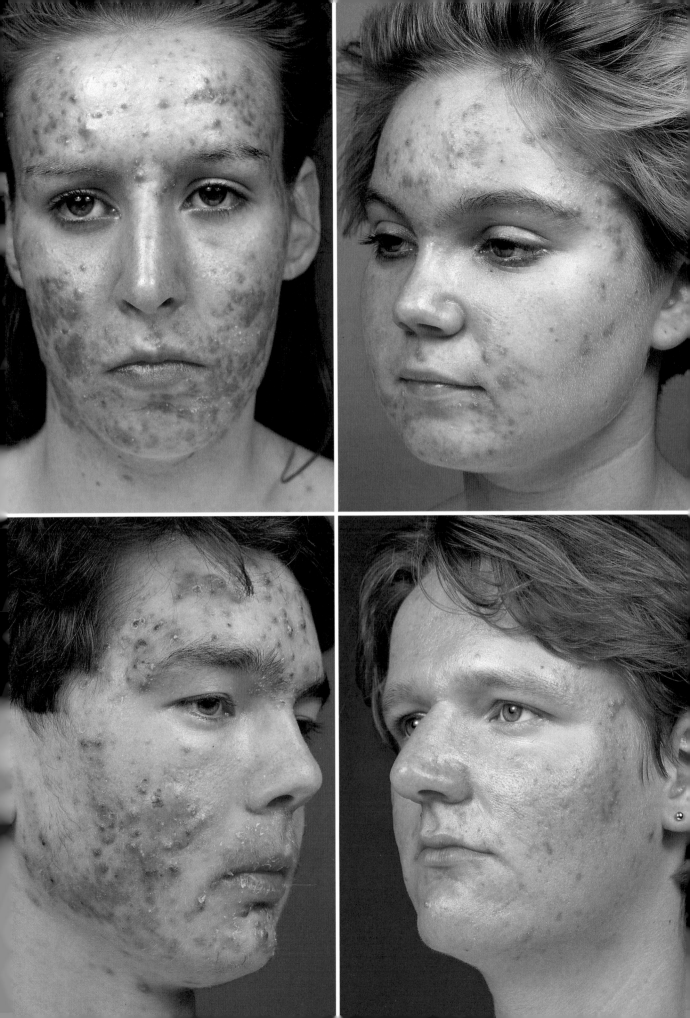

Acne Conglobata (Conglobate Acne)

The ultimate feral expression of acne is acne conglobata. It is a searing, scarring, spectacular disorder which is utterly devastating. The victims feel like and often act like lepers, viewing themselves as objects of the wrath of God. Once seen, acne conglobata is never forgotten.

The disease is found mainly in men with conspicuously oily skin. Histologic examination invariably reveals huge sebaceous glands. Lesions begin in early puberty. Severity increases over the years, culminating in late adolescence. Acne conglobata is much commoner in Whites than in Blacks.

In contrast to common belief, acne of this degree of severity does not subside after adolescence. Indeed, it characteristically persists, sometimes in a vivid and exuberant form, for many years, often into the individual's forties; in others it smolders lifelong. Subsidence is slow with periodic flares. Sometimes scars cover one third of the skin surface, and scattered lesions continue to appear episodically. Histologically, scarred skin often shows a remarkable degree of inflammatory activity with engorged vessels, mononuclear infiltrates, and foreign body granulomas.

The archetypical lesion of acne conglobata is the nodule – a large, succulent, tender, red, elevated, dome-shaped mass, at first firm, later becoming soft or even fluctuant. Nodules often fuse to form odd-shaped aggregates, sometimes several centimeters long. The lesions take many months to regress and invariably leave scars. They may evolve into draining sinuses, a labyrinth of tunnels, which periodically releases a serous or suppurative exudate at one or more openings. The draining sinuses typically remain active for years with occasional blow-ups.

Inflammatory lesions dominate. Nodules, of course, are conspicuous. There may be many persistent papules. Pustules are variable in number and usually not prominent. Open and closed comedones are curiously not common and never conspicuous. On the other hand, two types of secondary comedones are characteristic of long-standing acne conglobata: the whitish, firm cyst-like secondary comedones, and polyporous comedones which look like clusters of huge blackheads, actually scars.

Acne conglobata flourishes on the trunk, especially the back, and tends to be less violent on the face. Acne conglobata limited to the face is actually uncommon. In many patients, perhaps most, only the back is involved. It usually extends beyond the territory of acne. The buttocks and even the thighs are often afflicted. Lesions encroach on the neck, ear lobes, auditory canal, nape of neck, and within hairy scalp. Sometimes this fearful disease is generalized, with lesions occurring wherever there are follicles.

Scarring is inevitable and is rightfully dreaded. The full spectrum of scars can be found in any given patient. Atrophic scars, as thin as cigarette paper, often more than 3–5 cm wide with ectatic blood vessels shining through, may cover large areas. Hypertrophic scars may be intermingled: these are elevated, hard, fibrotic nodules of varying size, sometimes suggesting keloids. On the back these may occur as discrete, small, whitish, firm papular scars localized to follicles. These are frequently confused with closed comedones. When nicked with a sharp instrument, nothing comes out. On the face crateriform, ice-pick-like scars, troughs, tunnels, and other bizarre defects disfigure the surface. Sometimes inflammatory lesions blow up in old scars, e.g., pustules, papules, or nodules in either atrophic or hypertrophic scars.

Laboratory studies are generally not fruitful nor have endocrinologic investigations produced results. Delayed sensitivity responses are definitely decreased (mumps, tuberculin, contact allergens), but these findings are secondary to widespread inflammation. Immune deficiency cannot be blamed as an etiologic factor. The skin of these patients tends to be highly reactive to irritants such as croton oil. Local application of concentrated potassium iodide readily provokes pustules. "Fragile follicles" which burst soon after comedones begin to form are typical, but an explanation for this defect is lacking.

As regards treatment, our program is aggressive use of topical and oral drugs and in the meanwhile to provide generous hope and support. We often show before-and-after pictures of previous therapeutic success. This alone often greatly lifts the spirits and ensures cooperation.

Puhvel SM, Amirian D, Weintraub J, Reisner RM (1977) Lymphocyte transformation in subjects with nodulo-cystic acne. Br J Dermatol 97:205–211

Rajka G (1977) On cell-mediated immunity in acne conglobata. Acta Derm Venereol (Stockh) 57:141–143

Wilkins JW Jr, Voorhees JJ (1970) Prevalence of nodulocystic acne in white and negro males. Arch Dermatol 102:631–634

Acne Conglobata in an Adult

Acne does not always disappear in early adulthood, contrary to the common belief. Acne conglobata, in particular, can rage on for a lifetime, even into old age. This is the case in this 52-year-old man.

His back is a mess. Wide atrophic scars are everywhere, along with black polyporous comedones, papules, nodules, abscesses, and scars. The huge abscess on the neck is particularly painful, just by lying down. Movement is handicapped. Underwear and shirts are constantly soiled. This man became a social recluse. Nowadays, this fate can be avoided by vigorous therapy with isotretinoin.

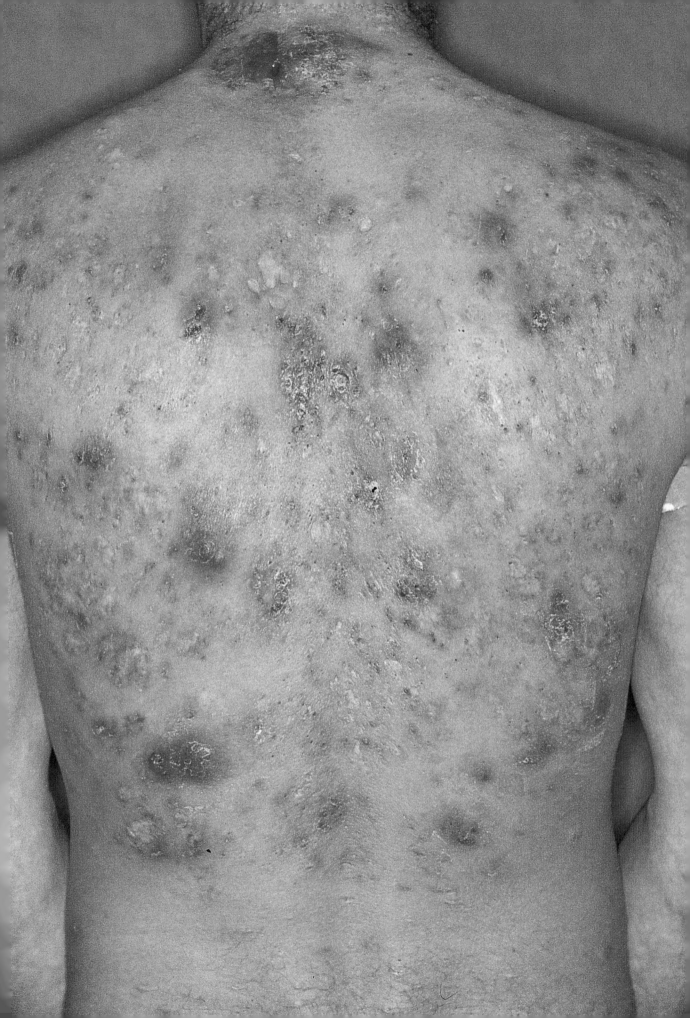

Acne Conglobata: A Skin Outrage

Acne lesions can be quite tender and painful, particularly when leaning against a chair, lying on the back or belly, sitting in a car, etc.

Above   This young man is battered by deep, hemorrhagic and confluent abscesses, wiping out wide territories of skin. There is a constant exudation of blood, serum, and pus, soiling underwear and clothes. Motion is painful

Below   Acne conglobata extends beyond the usual acne distribution, in this case down to the buttocks. In these patients, the follicles everywhere seem to be very fragile, rupturing readily from pressure and torsion. This picture could be mistaken for bacterial folliculitis except for the tell-tale lesions on the upper back

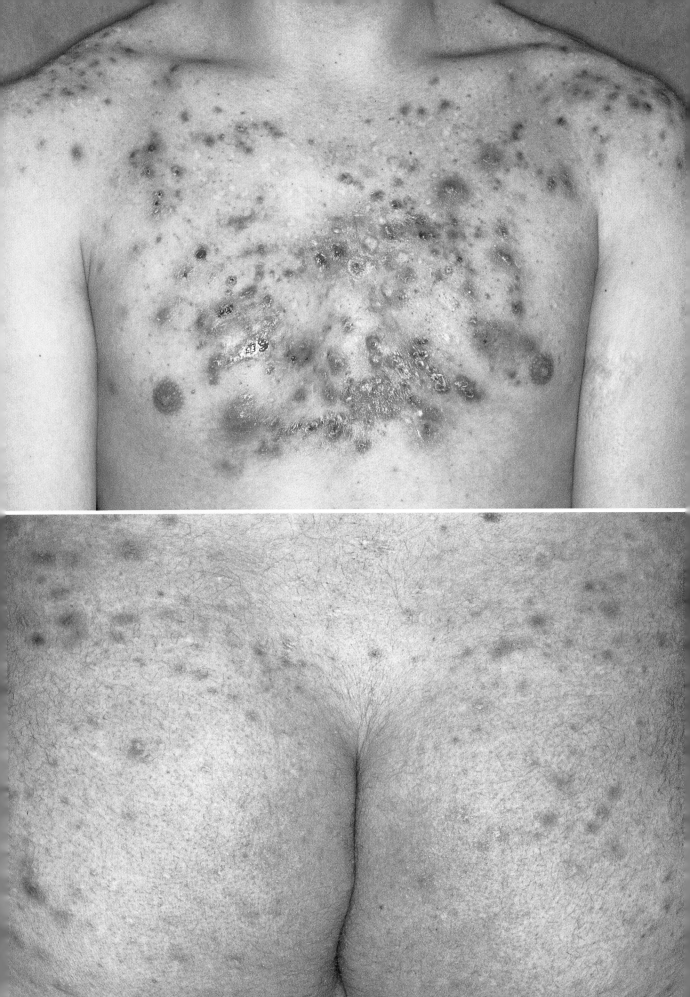

Unusual Localizations

Practically every region exept the palms and soles may be involved when acne is very severe.

Above   While the face and sholders are typical acne sites, the neck and the hairy scalp may also be seriously affected. Lesions on the neck are often very painful. Collars may aggravate the lesions mechanically. Here the lesions are mainly deep seated papulopustules and nodules, each one persisting for many months

Below

Left   The back of the ear, though hidden from view, is often involved to a surprising degree. Large open comedones on the ventral side of the ear may be numerous, as shown here

Right   Shoulder and upper arms are frequent locations in acne conglobata, with its numerous large inflammatory papules and pustules. Scarring is inevitable

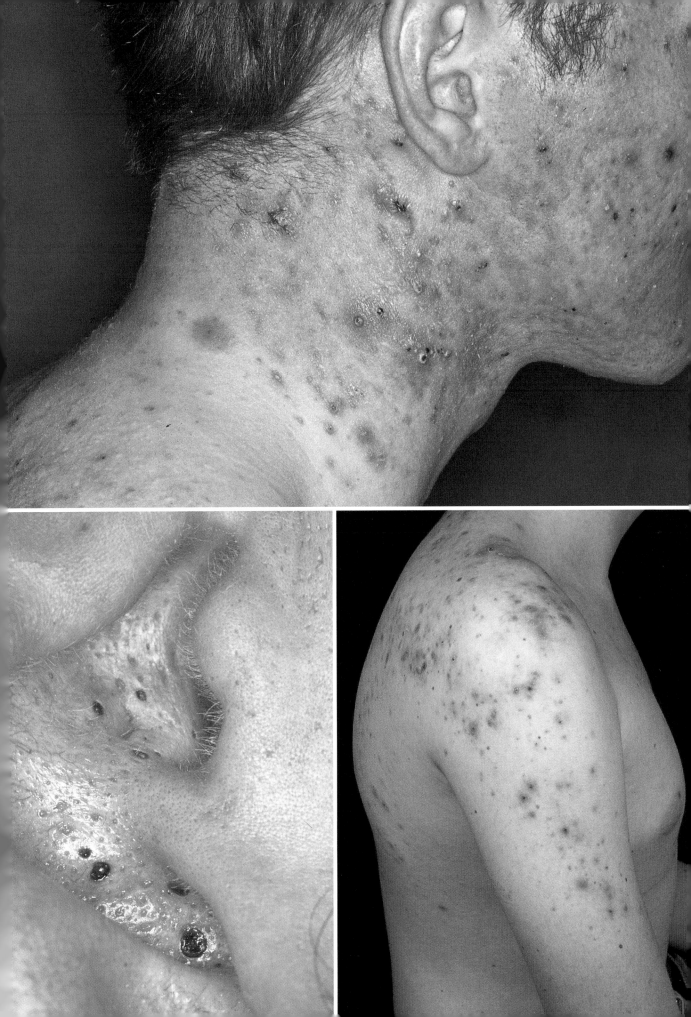

Odd Locations

In severe acne one frequently finds ectopic lesions in regions well outside the usual sites of acne.

Above   Acne in and behind the ears

Left   There are numerous, large, secondary, closed comedones behind the ear and over the mastoid. These persist for years and occasionally rupture, causing painful abscesses

Right   Open and closed comedones and a ruptured closed comedo, presenting as an abscess in the auditory canal

Below

Left   Papules, nodules, and scarring on the lower arms in a patient with acne conglobata

Right   While the trunk is the typical localization, the shoulders, nape, and hairy scalp may also show the savages of acne conglobata

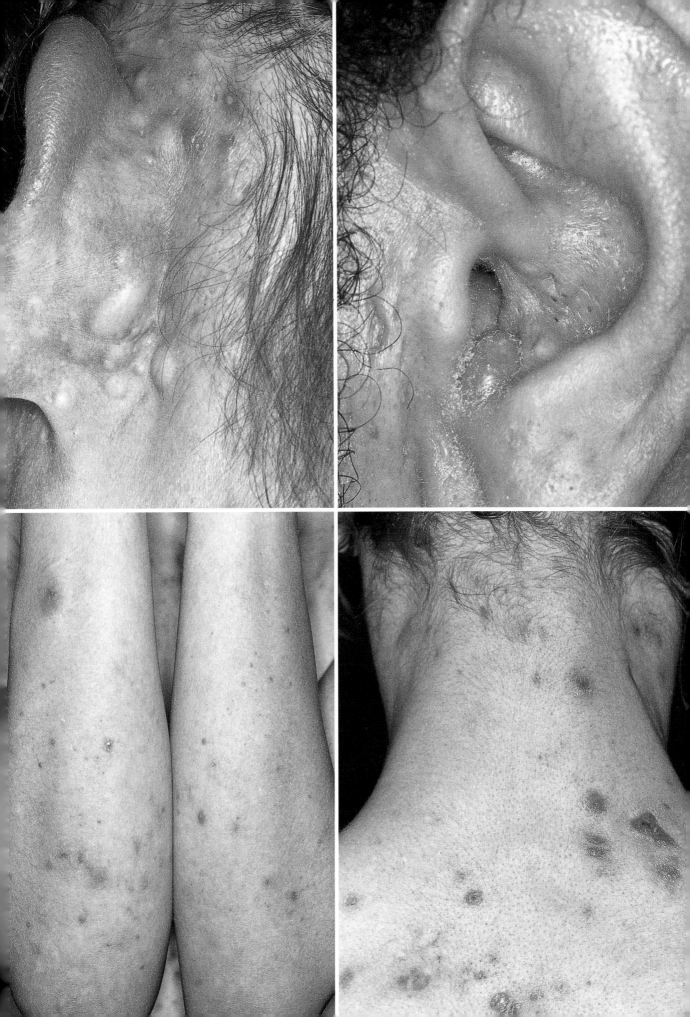

Victory Over a Terrible Disease: Acne Conglobata — Before Treatment

This 15-year-old boy had terrifying acne conglobata. A great mixture of inflammatory lesions and scars coexist. There are also linear draining sinuses alongside the nose, on the glabella, and nasolabial folds. In addition to disfigurement these lesions are tender and painful. The pitiful figure of Job depicted in the Bible could not have been more devastating.

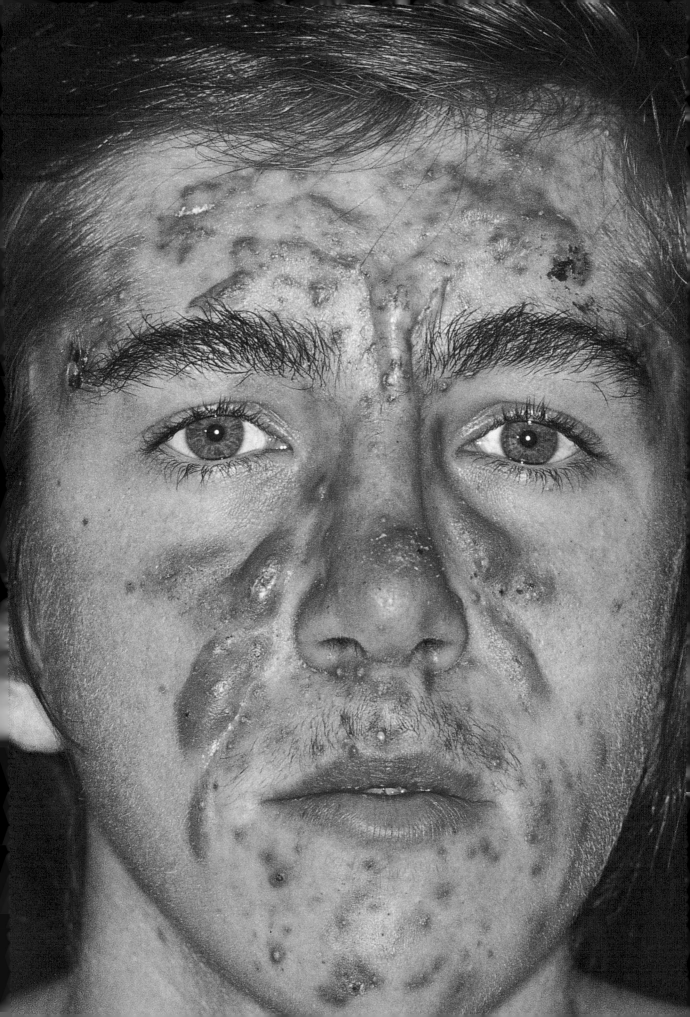

Four Months Later: Voilà!

Even before 1979, when isotretinoin first became available, acne conglobata could be successfully treated, as shown in this patient.

All that remains are some pustules. An all-out therapeutic attack was mounted in this horrendous case:

- Tretinoin was applied twice daily
- The nodules were injected with triamcinolone acetonide, some two or three times
- Dapsone (DDS), 100 mg daily, was given for 3 months
- This was accompanied by a full dose of tetracycline, 1000 mg twice daily, for several months

This patient has been satisfactory maintained on tretinoin alone.

Today one would start this patient on oral and topical corticosteroids and, followed within days, by isotretinoin

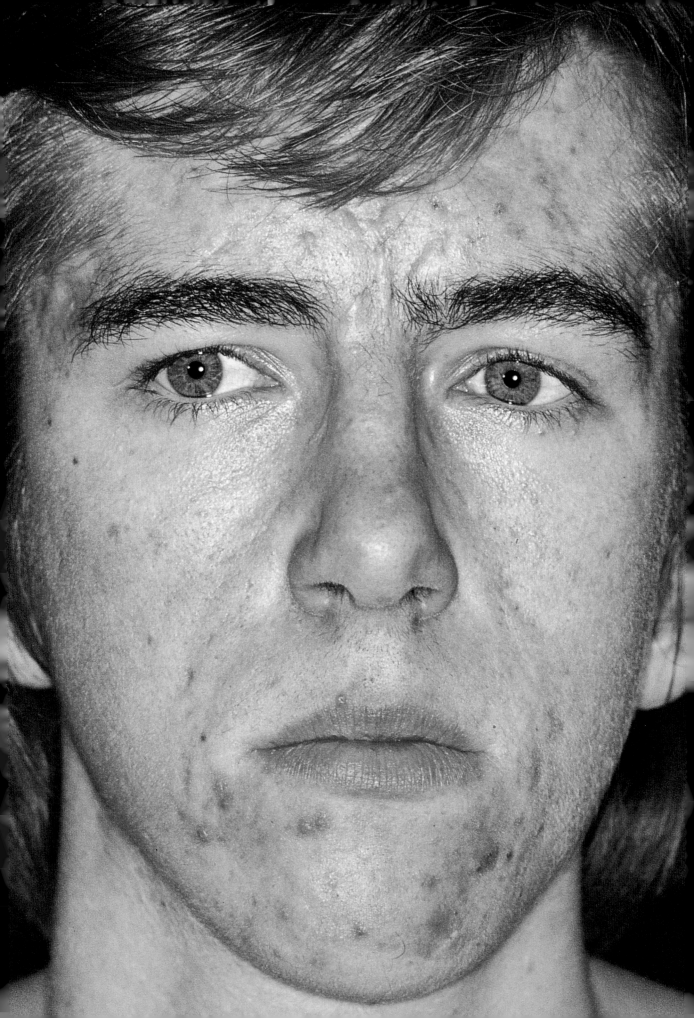

Acne Inversa

Unusual variants of a disease have generated considerable confusion regarding classification and pathogenesis. For instance it took a long time before it was understood that pustular psoriasis of von Zumbusch, pustular erythema annularis centrifugum, the inverse type of Barber-Königsbeck, and acrodermatitis suppurativa chronica of Hallopeau were all distinctive expressions of one disease: psoriasis vulgaris. The same can be said for certain variants of acne vulgaris, especially the condition described in this chapter, acne inversa.

What today we call acne inversa has lurked in the literature under several synonyms, namely, acne triad, acne tetrad, and hidradenitis suppurativa. It is time to flush out all out-dated synonyms and taxonomic ambiguities for this multifaceted disease.

Historical Background

Dissecting cellulitis of the scalp (perifolliculitis capitis abscedens et suffodiens) was described in 1907 by Hoffmann, but it was not connected with acne. Kierland wrote an influential paper on this entity in 1951. Unfortunately, he concluded that the target of the disease was the apocrine gland. A few years later in 1956 Pillsbury, Shelley, and Kligman coined the term "follicular occlusion triad" to encompass acne conglobata, hidradenitis suppurativa, and dissecting cellulitis. They argued that the central pathogenetic event, as in acne vulgaris, was follicular hyperkeratinization, distention of the infundibulum leading to rupture and colonization with a variety of pathogenic bacteria. They viewed retention hyperkeratosis as the primary event but, again, they thought that the vast destruction of tissue was a consequence of the involvement of the apocrine gland. To the original acne triad, we added another feature, the pilonidal sinus, to create the full picture of acne tetrad.

The important features of acne inversa are:

- Adults (not juveniles as in acne vulgaris) are affected
- Secondary comedones with multiple openings, linking two or more follicles
- Abscesses with communicating epithelium-lined channels (dissecting cellulitis)
- Draining sinuses in unusual locations, burrowing deeply into the skin of the groin, buttocks, perianal region, breast, and even the extremities
- Tendency towards deforming hypertrophic scars and contractures, particularly in the axillae and groin

Identifying Acne Inversa

Acne inversa is not rare, but frequently overlooked because of inadequate physical examination. The presence of one member of the tetrad indicates a search for lesions elsewhere. In some series there are more men than women, in others the

284

opposite. Typically the patients have fought this devastating disease for decades and have multiple areas of involvement. Acne conglobata is prominent in almost all patients, extending to the nape, retroauricular area, scalp, back, chest, mammary folds, axillae, groin, genitalia, perineum, anal fold, and buttocks. These ectopic lesions explain our term "acne inversa." The nape of the neck and the entire scalp can be affected, leaving scarring alopecia and tufted hairs protruding from the scalp. In women the submammary region can be involved bilaterally. The axillae and groin often display draining sinuses or extensive tissue destruction with monstrous scarring. Contractions may immobilize the arms. Pus draining from multiple foci creates a foul odor, an additional curse of this debilitating disease.

Sometimes the groin is involved. In extreme cases the entire anogenital region, including perineum, buttocks, anal fold, mons pubis, labia majora, and adjacent areas of the thighs may be devastated by sinuses and scars associated with pain and great discomfort. The draining sinus in the anal fold is synonymous with the familiar pilonidal sinus or pilonidal cyst. It can occur alone, of course, and this is also true for the other components of acne inversa. In some victims the disease progresses relentlessly. The sinuses can dissect deeply into tissue, far more than can be estimated clinically. Only radiologic imaging techniques and surgery uncover the massive penetration. Sinuses and abscesses make their way through muscles and fascia and bridge right and left sides of the body. The disease smolders wildly often for months and years. Painful and fluctuant furunculoid nodules signal new activity. These do not heal as they are part of the labyrinthian underworld of sinuses. The genitalia are not spared. Monstrous elephantiasis nostras-like swellings of penis, scrotum, or

vulva with total disruption of the genital anatomy are hellish outcomes.

Bacterial superinfection aggravates and propels the disease. A great variety of microorganisms can be isolated, often in combination. These include streptococci, gram-positive and gram-negative cocci and rods, and the full range of fecal bacteria. Usually these are not organisms of high virulence, such as β-hemolytic streptococci or *Staphylococcus aureus*. The microbiologic flora changes unpredictably. Early reports emphasized the role of bacteria, especially if virulent organisms were recovered. We regard bacterial infection as secondary to tissue destruction. In this milieu almost any organism can become invasive.

Excess body weight is not a primary although a complicating factor. Friction in wet intertriginous areas of course promotes follicular breakdown.

Abnormal levels of testosterone, androstendione, estrogen, and progesterone, along with menstrual irregularities and hirsutism have sometimes been reported, but the relevance of these abnormalities is questionable, and studies of androgen metabolism are inconclusive. It was only recently shown that apocrine glands are not targets of androgen metabolism.

Complications of Long-Standing Acne Inversa

Acne inversa is a disabling disease. Patients typically have consulted many physicians and received differing opinions regarding etiology and treatment. Many become desperate and depressed. The soiling of underwear, other clothing and bed linen, and an offending foul odor reduces all social and sexual contacts. Dermal contractions and painful inflammatory nodules finally turn them into outcasts. Hostility is frequent and understandable. The biblical afflictions of Job apply poignantly to acne inversa. Of course, none of these patients is healthy, variably suffering from fatigue, malaise, sleeplessness, etc.

Rarely the disease is life-threatening. Complications include squamous cell carcinoma (Marjolin ulcer) with metastases, a pitiful outcome which we have witnessed ourselves. Bacterial meningitis and systemic amyloidosis are rare but serious consequences.

Histopathology

Acne is a disease of the sebaceous follicles. Acne inversa localizes in nonfacial regions where there are terminal, pigmented, coarse hairs as in the axillae, groins, anal fold, mons pubis, and scalp. These regions tend to be rich in apocrine sweat glands, which are part of the apocrine–pilosebaceous unit. Thus it is understandable that the apocrine glands would also be engulfed in the necrotizing process. We regard apocrine involvement, serious as it might be, as a secondary event. The identical destructive process may occur in the absence of apocrine glands.

We have studied the histopathology of many patients with acne inversa. Control specimens were obtained from individuals undergoing surgical excision of axillary skin for the treatment of hyperhidrosis. The sections were cut stepwise, with particular attention paid to early histologic changes. The coiled, secretory portion of the apocrine sweat gland lies deeply in the subcutaneous fat. Apocrine sweat ascends through a long duct emptying into the infundibulum of the terminal hair follicle, just above the entrance of the sebaceous duct. Unlike eccrine glands, the secretory product is not delivered directly to the surface. It should be emphasized that apocrine sweat glands are characteristically found in body regions affected by acne inversa. This has confounded proper interpretion from the very start.

Acne vulgaris begins with retention hyperkeratosis of the infundibula of sebaceous follicles. The resulting comedo is the primary pathological event. Follicular rupture, inflammation, and re-encapsulation are secondary events. In contrast to acne vulgaris, acne inversa begins in terminal follicles, but the fundamental change is the same, namely, compact hyperkeratosis of the infundibulum giving rise to comedo-like horny impactions. The earliest inflammatory event is a segmental rupture of the follicular epithelium, spilling foreign-body material such as corneocytes, bacteria, sebum products, and hairs into the dermis. The dumping of foreign products excites first an infiltrate of granulocytes, followed by mononuclear cells, eventuating in a foreign-body granuloma. Epithelial strands try in vain to encapsulate the necrotic tissue. Secondary comedones are a conspicious picture of this disease.

In the earliest stage of follicular hyperkeratosis apocrine and eccrine sweat glands are not involved. Once rupture has occurred, the disease spreads rapidly, liquefying everything in its path. The reason for the rupture is unknown. Friction in intertriginous locations may be a contributory factor but cannot explain acne inversa on the nape of the neck and the hairy scalp. Secondary bacterial colonization in warm sweating armpits, anal fold, and groin certainly enhances and intensifies chronic inflammation. Far-flung abscesses dissecting through the dermis reach the subcutaneous fat and cause lobular and septal panniculitis. The abscesses engulf everything in their path, including eccrine and apocrine glands. One can easily observe how the inflammatory infiltrate gains access to the sweat gland apparatus. Pus migrates down through the ducts and engulfs the secretory coils. From there suppuration can dissect back to the skin surface. Draining sinuses may tunnel their way through fat and muscles. Similar events occur in dissecting cellulitis of the scalp and in the pilonidal cyst.

Acne inversa is a highly chronic disorder, but the understanding of its pathogenesis is still very limited. Apocrine glands do not bear increased numbers of androgen receptors. Abnormalities of the cellular or humoral immune system cannot be held to be responsible for the disease. Not unexpectedly, multiple laboratory abnormalities may be found, i.e., elevated erythrocyte sedimentation rate, leukocytosis, low serum iron, anemia, changes in serum electrophoresis pattern, etc. All of these are secondary phase-reaction events. Cell-mediated immunity may be depressed, but, again, this is secondary. Congenital α_1-antitrypsin deficiency has been reported, but could not be confirmed by us in a large series of patients.

In several patients there is a tremendous tendency toward dermal contractures, particularly in the armpits. Erysipelas is rare, but does occur in the genitoanal region; elephantiasis nostras-like swellings superimpose on acne inversa lesions.

Genetics

A genetic predisposition is well established in acne vulgaris. Seborrhea is the common background, an inherited trait. Heredity is probably also important in acne inversa but information is fragmentary. Familial occurrence of acne inversa has been reported. Acne conglobata occurs frequently in first-order relatives. A complete history should look into the family pedigree.

Differential Diagnosis

Acne inversa is often a diagnostic challenge. Even dermatologists are bewildered by odd variants of this disease. Sometimes one finds involvement of only one side of the groin or one axilla, or almost exclusive confinement to perineum, buttocks, and mons pubis. Secondary elephantiasis following streptococcal infection (elephantiasis nostras) with monstrous enlargement and distortion of external genitalia is rarely identified as an expression of acne inversa.

Furuncles in the axillae are commonly mistaken for acne inversa. Furuncles are *Staphylococcus aureus* infections with a distinct morphology and clinical course. Carbuncles must also be differentiated. These infections do not dissect through tissue and do not form sinuses. Other regional fistulating and granulomatous diseases have to be excluded. These include enteritis regionalis or ileitis terminalis (Crohn's disease), actinomycosis, tuberculosis, and granulomas. Finally, rectal fistulas have to be considered.

Treatment

A huge array of therapies has been tried. They range from X-rays including depilating doses to the armpits or the scalp, surgical excision with grafts, antiandrogens, vaccines, oral metronidazole, and antibiotics. None of these has been effective. Recently isotretinoin has been tried but with inconsistent results.

Acne inversa calls for a determined patient and a determined physician. The physician has to be both decisive and optimistic. Patients must be informed about the aggressive and progressive nature of the disease and the uselessness of waiting. Surgical treatment must be performed at the earliest recognized stage. This is crucial. All other measures such as antibiotics are complementary. Surgical plans should be discussed early on. Wide excision, well beyond the clinical borders of activity, is mandatory, regardless of the localization. Often it is necessary to operate stepwise on both axillae, the neck, perineum, mons pubis, and groins en bloc. Butterfly-shaped wide excisions in the genitoanal region may be indicated. Various techniques for plastic repair can be offered: (a) excision and allowance for granulation with secondary re-epithelization, (b) excision and allowance for temporary granulation with free grafting (full thickness, split or mesh) 7–14 days later, (c) excision and primary free grafting, (4) rotation flaps, or (5) even muscle flaps. Debridement of genital elephantiasis nostras has been performed with respectable results. In experienced hands, the results are surprisingly good. Scarring is inevitable, but the disease can be arrested.

should be used only after consultation with the surgeon and the anesthesist. Laser treatment has not been evaluated in this disease, but vaporization with a carbon dioxide laser might be useful in selected cases.

Outlook

Many patients with acne inversa drift away from society. The hardships may lead to unemployment, depression, alcoholism, divorce, and obesity. Nonsurgical therapies are a waste of time and allow the disease to worsen before the patient reaches the operating theater. Early diagnosis and a resolute approach with the scalpel bring gratifying rewards.

Pre- and Postoperative Adjuncts

Isotretinoin given daily for 3–4 months is an effective prelude to surgery. The drug has anti-inflammatory activity and can drastically reduce suppuration and edema. It also reduces the volume of the sebaceous glands. This pretreatment facilitates surgical excision and repair. To avoid new dissecting lesions, the drug can also be given postoperatively. The dose is individualized and ranges from 0.2–2.0 mg per kg body weight daily. The teratogenicity of isotretinoin has to be kept in mind for women of child-bearing age (p. 635). Isotretinoin generally results in improvement, sometimes impressively, but relapse is inevitable after withdrawal. We emphasize that surgery is the sine qua non of successful therapy.

We have also given corticosteroids systemically in addition to isotretinoin as another anti-inflammatory adjunct before operation in severely affected patients. The course is limited to a few weeks. Usually 1.0 mg prednisolone/kg body weight per day is given. Steroids

Barth JH, Kealey T (1991) Androgen metabolism by isolated human axillary apocrine glands in hidradenitis suppurativa. Br J Dermatol 125:304–308

Boyd AS, Zemtsov A (1992) A case of pyoderma vegetans and the follicular occlusion triad. J Dermatol 19:61–63

Brunsting HA (1952) Hidradenitis and other variants of acne. Arch Dermatol Syph 65:303–315

Burrows NP, Russell Jones R (1992) Crohn's disease in association with hidradenitis suppurativa. Br J Dermatol 126:523

Duperrat MM, Meunier, Pringuet R (1957) Acné conglobata fessière. Discussion d'une amylose secondaire. Bull Soc Fr Dermatol Syph 64:264–266

Fitzsimmons JS, Guilbert PR, Fitzsimmons EM (1985) Evidence of genetic factors in hidradenitis suppurativa. Br J Dermatol 113:1–8

Grösser A (1982) Surgical treatment of chronic axillary and genitocrural acne conglobata by split-thickness skin grafting. J Dermatol Surg Oncol 8:391–398

Harrison BJ, Mudge M, Hughes LE (1987) Recurrence after surgical treatment of hidradenitis suppurativa. Br Med J 294:487–489

Hughes LE, Harrison BJ, Mudge M (1989) Surgical management of hidradenitis – principles and results. In: Marks R, Plewig G (eds) Acne and related disorders. Dunitz, London, pp 367–370

Jemec GBE (1988) Effect of localized surgical excisions in hidradenitis suppurativa. J Am Acad Dermatol 18:1103–1107

Kierland RR (1951) Unusual pyodermas (hidrosadenitis suppurativa, acne congliobata, dissecting cellulitis of the scalp). A review. Minn Med 34:319–341

Lange W, Düring B, Osterloh B, Lepsien G (1992) Die chirurgische Therapie der Pyodermia fistulans sinifica (P.f.s.). Z Hautkr 67:341–344

Küster W, Rödder-Wehrmann O, Plewig G (1991) Acne inversa. Pathogenese und Genetik. Hautarzt 42:2–4

Mendonça H, Rebelo C, Fernandes A, Lino A, Silva LG (1991) Squamous cell carcinoma arising in hidradenitis suppurativa. J Dermatol Surg Oncol 17:830–832

Ostlere LS, Langtry JAA, Mortimer PS, Staughton RCD (1991) Hidradenitis suppurativa in Crohn's disease. Br J Dermatol 125:384–386

Pillsbury DM, Shelley WB, Kligman AM (1956) Bacterial infections of the skin. In: Dermatology, 1st edn. Saunders, Philadelphia, pp 482–484, 489

Plewig G, Steger M (1989) Acne inversa (alias acne triad, acne tetrad or hidradenitis suppurativa). In: Marks R, Plewig G (eds) Acne and related disorders. Dunitz, London, pp. 345–357

Quintal D, Jackson R (1986) Aggressive squamous cell carcinoma arising in familial acne conglobata. J Am Acad Dermatol 14:207–214

Rödder-Wehrmann O, Küster W, Plewig G (1991) Acne inversa. Diagnose und Therapie. Hautarzt 42:5–8

Schewach-Millet M, Ziv R, Shapira D (1986) Perifolliculitis capitis abscedens et suffodiens treated with isotretinoin (13-*cis*-retinoic acid). J Am Acad Dermatol 15:1291–1292

Weinrauch L, Peled I, Hacham-Zadeh S, Wexler MR (1981) Surgical treatment of severe acne conglobata. J Dermatol Surg Oncol 7:492–494

Whipp MJ, Harrington CI, Dundas S (1987) Fatal squamous cell carcinoma associated with acne conglobata in a father and daughter. Br J Dermatol 117:389–392

Yu CCW, Cook MG (1990) Hidradenitis suppurativa: a disease of follicular epithelium, rather than apocrine glands. Br J Dermatol 122:763–769

The Anatomy of Apocrine Sweat Glands

The topographic and histologic anatomy of apocrine sweat glands is presented here. Erroneously, apocrine sweat glands are thought to play an etiologic role in acne inversa (hidradenitis suppurativa).

Above Overview of normal axillary skin of a patient with hyperhidrosis. Beneath the epidermis is the bed of collagen (stained blue) with sebaceous follicles (—➤). Further below is the subcutaneous fat tissue, in which are embedded coarse terminal hairs (stained red), and a multitude of apocrine (o➤) and eccrine (●➤) sweat glands. (Trichromate)

Below Close-up view of the apocrine sweat gland apparatus of a patient with axillary acne inversa. The spatious cavities of the apocrine gland yield into one draining ampulla (✳), which merges into a straight ascending apocrine duct (—➤). This duct joins the follicular canal of the hair follicle (◇) a little further up. Unlike eccrine sweat ducts, which connect directly with the skin surface via the acroinfundibulum, apocrine sweat glands communicate only indirectly with the skin surface via follicular canals. There are very few exceptions. (Hematoxilin- and eosin)

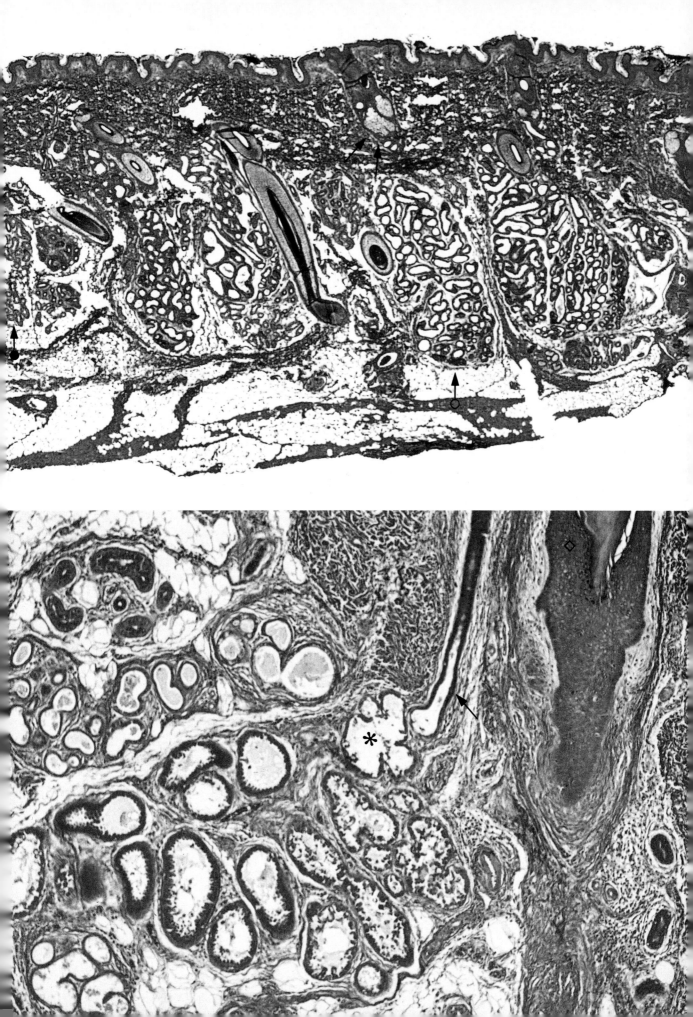

Acne Inversa: The Importance of Proper Biopsies

Like in many other diseases, much of what one sees and therefore interprets depends on the selection of histopathologic specimens. Biopsies from apparently normal skin or from very early inflammatory events, less than a few days old, and serial sections are prerequisites.

Above   Follicular hyperkeratosis

Left   In the armpit there are many terminal hair follicles, but only a very few sebaceous follicles. The earliest histologic changes one can find are micro-comedo-like impactions of keratinized material in terminal follicles. The hair is shown at the bottom

Right   A further development is a closed comedo-like structure, again, in a terminal hair follicle. The keratinizing portion of the apocrine duct entering the follicle (apocrine acrosyringium) is to the right (A). There is no inflammation yet

Below

Left   The apocrine gland (⟶), its draining ampulla (✱), and the stretched duct yielding above into the terminal hair follicle (T) with a keratinizing acrosyringium (A) all look intact

Right   Earliest inflammatory events can be located at the follicular epithelium of a terminal hair follicle, breaking wide open. The follicle becomes acanthotic. The apocrine duct (⟶) is still intact, though surrounded by inflammation. It shares a common exit (apocrine acrosyringium, A) with the terminal hair follicle, a rare variant of the topographic histology of apocrine glands

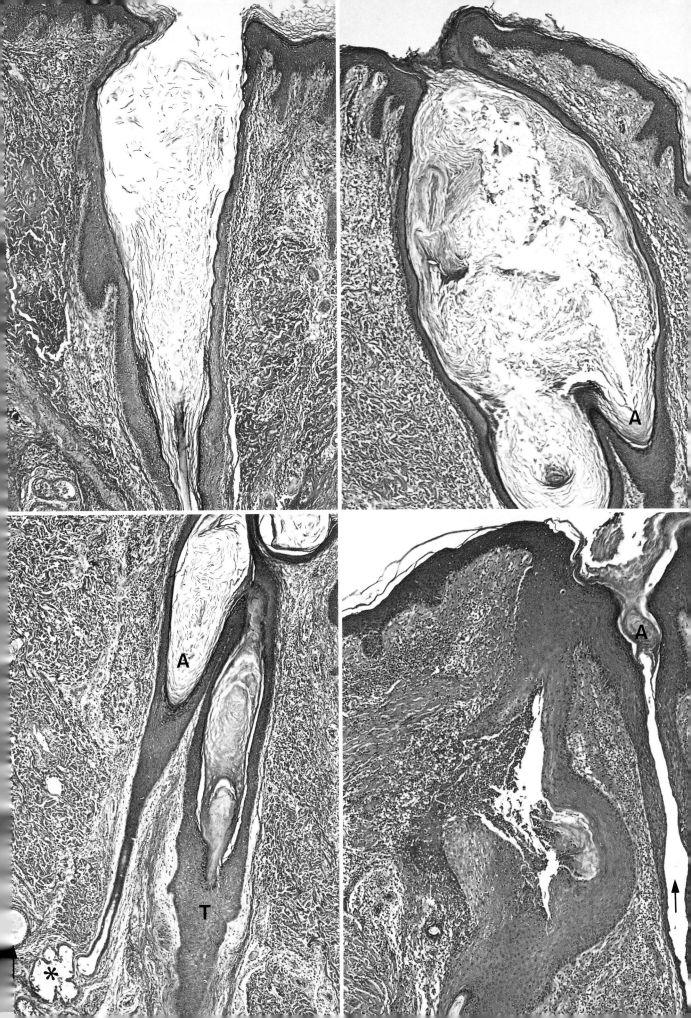

Acne Inversa – Devastating Inflammation

Above Early inflammatory stage of acne inversa in the armpit. The epidermis and upper corium look serene. The lower corium and adjacent subcutaneous fat, however, show widespread and dissecting abscesses destroying all anatomic structures

Below Acne inversa of the mons pubis. The entire dermis is filled by a widespread abscess, parts of which have been lost during histological preparation. Epithelial lined segments try to encapsulate the abscess. The final outcome will be a persistent, fistulating, epithelialized sinus tract

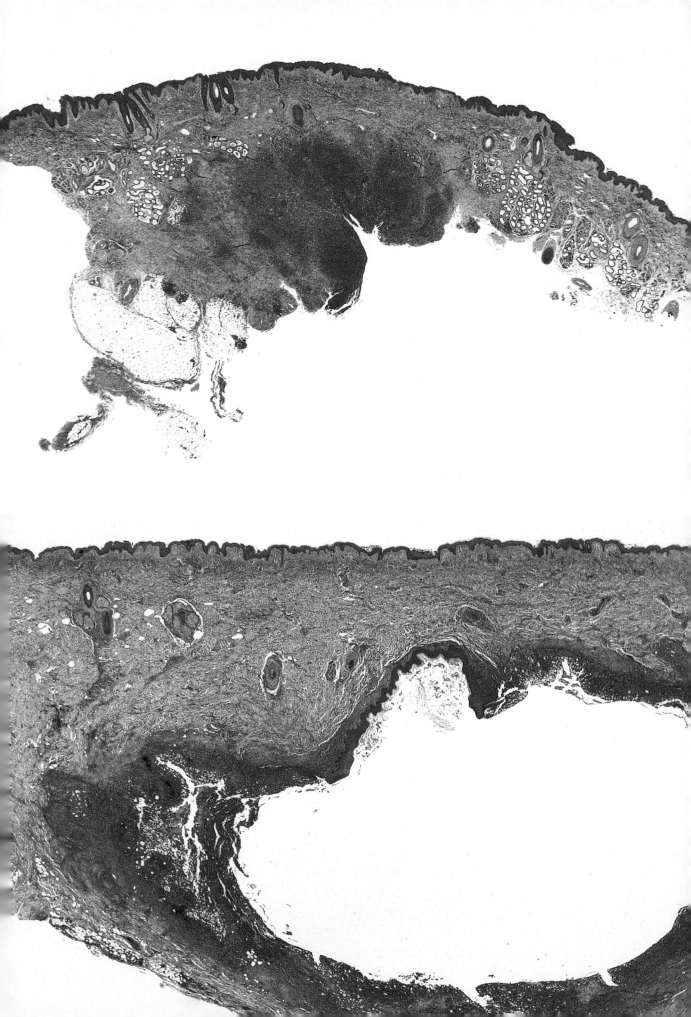

Dissecting Phenomena in Acne Inversa

Late stages in acne inversa are not amenable to pharmacological approaches. Once tunneled labyrinths have formed, only surgical approaches are meaningful.

Above   Acne inversa in the armpit. This overview tells the tragedy of the disease. Apocrine and eccrine sweat glands look serene, the trouble is deeper down. Epithelial lined dissecting tracts with vast inflammatory changes in their vicinity and lost strands of epithelium account for the chronicity of the disease

Below

Left   Acne inversa in the armpit. Again the sweat glands are not involved. A gigantic burrowing tract, furnished with restless epithelium, grows relentless into all directions. Fibrosis is in his neighborhood. The foul discharge in these patients is drained through such tracts towards the surface

Right   Acne inversa from the mons pubis. A fistulated tract, a draining sinus, has multiple openings, two of which are shown here. The entire dermis is scarred, the adnexa are wiped out

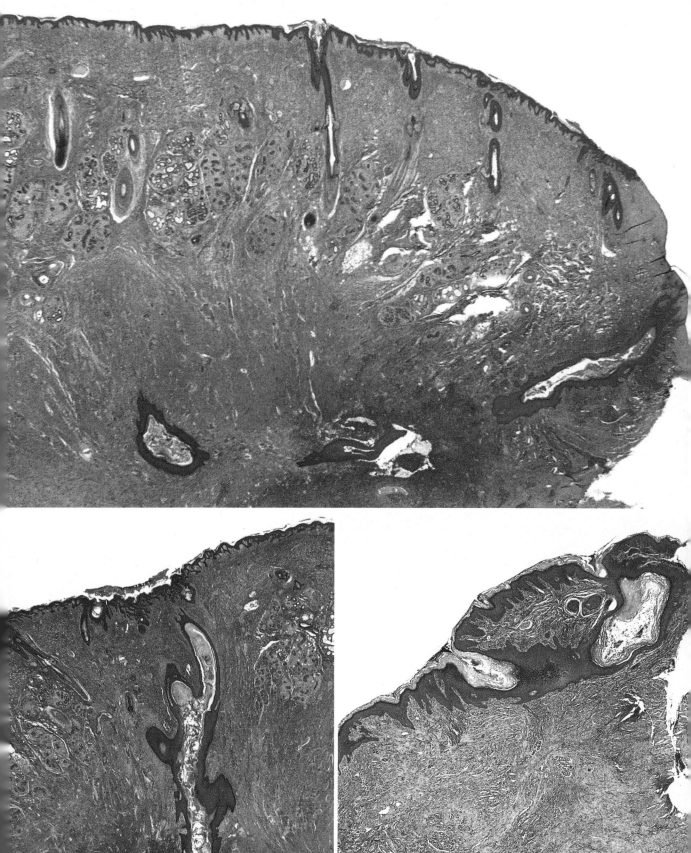

Dissecting Draining Sinuses in Acne Inversa

Not initial but late events in this variant of acne are horrible fistulating tracts. Once having seen this histopathology one can understand why the therapeutic approach cannot be based on drug treatment alone.

Above Acne inversa of the inguinal region. Wired canyons cut through all directions of the dermis. Fantastic patterns of epithelial islands, some of which line tracts, are embedded in a hemorrhagic abscess. All pre-existing structures have been eradicated

Below Acne inversa of the armpit. The initial events of the disease, e.g., follicular hyperkeratosis, can still be appreciated. Epithelial-lined, broad channels connect the skin surface with the subcutaneous fat and burrow into new territories, heralded by septal panniculitis

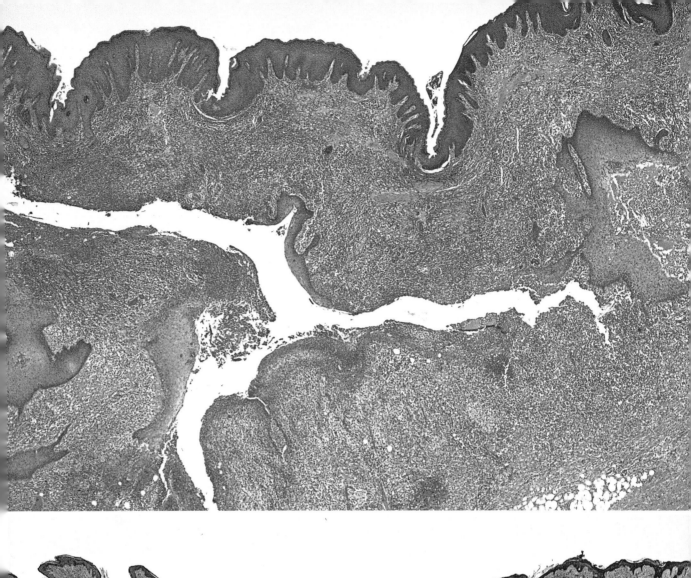
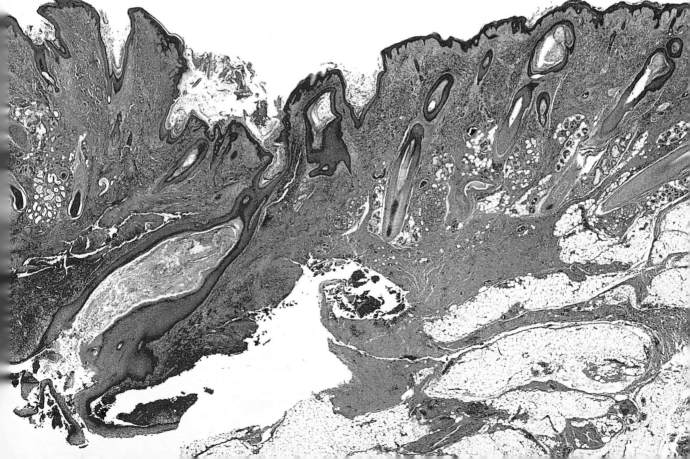

Acne Inversa: Violent and Generalized

Acne is everywhere on the body of this hapless man, particularly in the intertriginous areas.

Above   Both armpits, upper arms, and chest are covered with deep seated nodules, draining sinuses, and fistulated comedones. Fortunately there are as yet no dermal contractures. Superinfections by virulent organisms soil his clothing and produce offensive odors.

Below

Left   Scarring inflammatory lesions of the groin are painful. Some have left anetoderma-like atrophic scarring due to postinflammatory elastolysis

Right   The face is not spared. Nodules, papules, pustules, comedones, sebaceous gland hyperplasias, and, above all, multiple scars are late and disfiguring sequels of acne, lasting 35 years in this 49-year-old man. His facial expression is that of sadness

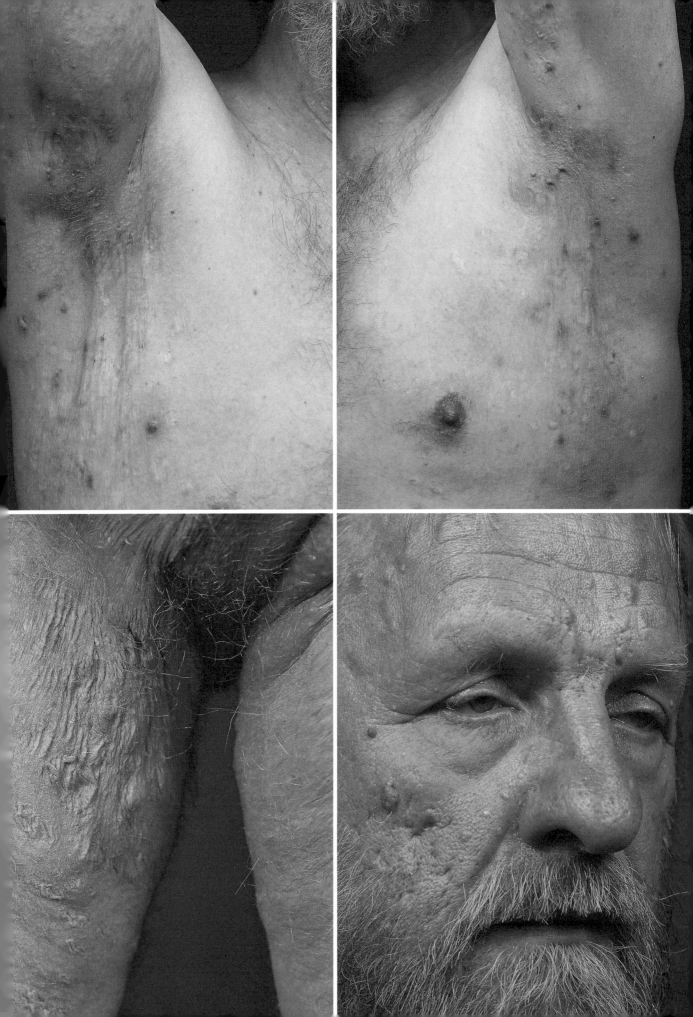

Acne Inversa: Differential Diagnosis

Diagnosis of acne inversa centers around a few diseases.

Above

Left   The small furuncles in the armpit represent a pyoderma. In this case *Staphylococcus aureus* can be recovered, a central necrosis is sloughed, and antibiotics induce prompt healing

Right   A tender furuncle in the armpit of a patient who suffers from chronically recurring furuncles (furunculosis). This man had also minor acne on his back, not shown here. *Staphylococcus aureus* was isolated from the furuncle

Below   In contrast to the furuncles shown above this is true acne inversa (*right* and *left*). Tunneled abscesses and dehiscing scars afflict both armpits. This condition requires quite different therapeutic strategies. The best is early surgical intervention with wide excision, primary closure, or grafting

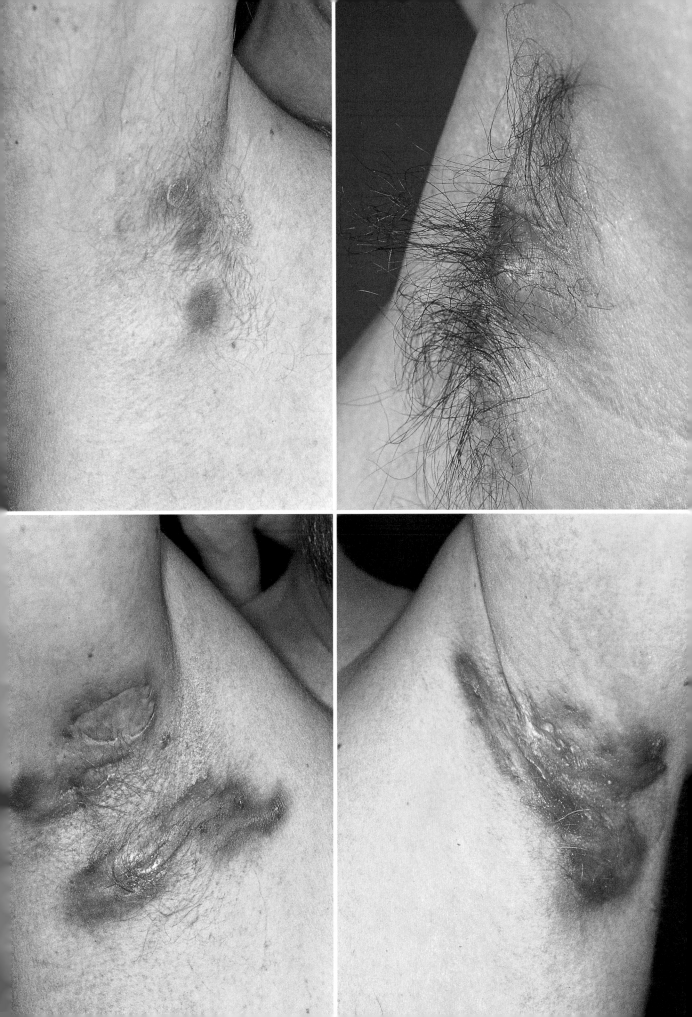

Acne Inversa: A Malicious Disease

Above   The disease at its worst. More than 30 years of abscesses in this 48-year-old man have bridged tunnels from right to left, through fascias and muscles, extending deep into the thighs. Amyloidosis and metastatic squamous cell carcinomas (Marjolin ulcer) with fatal outcome are feared complications, which we have witnessed in a few patients

Below

Left   This unfortunate women had a history of more than 35 years of ongoing mutilating disease with widespread abscesses of mons pubis, labia, inguinal folds, and buttocks

Right   The disease can encroach anywhere on the body. This is the same man as above, showing involvement of the popliteal space

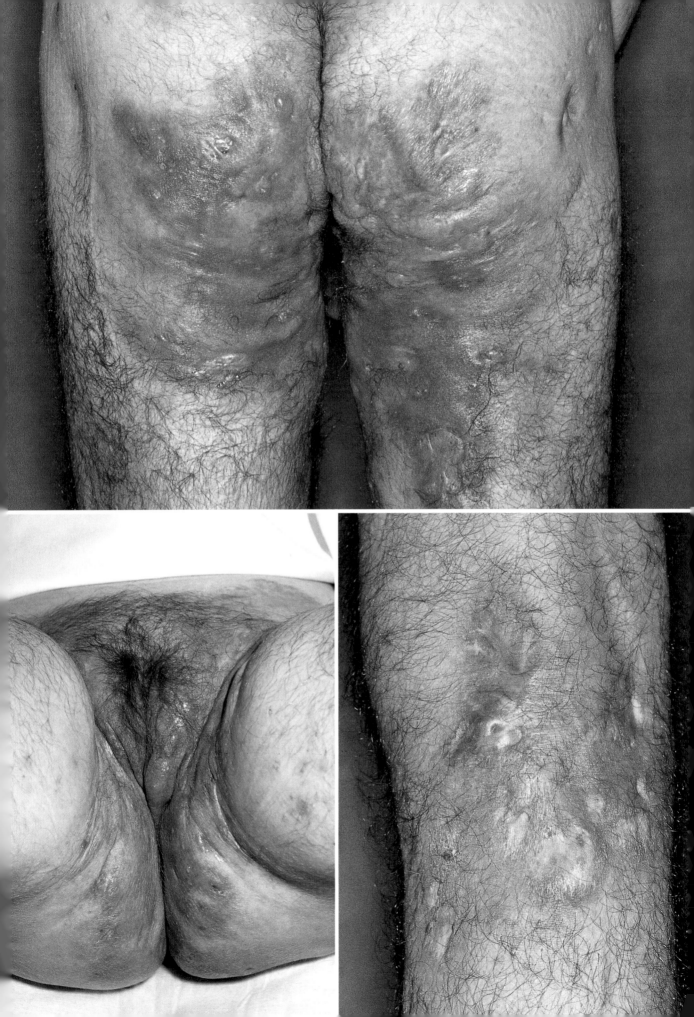

Dissecting Cellulitis of the Scalp

Above   Dissecting cellulitis of the hairy scalp is a terrible distructive disorder encompassing a variety of lesions. Fluctuant nodules and abscesses lead to a sclerosing alopecia accompanied by hemorrhagic suppuration and tufts of hair emerging from one distorted follicular orifice. The condition is quite painful. Pressure to any point of the scalp releases a foul smelling discharge. The final outcome is a burned-out hard fibrosis, with comedo-like scars

Below

Left   Close up the dissecting cellulitis showing bizarre-shaped areas of scarring which is hard and fibrotic

Right   This man has both acne keloidalis nuchae (shown here), still inflamed, with fresh satellite lesions in the periphery and dissecting cellulitis of the scalp (not seen here) and smoldering acne of the trunk

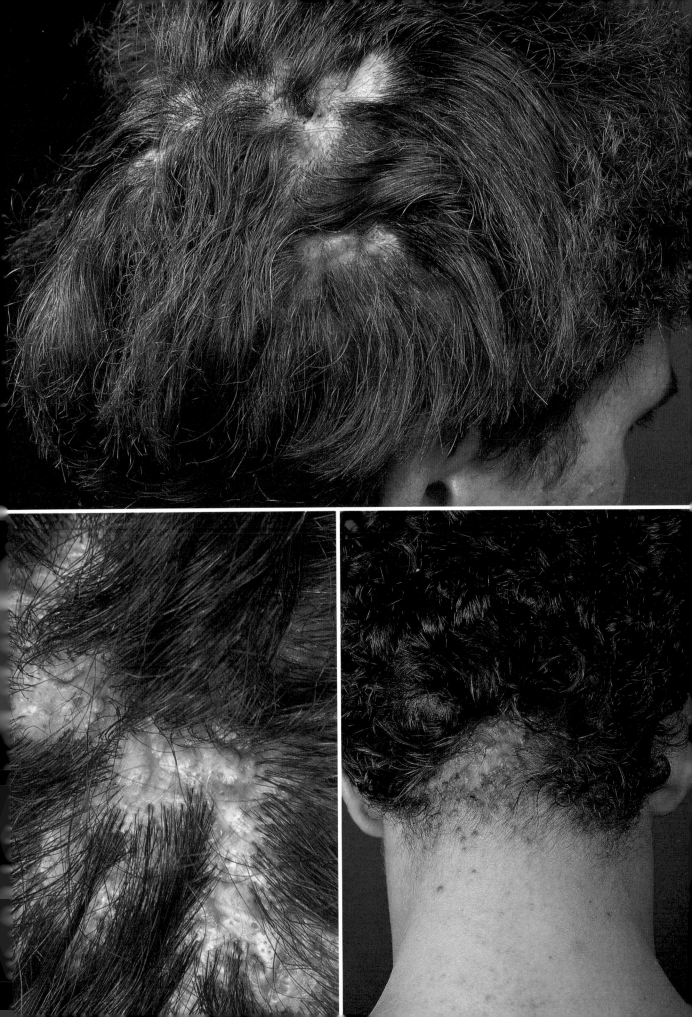

Acne Keloidalis Nuchae

Acne keloidalis nuchae is not a variant of acne. The pathogenesis is related to ingrown terminal hairs.

Above   Atrophic and hypertrophic scars have destroyed most of the hairy nape. Inflammation is still going on. This is a distressing condition which does not abate with time. Treatment of acne keloidalis nuchae is extremely difficult. Surgery is the only resource

Below   This excellent result was obtained by excision and primary closure. While some physicians favor destruction by laser or cryosurgery, incision with grafting yields the best final results and is curative. Pharmacologic approaches are useless

Herzberg AJ, Dinehart SM, Kerns BJ, Pollack SV (1990) Acne keloidales: transverse microscopy, immunohistochemistry, and electron microscopy. AM J Dermatopathol 12:109–121

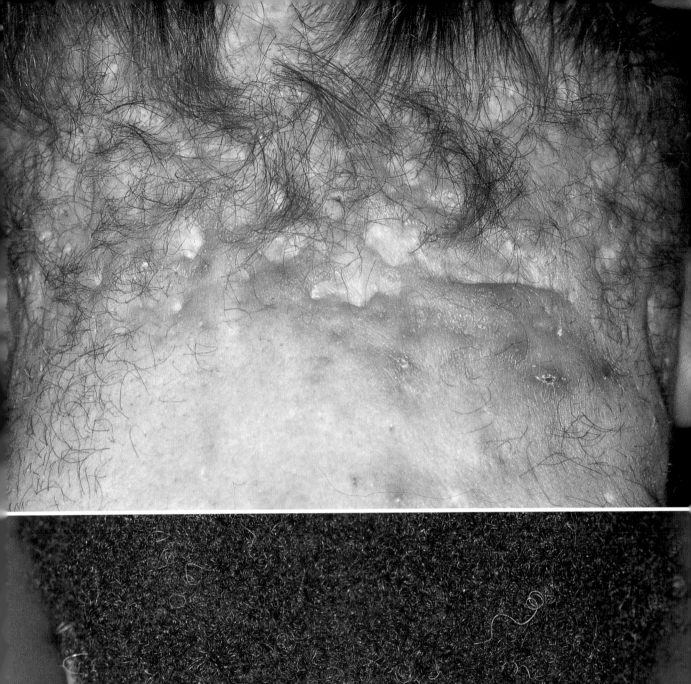
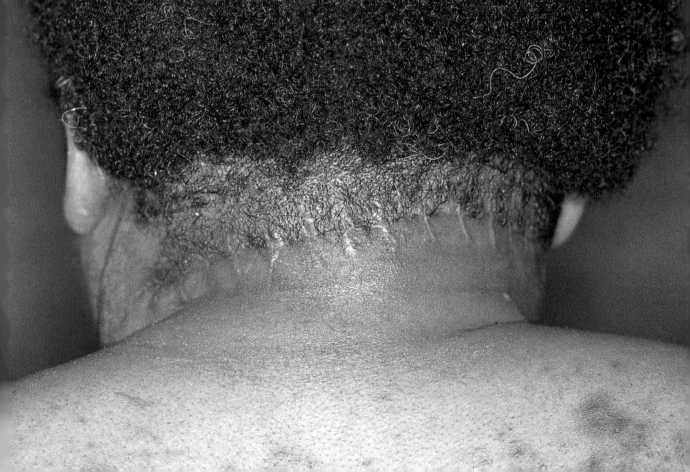

Hairy Problems

The scalp may be affected in acne patients.

Above

Left   Dissecting folliculitis has destroyed the topography of the hairy scalp. Chronic inflammation is still present with exudate, scales, crusts, and, above all, tufted hairs

Right   The gentleman has suffered from extensive dissecting folliculitis of the scalp, which has come to rest. A plaque on the nape is an example of acne keloidalis nuchae

Below   Acne keloidalis nuchae, still active with inflammation, follicular pustules, and tufted bushel-like hairs

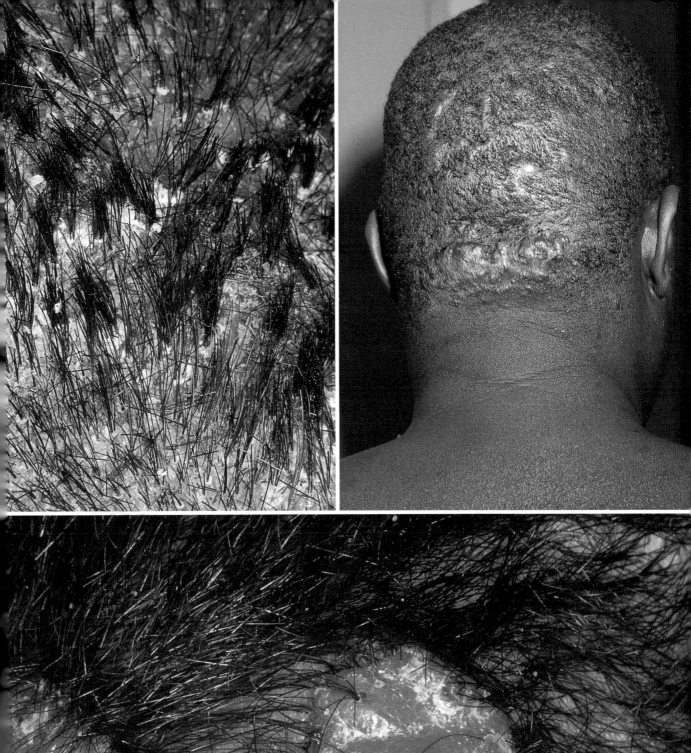
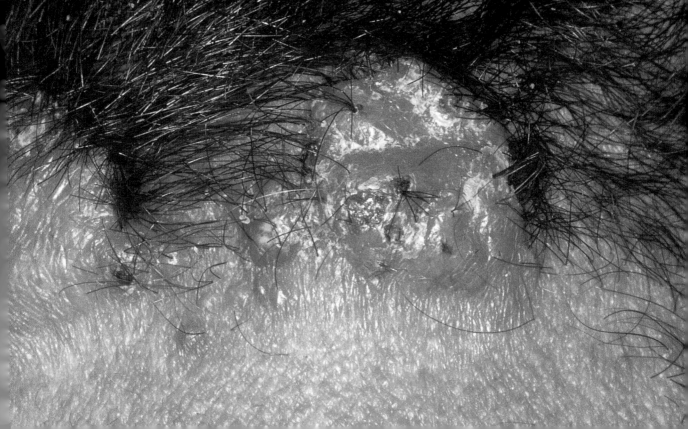

Acne Inversa

It is only recently that these monstrous intertriginous inflammatory, dissecting lesions were recognized as part of the multifarious acne spectrum. This and the following plates are meant to demonstrate the wide variety of skin lesions, body areas involved, extensiveness and intensiveness of skin destruction, therapeutic trials, and differential diagnosis.

Above Scars form bridges and canyons in the armpits; a foul-smelling fluid drains from multiple openings. Dermal contraction is extensive. Inflammatory, tender lesions have been present for decades

Below This patient was similarly afflicted. Shown here is the successful result of wide excisions down to the fascia followed by grafts. The patient is happy and completely resocialized

Below: Courtesy of Birger Konz, M.D., Munich, FRG

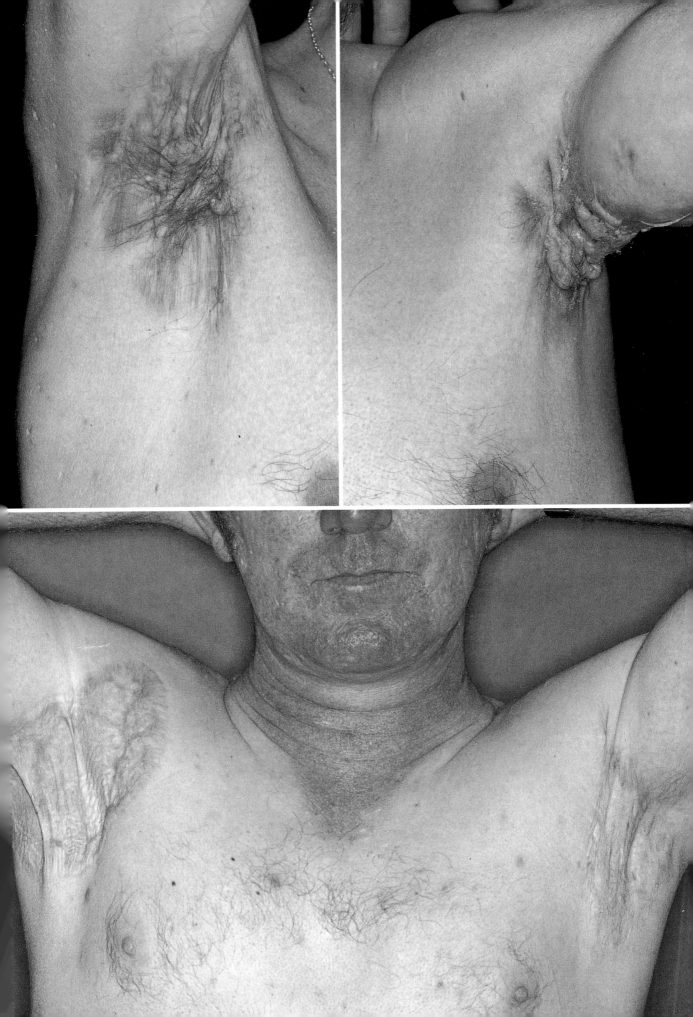

Acne Inversa: Genital Involvement

This man was constantly teased because of an apparent bulging mass in his pants. It was not what people thought, but rather a highly unusual manifestation of chronic inflammation, dissecting cellulitis, and scrotal and penile edema. Extensive acne inversa was found not only here but in both sides of the groin, anal fold, buttocks, and both axillae.

Serial reconstructions helped to relocate the penis and abandon the foul annoying smell emanating from body and clothes.

The operations were performed by Birger Konz, M.D., Axel Grösser, M.D., Department of Dermatology, and Professor Manfred Hofstetter, Department of Urology, University of Munich, FRG

Grösser A (1982) Surgical treatment of chronic axillary and genitocrural acne conglobata by split-thickness skin grafting. J Dermatol Surg Oncol 8:391–398

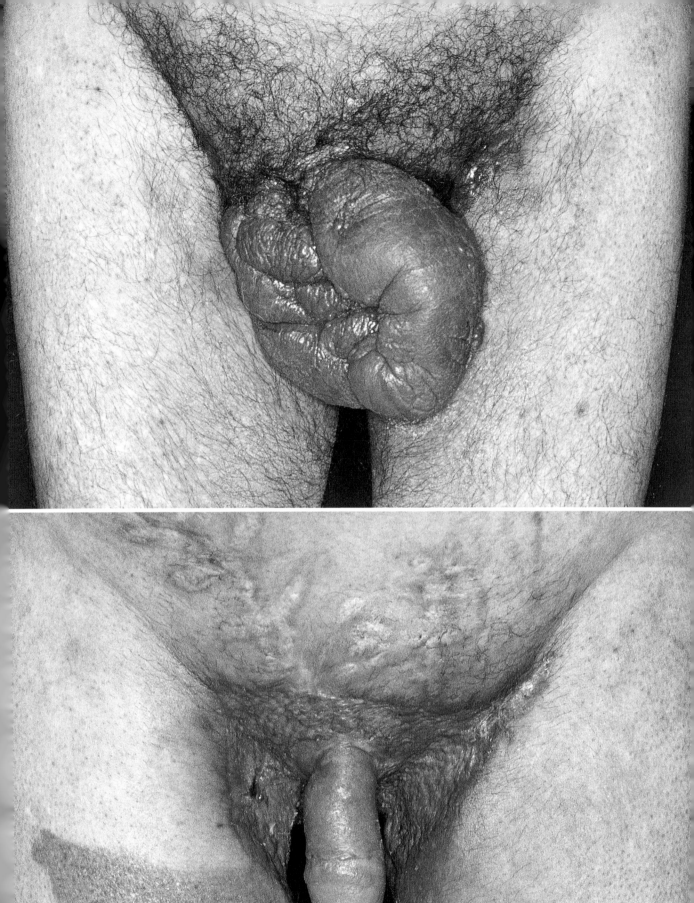

Acne Inversa: A Determined Surgical Approach

Axillary and in particular genital and inguinal involvement can be very successfully treated by wide surgical excision down to the fat tissue, and healing by secondary intention. The series of photographs was taken before (*above left*), at the end of the operation (*above right*), at 3 weeks (*below left*), and at 6 weeks (*below right*).

Courtesy of Michael Steger, M.D., Düsseldorf, FRG

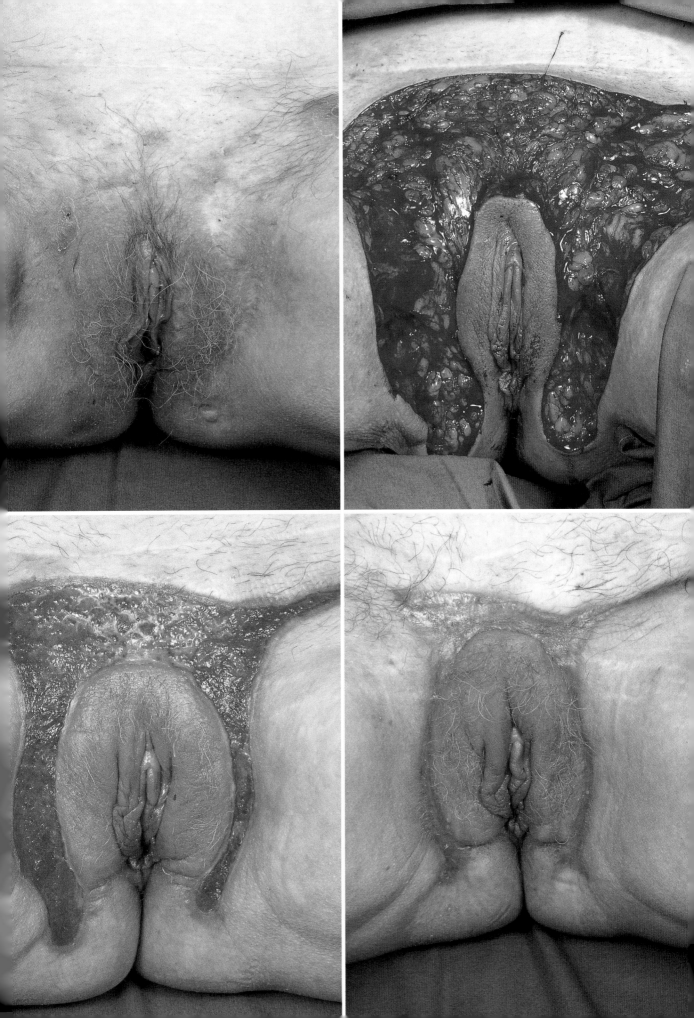

Acne Fulminans

This is a ferocious variety of acne with a typical set of clinical and laboratory findings, previously described under several designations such as acute febrile ulcerative conglobate acne with polyarthralgia, acute febrile ulcerative conglobate acne with leukemoid reaction, or acne maligna. It was renamed acne fulminans by us. Acne fulminans is an unforgettable disease. Once seen, it is instantly recognized. The uninitiated physician would regard it as horrendous acne conglobata. Earlier writers have done just that. It is important to avoid this error, for acne fulminans is more menacing to health, is not responsive to antibiotics, and must be treated in quite a different way.

The patients are boys, mostly between 13 and 16 years old, who usually have mild acne. Suddenly, without warning, in a matter of weeks, severe acne strikes like a bolt of lightning (*fulminare*, Latin = to flash). The diagnosis is easily made when the boys limp into the office, in bent-over posture, the shoulder girdle hanging down, reflecting a painful arthritis. Acne fulminans has been reported in siblings and monozygotic twins, suggesting a genetic component.

At first glance acne fulminans resembles acne conglobata because of the presence of numerous, highly inflammatory lesions on the upper chest and back with variable involvement of the face. The imprimatur of the disease, namely ulceration, is immediately evident. The distinctive feature of acne fulminans is the tendency of large nodules to collapse into ulcerative craters with overhanging margins. The base of the ulcer is a gelatinous, amorphous mass. The skin seems to die abruptly, forming large, confluent, exudative, necrotic plaques. The necrotic tissue is soft and jelly-like, into which a probe descends without resistance. Thick, rupia-like hemorrhagic crusts cover the ulcerations. If these are removed, fresh bleeding starts from below. Thick yellow pus drains from multiple holes. The lesions are excruciatingly tender. In contrast to acne conglobata, polyporous comedones and noninflammatory cysts are notably absent. The latter take time to develop. Acne fulminans is an explosive process. Ordinary comedones are hard to find. Without warning, rupture of microcomedones no longer results in a perifollicular abscess but in an extensive, spreading, liquefying necrosis engulfing neighboring follicles. If left untreated, healing, which is exasperatingly slow, always leaves extensive, deep fibrotic scars.

Acne fulminans is not solely a skin disease, but has profound systemic concomitant features. Typical findings include fever varying from low grade (38.5° C) to spiking (40° C) for days and weeks, leukocytosis of varying degree (9000–30000/μl) sometimes as extreme as to suggest granulocytic leukemia, increased sedimentation rate (up to 60 mm in the first hour, and to 100 mm or more in the second, Westergren method), anemia, circulating immune complexes, and proteinuria. The spleen may be enlarged. Sterile lytic bone lesions are not unusual when looked for, occurring mostly in the clavicles and metaphyses of long bones. Erythema nodosum may appear on one or both shins. A key feature is a variable polyarthritis of the large joints, usually without joint effusions. The joints involved are the sacroiliac, hips, knees, shoulders, elbows, and ankles. They account for the bent-over posture of these miserable, asthenic patients. Walking is painful.

The pathogenesis of acne fulminans is a mystery. Septicemia has been strongly suggested but has not been confirmed. The microorganisms in the lesions are not unusual, though *Staphylococcus aureus* can occasionally be recovered. High antistaphylolysin titers have been identified in some cases. It is not a pyoderma. Like patients with acne conglobata, delayed sensitivity reactions to ubiquitous antigens are depressed, but this is probably a nonspecific phase response. The basic defect remains unknown and existing speculations are not illuminating.

Androgen excess can initiate acne fulminans. This may happen iatrogenically to arrest excessive growth or be self-inflicted by power athletes. These cases are described elsewhere (pp. 352 and 353). Fortunately, acne fulminans is rare.

Differential Diagnosis

No other disease mimics the picture of acne fulminans. The knowledgeable physician can scarcely venture another diagnosis. The next best bets are acne tropicalis, severe acne conglobata, rosacea fulminans, pyoderma gangrenosum, and excess granulation tissue induced by isotretinoin therapy of acne conglobata.

Treatment

It is important to realize that acne fulminans does not respond to the convention-

al treatment for severe acne. Antibiotics are futile. It is easy to fall into therapeutic despair. Treatment can be very helpful when no stones are left unturned. Patients must be cautioned that there is no quick cure. The physician should be optimistic and confident. Bed rest is indicated and hospitalization is preferred.

Systemic. We prefer combination of isotretinoin and prednisone. The steroid is given first, for approximately 1 week at a dose of 1.0 mg/kg daily. Then isotretinoin is added at a dose of 0.5 mg/kg daily. After 2 or 3 weeks we taper the steroid. Isotretinoin is maintained as long as inflammatory lesions persist and all ulcers are completely epithelialized. This may take 3–4 months. The dose of isotretinoin can be adjusted to individual needs, in some an increase to 1.0 or even 2.0 mg, but in others a reduction to 0.2 mg/kg body weight daily might be necessary if pyogenic granuloma-like lesions erupt, a rare but frightening event. Antibiotics are not indicated unless there is evidence of secondary pyogenic infection. Antipyretics and nonsteroidal anti-inflammatory agents (NSAI) are rarely necessary in the early treatment phase. We prescribe analgesics in liberal quantities, as needed. The iron-deficiency anemia needs no supplementation, as it returns to normal with appropriate therapy. Psychotropic drugs are rarely needed but these may be helpful in depressed patients.

Topical. Frequent warm compresses with 20%–40% urea solutions are used in the acute phase to remove hemorrhagic crusts and debris. Urea is, in addition, a deodorant and antiseptic. Compresses with 20% urea cream can also be used. High potency corticosteroids are sometimes a helpful adjunct. We prefer clobetasole-17-propionate or β-methasone-17,21-dipropionate cream, liberally ap-

- Exclusively boys, usually aged 13–16 years, asthenic
- Acute onset within days or weeks
- Fever
- Leukocytosis
- Increased sedimentation rate
- Circulating immune complexes
- Arthritis, polyarthralgia of large joints, painful joint swellings, bent-over posture
- Widespread painful necrosis and ulceration covered with hemorrhagic crusts: back, chest, rarely face
- Granuloma pediculatum-like granulation tissue (synonyms: excess granulation tissue, inflammatory neovascular nodules) from ulcerated lesions, mostly on back or chest
  - Without isotretinoin therapy
  - Induced by isotretinoin therapy
- Erythema nodosum on one or both shins
- Proteinuria. If high, mimicking glomerulonephritis
- Osteolytic lesions (clavicles, ribs, etc.)
- Splenomegaly, painful
- Acne fulminans induced by isotretinoin (anecdotal reports)
- Acne fulminans induced by testosterone therapy in very tall boys or doping (body building or athletes

plied on all ulcerating lesions, regardless of their location, even in the face, twice daily for about 7–10 days and no longer. Topical corticosteroids reduce the intensity of inflammation and moderate ulceration.

Alternative Treatment. If isotretinoin is not acceptable for whatever reason, systemic treatment with dapsone (DADPS = diamino-diphenylsulfone, DDS) is started as soon as the explosive lesions are under control. The initial dose is 50 mg/day, which can be increased to 100 mg or 150 mg, rarely, 200 mg/day, according to tolerance. It is mandatory first to check for glucose-6-phosphate deficiency. The side effects of this drug (methemoglobinemia, sickle cell crisis, neuritis, etc.) must be kept in mind.

Prognosis

The prognosis is excellent. The active disease can fortunately be brought into remission but of course scarring is inevitable and can be quite disfiguring. We have never witnessed a recurrence or a later development of acne conglobata. All associated findings normalize, notably fever, erythrocyte sedimentation rate, leukocytosis, arthritis, anemia, proteinuria, swelling of spleen, osteolytic lesions, and erythema nodosum. If not properly diagnosed and adequately treated the disease smolders for a long time. We have seen boys who fought the disease for more than half a year before effective treatment was given.

Blanc D, Zultak M, Wendling D, Lonchampt F (1988) Eruptive pyogenic granulomas and acne fulminans in two siblings treated with isotretinoin. A possible common pathogenesis. Dermatologica 177:16–18

Camisa C (1986) Acute arthritis during isotretinoin therapy for acne. J Am Acad Dermatol 15:1061–1062

Darley CR, Currey HLF, Baker H (1984) Acne fulminans with arthritis in identical twins treated with isotretinoin. JR Soc Med 77:328–330

Elias LM, Gómez MI, Torrelo A, Boixeda JP, Ledo A (1991) Acne fulminans and bilateral seronegative sacroiliitis triggered by isotretinoin. J Dermatol 18:366–367

Engber PB, Marino CT (1980) Acne fulminans with prolonged polyarthralgia. Int J Dermatol 19:567–569

Goldschmidt H, Leyden JJ, Stein KH (1977) Acne fulminans. Investigation of acute febrile ulcerative acne. Arch Dermatol 113:444–449

Goldstein B, Chalker DK, Lesher JL Jr (1990) Acne fulminans. South Med J 83:705–708

Hartmann RR, Plewig G (1983) Acne fulminans. Tratamento de 11 patientes com o ácido 13-cis-retinóico. An Bras Dermatol 58:3–10

Jemec GBE, Rasmussen I (1989) Bone lesions of acne fulminans. J Am Acad Dermatol 20:353–357

Kellett JK, Beck MH, Chalmers RJG (1985) Erythema nodosum and circulating immune complexes in acne fulminans after treatment with isotretinoin. Br Med J 290:820

McAuley D, Miller RA (1985) Acne fulminans associated with inflammatory bowel disease. Report of a case. Arch Dermatol 121:91–93

Nault P, Lassonde M, St-Antoine P (1985) Acne fulminans with osteolytic lesions. Arch Dermatol 121:662–664

Orlow SJ, Watsky KL, Bolognia JL (1991) Skin and bones. II. J Am Acad Dermatol 25:447–462

Pauli SL, Valkeakari T, Räsänen L, Tuomi ML, Reunala T (1989) Osteomyelitis-like bone lesions in acne fulminans. Eur J Pediatr 149:110–113

Reizis Z, Trattner A, Hodak E, David M, Sandbank M (1991) Acne fulminans with hepatospenomegaly and erythema nodosum migrans. J Am Acad Dermatol 24:886–888

Reunala T, Pauli SL, Rasanen L (1990) Musculoskeletal symptoms and bone lesions in acne fulminans. J Am Acad Dermatol 22:144–146

Schaardenburg D van, Lavrijsen S, Vermeer BJ (1989) Acne fulminans associated with painful splenomegaly. Arch Dermatol 125:132–133

Sofman MS, Prose NS (1990) Dermatoses associated with sterile lytic bone lesions. J Am Acad Dermatol 23:494–498

Ström S, Thyresson N, Boström H (1973) Acute febrile ulcerative conglobate acne with leukemoid reaction. Acta Derm Venereol (Stockh) 53:306–312

Acne Fulminans

This 14-year-old boy is quite sick and has signs of systemic disease, notably fever and arthralgia. The distinguishing feature is the formation of highly inflammatory nodules and plaques which undergo swift suppurative degeneration leaving raggedy ulcerations whose base is filled with a gelatinous mush. The lesions are exquisitely tender and painful. Scarring is extensive.

Furthermore, the bent-over posture is typical. Walking is very painful.

Above   Hemorrhagic and necrotic confluent ulcerations with slow tendency to epithelialize. Horrendous draining sinuses are in both nasolabial folds and on the chin

Below   Close-up view from the chest during the explosive phase a few weeks earlier

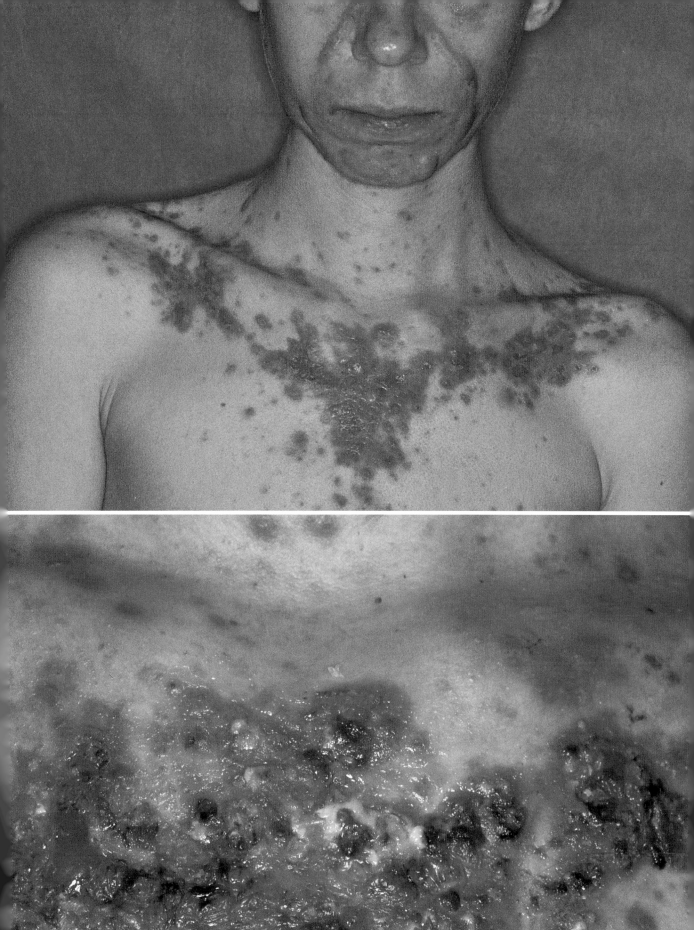

Acne Fulminans

Acne fulminans is a ferocious disease and strikes young men.

Above

Left   Pain can be read from the concerned expression of this boy. Within weeks he was attacked by fever, arthralgia, erythema nodosum ulcerating skin lesions, confluent nodules, and draining sinuses

Right   The appearance of this mushy, easily bleeding granulation tissue (detail from the patient to the lower left) is like raw meat

Below

Left   Acne fulminans destroys the back of this young man. Pyogenic-granuloma-like vascular proliferations make him feel very uncomfortable

Right   Erythema nodosum on the shins is sometimes seen in patients with acne fulminans

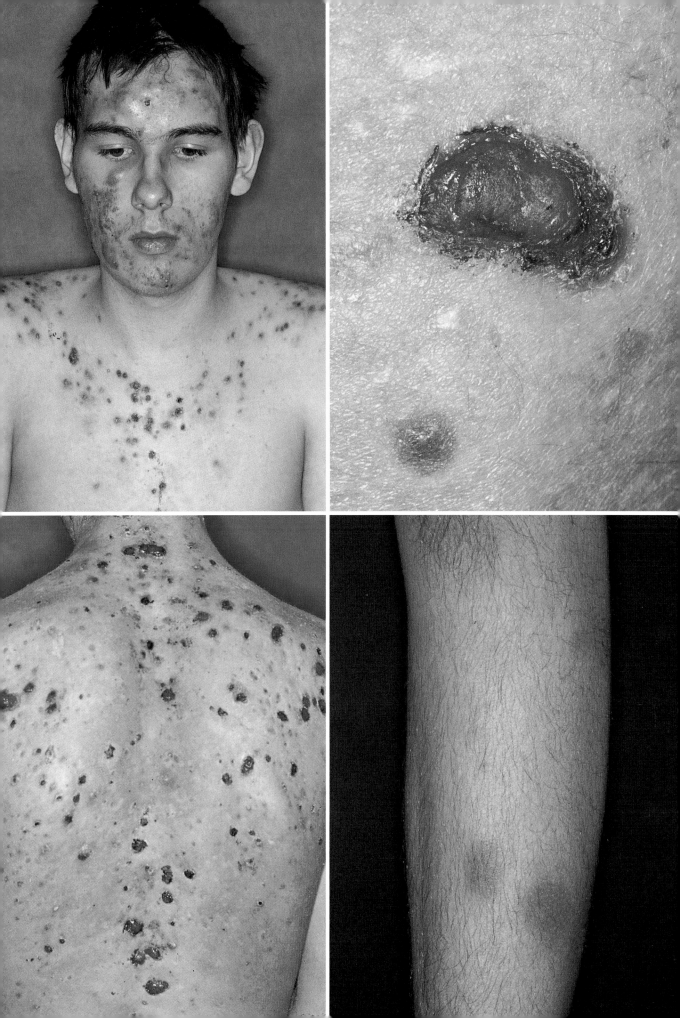

Hemorrhagic Skin Necrosis in Acne Fulminans

Ulceration is a typical sign of acne fulminans, preceded by bleeding into the skin.

Above The epidermis is totally necrotic. An infarct-like necrosis due to hyalinized thrombotic vessels and profuse bleeding, surrounded by a mixed granulocytic and lymphocytic infiltrate have caused havoc

Below Higher magnification of the gelatinous mass and dense inflammation. No wonder that bad scarring is inevitable

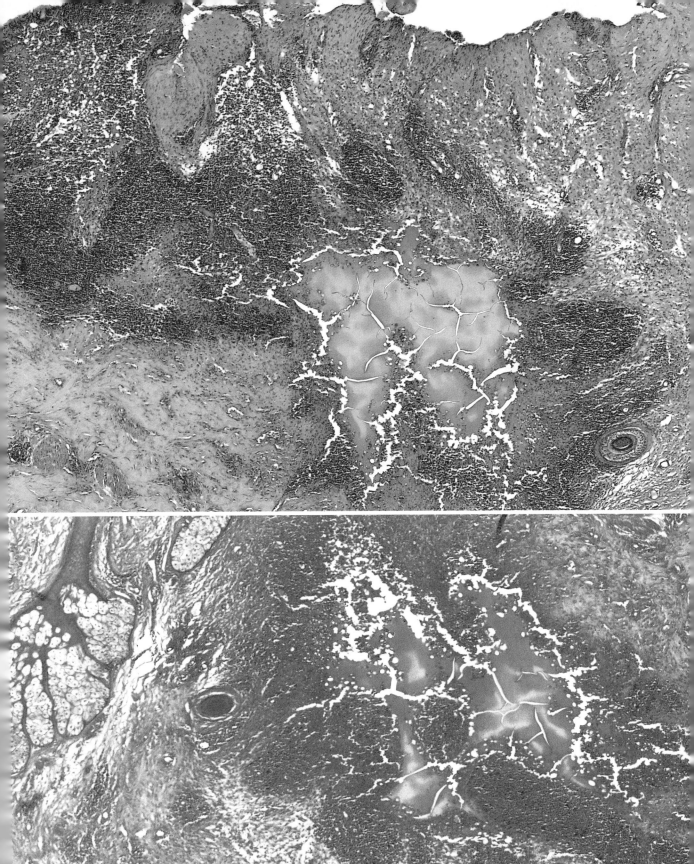

Solid Facial Persistent Edema of Acne Vulgaris

Nearly all experienced acneologists have seen solid facial persistent edema of acne vulgaris, this rare peculiar and serious complication of acne. However, it was not until a recent report from the Mayo Clinic, which gave it a name, that clinicians have become alerted to its occurrence.

Clinical Findings

Solid facial edema in adolescent sufferers of persistent acne occurs in both sexes. All patients have a history of acne which predates the edema by 2–5 years. Age of onset is in adolescence or early adulthood. Nothing is known concerning pathogenesis. Millions of youngsters have acne but only a few will develop this complication. A role for inheritance is suggested by its occurrence in 14-year-old identical twins. The clinical picture is alarming and quite characteristic and cannot be confused with anything else: there is a nonpitting, solid edema of the midthird of the face (centrofacial edema), but there is no scaling and no *peau d'orange* phenomenon. The skin does not indent when firmly pressed with a finger. There is little day-to-day variation. The edema is mainly localized on the forehead, upper eyelids, nasal saddle, nasolabial folds, and cheeks. It persists indefinitely, without fluctuation. Contrary to what one might think, it is low-grade acne that gives rise to solid, centrofacial edema, and not severely inflammatory papulopustular acne or acne conglobata.

Subjective complaints are slight, except for deformed facial contours. The appearance is grotesque, a grave threat to self-esteem. General symptoms like fever, elevated erythrocyte sedimentation rate, chills, pain, or increased local temperature are lacking. This is an important differential diagnostic criterion since at first glance the condition mimics streptococcal cellulitis; however, oral antibiotics are unavailing. The disease is stubborn and does not spontaneously involute.

Histopathology

The clinician, not the histopathologist, makes the diagnosis as histopathology is uncharacteristic. Only a few biopsies were obtained so far. A mild edema in the mid and deep dermis, ectatic lymph vessels, and occasionally a sparse to dense lymphohistiocytic perivascular infiltrate with remarkably many mast cells are features. There are no foreign-body granulomas.

Differential Diagnosis

To the *cognoscenti* solid edema is like no other condition. The Melkersson–Rosenthal syndrome comes to mind, but this cannot be sustained in the absence of scrotal tongue, lip edema, or peripheral facial nerve involvement.

A similar solid edema occurs in rosacea. Perhaps the pathogenesis is the same, related to lymphatic obstruction or fibrosis induced by mast cells. Again the cause is unknown. Rosacea tends to occur in an older age group and presents other signs.

Treatment

Treatment is highly unsatisfactory. Enterprising clinicians have tried almost everything imaginable, including X-rays and high doses of antibiotics. Compression garments are unwieldy and usually not effective. Daily lymph massage deserves more study as it might be valuable.

Systemic corticosteroids have been ineffective in our experience. Our tentative recommendation is low-dose isotretinoin, 0.1–0.2 mg/kg body weight daily over a period of many months. This is combined with an oral antihistamine given with the isotretinoin for several months thereafter. Preliminary results are encouraging. When desperate, clofazimine may be worth a trial (about 100 mg four times weekly). Of course, the underlying acne should be treated.

Comacho-Martinez F, Winkelmann RK (1990) Solid facial edema as a manifestation of acne. J Am Acad Dermatol 22:129–130

Connelly MG, Winkelmann RK (1985) Solid facial edema as a complication of acne vulgaris. Arch Dermatol 121:87–90

Djawari D (1990) Solides persistierendes Gesichtsödem als seltene Komplikation einer Acne juvenilis. Aktuel Dermatol 16:207–208

Friedman SJ, Fox BJ, Albert HL (1986) Solid facial edema as a complication of acne vulgaris: treatment with isotretinoin. J Am Acad Dermatol 15:286–289

Helander I, Aho HJ (1987) Solid facial edema as a complication of acne vulgaris: treatment with isotretinoin and clofazimine. Acta Derm Venereol (Stockh) 67:535–537

Humbert P, Delaporte E, Drobacheff C, Piette F, Blanc D, Bergoend H, Agache P (1990) Oedème dur facial associé à l'acné vulgaire. Efficacité thérapeutique de l'isotrétinoïne. Ann Dermatol Venereol 117:527–532

Tosti A, Guerra L, Bettoli V, Bonelli U (1987) Solid facial edema as a complication of acne vulgaris in twins. J Am Acad Dermatol 17:843–844

Acne Mechanica

Clinicians have long understood that various types of pressure and friction can intensify acne. The term chin acne acknowledges the deleterious effect of resting the chin on the hands for prolonged periods. When the influence of various traumas on acne subjects is examined, it is soon ascertained that many types of mechanical forces can aggravate existing acne. These include pressure, friction, stretching, rubbing, pinching, or pulling, indeed a whole gamut of mechanical stresses.

The likelihood of precipitating new lesions by trauma is proportional to the severity of acne. Usually mild acne is indifferent, but in highly inflammatory acne even moderate trauma can provoke crops of papulopustules and sometimes nodules. Mechanical forces, however, do not induce comedones. The worst expressions of acne mechanica have occurred in young boys with acne fulminans who had to use orthopedic casts.

Many patients rest their head on their hands in a very characteristic way while studying or reading, accompanied variably by rubbing and other manipulations. When the patient is thoroughly engrossed in various mental pursuits, hand pressure may act upon exactly the same spot, day after day. Watching television in an immobilized transfixed posture for hours each day provides another opportunity. The distribution will tell whether one or both hands are used and where they are placed. Such habits are largely unconscious. As soon as the aggravating role of the hands is spotted, the physician must try to stop the habit by making it conscious and issuing a cease-and-desist order with authority.

Other patients are rubbers and kneaders of a particular area of facial skin; they are often surprised when this activity is brought to their attention. These tic-like manipulations are difficult to stop, being so automatically performed. Students are especially likely to rub, stretch, manipulate, and knead a specific area of the skin when studying for examinations, a stressful time to say the least. Acne mechanica could legitimately be renamed acne traumatica.

We have made an inventory of acne mechanica according to location. Various habits and postures are very common sources of trouble. Physicians need to become more sensitive to many types of trauma that may worsen acne. Some forms of acne mechanica have received a specific designation such as fiddler's neck aptly named.

While we accept a contributory role of emotions in acne, attributed to anxiety, it can often be better explained by the activities of the hands rather than by the mysteries of the psyche.

The key diagnostic feature is an unusual distribution pattern. This immediately suggests external forces. A swath of inflammatory lesions across the forehead implicates a headband of some sort, perhaps a hat or a headdress. Symmetrical lesions over both shoulders enables one to state with Sherlockian sureness that

Face
  Supporting with hands
  Rubbing with hands or fingers
  Chin straps
  Football helmets
  Hockey and wrestling head and face guards
  Motorcycle face and head protectors
  Forehead bands – dress or athletic
  Hats

Neck
  Shirt collars
  Backpacks and straps
  Turtleneck shirts and sweaters
  Violin (fiddler's neck)

Shoulders
  Football pads
  Straps from backpacks
  Surgical tape
  Orthopedic casts

Arms and Legs
  Orthopedic casts
  Surgical tape

Back
  Backrest of chairs
  Seats – bus, car, truck, boat
  Orthopedic braces and casts
  Brassieres
  Confinement to bed
  Wide belts
  Packs and straps

Chest
  Wrestling
  Football pads
  Orthopedic casts

Buttocks
  Chairs
  Seats – bus, car, truck, boat

the patient plays American football. Likewise, certain patterns on the trunk or extremities will disclose a recent medical experience – a cast or occlusive bandages from injuries and operations.

The sovereign prescription is proscription – stop the mechanical force. Considerable ingenuity may be involved when, for example, the mechanical stress is occupational – a truck driver whose back is traumatized all day long by pressure against a hard, tall backrest.

It should be emphasized that acne mechanica is a complication of genuine acne; the underlying disease would be present in any event, of course in a much milder form. The additional physical forces merely intensify the disease precisely in the areas where these have been exerted. Acne patients have a special predisposition to develop lesions from all forms of chemical and physical stimuli. Accordingly, lesions may occur in unusual sites, for example, on the buttocks, an area one usually does not think of as the natural territory of the disease. Young acne patients who sit for long hours in one place will often show lesions exactly confined to pressure areas. A waistline distribution is a tip-off to the wearing of tight, wide belts.

A mechanical factor was clearly evident in tropical acne encountered in wartime in hot and humid climates. The disorder usually began and was most severe in pressure areas under heavy packs or where tight straps traumatized the skin.

Applying an occlusive, sticky tape to the skin for 10 or 14 days illustrates vividly how much harm friction can do. The new papulopustules which are thus provoked develop from the rupture of pre-existing microcomedones. The aggravating effect is not simply due to hydration, heat, maceration, or overgrowth of bacteria. Covering the skin with impermeable plastic film will not elicit new lesions except when used for many weeks. Some form of friction or tension is required to disrupt microcomedones.

Prophylactic measures against acne mechanica are very worthwhile, for the inflammatory lesions are often violent enough to leave scars in their wake.

Brun P, Baran R (1984) Une acné mécanique méconnue: la dermatite du cou des violoinistes. Ann Dermatol Venereol 11:241–245

Darley CR (1990) Acne conglobata of the buttocks aggravated by mechanical and environmental factors. Clin Exp Dermatol 15:462–463

Mills OH Jr, Kligman A (1975) Acne mechanica. Arch Dermatol 111:481–483

Acne Mechanica

Above

Left top Fiddler's neck is the pressure-induced folliculitis with fibrosis and secondary (fistulated) comedones where the violin contacts the skin. It is said that this peculiar response is more common in nervous musicians who sweat excessively. It develops in patients with a tendency to acne folliculitis or pseudofolliculitis barbae, but rarely in persons with dry smooth skin

Left bottom Acne mechanica of the buttocks, produced by rubbing against hard seats. As on the face the lesions comprise comedones, papules, and pustules and may heal with scarring

Right Hippie acne. Persons with a predisposition to acne vulgaris have fragile follicles which easily rupture from mechanical traumas. It should be understood that these persons already have acne vulgaris, though it may be mild. The trauma explodes microcomedones. This is acne mechanica on the forehead from wearing a tight headband. Hippie acne often decorates the brows of these individuals. The lesions are papulopustules. Times are changing, hippie bands are no longer in fashion in 1992

Below Acne mechanica due to a cast. This 16-year-old boy fractured his lower left arm, which was put in a cast for 8 weeks. Before the accident the boy had developed acne fulminans with typical lesions on face, chest, and back, but not on his arms. His fragile sebaceous follicles were mechanically irritated by the cast and moist–warm conditions which increase frictional forces. He developed an unusual crop of papules, pustules, and nodules. The right arm showed only a few papules

Above right: Courtesy of Otto H. Mills, Philadelphia, USA

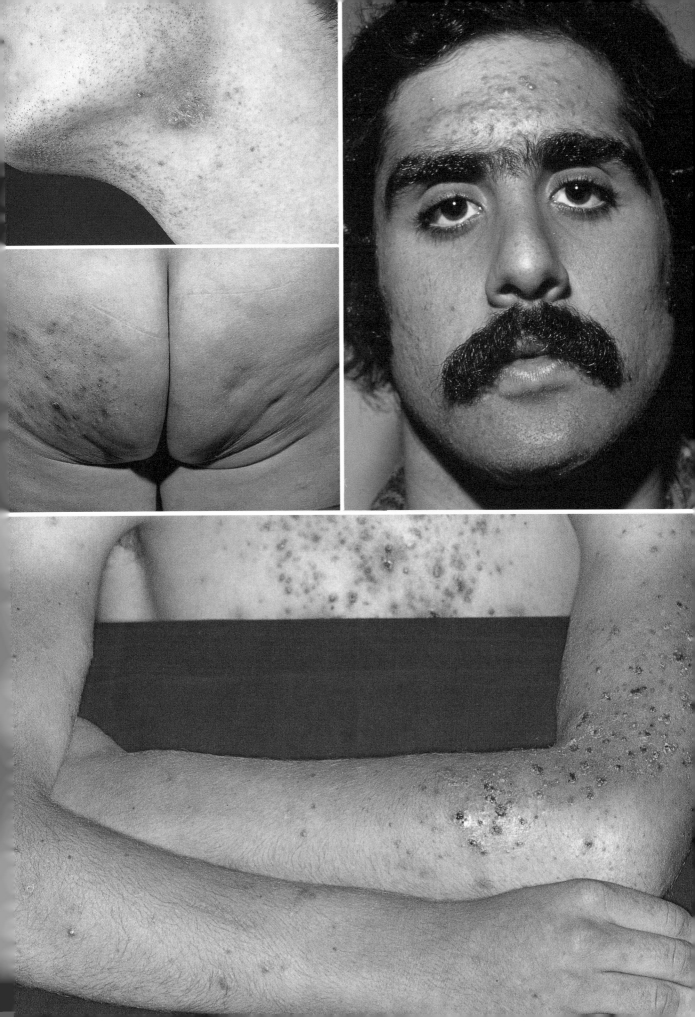

Back Acne

The literature contains no description of back acne, a rather common condition which we regard as a variant of acne vulgaris. Onset is in young adulthood, lasting indefinitely. Many, but not all, give a past history of acne of variable severity which has generally become quiescent when the back erupts. Almost all show shallow acne scars in the face. Hence, these are acne-prone people. The lesions are distributed on the upper back, extending sometimes onto the arms. They consist of scattered erythematous follicular papules and small nodules. Some enlarge to abscess-like lesions. Quite typical is their stubborn persistence, often for months and years with a fluctuating course. The indurated lesions usually do not discharge. Pustules are not numerous, while comedones are inconspicuous. Most patients show prominent follicular orifices which fluoresce brightly under Wood's light. Shallow scarring is common but moderate.

Back acne is predominantly a disease of men. We seem to encounter an increasing prevalence in women. Being out of sight, acne of the back is generally not brought to the attention of the dermatologist. Many patients simply live with the disease. Mechanical factors, such as leaning against the back of a chair for hours, aggravate the eruption or restless, fitful sleep produces a kind of acne mechanica. Occasionally larger nodules can become quite tender and cause pain when lying on the back. Back acne may last for decades with episodic flares. Minor expressions of back acne may occur in as many as 20% of healthy adult men, especially those with past acne.

Histologically the lesions are indistinguishable from deep papulopustules and nodules of inflammatory acne. Early lesions show infra- and perifollicular abscesses, usually associated with evidence of rupture. Older lesions display histiocytes and foreign-body cells, engulfing corneocytes and fragments of hair.

When the papules or nodules are nicked with a knife and the contents expressed, a horny kernel, often of surprisingly large size, can be identified in the necrotic material.

The sequence of events is entirely similar to that of acne: comedo formation, rupture, abscess, re-encapsulation, and histologic scarring.

The microflora is typical of acne. However, an abundance of the yeast *Pityrosporum orbiculare* in the apical region of some of the comedones has led to the separate nosologic designation *Pityrosporum folliculitis*. Classifying this eruption among the pityrosporoses, such as tinea versicolor, is a mistake in our opinion. Treatment deemed at the yeast is generally unavailing. The pathogenicity of *Pityrosporum orbiculare* has never been conclusively demonstrated in acne or acne-like disorders. Moreover, since almost all comedones are colonized by *Pityrosporum*, we see nothing unusual in their presence, except that they tend to be unusually abundant in back acne. There is no easy explanation for the localization and delayed onset of the disorder. We view adult acne of the back as simply one of the variants of acne. Their is evidence that sebaceous glands reach their peak size and function at different times in different regions. Back acne could reflect later maturation of the sebaceous glands in this area.

doses, as in youngsters, should be given until remission. Thereafter a lower maintenance dose should be found. Isotretinoin completely clears this long-lasting, smoldering fire on the back better than any other medication. The dose is from 0.1–0.5 mg/kg body weight for about 4 months.

Treatment

This is the same as for acne vulgaris. Topical or oral antifungal treatment with imidazoles does not ameliorate back acne.

Topical. Tretinoin is often effective when vigorously applied to tolerance. The assistance of another individual is usually required to achieve uniform application. In stubborn cases, combination therapy with benzoyl peroxide, azelaic acid, or topical antibiotics is quite helpful.

Systemic. Antibiotics are quite effective. Tetracycline-HCl, oxytetracycline, minocycline, doxycycline, or macrolids (erythromycin, josamycin) can be used. Full

Bergbrant IM, Faergemann J (1989) Seborrhoeic dermatitis and Pityrosporum ovale: a cultural and immunological study. Acta Derm Venereol (Stockh) 69:332–335

Bojanovsky A, Lischka G (1977) Pityrosporum orbiculare bei akneiformen Eruptionen. Hautarzt 28:409–411

Faergemann J, Johansonn S, Bäck O, Scheynius A (1986) An immunologic and cultural study of Pityrosporum folliculitis. J Am Acad Dermatol 14:429–433

Kieffer M, Bergbrant IM, Faergemann J, Jemec GBE, Ottevanger V, Skov PS, Svejgaard E (1990) Immune reactions to Pityrosporum ovale in adult patients with atopic and seborrheic dermatitis. J Am Acad Dermatol 22:739–742

Plewig G (1978) Pityrosporum in normal sebaceous follicles, comedones, acneiform eruptions, and dandruff. Mykosen (Suppl 1) 21:155–163

Acne Tropicalis (Tropical Acne)

Acne tropicalis is a terrible disease. It is acne conglobata times three. Knowledge stems mainly from observations among combat troops in tropical areas during World War II and in Vietnam. Nowadays acne tropicalis is a rarity. Relief is obtainable only by evacuation to a temperate climate. Except for this measure, the disease has unsurpassed stubbornness. The pathogenesis is still obscure. It unfolds against a background of heat and humidity. Skin infections thrive in the tropics, especially under the exigencies of warfare. As long as the individual remains in the tropics, and even if immobilized in the hospital, the disease rages on with unabated fury despite all topical and systemic measures.

Acne tropicalis is not an infectious disease. The victims usually have a history of mild acne in adolescence. They are acne prone but are generally in a quiescent state when tropical acne strikes. Fortunately very few patients develop this tropical variant. A tropical climate generally has no influence one way or the other on the course of pre-existing acne. There are no predictive indicators of the population at risk.

Most patients are past the peak of adolescent acne, about 25 years old on the average. Older men are by no means exempt. Acne tropicalis can also occur in teenagers.

The usual variety of acne conglobata lesions is found – pustules, papules, nodules, and draining sinuses. Cysts and polyporous comedones do not have enough time to form. The distribution is distinctive. The face tends to be spared; the lesions extend far beyond the boundaries of acne conglobata, spreading outwards and downwards to the lower back and abdomen. Involvement of the buttocks and thighs is frequent, even characteristic. One might call this disease acne generalisata.

The lesions tend to be very numerous, leaving very little trunk skin uninvolved. To make matters worse the nodules are larger and more succulent than in acne conglobata. They are very tender and commonly break down, giving forth a suppurative and often bloody discharge. The victims soil everything around them, feel very miserable and are disabled. Additionally they are a trial to those who must care for them.

The bacterial microflora is not unusual and does not explain the ferocity of the disease. *Staphylococcus aureus* is inconsistently recovered. Gram-negative bacteria are frequently isolated in small numbers and have no impact on the course of the disease. Antibiotics, including those active against gram-negative microorganisms, have little or no effect. Antibacterial therapy, local and systemic, is fruitless. Laboratory findings are merely those of severe inflammatory skin disease: elevated sedimentation rate, increased serum globulins, and a variable leukocytosis. Endocrinologic evaluations have not revealed significant abnormalities. Investigation of surface lipids, too, offers no illumination.

Mechanical factors, especially friction, operating on an overhydrated skin seem to play an essential role in provoking the eruption. Lesions are most likely to crop out under packs, in pressure areas (the buttocks), from the friction of wet clothing, etc. (p. 331). Thus, trauma is an unmistakable precipitating factor and helps to explain distribution.

Occupational Tropical Acne

Occupational tropical acne occurs in sweating workmen exposed to extremely hot conditions, e.g., coke ovens or furnace rooms in steel factories. Wearing fireproof or fire-resistant semiocclusive clothes aggravates the condition.

Differential Diagnosis

Acne tropicalis is a distinctive disorder which, because of its setting and devastating evolution, cannot be confused with any other disease. The disease matches acne fulminans in severity but the two are easily separated.

Treatment

There is but one thing to do – get out of the tropics or hot working conditions.

The disease rapidly abates spontaneously in a cool climate, with or without treatment.

Systemic. Though untried, oral isotretinoin would probably accelerate regression. Systemic corticosteroids would also make sense as in acne fulminans. Antibiotics are not warranted.

Topical. Once the acute phase of the disease is over one should look for secondary comedones. These would require comedolytic therapy with tretinoin.

Lamberg SI (1971) The course of acne vulgaris in military personnel stationed in Southeast Asia. Cutis 7:655–660

Lewis CW, Griffin TB, Henning DR, Akers WA (1973) Tropical acne: clinical and laboratory investigations. Letterman Army Institute of Research, report No. 16 (May 1973)

Novy FG (1949) A severe form of acne developing in the tropics. Arch Dermatol Syph 60:206–216

Sulzberger MB, Addenbrooke F, Joyce SJ, Greenberg S, Mack AG (1946) Tropical acne. Bull US Army Med Dept 6:149–154

Tucker SB (1983) Occupational tropical acne. Cutis 31:79–81

Postadolescent Acne in Women

According to dermatologic dogma acne vulgaris regresses in early adulthood. This is not true for women. Low-grade-acne may persist for decades past adolescence. Moreover, acne may spring up in women who more or less completely escaped adolescent acne.

Exact figures of prevalence are lacking since epidemiologic studies do not exist. Some dermatologists estimate that one third of adult women seen in practice have a pestilential, oscillating, persistent low-grade acne. Often, these women do not seek consultation for their acne, which they have learned to live with or to socially accept. Routine examination of the face regardless of the chief complaint will show that this is a rather common problem.

The importance of identifying this species of acne lies in that it may be misinterpreted as acne cosmetica, a common mistake. Originally it was thought that postadolescent acne was due to acneigenic substances in cosmetics and skin care products, especially moisturizers and sunscreens. As many as 50% of cosmetic products were found to be comedogenic in the rabbit ear assay. This neatly explained the limitation of the disorder to women. It turns out that cosmetic acne has been overdiagnosed. Cosmetics do not account for most of the cases of postadolescent acne in women. Experience has taught that withholding suspected cosmetics is largely unavailing. Furthermore, major manufacturers of cosmetics are very sensitive to safety issues and routinely test their products for acneigenic potential. Comedogenic cosmetics have virtually been eliminated. This clean-up has had no perceivable effect on the prevalence of postadolescent acne.

The distinguishing features of genuine acne cosmetica are fairly dense crops of closed and open comedones located in the areas of application. Papulopustules are also fairly numerous, sometimes without a preceding microcomedo (chemical folliculitis). Of course, it is not permissible to make a diagnosis of acne cosmetica in a woman who rarely or never uses cosmetics or who selects only brands made by reliable manufacturers. History is telling.

By contrast, in postadolescent acne, the lesions tend to be less numerous; the comedones are small and of the closed type. Papulopustules are scattered and generally show a pre-existing horny mass when the contents are expressed. Premenstrual flares and premenstrual tension syndrome are frequent. We view this as true acne vulgaris of endogenous origin.

The etiology is poorly understood. Most of these women are not housewives, but tend to be professionals who are competing frenetically with men in business. They are intense, ambitious people who are determined to be successful. The emotional cost is high. Many are lawyers, doctors, executives, and managers who are on their way up. When they are also keeping a husband and raising children the stress may be enormous. Our speculation is that a stress-related increased secretion of androgenic steroids by the adrenal gland could be responsible for this condition.

Treatment is simple and usually quite effective. Tretinoin alone is usually sufficient. In severe cases we sometimes add oral antibiotics.

Persistent Facial Acne in Women

Women with this type of nasty, therapy-resistant inflammatory acne warrant an endocrinologic work-up. Hyperandrogenic conditions, including polycystic ovary disease or adrenal hyperplasia, may lurk in the background. One should also inquire about intake of anabolic steroids. Usually, hormonal abnormalities are not uncovered in the absence of masculinization. Treatment should be aggressive nonetheless.

Above   The jawline is a typical area, where persistent inflammatory lesions predominate. This woman did not respond to conventional therapy. She was successfully treated with low-dose isotretinoin (0.2 mg/kg body weight) in combination with the antiandrogen cyproterone acetate prescribed as an oral contraceptive. Her face cleared completely in 7 months with no recurrence thereafter

Below   The woman is only 19 years old, but suffers miserably from closed comedones, scars, and confluent conglobate papules and nodules. Oral isotretinoin along with a contraceptive containing 2 mg of cyproterone acetate and 35 µg of ethinyl estradiol led to a permanent cure

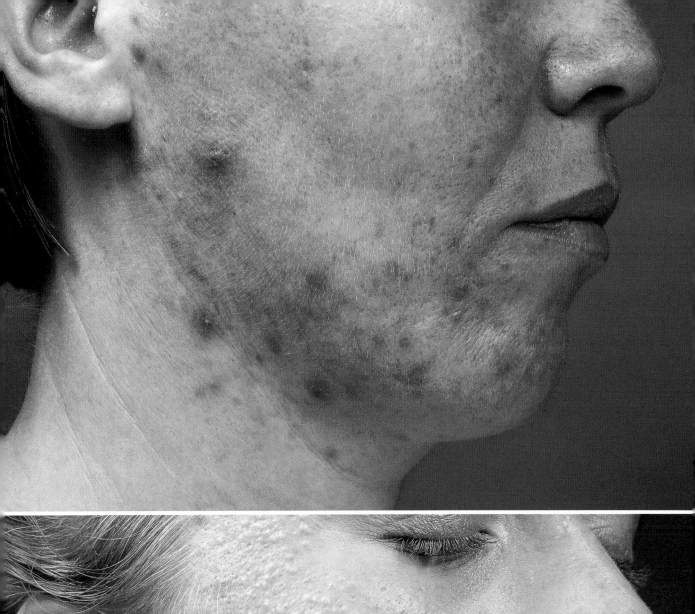
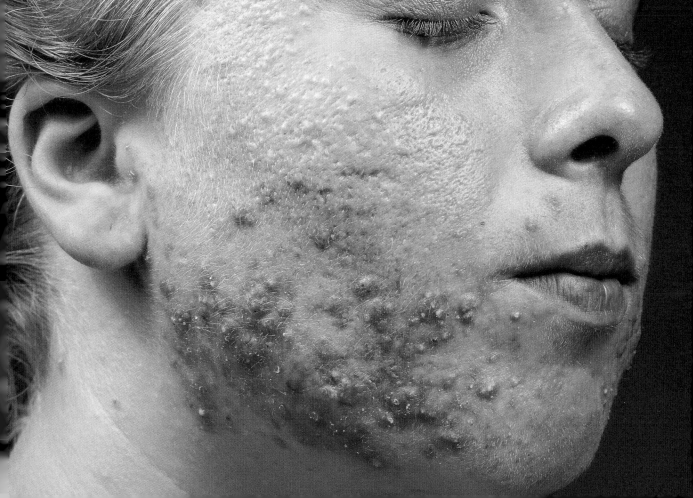

Premenstrual Acne

A variety of distressing symptoms occur in many women just prior to menstruation. Nervousness and irritability (premenstrual tension) are often attributed to psychologic influences. Objective changes also occur, such as weight gain and breast enlargement. These are not so easily passed off as having an emotional origin. Similarly, premenstrual exacerbation of acne is a genuine phenomenon, experienced by at least one third of patients. Some estimates range as high as 60%, not an improbable figure if one includes mild flares. Typically, the woman notices an increase in papulopustules about a week or so before menstruation. These spring up rapidly and like all other inflammatory lesions are mainly due to the rupture of invisible closed comedones (microcomedones). The phenomenon is most evident in comparatively mild papulopustular acne, far less so when numerous deep-seated papules are present. An outcropping of five to ten pustules more or less regularly every month is bound to be noticed, though the overall effect may not strike an outside observer. Some physicians have even doubted the existence of premenstrual acne. Although lesion counts rarely increase greatly, the fixed rhythm of the process can scarcely be overlooked. Fingering the lesions owing to heightened tension is not the cause though it may of course intensify the reaction. Indeed, there is no good explanation for the peculiar periodicity. There are unproved and we believe false claims that sebum secretion varies with the menstrual cycle, the increase occurring at just the right time to explain the flare. Others have been persuaded that free fatty acids in the surface lipids increase at this time. It is exceedingly unlikely that the amount or composition of sebum is affected by the menstrual cycle. Even so, such changes would not explain a sudden outcropping of inflammatory lesions.

An other observation, fanciful in our opinion, is that the follicular orifice becomes smaller between days 15 and 20 of the menstrual cycle. This supposedly impedes the outflow of sebum, laying the groundwork for an exacerbation 3–4 days later. There is preliminary evidence that progesterone mediates premenstrual acne in some unknown way. The omission of progestin in contraceptive regimens has avoided flares which otherwise occurred regularly.

Some believe that the flares occur only in those patients who show premenstrual weight gain. This too may be seriously questioned. Premenstrual flares often develop in women whose weight remains steady and whose breasts do not become edematous. It has been found that diuretics have no more prophylactic effect than placebos whether or not there is demonstrable weight gain.

We have no special treatment for premenstrual acne. We do not recommend diuretics. We take note of the phenomenon and treat the acne vulgaris according to its severity. When acne improves from contraceptive pills, preceeding menstrual flares generally diminish or disappear.

Pochi PE (1974) Acne in premature ovarian failure. Reestablishment of cyclic flareups with medroxyprogesterone acetate therapy. Arch Dermatol 109:556–557

Postmenopausal Acne

The dermatologic literature does not mention postmenopausal acne. Postmenopausal acne was discovered coincidentally in older women seeking medical counseling for a variety of facial problems, mainly hyperpigmentation, seborrheic keratoses, large pores, trichostasis spinulosa, wrinkles, and other signs of photodamage. Epidemiologic surveys do not exist, thus the prevalence of postmenopausal acne is not known. We think it is quite common as can be easily ascertained by questioning about breakouts.

Postmenopausal acne has the following characteristics:

- It affects women in their menopause, mostly within the first 2 years of ovarian failure. In fact, it may presage the last menstruation, often in association with other menopausal symptoms such as hot flashes. Perhaps it should be called *perimenopausal acne*. We propose the following explanation. As the ovaries no longer produce estrogens, but continue to synthesize androgens, as do the adrenals, a state of unopposed hyperandrogenism appears. Hormonal imbalance incites menopausal acne, thus making it a member of the expanding list of hyperandrogenic syndromes.
- Postmenopausal acne is low-grade acne with scattered small, closed comedones which become visible when the loose skin is stretched. Open comedones are rare, as small sparse papulopustules are not part of this picture.
- The disease smolders along over many years, an annoyance rather than a problem which threatens appearance. Exacerbations are uncommon. Eventually the low-grade acne burns out in the patient's seventies.
- Most of these women do not exhibit scarring from adolescent acne and do not give a compelling account of adolescent acne. They do have, however, large facial pores, especially on the nose and malar areas. A fair number complain of oiliness, but others insist that their skin is dry.

- Postmenopausal acne seems to be most common in Mediterranean people with thick, darker, oilier skin. We rarely encounter it in type I light-skinned, small pored, blue eyed, freckled Celts (Scottish-Irish).
- There seems to be an association with postmenopausal hirsutism of the chin and upper lip. Many ladies wax to remove unsightly hair or use bleaching agents. Vellus hairs of the beard area of the cheeks tend to be long, creating an unwelcome fuzz. Still, not all hirsute women have postmenopausal acne.
- Concomitant heavy use of cosmetics in this age group is uncommon. Thus perimenopausal acne is not likely to be confused with acne cosmetica; the latter shows a higher density of comedones and larger inflammatory lesions.
- Many of these women, being older, exhibit dermatoheliosis from chronic excessive exposure to sunlight for almost half a century. Many show the usual stigmata of photodamage, popularly called photoaging, e.g., wrinkles, blotches, growths, yellow leathery skin, etc.

Since comedones dominate the scene, tretinoin is the drug of choice. A 0.025% cream formulation is advised to begin with. Clearing of comedones can be anticipated within 4–5 months. As tolerance develops, usually in about 1 month, a 0.05% formulation is recommended.

Antimicrobial agents including benzoyl peroxide and topical antibiotics are rarely necessary.

These patients appreciate advice about their other cosmetic problems, particularly hirsutism for which we recommend electrolysis.

Balin AK, Kligman AM (eds) (1989) Aging and the skin. Raven Press, New York

Masculinizing Syndromes in Women

Polycystic Ovary Disease

Polycystic ovary disease (POD) is well known to the gynecologist, but rarely discussed in women with inflammatory acne. Women with POD have a variegate list of clinical and laboratory findings: menstrual irregularities, seborrhea, hirsutism, obesity, raised plasma concentrations of LH and testosterone, but normal values of FSH. Sometimes hyperprolactinemia is present. Androgen excess varies from study to study and is not easily defined in acne patients, as it not always correlates with the severity of the disease. The etiology of polycystic ovaries and POD is unknown.

Ultrasonography of the pelvic region is easily performed. Polycystic ovaries are defined according to the criteria of Adams as ten or more cysts, arranged peripherally in the ovary with a diameter of 2–8 mm, and an increased ovarian stroma and volume. The story is not so simple, though, as about 85% of women with acne were found to have deranged ovarian morphology by high-resolution ultrasound imaging and about 20% of women without acne. The presence of polycystic ovaries did not correlate with acne severity, infertility, menstrual abnormalities, hirsutism, and biochemical endocrinologic values.

What tests are recommended in suspected endocrinologic involvement of acne? This is difficult to answer, even for specialists of this subject, because virtually all of the reported endocrine studies on acne in women were done in severe or treatment-refractory cases.

When should hormone tests be ordered? It is only indicated in women with other signs of androgen excess than acne, e.g., hirsutism, menstrual abnormalities, androgenetic alopecia, etc. Laboratory studies should include total testosterone (TT), free testosterone (FT), and dihydroepiandrosterone-sulfate (DHEA-S). Testosterone is largely of ovarian origin, DHEA-S entirely of adrenal origin; thus the most likely source of increased androgen is determined. How often are elevated androgens discovered? Again this is sub judice, in no more than 20% of patients with severe acne, and probably much less if endocrinologic studies were done in all women with acne.

Treatment varies according to the recommendation of endocrinologists. The repertoire reaches from doing nothing to oral contraceptives, mainly of the antiandrogen type, low-dose oral corticosteroids, wedge-shaped resections of the ovaries as was recommended for women with the Stein–Leventhal syndrome.

Adams J, Polson DW, Franks S (1986) Prevalence of polycystic ovaries in women with anovulation and idiopathic hirsutism. Br Med J 293:355–359

Betti R, Bencini PL, Lodi A, Urbani CE, Chiarelli G, Crosti C (1990) Incidence of polycystic ovaries in patients with late-onset or persistent acne: hormonal reports. Dermatologica 181:109–111

Bunker CB, Newton JA, Conway GS, Jacobs HS, Greaves MW, Dowd PM (1991) The hormonal profile of women with acne and polycystic ovaries. Clin Exp Dermatol 16:420–423

Bunker CB, Newton JA, Kilborn J, Patel A, Conway GS, Jacobs HS, Greaves MW, Dowd PM (1989) Most women with acne have polycystic ovaries. Br J Dermatol 121:675–680

Peserico A, Angeloni G, Bertoli P, Marini A, Piva G, Panciera A, Suma V (1989) Prevalence of polycystic ovaries in woman with acne. Arch Dematol Res 281:502–503

Polson DW, Wadsworth J, Adams J, Franks S (1988) Polycystic ovaries – a common finding in normal women. Lancet 1:870–872

Androluteoma of Pregnancy

An androgen-producing tumor can turn an otherwise healthy person within weeks into a severely sick person. This woman had been working as a model until her first pregnancy. She was overwhelmed in the first trimester by unusual skin changes completely unknown to her: seborrhea, hirsutism on the face, chest, and abdomen, and eruption of papules, pustules, and abscesses, leaving behind unsightly scars. A masculinizing syndrome was suggested by deepening of her voice.

Her gynecologist suspected an androluteoma of pregnancy. Removal was followed by slow regression of all these lesions, leaving mild scars. A healthy boy was delivered several months later.

Androgenization of newborn girls is a worrisome complication of androgen excess.

Above

Left   Severe inflammation, seborrhea, and hirsutism disfigure this woman

Right   Acne conglobata-like hemorrhagic draining sinuses behind the earlobe

Middle

Left   The acne-prone area of the chest is also involved

Right   Increased hair growth and scattered papules and pustules on the abdomen are part of this disease

Below

Left   Inflammatory papules and pustules on the V-shaped area of the back

Right   Close-up of a highly inflamed papulopustule on the back

Below right: Courtesy of Professor Joseph Zander, Munich, FRG

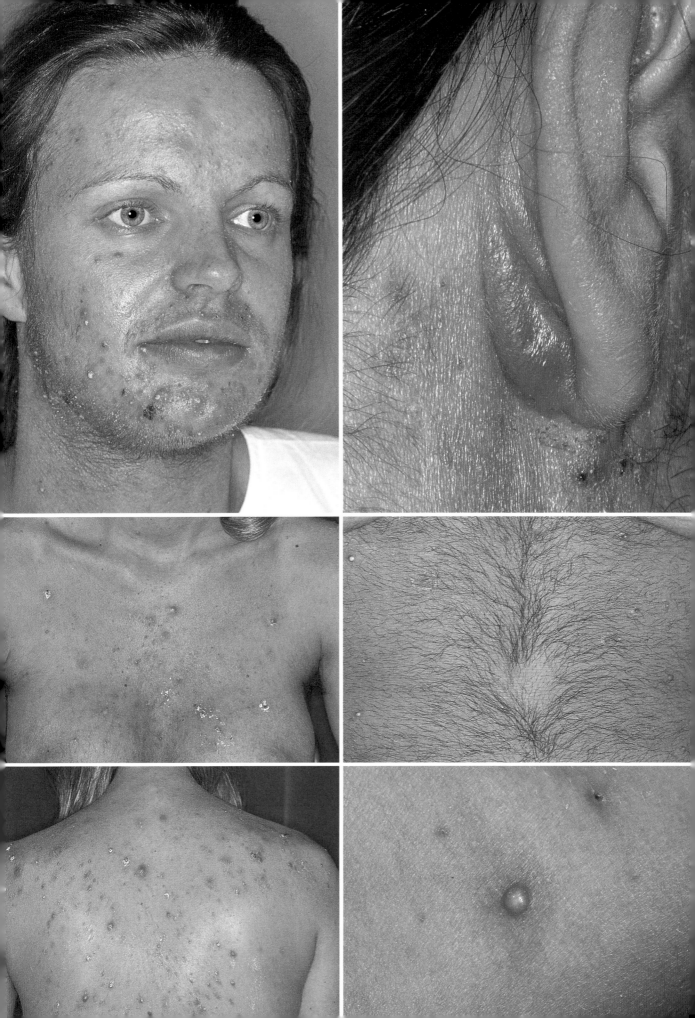

Androgen Excess in Men

XYY Acne Conglobata

Dermatologists are always delighted when skin lesions lead to the correct diagnosis of systemic disease or genetic disorders. It appears that acne conglobata is an important phenotypic feature of men with an extra Y chromosome. The XYY genotype first came to light in a penal survey of criminals and psychopaths. Three features were almost always present. Height was in excess of 180 cm, there was mental retardation or at least subnormal intelligence, and aggressive behavior. It later became known that some of these patients also had acne conglobata. The first investigators of this disorder were not dermatologists and could have overlooked skin lesions and scars. The incidence of XYY in newborn boys is about 1:1000 and that of acne conglobata in white adolescent men about 3%. In institutionalized juvenile delinquents the incidence of XYY was 1:35, twenty-four times the frequency in newborns. Furthermore one out of seven patients with XYY had severe inflammatory acne. In another outpatient survey the figure for acne conglobata was 2% in the white population. The prevalence in criminals was twice that figure. If aggressiveness is a true feature of this phenotype, the impulse to commit a crime will naturally be increased. However, caution is in order. Testosterone production and circulating levels of androgens have been found to be normal in these XYY patients. They do have very oily skin, a prerequisite for severe acne. It seems more likely that some persons with severe acne are emotionally traumatized by the unsightly, socially isolating affliction and are thus more likely to turn their hostility into antisocial behavior. This may be why the incidence of moderate to severe acne seems higher in prison populations.

XYY acne conglobata differs in no way from the same disorder in XY individuals. A clue may be the unusually early onset, even prepuberally, with peak severity in early adolescence. Severe acne in a very tall, not too bright boy calls for investigation. Fortunately the cytogenetic analysis is quite easy and does not require the preparation of chromosome maps. It turns out that the distal portion of the long arm of the Y chromosome binds strongly to quinacrine (atabrine) and can thus be readily identified by fluorescence microscopy. Leukocytes obtained by a finger prick will show two bright fluorescing dots. This is the exact counterpart of the Barr body which identifies the X chromosome in women.

The treatment is the same as for acne conglobata in XY subjects.

Gorlin RJ, Cohen MM Jr, Levin LS (1990) Syndromes of the head and neck, 3rd edn. Oxford University Press, New York, pp 61–63

Hook EB (1973) Behavioral implications of the human XYY genotype. Science 179:139–150

Jones KL (1988) Smith's recognizable pattern of human malformation, 4th edn. Saunders, Philadelphia, pp 64–65

Murken JD (1973) The XYY-syndrome and Kline-felter's syndrome. Investigations into epidemiology, clinical picture, psychology, behavior and genetics. Thieme, Stuttgart

Sosis AC, Panet-Raymond G, Goldenberg DM (1973) XYY chromosome complement in a patient with nodulocystic acne. Dermatologica 146:222–228

Voorhees JJ, Wilkins JW Jr, Hayes E, Harrell ER (1972) Nodulocystic acne as a phenotypic feature of the XYY genotype. Report of five cases, review of all known XYY subjects with severe acne, and discussion of XYY cytodiagnosis. Arch Dermatol 105:913–919

Body Building Acne

Excessive use, actually abuse, of androgens can induce acne vulgaris, acne conglobata, and even acne fulminans. It always aggravates pre-existing acne.

Body building acne is a dramatic variant of androgen-induced acne. The former belief that in postpubertal men sebaceous glands are maximally stimulated by circulating endogenous androgens is false. Exogenous androgens enhance seborrhea even in oily men.

Body building is a madness among men and women alike, especially in competitive international sports, e.g., weight lifters, swimmers, etc. Muscular teenagers, compared to whom Tarzan looks like a dwarf, greatly increase their muscular mass with high doses of androgens to attain a powerful figure according to their sense of beauty and health. Testosterone and its derivatives are usually not prescribed by physicians. They are easily accessible through illicit channels in many health- and athletics clubs. Sebum production increases rapidly, causing frank seborrhea in typical sites like the face, scalp, chest, and back. Severe inflammatory acne, including acne conglobata, can erupt within a few weeks of heavy dosing.

The worst complication is acne fulminans. Power athletes experience the same drastic afflictions.

Sometimes the situation is worsened by the addition of a super-vitamin bolus taken orally or injected: acneiform eruptions from high doses of vitamins B_1, B_6, and B_{12} are well known. Androgens eventually cause testicular atrophy and infertility, possibly only partially reversible. Athletic adolescents are usually uninformed concerning this. Of course, masculinization is inevitable in women. Usually violent expressions of acne rapidly developing in youngsters call for penetrating questioning. Denial is common. A urine test (doping test) for steroids may confirm a suspected diagnosis. Treatment consists of withdrawal from the anabolic steroids and vigorous therapy as for acne conglobata or acne fulminans.

In the USA several states have passed laws which prohibit a physician from prescribing, administering, or dispensing any anabolic steroid for the purpose of enhancing a person's performance in an exercise, sport, or game intending to increase muscle mass, strength, or weight without medical necessity. Violation results in suspension of the medical license and even imprisonment. Physicians should add their voice to the campaign by stressing the danger to health.

Heydenreich G (1989) Testosterone and anabolic steroids and acne fulminans. Arch Dermatol 125:571–572

Király CL, Collan Y, Alén M (1987) Effect of testosterone and anabolic steroids on the size of sebaceous glands in power athletes. Am J Dermatopathol 9:515–519

Király CL, Alén M, Korvola J, Horsmanheimo M (1988) The effect of testosterone and anabolic steroids on the skin surface lipids and the population of Propionibacteria acnes in young postpubertal men. Acta Derm Venereol (Stockh) 68:21–26

Knuth UA, Maniera H, Nieschlag E (1989) Anabolic steroids and semen parameters in bodybuilders. Fertil Steril 52:1041–1047

Merkle T, Landthaler M, Braun-Falco O (1990) Acne-conglobata-artige Exazerbation einer Acne vulgaris nach Einnahme von Anabolika und Vitamin-B-Komplex-haltigen Präparaten. Hautarzt 41:280–282

Acne Fulminans from Testosterone Therapy in Excessively Tall Boys

Over the past 30 years children everywhere have grown much taller than ever before. It is not rare to see teenagers taller than 2 m (7 ft.), while their forefathers were at least a head smaller. This explosion of growth rate is particularly evident in the asiatic races. Japanese and Korean children of today's generation sometimes look like giants compared to their parents. Good nutrition, protein-enriched diets, a surplus of minerals and vitamins act like fertilizer in agriculture and result in much heightened growth. Of course, there is also a genetic component. The increased growth rate is visible early, often at the age of 10–12 years. Alarmed parents sometimes ask for medical help to halt this excessive growth. One attempt is to administer testosterone and its derivatives to boys to control this process. The results are variable and the risks are great. The side effects include acne conglobata, acne fulminans, and all the other disagreeable expressions which anabolic steroids induce in power athletes.

Androgens cause hypertrophy of sebaceous follicles with marked seborrhea resulting in increased density of *Propionibacterium acnes*, ending in the worst kinds of inflammatory acne. The former concept that androgen-sensitive organs are under maximal stimulation in postpubertal boys is no longer acceptable. Treatment is the same as for acne fulminans.

Fyrand O, Fiskaadal HJ, Trygstad O (1992) Acne in pubertal boys undergoing treatment with androgens. Acta Derm Venereol (Stockh) 72:148–149

Hartmann AA, Burg G (1989) Acne fulminans bei Klinefelter-Syndrom unter Testosteron. Eine Nebenwirkung der Antihochwuchstherapie. Monatsschr Kinderheilkd 137:466–467

Klepzig K, Burg G, Schill WB, Knorr D, Tauber R (1986) Akne fulminans bei erhöhten Testosteronplasmawerten. In: Braun-Falco O, Schill WB (eds) Fortschritte der praktischen Dermatologie, vol 11. Springer, Berlin, pp 514–517

Mühlendahl KE von, Brämswig J, Traupe H, Happle R (1989) Akne fulminans nach hochdosierter Testosteronbehandlung bei hochwüchsigen Jungen. Dtsch Med Wochenschr 114:712–714

Traupe H, von Mühlendahl KE, Brämswig J, Happle R (1988) Acne of the fulminans type following testosterone therapy in three excessively tall boys. Arch Dermatol 124:414–417

Wild Outbreaks of Acne Following Testosterone Injections

Contrary to former belief, sebaceous glands in young adult men are not maximally stimulated by endogenous androgens. Excessive doses of androgens not only increases sebum production but can cause severe inflammatory acne.

Above Body building acne

Left This 21-year-old man had only mild facial acne since age 14 years. Two months ago he started a body building program together with illegal medication of anabolics and vitamin B cocktails. Face, chest, back, shoulders, and upper arms broke out with deep inflammatory papules, conglobate nodules, and pustules. Hypertrophic and keloidal scars were seen a year later. Thus doping caused acne conglobata

Right Close-up of left shoulder and upper arm showing the conglobate nature of the disease

Below Testosterone-induced acne fulminans. Testosterone injection is sometimes used in an attempt to arrest excessive growth in young boys. The iatrogenic therapeutic trial ended in a disaster. The 15-year-old boy received 250 mg testosterone propionate as a depot once weekly from March to September. In August he became seriously ill with malaise, fever, leukocytosis (24000/µl), elevated sedimentation rate (47/48 mm, Westergren method), and arthralgia. The skin on the chest, shoulders, upper arms, and back ulcerated and became crusted with hemorrhagic, easily bleeding and painful lesions.
The testosterone was stopped. Treatment with methyl prednisolone 40 mg/day for 1 week and isotretinoin 1.0 mg/kg body weight for many weeks abated the storm

Below: Courtesy of Kristina Klepzig, M.D., Tanja Merkle, M.D., and Professor Otto Braun-Falco, Munich, FRG

Klepzig K, Burg G, Schill WB, Knorr D, Tauber R (1986) Akne fulminans bei erhöhten Testosteronplasmawerten. In: Braun-Falco O, Schill WB (eds) Fortschritte der praktischen Dermatologie, vol 11. Springer, Berlin, pp 514–517

Merkle T (1990) Exazerbation einer Akne vulgaris nach Einnahme von Anabolika und Vitamin-B-Komplex-haltigen Präparaten. In: Braun-Falco O, Ring J (eds) Fortschritte der praktischen Dermatologie, vol 12. Springer, Berlin, ppo 546–547

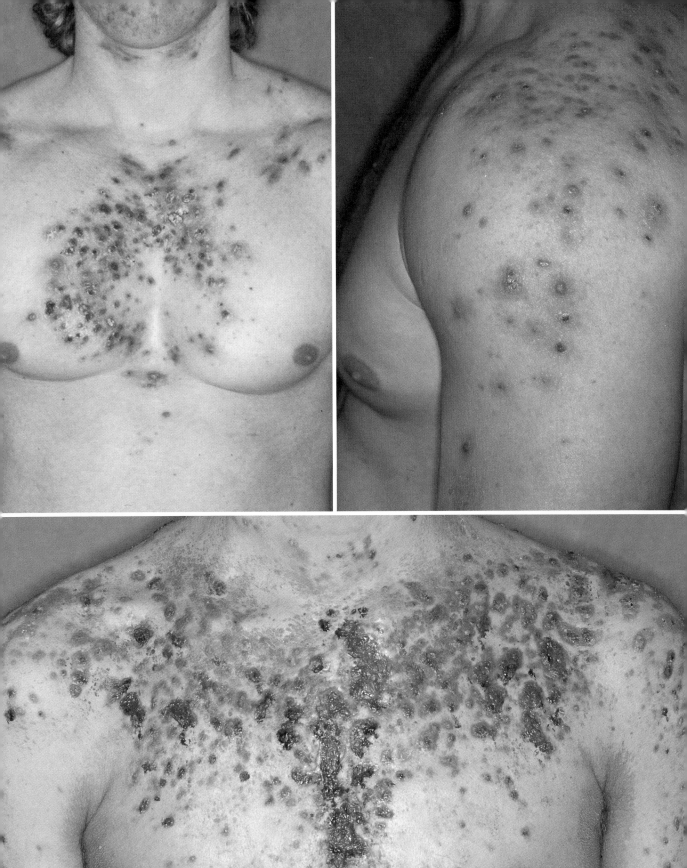

Excoriations

Dermatologists seem to delight in pedantic nomenclature. Textbooks refer to this disorder by its French name *acné excoriée des jeunes filles*. The ordinary term is excoriations in acne. These terms are confounded, however, by the fact that not all the patients have acne. Acne lesions are often just a pretext for manipulating the face.

Excoriations in Acne Patients

Excoriations usually begin in the teens when the patients start to see comedones or minor inflammatory lesions. Young women are especially susceptible, men rarely, perhaps because acne has less serious psychosocial consequences. Anxious subjects often cannot leave the lesions alone and attack them in different ways.

Ways of attack vary. Squeezing is most common. They take satisfaction in popping out comedones and suppurative material from inflammatory lesions, painful as this might be. Pickers are under less compulsion to manipulate and cause less damage. Others rub, but the really mecing maneuver is crushing between fingers, thereby dispersing the contents into the dermis.

Picking hours are either during the day when studying, reading or working, or during the morning or the evening toilet in front of a mirror. Magnifying mirrors turn even the slightest acne lesion into a deep crater.

Excoriations are diffusely distributed over the entire face which may have been severely disfigured. They are always polymorphic, including oozing excoriations, hemorrhagic crusts, and various forms of scars.

Excoriations in Patients Without Acne

The difference to the above-mentioned variant is that the patients do not have any obvious lesions, though they may have had acne in the past. They usually insist on the presence of prior lesions, which are no longer recognizable to the observer, having been obliterated by the fingers. Even careful inspection will not disclose acne lesions like open or closed comedones, papules or papulopustules. Every day the skin is gouged out with the fingernails, leaving broad, shallow, linear scars, preceded by a variable degree of crushing. It is easy to differentiate these linear self-induced scars from those due to acne itself.

Excoriations are not limited to the face, but are often found on the chest, breast, shoulder girdle, V-shaped area of the back, and lateral aspects of the upper arms as far as the fingers can reach. The damage is too great to be discounted as a kind of unconcious tic-like action. Some patients are disturbed in their psychosexual adjustments and have many unsolved problems which engender a variety of neurotic ways of acting. They may have no self-confidence and self-esteem, be emotionally labile, and self-piteous. The excoriating habit may go on for decades. The skin then becomes leathery, with a pebbled scarred surface and spotty pigmentation. This might be viewed as a form of cutaneous masochism.

Treatment

Topical therapy is ineffective. The most important thing is to explain the vicious cycle to the patient. Once excoriations are stopped, hemorrhagic scabs, stellate scars, and unpleasant hyper- and hypopigmentations will disappear. Often they have consulted many dermatologists who either missed the diagnosis or have a distaste for psychological confrontations. These patients have tried myriads of medicaments. They do not need a prescription but a frank consultation. Build a bridge; many will happily follow your advice.

We have two simple approaches. First we carefully count fresh and old excoriations and write down these figures in the presence of the patient. When the patient returns, we count them again. Usually the patient will be relieved by the gradually decreasing number of lesions. Secondly we take full facial photographs, en face and laterally, and show them on the next appointment.

No topical remedy is prescribed during the first consultation. If there is underlying acne, use appropriate topical therapy. The correction of scarring by dermabrasion or intralesional injection of collagen should not be considered until there is evidence that the patient has regained self-control.

When anxiety is high or depression is evident, it may be desirable to try sedatives and psychotropic drugs. If everything fails, referral to a psychiatrist is indicated. Behavioral therapy is sometimes helpful in stopping the manipulation. This disease can be mutilating to the skin and the psyche.

Arnetz BA (ed) (1991) Dermatological psychosomatics. Acta Derm Venereol [Suppl 156] (Stockh)

Fruensgaard K (1991) Psychotherapeutic strategy and neurotic excoriations. Int J Dermatol 30:198–203

Kent A, Drummond LM (1989) Acne excoriée – a case report of treatment using habit reversal. Clin Exp Dermatol 14:163–164

Kenyon FE (1966) Psychosomatic aspects of acne. Br J Dermatol 78:344–351

Molinski H, Rechenberger I (1977) Psychosomatik der Akne. Fortschr Med 95:2149–2153

Sneddon J, Sneddon I (1983) Acne excoriée: a protective device. Clin Exp Dermatol 8:65–68

Vogel PG (1974) Zur Acne excoriée des jeunes filles. Eine Symptomanalyse. Hautarzt 25:333–336

Excoriations

Patients sometimes have an irresistible urge to pick and scratch what they misinterpret as early acne lesions. The patients are mostly young women who do not have appreciable acne. This behavior reveals a neurotic preoccupation with the face.

Above

Left   Asymmetry is typical for excoriations. These are variable in size and shape and do not correspond to any natural distribution of disease, including acne. Hyperpigmentation is often a troublesome problem, particularly in dark-skinned people

Right   At first glance this looks like acne. However no comedones are present. All the lesions have been provoked by her own manipulations. Frenzies of ferocious picking may occur at times of stress

Below

Left   In addition to picking and squeezing, this patient has used her finger nails to scratch the skin. Linear, shallow lesions are diagnostic of excoriations

Right   This patient had severe acne in adolescence, at which time she became an obsessioned picker and squeezer. The habit deepened into severe attacks of the face after the acne cleared, leaving disfiguring scars. Psychosomatic or even psychiatric evaluation is indicated with self-destructive manipulations of this severity. Depression is common

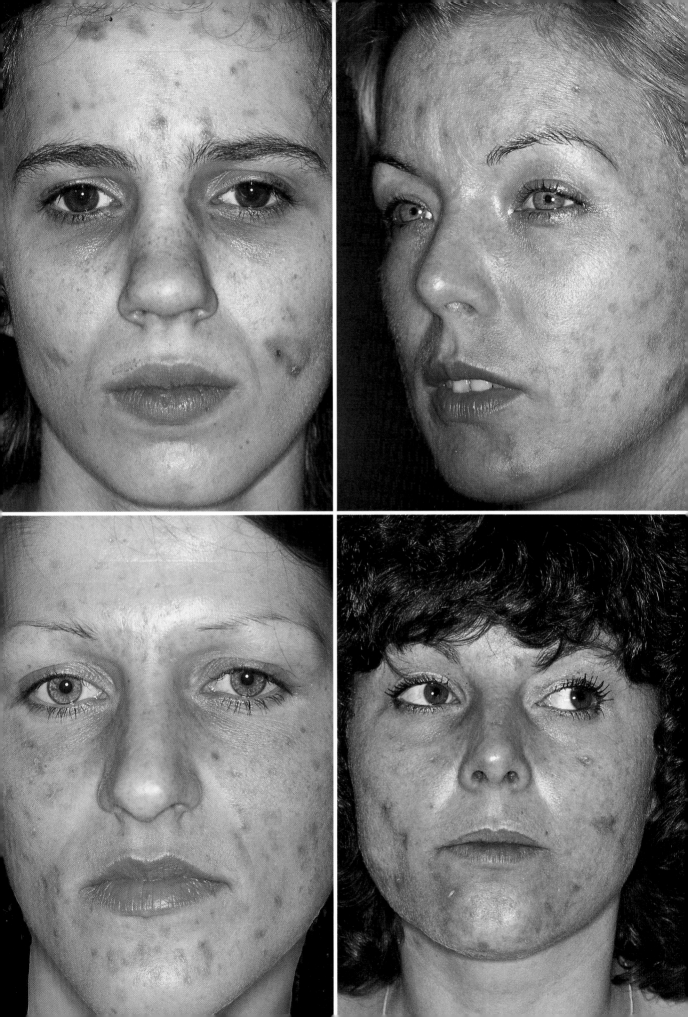

Acne Venenata

Venenum is Latin for poison. In this context it means poisonous for the sebaceous follicles. Acne venenata is contact acne, in most instances epicutaneous contact. Rarer routes of contact are by inhalation or ingestion; the latter are seen in some cases of chloracne. This will be dealt with in a different chapter.

Contact with a great variety of substances can produce a follicular eruption which ranges in expression from trivial to terrible. The initiating event is the formation of a comedo. Acne venenata is therefore a species of true acne, not an acneiform eruption.

Cosmetics, toiletries, and grooming agents are the sources of acneigenic substances which cause the commoner types of acne venenata. Certain variants of acne venenata are separately named because of their distinctive localizations and causes, e.g., cosmetic acne, pomade acne, etc.

The most extensive and most severe cases occur in the industrial setting. These comprise the occupational acne venenatas. Ferocious outbreaks of generalized acne leaving hardly a follicle untouched have been recorded in certain manufacturing plants in the past 50 years. Now that acneigenic chemicals can be identified by the rabbit ear test one would think that such disasters would be unlikely to occur anymore. This is not true. Chloracne is still with us; there are still outbreaks.

One must appreciate that extensive eruptions of acne venenata can occur not only from external contact but also by inhalation or even by accidental ingestion of acneigenic chemicals. Dramatic instances of the latter have been reported in Japan, Taiwan, and Spain where chlorinated hydrocarbons accidentally contaminated rice oil and other food products. These epidemics were associated with systemic toxicity associated with anorexia, vomiting, asthma, swelling of limbs, neuropathies, as well as the whole spectrum of acne lesions, not only in typical locations but also on the axillae, penis, extremities, nipples, and eyelids. Comedones and cysts develop everywhere there are follicles.

Other epidemics clearly implicate a contactant, for example, among ethnic groups who regularly treat their scalps with oils. Numerous comedones develop on the face, especially in areas adjacent to the scalp. The oils used were cheap-grade products containing comedogenic impurities.

Comedones, especially blackheads, are the hallmarks of acne venenata. Cysts and extensive inflammatory lesions occur only with the more potent materials. Typically the lesions occur in hordes. The best known varieties of acne venenata are acne cosmetica; pomade acne; the occupational acnes: petroleum oil acne and oil, tar, and pitch acne; and chloracne.

The Occupational Acnes

Petroleum Oil Acne. Oilfield and refinery workers can acquire an extensive eruption of acne lesions. Face, neck, ears, and forearms are the sites of predilection. When working outdoors in sunny regions acne venenata may be greatly aggravated by ultraviolet (UV) radiation, an example of photocomedogenicity.

Oil, Tar, and Pitch Acne. Coal tars and pitches are well-known acneigens that can cause massive eruptions in road workers, roofers, and other occupations. Phototoxic reactions complicate the picture and are sometimes responsible for horrendous exacerbations. Substances which are both comedogenic and phototoxic cause the worst eruptions, e.g., coal tar.

Cutting Oil Acne. A wide variety of cutting oils are used throughout the world. Many of them are mixtures of paraffin oils, with antioxidants and antimicrobials added. The composition of cutting oils varies greatly with manufacturers. Because of their extensive use they constitute the commonest cause of occupational acne. Cutting oil acne occurs especially where occupational standards and federal regulations are lax or absent. Standards require shields on the mechanical equipment to prevent splashing. Helmets, goggles, screens, and long-sleeved garments are of course protective.

Cutting and drilling oil acne occurs where splashings of these fluids repeatedly come into contact with the skin. Three body sites are particularly at risk: face, forearms, and thighs. Direct contamination of the unprotected face, or soiling of working clothes, wearing them for several days without proper cleaning, provokes this contact acne.

At first densely studded closed and open comedones develop within a few months.

The apex of the prominent pores is of dirty gray-black color. Inflammation follows as a secondary event, creating deep-seated and painful nodules, sometimes mimicking the picture of acne conglobata. Less often the lesions are inflammatory to begin with showing a pustular folliculitis. Inevitably, comedones follow with dense crops of blackheads.

Treatment

The key requirement, of course, is to stop the exposure. This alone is not sufficient, for serious cases take a long time to resolve, sometimes several years. Apparently high tissue concentrations of insoluble acneigenic substances, notably chlorinated hydrocarbons, are responsible for this persistence. Enforced safety standards at work are an important task of occupational dermatology. Freshly laundered working clothes should be provided.

For most cases the treatment of choice is tretinoin. Comedones are typical of acne venenata, and no other exfoliant is as effective as tretinoin. Antibiotics are generally not required.

Suncreens are recommended for outdoor laborers in contact with comedogenic substances, especially oils and tars.

Braun W (1955) Chlorakne. Akneartige Hautveränderungen durch chlorierte Kohlenwasserstoffe. Editio Cantor, Aulendorf

Crow KD (1970) Chloracne: a critical review, including a comparison of two series of cases of acne from chlornaphthalene and pitch fumes. Trans St. Johns Hosp Dermatol Soc 56:79–99

Kaidbey KH, Kligman AM (1974) A human model of coal tar acne. Arch Dermatol 109:212–215

Tindall JP (1985) Chloracne and chloracnegens. J Am Acad Dermatol 13:539–558

Contact Acne

This man sharpened dental tools using oils which contained chlorinated hydrocarbons. These drilling oils contaminated his entire face. He had many large open comedones especially on the cheeks where sebaceous follicles are abundant. Sparing of the nose is typical. Nasal follicles have thick, sturdy horny layers which impede transport of acneigenic materials. Dense and large blackheads are the hallmarks of chloracne. Treatment of choice was tretinoin, which completely cleared the ugly comedones.

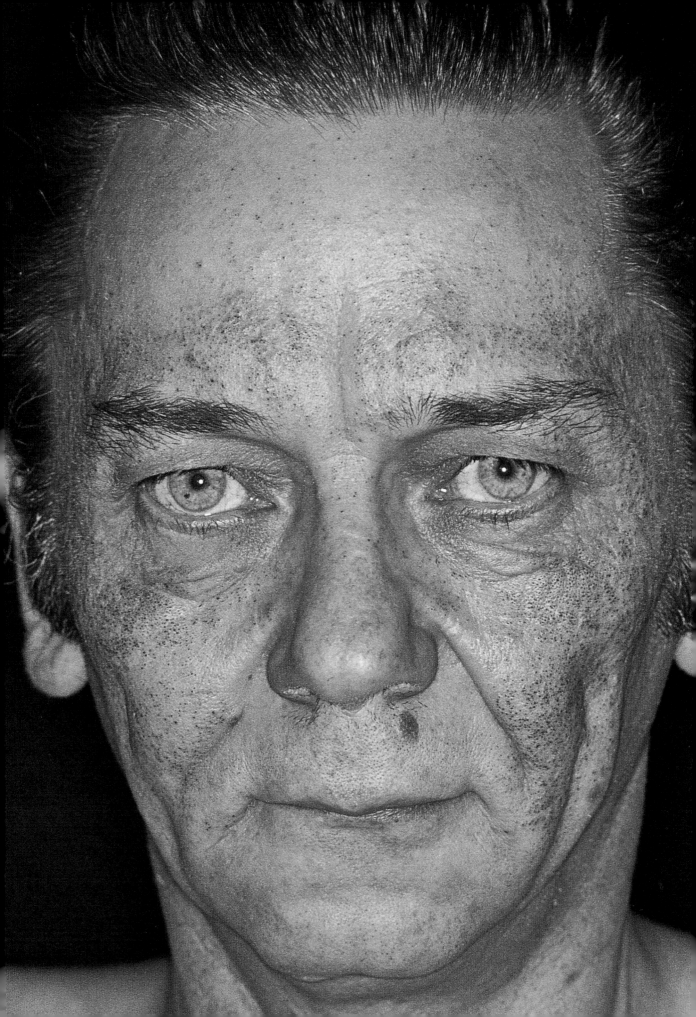

Oil Acne and Chloracne: Industrial Hazards

Contamination of the skin with acneigenic (comedogenic) cutting oils, greases, tars and other petroleum distillates or halogenated aromatic hydrocarbons may cause contact acne. Predilection sites are thighs, lower arms, and shoulders. Almost every follicle is involved. Mostly noninflammatory comedones in a monomorphic pattern evolve; inflammation is always secondary.

Above   Oil acne in mechanics

Left   Oil acne on the thigh of an automobile mechanic. Soon after microcomedones have formed they turn into papulopustules

Right   Oil acne in an industrial worker. Every follicle is accentuated by a small keratotic plug (comedones). A few lesions became inflamed

Below   Histopathology of chloracne. After exposure to penta- and hexachloronaphthalene chloracne developed. All follicles are involved, typical for chloracne. Dense layers of coneocytes form compact comedones. Bacteria are notably absent, probably because of the toxic (bacteriostatic) effects of the chemical. All sebaceous glands are regressed; the pilary units are intact

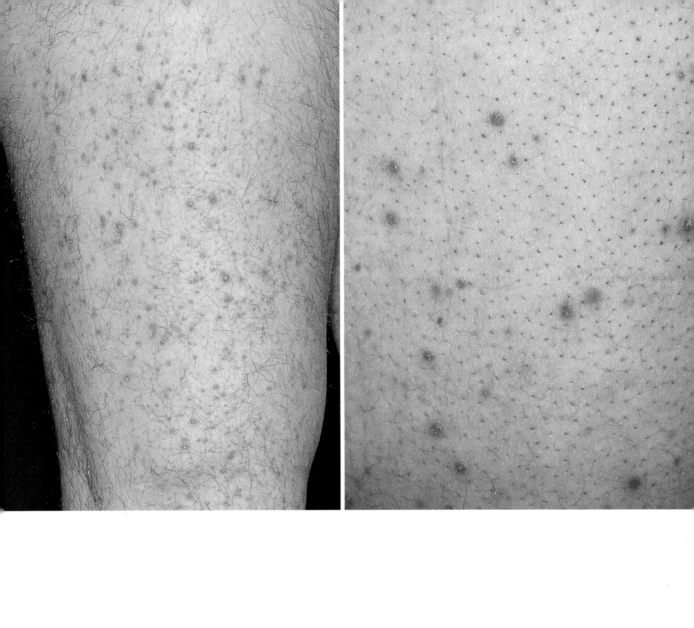
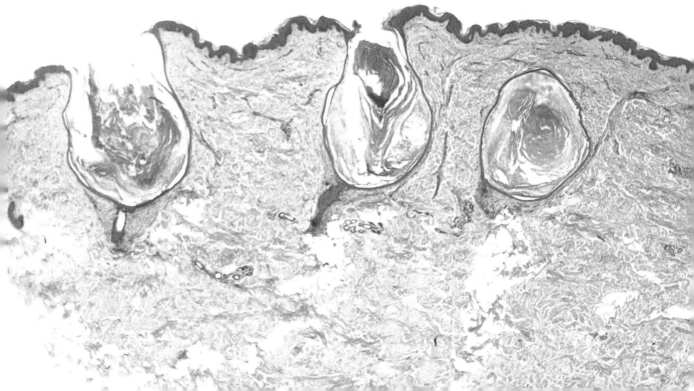

Pitch Acne

Above   The comedones on forehead, temple and nose are a result of prolonged exposure to tars and pitch in a road worker

Below   The histopathology of comedones induced by tars and other potent occupational acneigens is different from comedones of acne vulgaris. The epithelial lining is thicker rather than thinner. Bacteria are notably absent because tars contain bacteriostatic substances. All sebaceous glands have totally regressed. Minute epithelial buds at the bottom of the comedones tell where the sebaceous acini were once attached

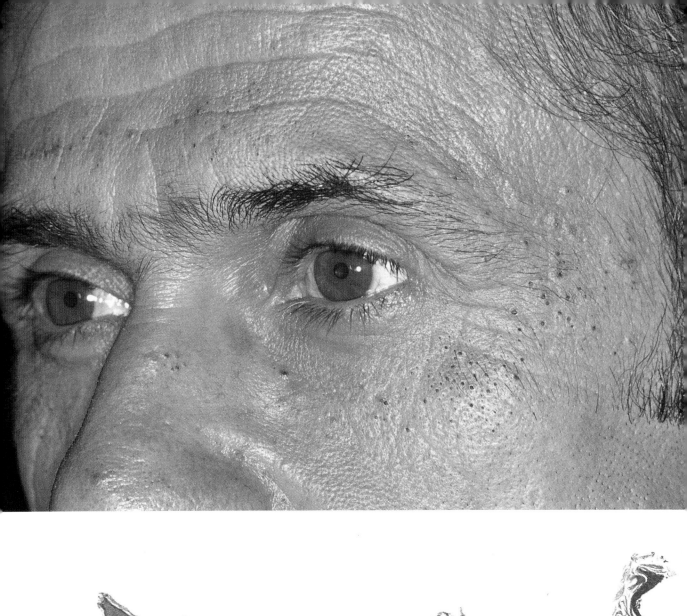
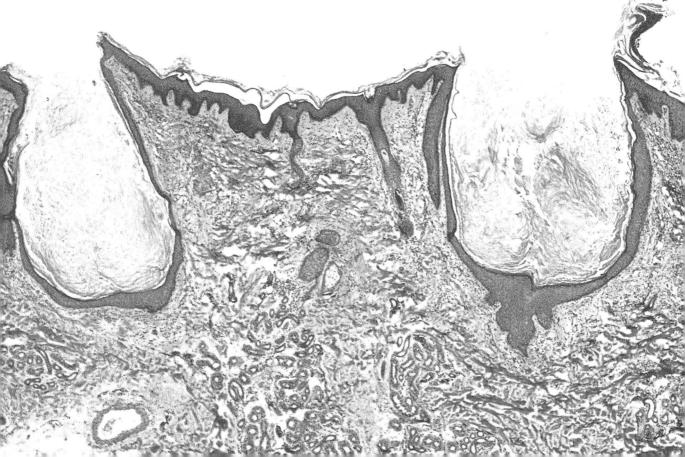

Acne Cosmetica

Acne cosmetica is another variant of acne venenata. The patients are women who tend to have been enthusiastic users of cosmetics for years and decades. We use the term cosmetics in the broadest sense to include all the practices relating to cleansing and self-adornment. A pertinent history encompasses questioning about the use of moisturizers, foundation creams, cleansers, toners, abrasives, anti-wrinkle creams, sunscreens, blushers, etc. The longer the list, the greater the likelihood of trouble. Even hair care products such as conditioners and shampoos, become suspect when the eruption borders the scalp.

Women often do not see a connection between cosmetic usage and their facial lesions. Afflicted women will often run from one cosmetic counter to another randomly, haphazardly switching products in search of clear skin. Then, too, applications tend to become heavier to mask papulopustules. Flushers and blushers often prefer camouflage, but the pigments in masking preparations are often compacted in a matrix of comedogenic oils and are predictably aggravating.

Moreover, certain over-the-counter anti-acne medicaments are actually comedogenic, especially those containing sulfur. Paradoxically, concentrations of some benzoyl peroxide formulations worsen acne. Benzoyl peroxide is mistakenly viewed as comedolytic when it is actually comedogenic. The vehicles of certain topical antibiotics are also comedogenic and may account for puzzling differences in efficacy of products of equal concentrations of the same antibiotic. A high level of suspicion must be maintained when acne unaccountably persists.

We emphasize that a variety of irritants can aggravate acne. First of all, irritating chemicals contained in soaps, cleansers, astringents, and toners definitely enhance the activity of comedogenic substances. They are not comedogenic in their own right but act as promoters. Among irritants which are common components of facial products, one has to list cationic surfactants, often used as preservatives, certain fragrances, and even propylene glycol. These affects are concentration dependent. A mere presence is not sufficient.

The question of comedogenicity is much more complex than we originally presented in our acne paper on comedogenicity (1975). The term comedogenicity has thus to be qualified and expanded conceptionally. It turns out that a horny kernel cannot be demonstrated in all papulopustules as is usually the case in acne vulgaris. Irritants by themselves can damage the follicular epithelial lining, allowing sebum, an irritating oil, to seep into the skin, provoking a toxic inflammatory lesion. This may be regarded as a type of chemical folliculitis, which skips the horny impaction state. Furthermore, while true acne localizes in sebaceous follicles, chemical folliculitis frequently involves the smaller, more numerous vellus follicles. This unusual localization may be suspected when there are myriads of densely distributed small pustules. Formerly we explained a surface studded with tiny pustules by diagnosing miliaria, a sweat disorder. Histologic investigation, however, clearly points to vellus follicles. Sometimes, a mild sub-sunburn will precipitate a chemical folliculitis. One always has to keep in mind the tremendous physical and chemical assaults the facial skin receives every day. These have cumulative effects.

The term we now prefer is acneigenicity, which encompasses noncomedonal inflammatory lesions (chemical folliculitis) in contrast to agents which are purely comedogenic (comedogenicity). The two are often combined.

Clinical Findings

At first glance the appearance of acne cosmetica may resemble acne vulgaris. In fact, many of these women can be recognized as acne prone by a history of acne during adolescence. In such cases, acne cosmetica is superimposed on acne vulgaris. However, prior acne is not a prerequisite to the diagnosis. The disorder may first appear in the patient's twenties and thirties following changes in cosmetic practices.

A helpful clue to the diagnosis is the high density of the lesions which crowd the surface. There may be numerous closed comedones with a scattering of papulopustules; or most of the lesions may be small papulopustules or any combination thereof. Open comedones are also found but are usually not numerous or large. Premenstrual flares are not characteristic. Severe inflammatory acne is never due to cosmetics.

Localization patterns implicate cosmetics. For example, numerous acneiform lesions on the cheeks suggest blushers and bronzers. A feature that has not been suf-ficiently emphasized is the fairly frequent accompaniment of perioral dermatitis, which we attribute mainly to external contactants (p. 479).

In the original paper on acne cosmetica it was categorically stated that "an automatic diagnosis of acne cosmetica in a woman with a mild acneiform eruption would be correct 95% of the time." We found that about 50% of facial creams and lotions randomly sampled were comedogenic in the rabbit ear assay. Thus, the circumstantial evidence implicating cosmetics and toiletries in acne cosmetica was very compelling. After all, most women use cosmetics and postadolescent acne occurs in at least a third of adult women, but not at all in men. The idea was logical and was swiftly endorsed by dermatologists.

While acne cosmetica is a reality, however, times have changed and cosmetics can no longer be regarded as the principal cause of postadolescent acne in women. The reasons are as follows:

- Major producers of cosmetics routinely test their products in the rabbit ear assay which, whatever its failings, excludes moderately acneigenic compounds.
- Complete withdrawal of all cosmetics too often fails to result in clearing. Partial remissions are commonly followed by flares.
- Astonishingly, the deliberate use of known acneigenic products, applied daily and liberally for up to 3 months, did not aggravate acne in acne-prone subjects. Most experienced no worsening. The sample size was small and the exposure time short.
- By contrast, in classic forms of acne cosmetica with densely studded lesions of small comedones and small papulopustules accompanied by an incriminating history, withdrawal of the suspected agents is indeed followed by gradual clearing within 3–4 months.

What then is the cause of low-grade acne in adult women? We propose an alternative explanation in which we inculpate emotional stress as a dominant causative factor.

As regards treatment, in bona fide cases withdrawal of suspected acneigenic agents is sufficient by itself. A list of nonacneigenic products should be supplied. Actually, a wide choice is now available, especially if one sticks to major manufacturers who follow current guidelines for avoiding acneigenic formulations.

Regression of lesions can be accelerated by topical tretinoin, starting with the lowest concentration to keep down irritancy. Oral antibiotics are also helpful to achieve a fast response.

Kligman AM, Mills OH Jr (1972) "Acne cosmetica". Arch Dermatol 106:843–850

Kligman AM (1988/89) A critical look at acne cosmetica. J Cutan Aging Cosmet Dermatol 1:109–114

Contact Acne

A wide variety of compounds can cause acne, initially often not suspected by the patients and physician.

Above

Left Acne cosmetica due to a comedogenic cosmetic series, heavily used by this lady

Right Steroid acne. Years ago steroid-containing antiacne drugs were still available. Today some patients use corticosteroids to improve skin blemishes of all kinds. Initially the drug works well, but sooner or later new lesions will spring up. If used for many months, results like this emerge with hundreds of brown-red papules, comedones, and telangiectases

Below

Left Acne cosmetica in a typical distribution. Several cosmetics, moisturizers, day and night cremes etc. were used. Pattern and morphology of lesions are indicative of comedogenic cosmetics

Right Hundreds of tiny closed comedones, papules, and pustules cover the entire face of this young girl, who probably started with a very minor acne problem, followed by intensive and extensive use of cosmetics. Once diagnosed the best recommendation is abstinence of cosmetics and a good peel with tretinoin

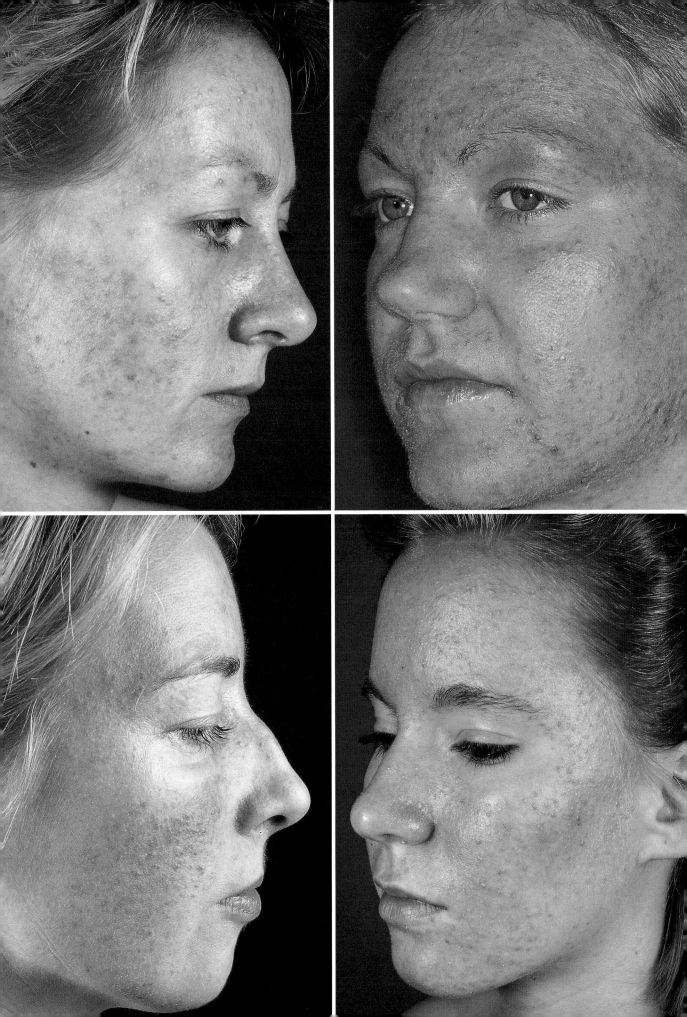

Chap-Stick Acne

Acne cosmetica is common in women who use comedogenic products. The culprit ingredients are identified, e.g., in the rabbit ear model.

Lip balsam can cause comedones very similar to what is known as pomade acne. Repetitive applications of a lubricating lip stick (Chap-Stick is a US brand name) associated with the appearance of a single row of open and closed comedones along the vermillion border of the upper lips and the oral commisures of two black women. Therapy consists of elimination of the offending comedogenic lubricant and expression of visible comedones.

Shelley WB, Shelley ED (1986) Chap-Stick acne. Cutis 37:459–460

Pomade Acne

Pomade acne is a prototype of acne venenata, and therefore a true member of the acne family. It was very common and still is in some cultures and among certain ethnic groups. It is not surprising that the cosmetic-conscious French first identified acne venenata due to brilliantines applied to the scalp and face. Impurities in cheap products were incriminated. The situation has changed. Pomade acne is nowadays more likely to be caused by more expensive formulations with high-grade ingredients. In America pomade acne is almost exclusively a problem of adult Blacks, especially men. It also occurs in women and teenagers who apply various greases and oils to the scalp as hair-grooming aids. Some inexplicably rub the pomade over the face as well. The prevalence in Black men may be as great as 25%, at least in a mild forehead form.

The lesions consist mainly of closely set, uniform, small, closed comedones, often in dense crowds. The comedones are chiefly located on the forehead and temples. These are the areas of drainage from the scalp. The cheeks and chin may also be involved when the pomade is rubbed over the entire face. In the most affected areas almost every follicle is involved. From time to time a few pustules may be present. Open comedones are rare and never large.

Puncture releases a small whitish kernel of horny material, proof that the lesion is in fact a comedo. Histopathology reveals comedones identical to those of acne vulgaris.

Test Procedure. Comedogenicity of various pomades has been assayed in the rabbit ear model. For details see p. 234. The rank order of comedogenic potency correlates well with the clinical data. Simple hydrocarbons, such as mineral oil and petrolatum in their refined forms, are inactive. These are sometimes contaminated with other ingredients. It is wise to check the label. The more complex pomades are nicer but more expensive and more comedogenic. Sometimes hair conditioners and exotic shampoos are comedogenic and can create a disorder mimicking pomade acne.

It must be emphasized that pomades and cosmetics are weak comedogens. They become significant only because of daily use for years, still not every user develops comedones. Persons with past acne or still ongoing acne, seborrhea, and prominent follicular pores are particularly at risk. We found that comedones are more readily provoked in Blacks than in Whites. The follicles of the former are genetically primed toward hyperkeratosis. This predisposes Blacks to acne venenata. Blacks also have a greater tendency to develop chloracne.

Differential Diagnosis. Pomade acne is easily recognized in adults past the acne age. History is telling. In adolescents the peculiar localization in areas contiguous to the scalp plus the high number of closed comedones helps to differentiate pomade acne from acne vulgaris. Still the two conditions may resemble each other and of course may coexist. When external acneigens can be excluded the diagnosis is acne vulgaris. Other variants of contact acne, such as oil, tar, and cutting oil acne, are easily sorted out by occupational history.

Treatment. Treatment is obvious: stop application of the offending agent. There is a wide variety of noncomedogenic grooming agents. Topical tretinoin is the treatment of choice for clearing comedones.

American Academy of Dermatology Invitational Symposium on Comedogenicity (1990) J Am Acad Dermatol 20:272–277

Berlin C (1954) Acne comedo in children due to paraffin oil applied on the head. Arch Dermatol Syph 69:683–687

Kligman AM (1989) Updating the rabbit ear comedogenic assay. In: Marks R, Plewig G (eds) Acne and related disorders. Dunitz, London, pp 97–106

Plewig G, Braun-Falco O (1971) Behandlung von Comedonen bei Morbus Favre-Racouchot and Acne venenata mit Vitamin A-Säure. Hautarzt 22:341–345

Plewig G, Fulton JE, Kligman AM (1970) Pomade acne. Arch Dermatol 101:580–584

Chloracne

Definition

Chloracne is a form of acne which is induced by contact with halogenated hydrocarbons. Some of these are superpotent toxins. Industrial accidents worldwide have been associated with catastrophic epidemics of poisoning and became a source of major legal battles regarding compensation. High levels of exposure result in systemic toxicity involving the liver (porphyria) and central nervous system. Deaths have been reported. Chloracne is a dermatologic disaster. Generally it is caused by external contact as well as from inhalation in occupational settings. Chloracne may even result from ingestion, although such events are uncommon. Poor hygiene is a contributing factor.

Chloracne has been experimentally induced in rabbits and humans. Microgram quantities can evoke the follicular eruption.

Chemistry

Not the number of chlorine atoms but their position and their isomerization on the hydrocarbon ring determines toxicity. The major chloracneigens are polyhalogenated naphthalenes, polyhalogenated biphenyls, polyhalogenated dibenzofurons, dioxins, and azobenzenes and azoxybenzenes.

Polyhalogenated Naphthalenes. Penta- and hexachloronaphthalenes are the principal offenders. The trade name for these materials is Halowax. This material has been used extensively in ship building, for insulating electrical wires, wood preservatives, sealing compounds, and dielectrics for condensors. The role of Halowax in the causation of chloracne is so prominent that Halowax acne has become a synonym for chloracne.

Polyhalogenated Biphenyls. Polychlorinated biphenyls (PCBs) and polybrominated biphenyls (PBBs) have been used in industrial processes since 1929, but were recognized as ubiquitious contaminants decades later. They are often found together with hexachloronaphthalenes and polychlorodibenzofurans. Today the polyhalogenated biphenyls are permitted only for closed systems, e.g., electrical transformers and capacitors. Unfortunately accidental explosions can generate very toxic polychlorinated dibenzodioxins (PCDD) or TCDD.

Polyhalogenated Dibenzofurans. These are contaminants in chlorinated phenols. Polychlorinated dibenzofurans (PCDF), e.g., penta- and hexachlorodibenzofurans, are major chloracneigens and are hepatotoxins. Polybrominated dibenzofurans (PBDF) have also caused outbreaks of chloracne.

Dioxins. Dioxin is 2,3,7,8-tetrachlorodibenzo-*p*-dioxin (TCDD). Although there are many isomers of dioxin, the term dioxin is applied generally to this class of hydrocarbons. There is no industrial need for the manufacture of dioxins. Dioxins are unwanted by-products from the production of chlorinated phenols or 2,4,5-T (trichlorophenoxyacetic acid), compounds which have many uses as weed killers, etc. Dioxins may also be generated by combustion processes.

Three compounds are of major concern: TCDD; hexachlorodibenzo-*p*-dioxin, HCDD; 2,3,7,8-tetrachlorodibenzofuran, TCDF.

Azobenzenes and Azoxybenzenes. Chloracne has occurred in relation to the manufacture of 3,4-dichloroaniline and related herbicides. Of importance is 3,4,3',4'-tetrachloroazoxybenzene (TCAOB) and 3,4,3',4'-tetrachloroazobenzene (TCAB); these are contaminants in the production of dichloroaniline. The pesticides and herbicides propanil and methazole belong to this family.

A Synopsis of Major Epidemics of Chloracne

Trichlorophenol Accident in Ludwigshafen, FRG, 1953. An explosion in a BASF plant liberated 2,4,5-trichlorophenol and its derivatives and contaminants. Forty-two laborers became ill with the full-blown picture of widespread acne and systemic toxicity. We have witnessed acne conglobata-like chloracne from this accident almost 40 years later.

Yusho Poisoning in Japan 1968. Rice oil became contaminated with large amounts of tetrachlorobiphenyls and chlorodibenzofurans. It afflicted 1665 persons! Fifty-one died from this unprecedented exposure.

Firemaster Flame Retardant, Michigan, USA, 1973. Hundreds of pounds of hexabrominated biphenyl flame retardant (Firemaster BP-6) were accidentally mixed with cattle feed. Thousands of animals died. Humans became exposed through contact with contaminated feed or from consumption of dairy products. Prompt public health measures limited the damage. There were no deaths.

Pesticide-Herbicide Production in Ohio, USA, 1972–1973 and Arkansas, USA, 1974–1977. Forty-one workers developed chloracne due to 3,4-dichloroaniline and its derivatives azo- and azoxybenzenes.

TCDD Poisoning in Seveso, Italy, 1976. Following the explosion of a reactor vessel at least 600 kg of 2,4,5-trichlorophenate contaminated with an unknown amount of TCDD were dispersed over a wide area. People had to be evacuated from their homes. Soil, agricultural products, and cattle were contaminated. Biodegradation of these chemicals is very slow. From this tragedy 447 persons developed severe acne, and 193 showed late sequels.

PCB Poisoning in Taiwan, 1979. The source of PCB poisoning was contaminated rice bran oil, which had been ingested by a large number of people. PCB was incriminated. More than 1000 persons became ill, more than half with chloracne.

The Spanish Oil Catastrophe, 1981. Adulterated oil was fraudulently sold to the public as pure olive oil. Several deaths, including infants, resulted from this criminal act of commerce.

Chemical Warfare and Chloracne. In the late 1980's during the Iran–Iraq war, reports of massive outbreaks of chloracne were reported in the media from reliable sources. The causative hydrocarbons were not identified. We have personally seen dramatic examples of severe chloracne in soldiers from this battle zone.

Agent Orange. Two herbicides are widely used for brush and weed control throughout the world: 2,4,5-trichlorophenoxyacetic acid (2,4,5-T) and 2,4-dichlorophenoxyacetic acid (2,4-D). More than 400 million liters were sprayed during 1965 to 1970 in Vietnam to destroy covering vegetation in strategically important areas. No chloracne was ever reported, but many vague systemic complaints arose. Thousands of soldiers have sought compensation, but no instance of harm has been proved after extensive investigations. In the Operation Ranch Hand of the Air Force more than a thousand men were engaged in handling herbicides from 1961 to 1971 in Vietnam. The mysterious complaints were never traced to one of the known halogenated hydrocarbons. All these cases are suspect in the absence of the characteristic skin eruptions, the most sensitive indicator of exposure.

The Route of Contamination

Dioxin and other acneigenic hydrocarbons can cause toxicity by direct contact with the skin and mucous membranes (percutaneous absorption), by inhalation of dust and fumes, or by ingestion (contaminated food, small children swallowing contaminated dust and soil). Tiny quantities of these superpotent poisons are sufficient to provoke chloracne. It is estimated that about 50 µg of dioxin or 100 µg of TCDD per kilogram body weight are lethal for humans.

Usually chloracne is a result of accidents such as explosions. Poor ventilation in the work place may be also a contributing factor. Next most hazardous is inadvertent contact with fluids in transformers and heat exchange fluids. Another risk stems from pyrolysis by accidental or deliberate fire, generating mainly PCDD and PCDF. Municipal incinerators burning halogenated hydrocarbons are another source. Finally eating contaminated food like fish with high levels of dioxin or dibenzofuran or contaminated cooking oils can cause serious outbreaks.

The molecular basis of the toxic effects is most probably the induction of drug-metabolizing enzymes. These need metabolic activation by cytochrome P450-dependent microsomal mono-oxygenases to exert their toxic activities. TCDD is the most potent inducer of P450. In the liver the halogenated hydrocarbons probably bind to cell membrane receptors that activate enzyme systems, for instance δ-aminolevulic acid synthetase in liver microsomes. Furthermore, the enzyme uroporphyrinogen decarboxylase is inhibited, causing hepatic porphyria, a common feature in some epidemics.

Clinical Findings

Clinical Findings vary greatly depending on the nature and intensity of the exposure.

Acute Chemical Burn. Erythematous patches develop within hours on uncovered body sites, such as face, neck, arms, and legs. These may crust and slough off, leaving shallow scars. These sites become hyperpigmented and studded with typical comedones.

Comedones. Comedones are the hallmark of chloracne. Whenever the skin is contaminated, nearly every follicle is involved, especially the sebaceous and vellus follicles of the face. Crowds of comedones densely occupy the surface. The main sites of predilection are the face, neck, axillae, scrotum, and penis. On the face favorite locations are the cheeks and forehead, but also notably the area behind the ear. Often the nose is curiously spared. With heavy exposure the entire surface is involved, exempting only areas free of follicles, namely, palms and soles. After a period of about 1–2 months noninflammatory closed comedones develop. These slowly enlarge and may become large open comedones. Some grow to cystic lesions more than 5 cm in diameter. Inflammation with tender large papules and abscesses is a secondary and frightening event. Mechanical factors like pressure, stretching, or rubbing may cause rupture of closed comedones and large cysts. This sequence goes on for months and years with repeated explosions of severe inflammation. The victims are plagued by relentless crops of all types of acne lesions; the worst are acne conglobata-like inflammatory nodules. Draining sinuses develop by fusion of epithelialized channels; debris becomes trapped, and large areas of skin ooze pus and blood, a horrible sign. This trouble can go on for years, even decades. The indefinite, long course of severe chloracne gives this disorder its dreaded reputation.

Milder cases in which comedones predominate disappear spontaneously. Widespread atrophic and hypertrophic scars mark the end stage of this ferocious disease.

The Meibomian glands of the eyelids may become involved, developing comedo-like cystic lesions with cheesy contents. Conjunctivitis, lid edema, and chronic inflammation also occur (ophthalmic chloracne).

Histopathology

Many studies have provided histopathologic details. Moreover, comedones can be quickly induced in the pinna of rabbits, providing a useful animal model for screening comedogenic chemicals. In the rabbit the process stops at the comedonal stage. Chloracne comedones are quite distinctive and look different from those in acne vulgaris. The first event is the disappearance of sebaceous glands with transition of the sebocytes into keratinizing cells. The acneigen stimulates the turnover of the follicular epithelium. The entire pilosebaceous follicle produces masses of coherent dense corneocytes, distending the follicular canal and rapidly giving rise to conspicuous comedones. It is noteworthy that the comedones, unlike in acne vulgaris, are sterile. Bacteria and yeasts cannot survive in this milieu, probably due to the toxicity of the hydrocarbons. Moreover, the complete absence of sebaceous lipids withdraws the energy source for the microflora. Inflammatory lesions of chloracne are indistinguishable from those of acne conglobata.

Other Dermatological and Nondermatological Manifestations

Severe exposure commonly leads to liver disease with hepatitis and porphyrias of the hepatic type, mainly porphyria cutanea tarda. Associated findings are hyperpigmentation, hypertrichosis, bulla formation on sun-exposed skin, milia, and scars. Nausea, vomiting, and diarrhea are signs of acute poisoning. Musculoskeletal pains with bursitis have been mentioned. The pulmonary system may be affected with bronchitis and dyspnea. The central nervous system is sometimes a target. Victims complain of fatigue, headaches, sleeplessness, irritability, impotence, and loss of libido. The peripheral nervous system may also be involved. Neuropathy has been well documented with motor and sensory loss.

Teratogenicity, well known from animal studies, awaits confirmation in humans. Proof of carcinogenesis in humans has not been unequivocally established, although in the Yusho accident an increased rate of malignant neoplasms was seen.

Treatment

The dramatic outbreaks have given ample opportunity to test everything available in the repertoire of acne therapies. Topical comedolytics like salicylic acid are not effective. Neither are other old-fashioned drugs such as sulfur and resorcinol. Benzoyl peroxide is futile. Though experience is limited, vigorous application of tretinoin is valuable, at least in removing comedones and sometimes in hastening involution of inflammatory lesions. Surgical intervention may be necessary to eliminate large lesions, using the scalpel, curette, or electrosurgery. Topical or systemic antibiotics are ineffective.

Orally given isotretinoin, owing to its comedolytic and anti-inflammatory actions, may be helpful according to our preliminary experience. High doses should be used. We emphasize prophylactic administration early in the course of the disease.

Caputo R, Monti M, Ermacora E, Carminati G, Gelmetti C, Gianotti R, Gianni E, Puccinelli V (1988) Cutaneous manifestations of tetrachlorodibenzo-*p*-dioxin in children and adolescents. Follow-up 10 years after the Seveso, Italy, accident. J Am Acad Dermatol 19:812–819

Dunagin WG (1984) Cutaneous signs of systemic toxicity due to dioxins and related chemicals. J Am Acad Dermatol 10:688–700

Gladen BC, Taylor JS, Wu YC, Ragan NB, Rogan WJ, Hsu CC (1990) Dermatological findings in children exposed transplacentally to heat-degrated polychlorinated biphenyls in Taiwan. Br J Dermatol 122:799–808

Goldmann PJ (1973) Schwerste akute Chloracne, eine Massenintoxikation durch 2,3,6,7-Tetrachlordibenzodioxin. Hautarzt 24:149–152

Herxheimer K (1899) Über Chlorakne. Münch Med Wochenschr 46:278

Moses M, Prioleau PG (1985) Cutaneous histologic findings in chemical workers with and without chloracne with past exposure to 2,3,7,8-tetrachlorodibenzo-*p*-dioxin. J Am Acad Dermatol 12:497–506

Passi S, Nazzaro-Porro M, Boniforti L, Gianotti F (1981) Analysis of lipids and dioxin in chloracne due to tetrachloro-2,3,7,8-*p*-dibenzodioxin. Br J Dermatol 105:137–143

Plewig G (1970) Zur Kinetik der Comedonen-Bildung bei Chloracne (Halowaxacne). Arch Klin Exp Dermatol 238:228–241

Plewig G (1970) Lokalbehandlung der Chloracne (Halowaxacne) mit Vitamin A-Säure. Hautarzt 21:465–470

Seghal VN, Ghorpade A (1983) Fume inhalation chloracne. Dermatologica 167:33–36

Taylor JS, Lloyd JM (1982) Chloracne from 3,3′,4,4′-tetrachloroazobenzene: update and review. In: Hutzinger O (ed) Chlorinated dioxins and related compounds. Pergamon, Oxford, pp 535–544

Tindall JP (1985) Chloracne and chloracnegens. J Am Acad Dermatol 13:539–558

Urabe H, Kodak H (1976) The dermal symptomatology of Yusho. In Higuchi K (ed) PCB poisoning and pollution. Academic Press, New York, pp 105–123

Wong CK, Chen CJ, Cheng PC, Chen PH (1982) Mucocutaneous manifestations of polychlorinated biphenyls (PCB) poisoning: a study of 122 cases in Tawan. Br J Dermatol 107:317–323

Chloracne in Children

The Seveso accident is narrative of the acute toxic phase of chloracne as well as some of its late residues on the skin.

Above   The toxic rash on arms and face with urticarial and confluent papules appears on body sites unprotected by clothes

Below

Left   Exposed skin is heavily afflicted by confluent papules on face and chest and more prominent plaques on the arms. The latter resemble erythema elevatum et diutinum

Right   The follicular bound papules, the better known morphology of chloracne, appear within weeks and turn into variable other lesions, particularly pustules, deep and persistent nodules, and secondary comedones. Inflammation is long standing, scarring unavoidable

Below right: Courtesy of Professor Rugero Caputo, Milan, Italy

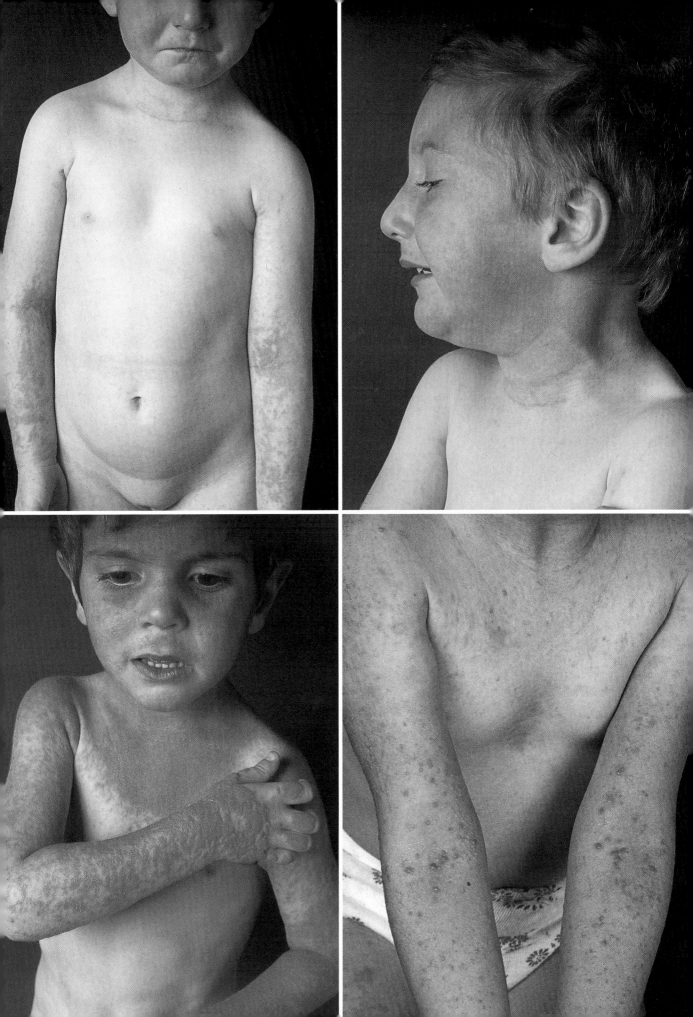

Chloracne in Children

The potency of dioxin is vividly documented in this series of children, who were among the victims of the Seveso poisoning.

Above   The child is miserable with the extensive chloracne in his face, arms, and armpits. One can literally hear his cries. Fortunately there was no permanent internal organ involvement reported in this chloracne series

Below   The facial skin of this young girl is studded with papules, pustules, and closed comedones. Inflammation raged for a long while, leaving a network of disfiguring scars behind (2 years later, *right*)

Below: Courtesy of Professor Rugero Caputo, Milan, Italy

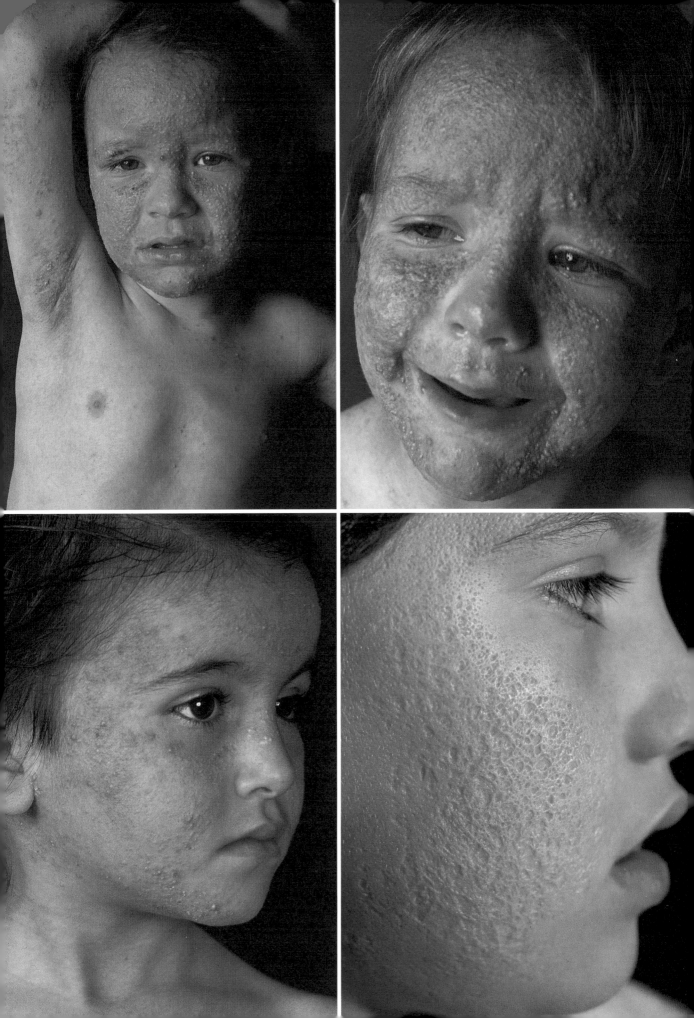

Chloracne

The Seveso catastrophe left in its toll long-lasting, large, open comedones associated with ongoing inflammation. This plate shows the histopathology.

Above Chloracne starts with a retention hyperkeratosis in every sebaceous follicle, along with epidermal hyperkeratosis. The eccrine sweat glands are similarly involved with ductal and acrosyringeal obstruction. The sebaceous glands have regressed or have been destroyed. An inflammatory component is notable with widespread perivenular infiltrates. Additionally, there is a mixed lymphocytic, granulocytic, and fibroblastic reaction

Below

Left High magnification of the cross-section of a sweat duct. The canal is filled with an accumulation of keratotic and parakeratotic debris, pointing to cell necrosis of the inner tubular cells

Right High magnification of the distal portion of an eccrine sweat duct just before entering the epidermis (acrosyringium). The lumen is completely blocked by a cast of hyaline-like keratotic debris. Cell wall necrosis and leakage of chemoattractants have lured polymorphonuclear cells to the site. Hyperkeratosis is not limited to the follicles

Below: Courtesy of Professor Rugero Caputo, Milan, Italy

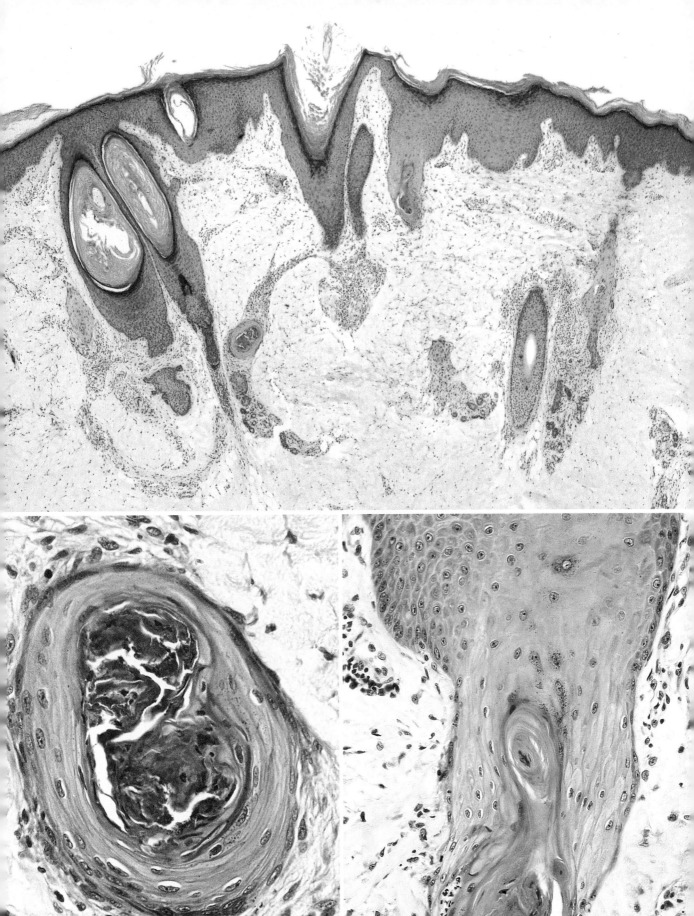

Chloracne: The Reverse Side

No other portrait illustrates the aggressiveness of chloracne better than this view of the neck, shoulders, and upper back. It is the same man as in the following plate. A variety of scars on the back – flat, atrophic, crateriform, ice pick, polyporous – tell where the inflammatory storm raged. There is still inflammation, especially notable by histology. The neck shows huge cyst-like structures, 10×5 cm in size, suppurating from various openings. They are tender and painful.

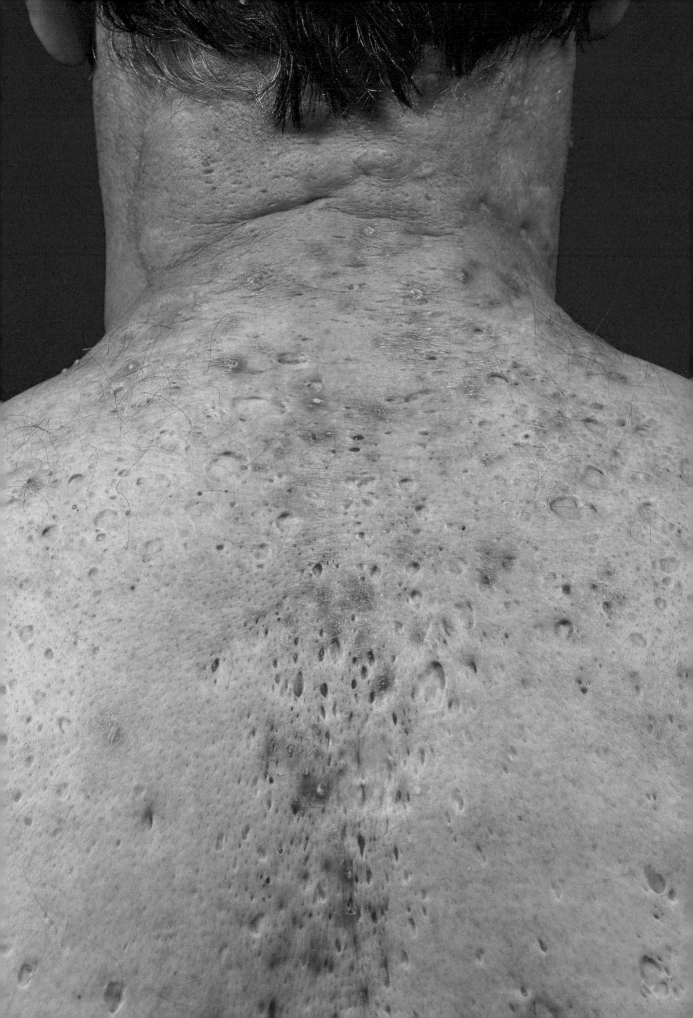

Chloracne: Terrible and Lifelong

Intense exposure to potent polychlorinated aromatic hydrocarbons induces severe chloracne which terminates in a variety of horrendous scars.

This man helped to clear up the BASF plant after the explosion in 1957, spending a few days in the demolished factory. He became acutely ill with systemic signs and later developed chloracne. Decades after this catastrophe he still shows the stigmata of ongoing chloracne. Hydrocarbons stored in the subcutaneous fat probably contribute to the persistence of active lesions.

Above   Draining sinuses and deep-seated nodules periodically erupt like volcanos. Both armpits, inner sides of upper arms, and chest are studded with smoldering lesions

Below

Left   Both buttocks, the anal fold, thighs, and knee pits are covered by fistulated polyporous scars, accompanied by varying degrees of inflammation

Right   Even the kneepits are involved, with fistulated scars and periodic forming of abscesses

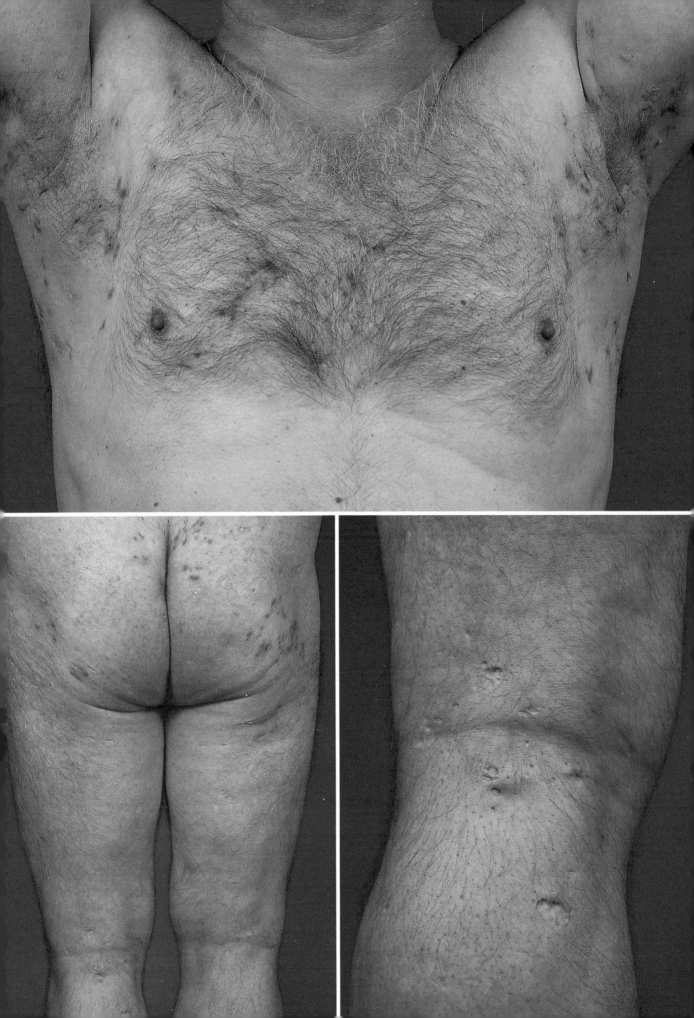

Chloracne

The most horrendous expressions of acne are seen in severe cases of chloracne. Chloracne was fairly common in the earlier part of the century, but it is still with us. This and the next plate are examples of chloracne seen in 1989 in a soldier engaged in a war in the middle East. The source was never identified, but the reports mention gas exposure in chemical warfare.

Chloracne covers this man from top to bottom except where there are no sebaceous follicles on palms and soles. The lesions start as small, noninflamed, closed comedones, which either slowly enlarge to open comedones, or sooner or later rupture, leaving variously shaped and sized abscesses. The largest closed comedones are actually true epithelial cysts, some of them several centimeters in diameter. Scarring is inevitable with fistulated comedones prevailing.

Above   Numerous closed comedones and larger cysts on face and neck

Below   Close-up of open and closed comedones

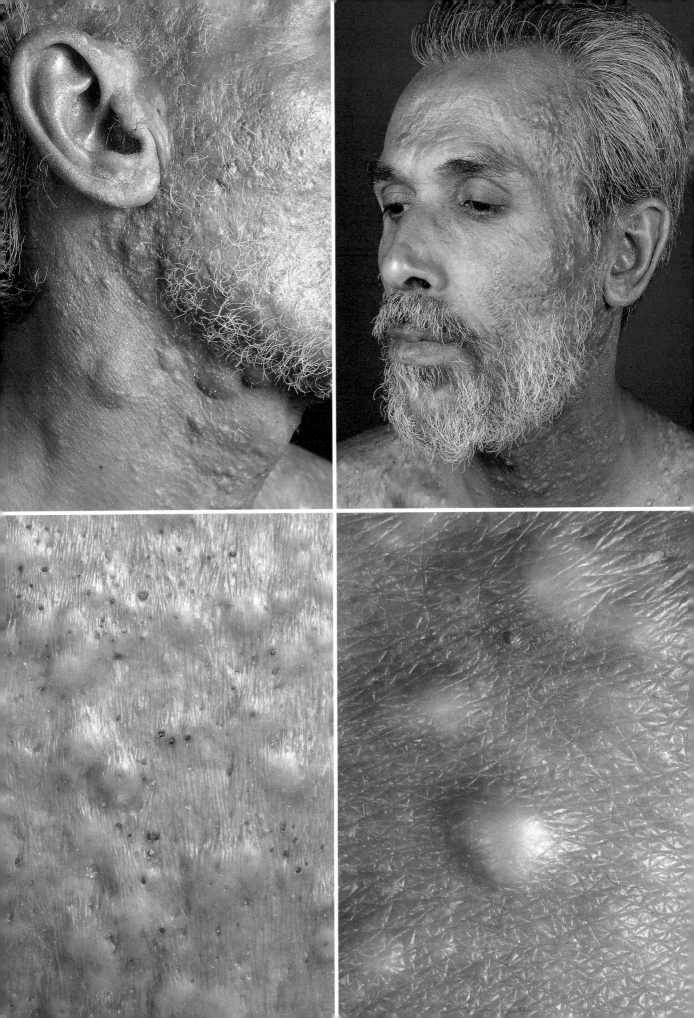

Chloracne

Above

Left   One could call this "acne universalis." Acne is everywhere

Right   Even the legs are involved, with abscesses in the intertriginous areas of the kneepits

Below   Halowax acne on the back. Almost every follicle is involved. Closed and open comedones, papules, and pustules are conmingled. The disease bothered this man for many years

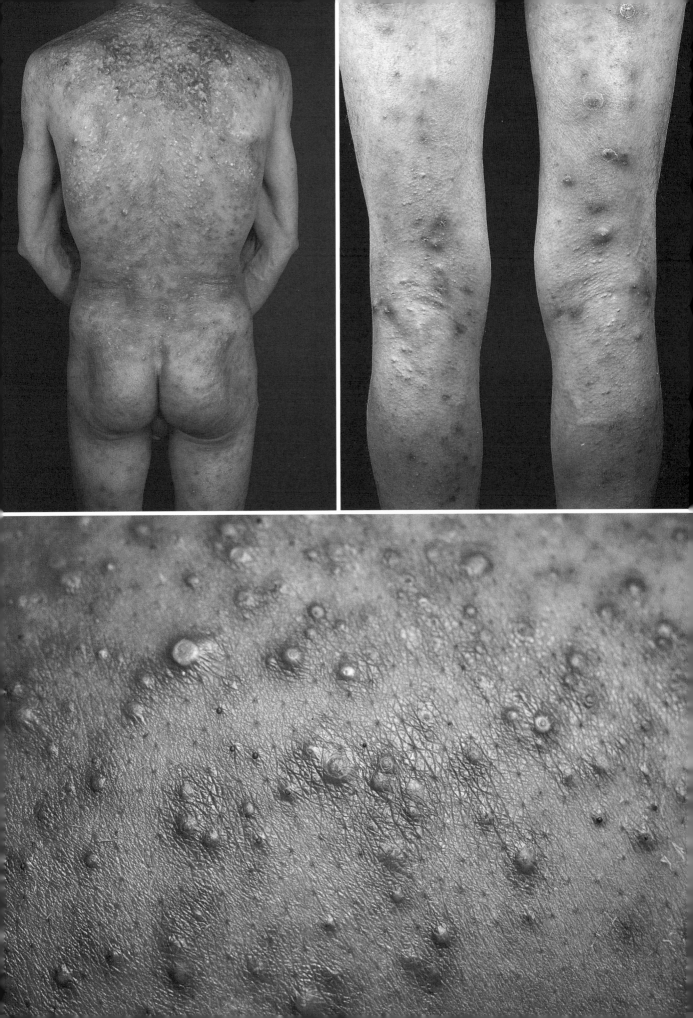

Solar Comedones (Favre-Racouchot's Disease)

Open and closed comedones, particularly around the eyes and on nose, cheeks, and forehead of Caucasian subjects, are but one of the many pathologic changes caused by excessive exposure to sunlight. They are also called senile comedones, an ungracious term. The peak occurrence is from age 60 to 80, but if there is enough occupational or recreational UV exposure these comedones can disfigure the face of adults in their forties. Men are much more often affected than women. Solar comedones often start with small closed comedones. With time these develop into big, open, often dark comedones which are found on a background of yellow, thickened, elastotic skin. When exuberant, this condition is also designated Favre–Racouchot's disease, in which the lesions are described as cysts and comedones. The former is erroneous. They are merely tightly closed comedones intermingled with large open comedones.

Histopathology

The histopathologic picture is distinctive and not easily confused with other conditions. Small and large, open and closed comedones with densely packed corneocytes are typical. The epithelium is thinned out, sometimes showing restless growths with variable hyperplastic sprouts, which may be remnants of undifferentiated sebaceous acini. As in acne comedones, the sebaceous glands are shrunken, and even absent in these enormous comedones. Another characteristic is the sparsity or absence of *Propionibacterium acnes*. *Pityrosporum* yeasts are frequently found around the periphery, mostly in the spaces between corneocytes. Solar comedones are neither clinically nor histologically inflamed. The comedones are always embedded in heavily elastotic skin, best seen in tissue stained for elastic fibers. Telangiectatic blood vessels and lymphatic vessels complete the picture. No matter how large the comedones, they never lead to scars. The lesions slowly get larger and larger with time and do not disappear spontaneously. Though completely unrelated, trichostasis spinulosa is often an incidental finding, also caused by actinic damage.

Treatment

Manual extraction is possible but difficult. The comedones are hard, deeply rooted, and painful to extract. Our approach is to use tretinoin aggressively, increasing to the highest concentration as hardening develops. Small open comedones fall out in 2–3 months, while closed ones take much longer. The extremely large comedones become loosened from their anchorage and can then be easily extracted. A side benefit of tretinoin is its ability to partially reverse many of the changes of photodamaged skin. Patients may want to take advantage of improving their appearance by long-term use of tretinoin, even after the comedones have disappeared. Dermabrasion, recommended in the past, is no longer an option. Plastic surgeons may be called for face lifts and blepharoplasty. Another option is oral isotretinoin. The dose should be low, 0.2 mg or even less, e.g., 0.05–0.1 mg/kg per day. Very low doses, 2.5 mg–5.0 mg once daily without regard to body weight, have given quite good results. Open and closed comedones slowly fall out and are not replaced by new ones. Likewise, circumscribed sebaceous gland hyperplasias, very common in this patient cohort, melt down. Trichostasis spinulosa disappears, too. A smooth, clean facial complexion can be brought about. Duration of treatment is 4–6 months and longer if desired. The 5-mg dose is not associated with systemic toxicity, and laboratory values remain normal. Beneficial effects can be enhanced by concomitant use of topical tretinoin.

Broad-spectrum sunscreens of SPF 15 or more are recommended to every patient with solar comedones.

Favre M, Racouchot J (1951) L'élastéidose cutanée nodulair a kystes et a comédons. Ann Dermatol Syph 78:681–702

Gloor M, Friederich HC (1974) Über die Zusammensetzung der Comedonenlipide bei Morbus Favre–Racouchot. Hautarzt 25:439–441

Kligman LH, Kligman A (1987) Photoaging. In: Fitzpatrick TB, Eisen AZ, Wolff K, Freedberg LM, Austen KF (eds) Dermatology in general medicine. 3rd edn. McGraw-Hill, New York, pp 1470–1475

Mohs E, McCall MW, Greenway HT (1982) Curettage for removal of the comedones and cystes of the Favre-Racouchot syndrome. Arch Dermatol 118:365–366

Plewig G, Braun-Falco O (1971) Behandlung von Comedonen bei Morbus Favre–Racouchot und Acne venenata mit Vitamin A-Säure. Hautarzt 22:341–345

Sharkey MJ, Keller RA, Grabski WJ, McGollough ML (1992) Favre-Racouchot syndrome. A combined therapeutic approach. Arch Dermatol 128:615–616

Turner E, Grube C (1990) M. Favre–Racouchot – unilaterale Variante. Aktuel Dermatol 16:286–287

Solar Comedones – Favre-Racouchot's Disease

Above   These open and closed comedones around the eyes and on the cheeks of aging Caucasians, ungraciously called senile comedones, are but one of many pathologic changes caused by excessive exposure to sunlight. In the elderly they become large enough to look like cysts situated on a background of yellow, thickened elastotic skin

Below   The oval lesion on the far left is a horn-filled cyst lined by a thin epithelium. With serial sectioning, an opening is always found as in two other comedones. These are simply closed and open comedones. They are hard to pressed out, contain fewer bacteria than acne comedones, and the sebaceous acini regressed to epithelial buds and sprouts usually restless with variable hyperplastic growths

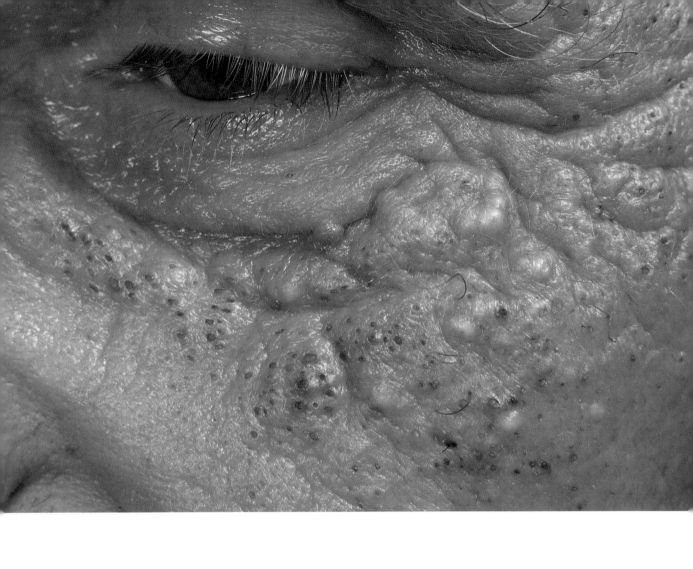

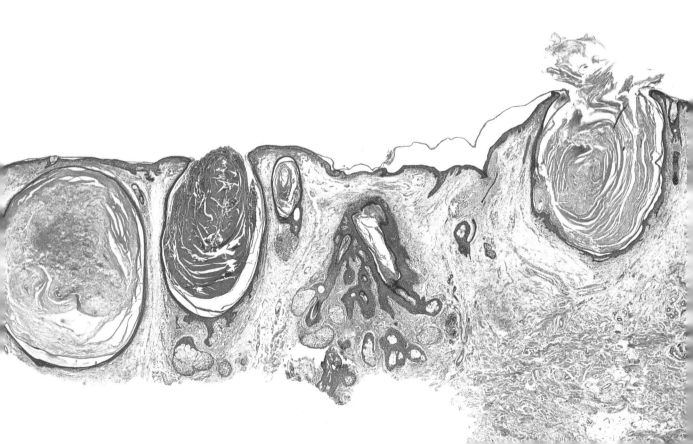

Acne Aestivalis (Mallorca Acne)

This variant in the repertoire of acneiform eruptions is a stranger in every aspect. Everything about it is unusual and indeed inexplicable. An undisputed etiologic factor is UV radiation, either from solar exposure or artificial sources.

Acne aestivalis is a seasonal disorder. It starts in spring, peaks in summer, and disappears completely in fall. The key features have been well described in the original publication by Hjorth and co-workers. After a long dark winter, sun-hungry Scandinavians flew into the bright Mediterranean sun in spring (mostly to the island of Mallorca). Enthusiastic sunbathing provoked an acneiform eruption which persisted throughout their vacation and in the weeks thereafter at home. The victims are equally women and men, between 20 and 40, generally with no prior history of acne vulgaris.

The distribution is unusual. The face is mostly spared; the lesions concentrate on the lateral aspects of upper arms, shoulder girdle, back, and chest. The typical lesions are numerous, dull red, dome-shaped, hard, small papules, usually not more than 2–4 mm in diameter. Comedones and pustules are generally absent. The papules spring up suddenly within 1–3 days and last for many weeks, finally involuting without scar formation.

Clinically and histologically the lesions resemble steroid acne and evolve in the same way. A segment of the follicular epithelium becomes necrotic, and a sharply limited abscess develops at the site of rupture. Following epithelial re-encapsulation of the abscess, the follicle becomes hyperkeratotic, but the quantity of corneocytes is generally too small to be visible as a comedo.

An eruption identical with Mallorca acne has occurred in patients receiving total body UV-A radiation for the phototherapy of chronic dermatoses, or undergoing treatment with 8-methoxypsoralen and UV-A radiation (PUVA). This suggests that the action spectrum lies in the long-wave ultraviolet region. How or why this happens only in certain individuals is a mystery. One suggestion is that UV-A activates porphyrins produced by *Propionibacterium acnes* residing in sebaceous follicles.

Sunscreens and body lotions used during sunbathing have sometimes been incriminated but proof of this etiology for Mallorca acne is lacking. While some sunscreens are photocomedogenic, Mallorca acne explodes suddenly even in the absence of comedones. Like patients with polymorphic light eruption, subjects prone to acne aestivalis react the same way year after year. The disease eventually abates after many years, perhaps because of less intensive sunbathing.

Prevacation prophylaxis can be offered by carefully and gradually increasing exposures to full body artificial UV radiation, UV-B and/or UV-A or even PUVA therapy prior to the first exposure to natural sunlight. Few patients will go to this trouble.

Treatment

The disease is rather stubborn. Topical tretinoin vigorously applied is the treatment of choice. Benzoyl peroxide is an alternative. Topical steroids should be avoided, since they aggravate the disease. There is no systemic treatment.

Hjorth N, Sjølin KE, Sylvest B, Thomsen K (1972) Acne aestivalis – Mallorca acne. Acta Derm Venereol (Stockh) 52:61–63

Hofmann C, Plewig G, Braun-Falco O (1977) Ungewöhnliche Nebenwirkungen bei oraler Photochemotherapie (PUVA-Therapie) der Psoriasis. Hautarzt 28:583–588

Mills OH, Kligman AM (1975) Acne aestivalis. Arch Dermatol 111:891–892

Sjølin KE (1979) Acne aestivalis. A histopathological study. Acta Derm Venereol (Stockh) [Suppl 85] 59:171–176

Acne Aestivalis (Mallorca Acne)

For unknown reasons some people react to intensive sun exposure in spring or summer with an acneiform eruption, called Mallorca acne. The lesions are monomorphic, follicular papules containing a small central core of horn with a surrounding inflammatory reaction. The lesions feel firm on palpation, and last for several weeks.

Above

Left   Inflammatory keratotic papules on the right upper arm

Right   Scattered follicular bound inflammatory papules on the back

Below   Widely scattered acne aestivalis on the right and left arm

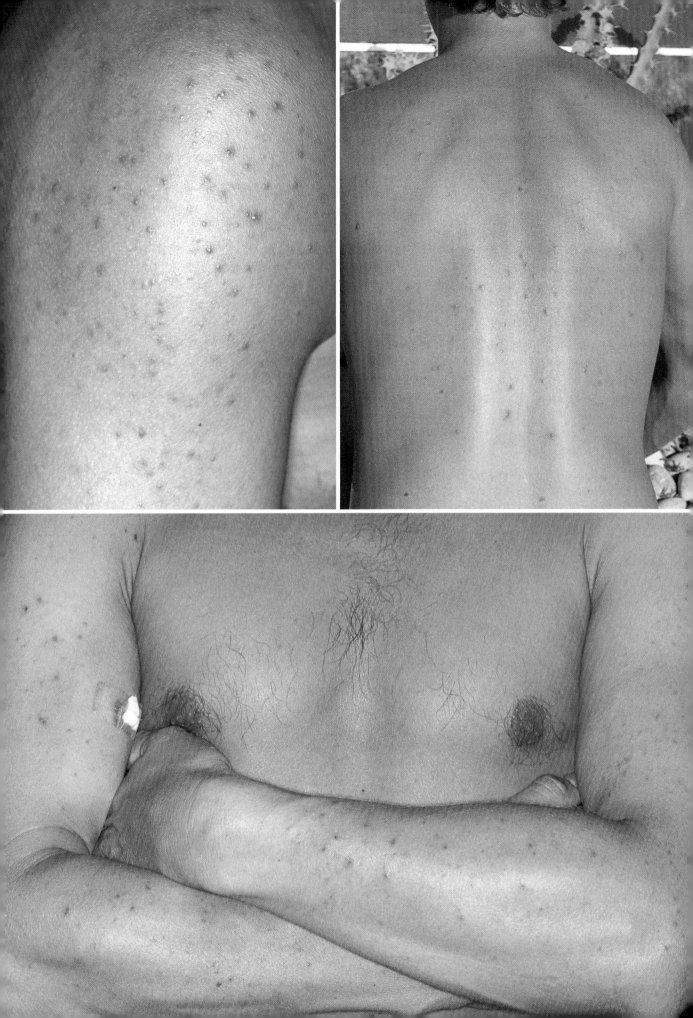

Radiation-Induced Comedones

Physical agents can cause comedones. Solar comedones in photoaged skin are quite common. Additionally, ionizing radiation for the treatment of malignancies frequently induces striking comedones.

Soft X-ray therapy, e.g., for basal cell carcinoma on the nose or cheeks, is sometimes followed weeks to months later by densely studded, pigmented, open comedones. These develop after the acute phase of radiation dermatitis abates and are strictly confined to the irradiated field. There is no differential diagnosis. The patient knows the cause. The comedones generally disappear spontaneously after many months. This can be hastened by topical tretinoin.

Other radiation sources can cause a similar picture, e.g., cobalt radiation. The penetrating ionizing radiation induces metaplasia of the follicular epithelium, which then produces corneocytes that do not slough.

For comedones following ultraviolet radiation, see the chapters "Acne Aestivalis" (p. 400) and "Solar Comedones" (p. 396).

Hartman MS (1950) Postradiation comedos. Arch Dermatol Syph 62:440–441

Stein KM, Leyden JJ, Goldschmidt H (1972) Localized acneiform eruption following cobalt irradiation. Br J Dermatol 87:274–279

Trunnell TN, Bayer RL, Michaelides P (1972) Acneform changes in areas of cobalt irradiation. Arch Dermatol 106:73–75

ACNEIFORM DISEASES

Acneiform Eruptions

The term acneiform eruption is used too carelessly. It denotes conditions which resemble acne. The extent to which things look alike depends on the knowledge and experience of the observer. To some, all forms of papules and pustules are the same. Without an explicit definition the subject of acneiform eruptions becomes smothered in a semantic smog. Only an undisciplined imagination can include acne necrotica miliaris (scalp pustules) among the acneiform eruptions: The only resemblance it bears to acne vulgaris is the word acne. Similarly, acne rosacea (an outdated terminology) and acne keloidalis nuchae have only a phonetic connection with acne. We distinguish true acne from acneiform eruptions according to the following.

Acne

True acne is a follicular eruption which begins with a horny impaction, the comedo. Rupture of the comedo provokes a foreign body inflammatory reaction which takes the form of papules, pustules, and nodules. Thus the morphologic expressions are highly variable, depending on the stage and severity. The disease has a wide spectrum from minor to major. Acne vulgaris is predominantly a disease of adolescents, but some variants begin or extend into adult life and even old age. Failure to recognize this results in many missed diagnoses.

Acneiform Eruptions

Acneiform eruptions, like acne, originate in follicles, but the initial lesion is inflammatory, typically a papule or pustule. Comedones are later secondary lesions, a sequel to encapsulation and healing of the primary abscess. The earliest histologic event is spongiosis, and this is then followed by a break in the follicular epithelium, allowing the contents of the canal to spill into the dermis and provoking a nonspecific neutrophilic infiltration.

Acneiform eruptions are almost always drug-induced. The most common drugs are listed in the table (p. 408).

Acneiform eruptions can usually be distinguished on clinical grounds. Important clues are:

- Sudden onset, within days
- Often widespread involvement
- Unusual localizations, e.g., forearms, buttocks
- Occurrence beyond the acne age
- Monomorphic lesions: papules or papulopustules at the same stage of development
- Systemic signs of drug toxicity with fever and malaise
- Clearing of the inflammatory lesions after the drug is stopped, sometimes leaving secondary comedones

Acneiform eruptions are usually iatrogenic, i.e., they arise as a side effect of therapy. Corticosteroids are superpotent acneigens and are therefore used to re-

The distinction between acne and acneiform eruption

	Acne	Acneiform eruption
Site	Sebaceous follicle	Sebaceous follicle
Causation	Multifactorial: Androgens Sebum Propionibacterium acnes Follicular keratinization Heredity	Drugs, foodstuff
Primary lesion	Comedo (noninflammatory)	Papule, papulopustule (inflammatory)
Secondary lesion	Papules Papulopustules Nodules Cysts Draining sinuses	Secondary comedones
Scarring	Inevitably after inflammation, shallow to deep	Usually absent or minimal
Onset	Slow, months to years	Sudden, days to weeks
Age of onset	Adolescence	Adulthood and later
Course	Prolonged, years	Short, after withdrawal of the cause
Therapy	Depends on severity: topical, systemic	Not necessary after withdrawal of offending agent

produce the disease. Most information on the pathogenesis and histopathologic events stems from studies of experimental steroid acne.

Oral iodides and bromides given over months in moderate doses have a well-deserved reputation for being able to cause acneiform eruptions. Topical application of potassium iodide can also provoke papules and pustules.

Modern fads bring new hazards. The biotrip has put many so-called health products on the market. A kelp diet is popular among certain health enthusiasts. Kelp is an alga rich in iodides. We now recognize Kelp acne.

In all acneiform eruptions the responsible agent becomes known by taking a detailed history. Large doses of iodides, e.g., 15 drops of saturated potassium iodide (Lugol's solution), which is used for its effect on the thyroid gland, can precipitate an eruption in about 1 week, especially in acne-prone individuals. Hidden sources of iodides include vitamin and mineral preparations, remedies for asthma and colds, hypnotics, sedatives, thyroid prescriptions, and radiopaque materials. Absorption from nasal remedies, douches, and suppositories are exotic sources. Bromides occur in sedatives, analgesics, and cold remedies.

On the other hand, physicians have greatly exaggerated the capacity of iodides in the normal diet to aggravate acne. It is silly and irrational to exclude iodized salt from the diet. Such miniscule amounts can never induce an acneiform eruption.

Acneiform Eruptions

Synopsis of the acneiform eruptions, and various examples of the forms, e.g., steroid acne, and variations thereof, e.g., from topical or systemic corticosteroids

Steroids
  Topical corticosteroids
  Systemic corticosteroids: enteral, parenteral, inhalation
  Adrenocorticotrophic hormone

Antiepileptics
  Trimetadione
  Phenytoin

Antidepressants
  Lithium
  Amineptine

Tetracyclines
  Tetracycline·HCl
  Oxytetracycline
  Doxycycline
  Minocycline

Isonicotinic Acid Hydrazide (INH)

8-Methoxypsoralen + UVA (PUVA)

Phenobarbiturates

Thyroid Preparations
  Thiourea
  Thiouracil

Vitamins
  Vitamins B_1, B_6, B_{12}, D

Halogens
  Iodides
  Bromides

Disulfiram

Quinine

Imuran

When acne worsens or fails to respond to sound therapy, one should inquire about concomitant drug intake, health care products, health supplements, or dietetics. Acneiform eruptions induced by agents used to treat acne are very rare, but it is important to recognize them. Oral tetracyclines, for example, can induce a pustular eruption.

Braun-Falco O, Lincke H (1976) Zur Frage der Vitamin-B_6/B_{12}-Akne. Münch Med Wochenschr 118:155–160

Harrell BL, Rudolph AH (1976) Kelp diet: a cause of acneiform eruption. Arch Dermatol 112:560

Heng MCY (1982) Lithium carbonate toxicity. Acneform eruption and other manifestations. Arch Dermatol 118:246–248

Hitch JM (1967) Acneform eruptions induced by drugs and chemicals. JAMA 200:879–880

Labeille B, Westeel PF, Andrejak M, Denoeux JP (1989) Acné kystique profuse induite par le Survector®: une nouvelle observation. Nouv Dermatol 8:28

Lantis SH (1969) Acneform eruptions. J Am Med Wom Assoc 24:305–309

Plewig G (1978) Pityrosporum in normal sebaceous follicles, comedones, acneiform eruptions, and dandruff. Mykosen (Suppl) 1:155–163

Plewig G (1986) Akneiforme Arzneireaktionen und provozierte Akne. In: Braun-Falco O, Schill WB (eds) Fortschritte der Praktischen Dermatologie und Venerologie, vol 11. Springer, Berlin Heidelberg New York, pp 272–279

Plewig G, Strzeminski YA (1985) Jod und Hauterkrankungen. Dtsch Med Wochenschr 110:1266–1269

Schmoeckel C, von Liebe V (1983) Akneiformes Exanthem durch Azathioprin. Hautarzt 34:413–415

Thioly-Bensoussan D, Edelson Y, Cardinne A, Grupper C (1987) Acné monstrueuse iatrogène provoquée par le Survector®: première observation mondiale à propos de deux cas. Nouv Dermatol 6:535–537

Yoder FW (1975) Acneiform eruption due to lithium carbonate. Arch Dermatol 111:396–397

Acneiform Eruptions

Sometimes acneiform eruptions mimic true acne. There are clues to separate the two conditions. In contrast to acne, the eruption is monomorphic, and there is always a drug history. Once the offending drug has been withdrawn the condition clears spontaneously.

Above

Left   This comes close to acne papulopustulosa; comedones are absent. Minocycline was the causative drug

Right   The location and distribution is as in acne, but the quality of the lesions is different. Monomorphic papules erupted soon after the oral intake of a corticosteroid

Below

Left   Dense distribution of juicy papules and pustules on a slightly erythematous background and the history of lithium use lead to the correct diagnosis

Right   Close-up of acneiform pustules due to azathioprine with an inflammatory halo. Sometimes secondary comedones evolve, particularly in steroid acne

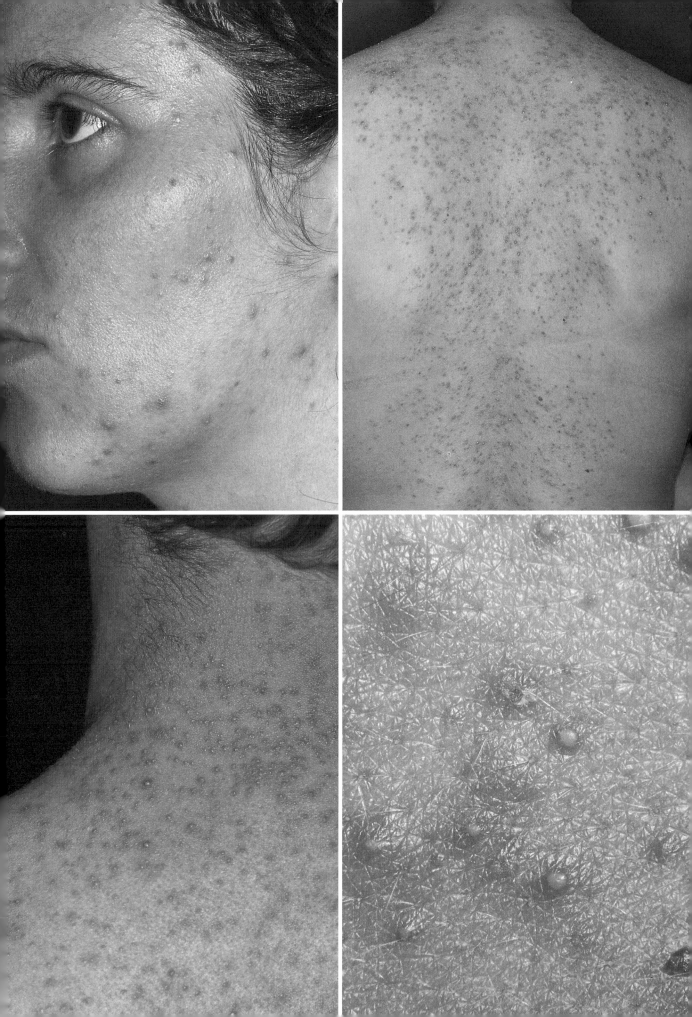

Halogens Are Proinflammatory Agents

Iodides and bromides when given for diagnostic or therapeutic reasons can cause unusual inflammatory skin reactions which generally originate in follicles. The provocation of these eruptions requires very large doses. Dietary iodides are harmless.

Above

Left   An acute flare-up of a pseudofolliculitis barbae-like pattern occurred in this man, who received saturated iodide solution (Lugol's solution) for less than 1 week

Right   Iododerma presenting as asymmetrically distributed abscesses and deep seated nodules in an adult, who was treated with an iodide-containing medication. Crops of pustules or inflmmatory nodules are a common expression of iodide folliculitis

Below   Three examples of bromoderma on the leg and the nape of the neck in patients on bromide-containing sedatives. There is a rough resemblance to acne conglobata. Blood levels of halogens confirm the diagnosis, which may be suspected from the morphology alone and, of course, from a history or drug intake

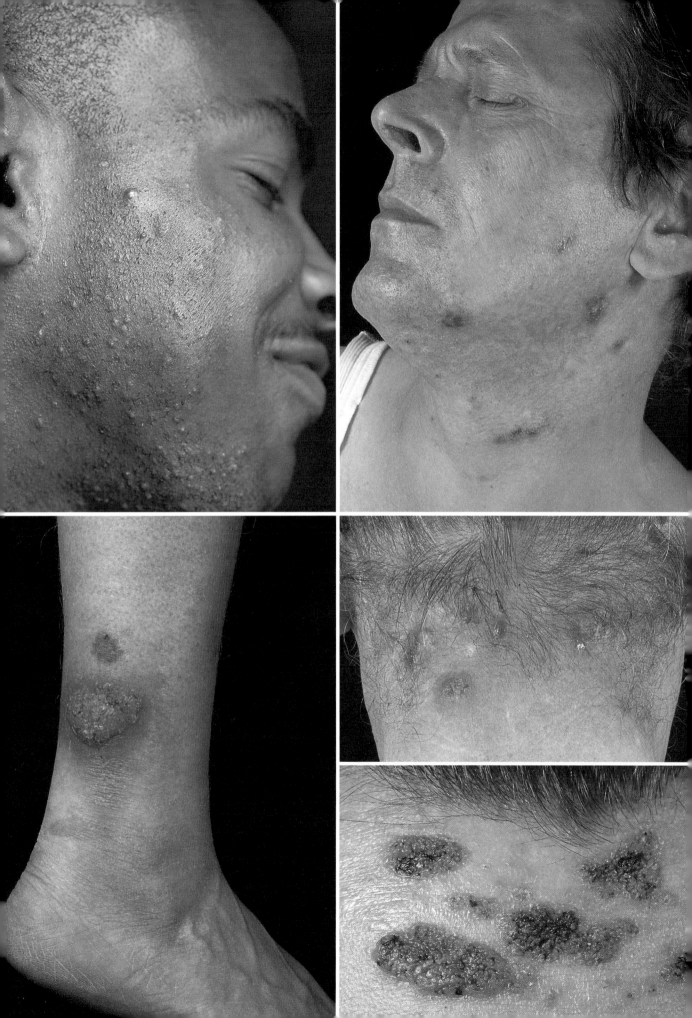

Steroid Acne

Steroid acne is the acneiform eruption par excellence. Clinical findings and histologic events show exactly what is meant by an acneiform eruption. Steroid acne from topical applications is nowadays a rarity. Most doctors have learned not to apply steroids to the face. This contrasts with oral administration.

Steroid-induced acneiform eruptions have become commonplace because of the extensive and justifiable use of steroids to treat autoimmune diseases and to prevent allograft rejection, e.g., after kidney or bone marrow transplants. ACTH has the same potential but is rarely used. Identical lesions are provoked by topical corticosteroids. Rarely acne occurs due to inhaled corticosteroids.

Systemic Steroid Acne

The eruption has the following characteristics:
- Rather abrupt onset as early as 1–2 weeks after high doses; delayed onset with lower doses, usually after 3–6 weeks.
- Affected areas are the face, forehead, V-shaped areas of chest and upper back, shoulder girdle, and lateral aspects of upper arms. Rarely the scalp, buttocks, and thighs are involved. Thus, the distribution resembles that of severe acne vulgaris.
- Numerous monomorphic lesions of uniform size and shape and at the same stage of development crop up. They are dull red, smooth, dome-shaped papules, sometimes topped by a soft abscess. The inflammatory lesions are not deep seated and never attain the size of nodules; scarring is minimal. Comedones are absent during the evolving eruption.
- Subsequently, in a matter of months, closed and finally open comedones will replace inflammatory papules. These are properly classified as secondary comedones.
- In the final stage the skin may be studded with large, ugly blackheads.
- Neither children nor the elderly are very susceptible to steroid acne. Nevertheless, children can sometimes develop it, usually those who receive polychemotherapy including corticosteroids for leukemia.
- Patients with a past history of acne, seborrhea, or still ongoing acne are particularly at risk.
- Blacks have sturdier follicles and are less susceptible than whites.

Histopathology. The first change is focal necrosis of a segment of the follicular epithelium. The contents of the follicular canal become dispersed into the perifollicular connective tissue. In this way corneocytes, sebum, *Propionibacterium acnes, Staphylococcus epidermidis, Pityrosporum ovale, Demodex folliculorum* mites (when present), and vellus hairs are dumped into the dermis, calling forth neutrophils and lymphocytes to form a perifollicular abscess. Tongues of follicular eptihelium quickly encapsulate the abscess. Due to the anti-inflammatory activity of the steroid only a small strictly localized abscess develops at the site of the rupture. The clinical lesions are "cool" and nontender for the same reason. After re-encapsulation a comedo begins to form, accompanied by massive proliferation of *Propionibacterium acnes*. Thus the sequence is the very opposite of acne vulgaris. An inflammatory lesion is the first change, and comedo formation a later event. Acne vulgaris and steroid acne are quite different processes, although the comedones may be clinically indistinguishable. Histologically, fibrosis betrays the earlier inflammatory event in steroid acne in contrast to the primary comedo in acne vulgaris. Systemic steroids have no obvious effect on the sebaceous glands or sebum output. This contrasts to topical usage, which can produce atrophy of the gland.

Topical Steroid Acne

Occlusive application of potent steroids uniformly and rapidly provokes the typical eruption. This often happens during occlusive therapy for psoriasis vulgaris, chronic eczema, lichen planus, or discoid lupus erythematosus, especially in acne-prone areas. On topical application of potent steroids, even without occlusion, steroid acne is readily induced on the face, upper back, and paravertebrally. Dome-shaped follicular papules erupt within 2–3 weeks with highly potent steroids. Persons with still active acne vulgaris or a past history of it, with oily, large-pored skin are particularly at risk. Topical steroid acne resembles the systemic variety in all particulars except for atrophogenic changes of the epidermis, dermal thinning, and shrinkage of sebaceous glands.

The ability of topical steroids to induce acne is directly related to the potency class based on therapeutic efficacy. Clobetasol-17-propionate, betamethasone-17,21-dipropionate, and fluocinolone acetonide are at the head of the list, while dexamethasone is much weaker and hydrocortisone is marginal. Nontheless, hydrocortisone and its nonfluorinated derivatives may, after long usage, induce low-grade acne in the face of susceptible persons.

Unfortunately, many women are foolish enough to apply corticosteroids, even potent ones, to the face. This is due mainly to the misconception that this miracle drug will improve the complexion. They may have some minor skin changes, perhaps a few papulopustules, wrinkles, dryness, or early signs of photoaging or perioral dermatitis, and will get steroids, often illicitly, to overcome their cosmetic problems. Because of the long latency period everything may go smoothly at first, inspiring confidence in the treatment. When new lesions begin to spring up in abundance the alarmed patient is just as likely to redouble her efforts, applying larger quantities with increasing frequency. Withdrawal at this stage will provoke a full-blown rebound eruption, a true cosmetic nightmare.

Another side effect of corticosteroid treatment is steroid dermatitis. It occurs without a background of acne or rosacea. Many elements are intermingled: epidermal atrophy, telangiectasias, folliculitis, papulopustules, and a rebound flare after stopping.

Steroid rosacea is another tragedy resulting from improper use. It occurs in persons who blush easily; they have the rosacea tendency. These patients develop steroid rosacea with bright red cheeks, follicular pustules, and then atrophic skin through which many telanciectatic vessels can be seen.

Treatment

Steroid acne is not easy to treat. The response is slow and patients may agonize for many months. Patients need counselling and strong support during withdrawal. Of course topical corticosteroids must be stopped immediately. We do not share the view of some colleagues who use low potency steroids in lesser concentrations to avoid the very unpleasant rebound phenomenon. Even hydrocortisone will postpone the time required to reach the steroid-free state. Mild noncomedogenic moisturizers are permitted, but only if urgently requested by the patient.

Once the storm has abated, one may try the lowest strength of tretinoin cream, 0.025%, to eliminate comedones, starting with nightly applications every other day. Topical antibiotics are useless, and benzoyl peroxide may delay the return to normal. Systemic agents are usually not required. Still, there is fairly good evidence that full courses of tetracyclines, especially lipophilic minocycline, 100 mg daily, help to resolve inflammation and to provide general relief. Isotretinoin is also effective. We recommend a low dose, 5 mg per day, not adjusted to body weight, for about 3 months. This is sufficient to clear the lesions. Of course the teratogenic potential has to be considered in women of reproductive age (p. 635).

Hurwitz RM (1989) Steroid acne. J Am Acad Dermatol 21:1179–1181

Kaidbey KH, Kligman AM (1974) The pathogenesis of topical steroid acne. J Invest Dermatol 62:31–36

Layton A, Monk B, Rhodes DJ, Cunliffe WJ (1992) Acne due to inhaled corticosteroids. Br J Dermatol 127 (Suppl 40):30–31 (Abstract)

Lehmann P, Zheng P, Lavker RM, Kligman AM (1983) Corticosteroid atrophy in human skin. A study by light, scanning, and transmission electron microscopy. J Invest Dermatol 81:169–176

Plewig G, Kligman AM (1973) Induction of acne by topical steroids. Arch Dermatol Forsch 247:29–52

Zheng P, Lavker RM, Lehmann P, Kligman AM (1984) Morphologic investigations on the rebound phenomenon after corticosteroid-induced atrophy in human skin. J Invest Dermatol 82:345–352

Steroid Acne

Once seen this picture is memorable. Unlike acne vulgaris the lesions are remarkably uniform, consisting of dome-shaped, inflamed, sharply circumscribed papules. The distribution pattern is typical.

Above   The V-shaped eruption took the chest and shoulders about 4 weeks after corticosteroids were administered orally to a patient with arthritis. High doses, in this case 100 mg prednisolone, are required to precipitate so intensive a reaction in so short a time

Below

Left   The same patient as above. Widespread papulopustules cover most of the back, wherever there are sebaceous follicles

Right   Steroid acne on the upper arm of a young man, who also received corticosteroids orally. Later these lesions may transform into comedones

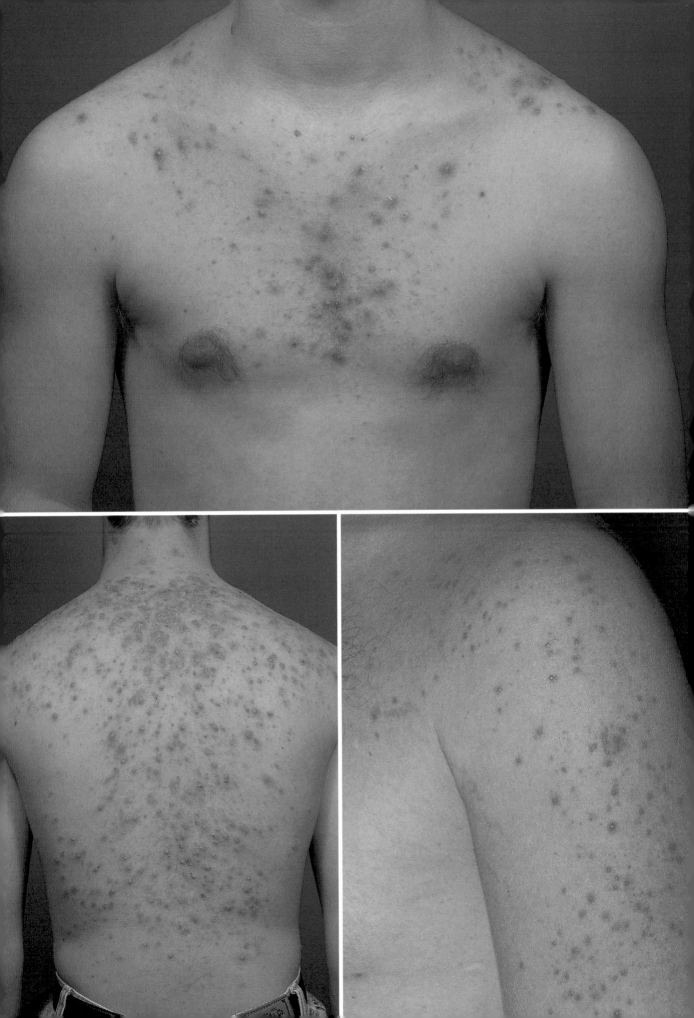

How Steroid Acne Develops

Steroid acne is the best studied model of acneiform eruptions. Regardless of what drug causes acneiform eruptions, the histologic events are very similar. The same applies for topical or systemic administration of the offending medicament.

Above

Left   The earliest detectable event is a focal necrosis of the mid-portion of the infundibulum of the sebaceous follicle. There is no comedo. Lymphocytes and some granulocytes are at the breach

Right   The next step is the migration of the follicular epithelium, engulfing the localized abscess like tongues

Below

Left   An asymmetrical closed comedo is in the process of being formed; the sebaceous acini are still present but small. Parts of the engulfed debris and inflammatory cell population have been trapped and condensed in the comedonal kernel

Right   An older, closed comedo with a compact kernel and parakeratotic cells in the center. Asymmetry and pericomedonal fibrosis can be mentioned. The comedo wall is thin, the sebaceous glands became atrophic, and the pilary portion is intact. The apical pore is tightly closed

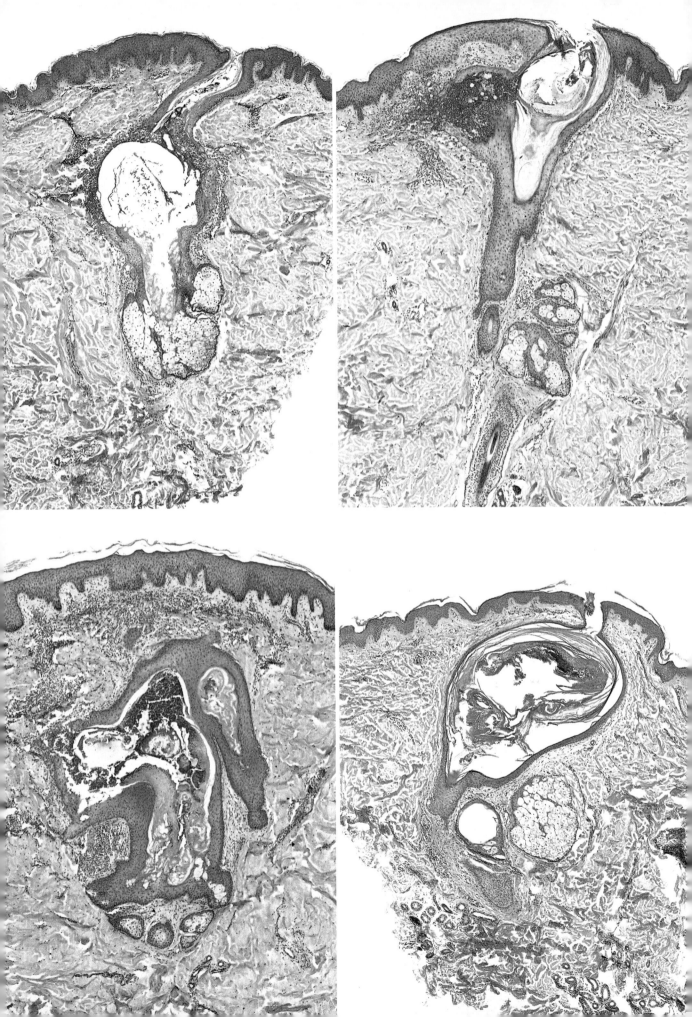

Steroid Acne

Sebaceous follicles of the face, upper chest, and back are particularly prone to react with steroid acne. Both the topical and systemic routes of application cause very similar events. In general, topical application of corticosteroids causes less inflammation than the systemic. This plate documents early and late events of experimentally induced steroid acne from topical administration alone.

Above Two neighboring sebaceous follicles in different stages of comedo formation. The one to the left is an early open comedo, just past the stage of a micro-comedo. The sebaceous glands are still large. The one to the right is much more advanced, of the closed type, with colonization of bacteria, keratinization of the sebaceous duct, and involution of sebaceous glands. Asymmetry is usually a sign of earlier rupture and re-encapsulation, though not accompanied here by pericomedonal fibrosis

Below Late stage of steroid acne. The two large closed comedones, more than six months old, are almost indistinguishable from comedones seen in genuine acne vulgaris. Their wall is extremely thin; the sebaceous glands have all regressed to minute epithelial buds at the bottom. Slight asymmetry and pericomedonal fibrosis fall of earlier inflammatory events.

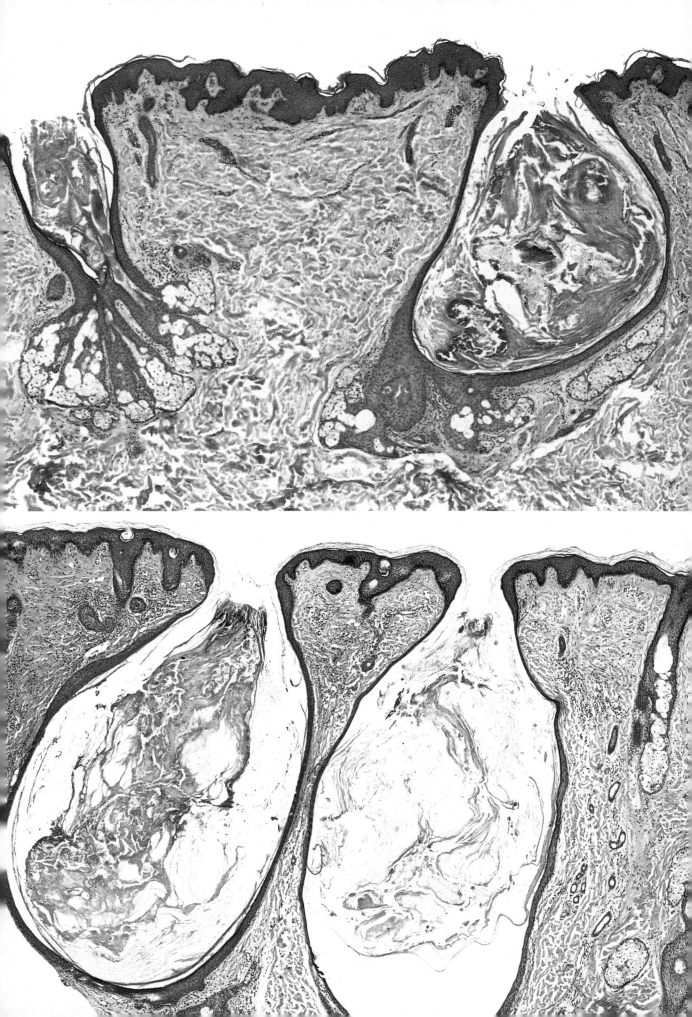

Amineptine Acne

Next to chloracne the most horrendous form of exogenous acne is due to chronic overdosage with the tricyclic amineptine, a widely used antidepressant available since 1978. The recommended dose is 100–200 mg/day. Acute hepatitis may appear in the first weeks of treatment, even with therapeutic doses. Dermatologic side effects were not reported until 1987.

In 1987–1988 about 20 cases of severe acne were brought to the attention of the Paris Poison Control Center. Most were women between 30 and 60 years of age, often heroin addicts or alcoholics. Having discovered the pleasant mood-enhancing and relaxing effect, the victims recklessly increased the doses to enormous amounts, up to 6000 mg a day. Amineptine illustrates the serious and unexpected hazards which arise from the misuse of valuable drugs.

The face, neck, earlobes, chest, upper back, extremities, and occasionally the perianal region become studded with hundreds, even thousands, of relatively large closed comedones, 3–5 mm in diameter. These may slowly enlarge to form huge cyst-like structures. Rupture gives rise to papules, nodules, and fluctuating abscesses 1–2 cm in diameter. The patients feel miserable and are disgusting to behold. Urine analysis reveals amineptine metabolites. The disease persists indefinitely unless the drug is discontinued. After stopping, the acne resolves slowly over a period of many months.

Topical tretinoin is effective but works slowly. It should be used aggressively, preferably twice daily. Careful supervision is recommended for these notably non-compliant patients, especially drug abusers. Isotretinoin 1.0 mg/kg body weight per day was ineffective for the myriads of comedones in the few patients treated this way. Withdrawal is the sovereign remedy.

Thioly-Bensoussan D, Edelson Y, Cardinne A, Grupper C (1987) Acné monstrueuse iatrogène provoquée par le Survector: première observation mondiale à propos de deux cas. Nouv Dermatol 6:535–537

Vexiau P, Gourmel B, Castot A, Husson C, Rybojad M, Julien R, Fiet J, Hardy N, Puissant A, Cathelineau G (1990) Severe acne due to chronic amineptine overdose. Arch Dermatol Res 282:103–107

Amineptine Acne

The first report of this extraordinary drug-induced acne was from Paris. A series of patients misused this antidepressant and, unfortunately, developed extensive acne.

Above

Left   Closed comedones, a few of them having ruptured already, stud this face

Right   A look behind the ear discloses confluent cystic lesions in the same woman

Below   Numerous small and large closed comedones, somehow mimicking solar comedones, are another manifestation of this potent acne-promoting drug

Below: Courtesy of Patrick Vexiau, M.D., Paris, France

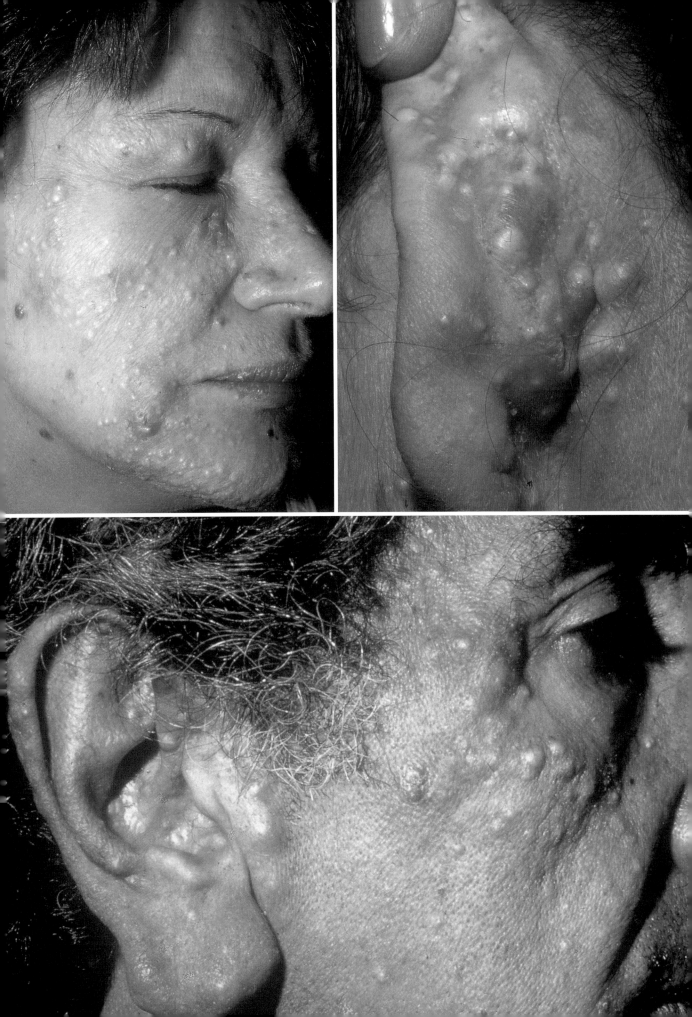

Horrendous Amineptine-Induced Acne Conglobata

The antidepressant amineptine, self-administered in very high doses to achieve emotional nirvana, precipitates a vicious form of inflammatory acne. This eruption may be viewed as acne conglobata times three.

Above   The frightened face of an addict, presenting unusually dense aggregations of closed comedones, and boil-like abscesses on forehead, glabella, and upper eyelids

Below   The back is a total mess of open and closed large comedones. Some of these have ruptured to form deep, wide fluctuant abscesses, which inevitably scar. Tissue destruction is enormous. The picture is reminiscent of chloracne

Below: Courtesy of Patrick Vexiau, M.D., Paris, France

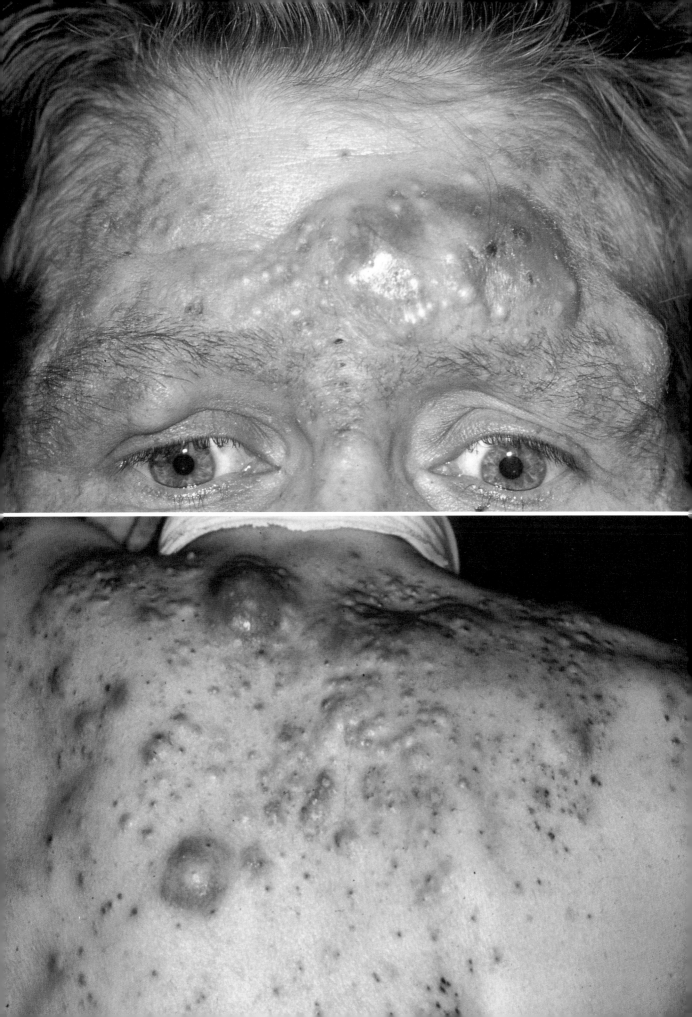

ROSACEA

Rosacea

The disease was originally called acne rosacea, an inept term which unfortunately still persists. Rosacea is easily confused with acne and may coexist with this disease.

Description

Papules and papulopustules occur in the central region of the face against a vivid erythematous background with telangiectases. Later, diffuse hyperplasia of connective tissue with enormously enlarged sebaceous glands may occur. The disease evolves in stages. The early signs are recurrent episodes of blushing which finally become persistent dark red erythema, particularly on the nose and cheeks, often before the age of 20. These persons are the so-called flushers and blushers. Rosacea is common in the third and fourth decades of life and peaks between the ages of 40 and 50 years. In the worst cases, disfiguring dermal hypertrophy, particularly of the nose (rhinophyma), may develop after many years.

Rosacea is a relatively common disease, especially in fair-skinned people. It has been called the curse of the Celts. It is rarer in dark-skinned people, particularly so in American and African Blacks, though in sunny countries such as Italy rosacea is surprisingly common. Women are more often affected than men, although the grotesque tissue and sebaceous gland hyperplasia leading to rhinophyma occurs mostly in men. Rosacea can cause severe emotional distress owing to its chronic course.

The importance of sun-damaged skin as the background of rosacea cannot be stressed enough. Rosacea is always associated with solar elastosis and heliodermatosis. It is superimposed on actinically damaged skin. Sun sensitivity is a frequent feature of rosacea in type I, fair-skinned patients. Many burn easily and tend to avoid sunbathing.

Rosacea also exhibits a wide spectrum of manifestations. Especially in young patients there may be preceding history of acne leading to a hybrid status in which rosacea coexists with acne. It is important to recognize those acne patients who are flushers and blushers as they may develop rosacea later on. Such patients are therapeutic challenges. As a rule acne peaks in adolescence, years before papulopustular rosacea makes its insidious appearance.

Pathogenesis

Virtually nothing is known about causation. Possibilities which have been discussed include gastrointestinal disease, hypertension, *Demodex folliculorum* mites, emotional stress, etc. None of them has been proved. Rosacea patients are constitutionally predisposed to blushing and flushing. Sunlight and heat are definitely contributing factors. The influence of heredity is moot, as is almost everything that has been written about etiology.

Rosacea is considered by some to be a seborrheic disease. However, seborrhea is not a consistent feature. Rosacea is not primarily a disease of sebaceous follicles, in contrast to acne vulgaris. Comedones are absent. Nevertheless, rosacea may resemble acne.

Clinical Findings

Rosacea is a centrofacial disease. It is localized on the nose, cheeks, chin, forehead, and glabella. Rarer localizations usually overlooked are the retroauricular areas, the V-shaped area of the chest, the neck, the back, and even the scalp.

The hallmarks of rosacea are papules and papulopustules, vivid red erythema, and telangiectases, preceded by episodes of flushing. Comedones are notably absent. If present, they are of other origin, e.g., from concomitant solar comedones (Favre–Racouchot's disease) or contact acne (acne cosmetica). Rarely papules are numerous enough to be nearly confluent. Granulomatous changes can emerge in later stages, sometimes receiving special designations such as lupoid rosacea. Rhinophyma and other phymas are the ultimate tissue reaction in males.

Rosacea evolves in stages over a period of decades.

Episodic Erythema (The Rosacea Diathesis)

Rosacea patients characteristically react with erythema on the central areas of the face, less often the neck, and the V-shaped area of the chest. These individuals are constitutionally predisposed to blushing and flushing, evoked by numerous nonspecific stimuli: ultraviolet radiation, heat, cold, chemical irritants, emotions, alcoholic beverages, hot drinks, spices. It is a mistaken belief that these

The many faces of rosacea

Classical expressions

- Episodic erythema: rosacea diathesis
- Stage I: Persistent moderate erythema with scattered telangiectases
- Stage II: Persistent erythema, numerous telangiectases, papules, and pustules
- Stage III: Persistent deep erythema, dense telangiectases forming sprays of vessels, especially on the nose; papules, pustules, nodules with variable plaque-like edema

Variants

- Persistent edema
- Ophthalmic rosacea with blepharitis, conjunctivitis, iritis, iridocyclitis, hypopyoniritis, and keratitis
- Lupoid or granulomatous rosacea
- Steroid rosacea
- Gram-negative rosacea
- Rosacea conglobata
- Rosacea fulminans (alias pyoderma faciale)
- Halogen-aggravated rosacea
- Phymas in rosacea: rhinophyma, gnathophyma, metophyma, otophyma, blepharophyma

persons flush when they drink tea and coffee. In fact the specific stimulus is heat. Cold tea and coffee have no effect. Flushing is more intense and lasts longer than in those who tend to blush when embarrassed. Eventually flushing and blushing lead to permanent erythema.

Different mediators including substance P, histamine, serotonin, prostaglandins, and others have been proposed to be implicated in the erythematous response. Experimental reproduction of the typical flush has not been achieved. Hence, the mechanism is still speculative.

Stage I Rosacea

The erythema may persist for hours and days, hence the old term erythema congestivum. Erythema lasting only a few minutes is not early rosacea. Telangiectases become progressively prominent, forming sprays on the nose, nasolabial folds, cheeks, and glabella. Most of these patients complain of sensitive skin that stings, burns, and itches after application of a variety of cosmetics, especially certain fragrances and sunscreens. Trauma from abrasives and peeling agents readily induces long-lasting erythema. Thus the facial skin is unusually vulnerable to chemical and physical stimuli.

Stage II Rosacea

Inflammatory papules and pustules crop up and persist for weeks. Some papules show a small pustule at the apex, justifying the term papulopustular. The lesions are always follicular in origin, mainly in sebaceous follicles but also in the smaller and more numerous vellus follicles. Comedones do not occur. The deeper inflammatory lesions may heal with scarring, but scars are inconspicuous and tend to be shallow. Facial pores become larger and prominent. If there has been much solar exposure over decades, the stigmata of photodamaged skin become superimposed, namely yellowed, leathered skin (elastosis), wrinkles, and solar comedones. The papulopustular attacks become more and more frequent. Finally, rosacea may extend over the entire face and even spread to the scalp, especially if the patient is balding. Itchy follicular pustules of the scalp are typical. Eventually, the sides of the neck as well as the retroauricular and presternal area may be affected. Papular rosacea of the back is not rare and is often overlooked. It is helpful to have rosacea patients get undressed for examination of the entire integument. Even the palms may show persistent erythema. Rosacea principally strikes the face but it may be a generalized disease. Bacteriologic studies of papulopustules have revealed nothing of interest. Usually only small numbers of the resident microflora are recovered, or none at all. Bacteria cannot be inculpated in the causation of rosacea.

Stage III Rosacea

A small proportion of patients goes on to develop more serious expressions of the disease, namely large inflammatory nodules, furunculoid infiltrations, and tissue hyperplasia. These derangements occur particularly on the cheeks and nose, less often on the chin, forehead, or ears. The facial contours gradually become coarse, thickened, and irregular. Curiously, patients may not notice these disfigurements. The deranged appearance becomes evident when photographs from previous years are reviewed. Finally, the patient shows diffusely inflamed, thickened, edematous skin with large pores, resembling the peel of an orange (*peau d'orange*). These coarse features are due to extensive inflammatory infiltration, connective tissue hypertrophy, massive fibrosis and elastosis, diffuse sebaceous gland hyperplasia, and extreme enlargement of individual sebaceous glands forming dozens of yellowish umbilicated papules on the cheeks, forehead, temples, and nose. Thickened folds and ridges may create a grotesque appearance mimicking leonine facies of leprosy or leukemia. The ultimate deformity is the phymas, of which rhinophyma is the prototype.

Variants of Rosacea

Classic rosacea is easily diagnosed; its variants are often not recognized or misdiagnosed.

Persistent Edema of Rosacea

This feature is not common but is typically overlooked. In fact, the literature hardly mentions this distressing variant. A hard nonpitting edema is found on involved areas, mainly on the forehead, glabella, nose, or cheeks. This unusual manifestation may lead to other wrong diagnoses that delay proper treatment. A similar edema occurs in patients with persistent inflammatory acne and in the Melkersson–Rosenthal syndrome. Thus this edema is nonspecific and develops on the background of chronic inflammation.

Ophthalmic Rosacea

Eye involvement in rosacea is surprisingly common. Indeed, the disease may begin in the eye and escape diagnosis for a long time, resulting in ineffective and even harmful treatments. The ophthalmic signs are exceedingly variable, including blepharitis, conjunctivitis, iritis, iridocyclitis, hypopyoniritis, and even keratitis. The term ophthalmic rosacea covers all these signs.

The prevalence is not known, but about 40% of a large number of rosacea patients participating in our cooperative isotretinoin trial were diagnosed by ophthalmologists as having some kind of inflammatory eye involvement. Blepharitis and conjunctivitis were most common.

The ophthalmic complications are independent of the severity of facial rosacea. Rosacea keratitis has an unfavorable prognosis, and in extreme cases can lead to corneal opacity with blindness. The most frequent sign, which may never progress, is chronically inflamed margins of the eyelids with scales and crusts, quite similar to seborrheic dermatitis, with which it is often confused. Pain and photophobia may be present. It is instructive to ask rosacea patients how their eyes react to bright sunlight. All patients with progressive rosacea should be seen by an ophthalmologist for a thorough examination to detect early subclinical complications. Indeed, cooperation between the dermatologist and the ophthalmologist is the ideal arrangement for the management of rosacea patients.

Lupoid or Granulomatous Rosacea

Some patients develop lupoid epitheloid granulomas in a diffuse pattern. One sees dozens of brown-red papules or little nodules on a diffusely reddened, thickened skin, frequently involving the lower eyelids. Diascopy with a glass slide best reveals the soft nodules. Histopathology shows perifollicular and perivascular epitheloid granulomas without foreign body components, giving rise to the archaic term lupoid granulomas, in reference to lupus vulgaris. The course is chronic and unremittent. The diagnosis is often missed. Differential diagnoses include lupoid perioral dermatitis, lupoid steroid rosacea, small nodular sarcoidosis, and lupus miliaris disseminatus faciei.

Steroid Rosacea

When a rosacea patient is erroneously treated for a prolonged time with topical steroids the disorder may at first respond, but inevitably the signs of steroid atrophy emerge with thinning of the skin and marked increase in telangiectases. The complexion becomes dark red with a copper-like hue. Soon the surface becomes studed with round, follicular, deep papulopustules, firm nodules, and even secondary comedones. The appearance is shocking with a flaming red, scaling, papule-covered face. Steroid rosacea is an avoidable condition which in addition to disfigurement is accompanied by severe discomfort and pain. Withdrawal of the steroid is inevitably accompanied by exacerbation of the disease, a trying experience for patient and physician.

Gram-Negative Rosacea

This is a newcomer among gram-negative infections, not likely to be diagnosed unless one has been informed of its existence. Clinically it looks like stage II or III rosacea. Multiple tiny yellow pustules increase suspicion. Neither oral antibiotics nor metronidazole will control the disease. The diagnosis rests on demonstration of gram-negative organisms by culturing the contents of several pustules. The disease is analogous to gram-negative folliculitis which frequently develops in acne patients on long-term antibiotics. The organisms identified include *Klebsiella*, *Proteus*, *Escherichia coli*, *Pseudomonas*, *Acitenobacter*, and others.

Rosacea Conglobata

Rarely a patient with severe rosacea shows a reaction which mimics acne conglobata with hemorrhagic nodular abscesses and indurated plaques. The course is progressive and chronic. This variant mainly occurs in women. Diagnosis is based on recognizing preexisting rosacea, limitation to the face, and no other signs of acne conglobata on the back, shoulders, chest, or extremities.

Rosacea Fulminans

This variant was first described by O'Leary and Kierland under the designation pyoderma faciale. It has been a matter of controversy ever since. One can say with certainty that it is neither a variant of acne nor a pyoderma. We interpret it to be an extreme form of rosacea conglobata. In analogy to its acne counterpart, acne fulminans, we opt to call it rosacea fulminans.

This is a conglobate, nodular disease springing up abruptly on the face of young women. It does not occur in men. Rosacea fulminans is confined to the face. Once seen it is never forgotten. The appearance is horrendous. Monstrous coalescent nodules and confluent draining sinuses occupy most of the face. The main locations are the chin, cheeks, and forehead. Ripe abscesses form with multiple pustules riding on top of the carbunculoid nodules. The face is diffusely reddened. Seborrhea is a constant feature but may be overlooked. When questioned closely, patients will often describe the development of oiliness before the explosion. The disease is both embarrassing and debilitating.

The history is uniform. The skin is ferociously attacked within a few days to weeks. Prior rosacea is sometimes denied, but we perceive a connection since signs of rosacea may make their appearance later. Some patients, too, have been flushers and blushers.

The etiology remains obscure. Severe emotional stress, like the death of a family member, divorce, loss of a lover, accidents, etc., is often blamed. Other patients deny preceeding stress. The exact importance of stress is another controversial aspect of this mysterious disease.

The prognosis is excellent. Once the disease has been brought under control with isotretinoin and systemic steroids it does not recur. We do not refer these unfortunates to psychiatrists.

The differential diagnosis includes acne conglobata (young patients, mostly men, longer history, other signs of acne, comedones, scars, seborrhea, no flushing or blushing), acne fulminans (only seen in teenage boys), bromoderma, and iododerma.

Phymas in Rosacea

Phyma is the Greek word for swelling, mass, or bulb. Phymas occur in various areas of the face and ears. Rhinophyma is the commonest among these and the best known. Other phymas cause difficulties in diagnosis.

Rhinophyma

Rhinophyma (*rhinos*, Greek = nose) occurs exclusively in men. Fortunately, only a few rosacea patients develop this complication. The bulbous nose develops over many years as a result of progressive increase in connective tissue, sebaceous gland hyperplasia, ectatic veins, and chronic deep inflammation. Rhinophyma may accompany stage III rosacea. Surprisingly, in other patients the signs of rosacea on the rest of the face may be rather mild.

Four variants of rhinophyma can be recognized although, of course, these are arbitrary divisions and most cases are mixtures:

Glandular Form. The nose is enlarged mainly because of enormous lobular sebaceous gland hyperplasia. The surface is pitted, with deeply indented and distorted follicular orifices. The tumorous expansions of the nose are often asymmetrical and of varying size. Lumps and sulci occur. Sebum excretion is increased. Compression by the fingers yields a white pasty substance consisting of an amalgam of corneocytes, sebum, bacteria, and sometimes *Demodex folliculorum* mites.

Fibrous Form. Diffuse hyperplasia of the connective tissue dominates this picture. A variable amount of sebaceous hyperplasia may be seen.

Fibroangiomatous Form. The nose is copper red to dark red, greatly enlarged, edematous, and covered by a network of large ectatic veins. Pustules are frequently present.

Actinic Form. Nodular masses of elastic tissue distort the nose but not to the extremes exhibited by classic rhinophyma. These are similar to the elastomas that occur in older individuals with markedly photodamaged skin as a result of overexposure to sunlight. This variety is mainly observed in subjects of Celtic origin who burn easily and tan poorly.

Other Phymas

Gnathophyma (*gnathos*, Greek = jaw) designates swelling of the chin.
Metophyma (*metopon*, Greek = forehead) refers to cushion-like swellings on the forehead above the saddle of the nose.
Otophyma (*ota*, Greek = ear) is a cauliflower-like swelling of the earlobes.
Blepharophyma (*blepharon*, Greek = lid) refers to chronic swelling of eyelids, mainly due to sebaceous gland hyperplasia.

Histopathology

The histopathology varies with the stage and quality of the disease. It must be admitted forthrightly that the changes are not diagnostic. Usually the clinical picture determines the diagnosis. Clinicians rarely biopsy the diverse lesions of rosacea. Histopathologists take their clue from the clinicians and find that the picture is "compatible with rosacea." Elastosis from photodamage is a constant feature and constitutes the terrain in which rosacea emerges.

In stage I rosacea there are mainly ectatic venules and lymphatics, slight edema, and sparse lymphatic perivascular infiltration. Moderate hyperplasia of the elastic tissue is present with increased curled, thickened elastic fibers (elastosis).

In stage II rosacea there is increasing lymphohistiocytic perivascular and perifollicular infiltration. Intrafollicular collections of neutrophils are often found, invariably when pustules are biopsied. The veins are thickened and grossly dilatated. Elastosis is more advanced.

In stage III rosacea there is diffuse hypertrophy of the connective tissue, accompanied by hyperplasia of sebaceous follicles with long, deformed follicular canals, and large, irregular sebaceous acini. Epithelialized tunnels undermine the hyperplastic tissue and are filled with inflammatory debris. Elastotic changes are prominent, often evident as amorphous masses of degenerated elastic tissue.

Demodex folliculorum mites are often found in all types of rosacea, usually in small numbers, within the follicular infundibula and sebaceous ducts. They are merely commensals and do not play an etiologic role in rosacea as formerly believed. This is different from *Demodex folliculorum* folliculitis, a true demodicosis.

Epitheloid granulomas of the noncaseating type with multiple foreign body multinucleated cells are the histopathologic equivalent of lupoid rosacea.

Rupture of follicles creates many confusing pictures. Far-flung abscesses with pseudoepitheliomatous hyperplasia, widespread necrosis, and lakes of granulocytes are characteristic of rosacea fulminans.

Immunofluorescence and immunohistochemical techniques have not contributed to the histopathologic identification of rosacea, nor to an understanding of its pathogenesis. Immunoglobulins are often demonstrable, especially at the dermoepidermal junction, but these reflect mainly photodamage and chronic inflammation.

Treatment

Rosacea is not curable. Nonetheless it is a treatable condition which can be moderated by the informed physician. Caring for rosacea patients requires a dedication on the part of the clinician and the patient. Naturally treatment schedules are determined by the stage and severity of the disease.

Topical

Rosacea patients have skin which is unusually vulnerable to chemical and physical insults. All sources of local irritation such as soaps, alcoholic cleansers, tinctures and adstringents, abrasives and peeling agents must be avoided. Only very mild soaps or properly diluted detergents are advised. Liquid detergents are available which are usually mild.

Protection against sunlight must be emphasized. Sunscreens are a must, though not sufficient in themselves. For some it may be hard to find a sunscreen which is tolerated without burning or irritation. In this regard one can recommend a new type of sunscreens; these incorporate highly micronized zinc oxide and titanium oxide, the particles of which are in the 20- to 50-nm range. They contain no chemical sunfilters and are very bland. They absorb photons and are completely different form the opaque particulate sunscreens which scatter and reflect ultraviolet radiation. Otherwise one can recommend broad spectrum sunscreens with an SPF of 15 or more, selecting those which provide protection against UV-B and UV-A.

Topical antibiotics as used in acne are sometimes effective. Erythromycin in a nonalcoholic base seems to be the best choice. Metronidazole is a newcomer in the anti-rosacea repertoire. In the USA a 0.75% gel (MetroGel) is available. Its efficacy has been proved beyond doubt. The gel is applied twice daily and has its greatest effect in papular and pustular rosacea. The mode of action is unknown. It does not alter erythema, telangiectases, or flushing. Where not available extemporaneous formulas may be employed. In Europe, e.g., where there is no registered preparation yet, we recommend a 2% lotion:

Rp. Metronidazole   2.0
     Eucerin lotion   ad 100.0

The antifungal imidazoles are also gaining popularity but their efficacy has not been tested against metronidazole. Ketoconazole cream (Nizoral) seems to be effective. The imidazoles perhaps work as an anti-inflammatory agent, but information is limited. Ciclopirox is another antifungal (Batrafen, Loprox) that seems to be promising as a treatment.

Old-time remedies should not be forgotten. Drying lotions fall into this category. Either use a commercial precipitated sulfur lotion or prescribe an extemporaneous product:

Rp. Hydragyrum sulfur. rubr.   0.5
     Sulfur praecipitati   2.0
     Lotio zinci   ad 100.0

Isotretinoin may have a place but has not been well studied. We have preliminary evidence that 0.2% isotretinoin in a bland cream is helpful. It is less irritating than tretinoin, and seems to supress inflammatory lesions in stage II and III rosacea.

Demodex folliculorum mites are no longer considered to play an etiological role in rosacea. It is good advice, though, to check for mites. This is best done with the skin surface biopsy technique using a drop of cyanoacrylate on a glass slide, then covered with immersion oil and viewed under ×10 magnification. Massive infestations of *Demodex folliculorum* mites may sometimes aggravate rosacea. The mites are satisfactorily controlled with lindane (γ-hexachlorocyclohexane), crotamitone, permethrin, or benzoyl benzoate. Treatment is once daily for 2–5 days. Intermittent schedules of application, including weekend doses every 2–3 weeks, can keep the mite population under control.

Obliteration of ectatic vessels, particularly on the nose, can be achieved by intravascular insertion of a fine diathermy needle or by light electrocoagulation of the surface. In expert hands these physical modalities are very effective and practical. When the ectasias are numerous and large, the laser is the method of choice. The argon laser and tunable pulsed-dye lasers give the best results.

Corticosteroids should never be used. The only exception is rosacea fulminans. In these women short courses of oral and topical corticosteroids are a reasonable option.

Systemic

The most agreeable feature of rosacea is that it generally responds well to oral antibiotics.

Tetracycline HCl, oxytetracycline, doxycycline, and minocycline are usually quite effective in controlling papulopustular rosacea and even reducing erythema. It is important to start with full doses, e.g., 1.0–1.5 g tetracycline HCl or oxytetracycline per day. Likeweise, 50 mg minocycline or doxycycline twice daily can be given. As soon as full control of papulopustules is achieved, usually after 2–3 weeks, maintenance doses of 250–500 mg tetracycline HCl or oxytetracycline or 50 mg minocycline or doxycycline per day are generally sufficient. Rosacea patients often know how to titrate disease activity and vary dosage accordingly. Patient input should be encouraged. Some get by with 250 mg tetracycline HCl every other day. Erythromycin is also effective but mostly used as a backup drug when tetracyclines are not tolerated or seem to be ineffective.

Antibiotic therapy in rosacea is often not sufficiently well monitored. The disease has its ups and downs. Too often patients are put on a fixed dose for many years. The situation should be periodically controlled, since topical drugs may be sufficient during inactive periods. Some patients may become addicted to oral antibiotics and find ways to get them without prescription.

Isotretinoin (13-*cis*-retinoic acid) is an excellent drug for severe forms of rosacea. Isotretinoin is indicated for all forms of severe or therapy resistant rosacea, especially the variants which are unresponsive to antibiotics, e.g., lupoid rosacea, stage III rosacea, rosacea conglobata, gram-negative rosacea, and rosacea fulminans. It is particularly helpful in patients who have oily, wide-pored skin and multiple, often many dozens of sebaceous gland hyperplasias. Furthermore, many forms of phymas respond to this drug. The dose required for the control of severe rosacea varies. We emphasize that isotretinoin is a rescue drug, not the one of first choice.

- Standard dose: 0.5–1.0 mg/kg body weight per day as used in acne. Side effects on the eyes make this dose unbearable for many patients. Ophthalmic rosacea may get worse, complaints of dry eyes can increase, and so can blepharitis. This may lead to the inability to use contact lenses. The high dose is only used in rosacea fulminans, or preoperatively for a couple of months to shrink rhinophyma before surgical reduction of the bulbous nose.
- Low dose: A low dose of 0.1–0.2 mg/kg body weight per day is usually effective in severe rosacea. This is really quite low, e.g., 7.5–15.0 mg daily for a patient weighing 75 kg. Side effects are greatly reduced. This dose is preferred for all forms of rosacea with ocular involvement.
- Minidose: For troublesome, stubborn, moderate rosacea we have achieved quite satisfactory results with 2.5–5.0 mg daily (not adjusted to bodyweight). 2.5-mg capsules are available in Europe. This dose is surprisingly helpful in many forms of the disease, excluding severe cases. Side effects on the eyes are minimal. Duration of therapy is longer than with the other doses, generally about 6 months. The cumulative dose, however, is extraordinarily low.
- Precautions with isotretinoin: The usual precautions have to be applied as in the therapy of acne (p. 625). Isotretinoin is a teratogen, and is therefore contraindicated for women of childbearing age unless the patient meets all the requirements printed in detail in the package label.
- Laboratory monitoring of SGOT, SGPT, cholesterol, and triglycerides before therapy and at monthly or bimonthly intervals thereafter. It is noteworthy that with minidose isotretinoin no changes in laboratory parameters have been observed, particularly cholesterol and triglycerides.

Rosacea fulminans requires special care. Treatment starts with oral corticosteroids, e.g., prednisolone 1 mg/kg body weight per day, for 1 week to cool down the fire. Then isotretinoin is added, at around 0.2–0.5, rarely 1.0 mg/kg body weight per day, with a slow tapering of the corticosteroid over the next 2–3 weeks. Isotretinoin is continued until all inflammatory lesions have disappeared. This may require 3–4 months. Draining abscesses should not be incised. Concomitant treatment in the first 2 weeks may consist of warm compresses and topical application of a potent corticosteroid cream. This is the only indication for topical and systemic corticosteroids in the treatment of rosacea.

Metronidazole is a chemotherapeutic agent registered for the treatment of infections caused by *Trichomonas vaginalis*, *Entamoeba histolytica*, or *Giardia intestinalis*. The usual dose is 500 mg two times daily for 6 days. Oral metronidazole is generally effective in the treatment of most types of moderate rosacea, including stages II and III. However, it may require 20–60 days to achieve control with a daily dose of 500 mg. The drug is not without side effects. It should be pointed out that rosacea is not an approved indication. The mechanism of action in rosacea is unknown. It is questionably mutagenic. Accordingly, oral metronidazole should be considered a second-line drug, to be tried when other methods have failed.

Miscellaneous

Facial massage has long been recommended. This is the so-called Sobye's massage. Its value is uncertain, and controlled studies are lacking. Twice daily gentle circular massage is given for several minutes to nose, cheeks, and forehead. The mechanism of action may be accelerated lymphatic drainage with reduction of edema.

There is no specific *rosacea diet*. Dietary limitations relate only to factors which provoke erythema, flushing, and blushing like alcoholic beverages, hot drinks, and spicy food. Encourage the patients to find out which dietary items are troublesome.

Surgical treatment of rhinophyma is a very successful approach. Excellent cosmetic results can be obtained. A variety of techniques are available, including scalpel or rasor modeling, electrocoagulation, argon laser, CO_2 laser, pulsed dye lasers, etc. Much depends on the training and the skill of the surgeon. Isotretinoin may be used very effectively before the operation to shrink down hypertrophic tissue, especially the huge sebaceous glands. This is strongly recommended.

Bleicher PA, Charles JH, Sober AJ (1987) Topical metronidazole therapy for rosacea. Arch Dermatol 123:609–614

Braun-Falco O, Korting HC (1983) Metronidazoltherapie der Rosacea. Medikament und Indikation. Hautarzt 34:261–265

Burton JL, Pye RJ, Meyrick G, Shuster S (1975) The sebum excretion rate in rosacea. Br J Dermatol 92:541–543

Clark DP, Hanke CW (1990) Electrosurgical treatment of rhinophyma. J Am Acad Dermatol 22:831–837

Dupont C (1986) How common is extrafacial rosacea? J Am Acad Dermatol 14:839

Gamborg Nielsen PG (1983) A double-blind study of 1% metronidazole cream versus systemic oxytetracycline therapy for rosacea. Br J Dermatol 109:63–65

Greenbaum SS, Krull EA, Watnick K (1988) Comparison of CO_2 laser and electrosurgery in the treatment of rhinophyma. J Am Acad Dermatol 18:363–368

Guarrera M, Parodi A, Cipriani C, Divano C, Rebora A (1982) Flushing in rosacea: a possible mechanism. Arch Dermatol Res 272:311–316

Gudmundsen KJ, O'Donnell BF, Powell FC (1992) Schirmer testing for dry eyes in patients with rosacea. J Am Acad Dermatol 26:211–214

Haneke E (1986) Klinik und Therapie der Rosazea. In: Macher E, Knop J, Czarnetzki BM (eds) Jahrbuch der Dermatologie. Regensberg und Biermann, Münster, pp 151–164

Hoting E, Paul E, Plewig G (1986) Treatment of rosacea with isotretinoin. Int J Dermatol 25:660–663

Irvine C, Marks R (1989) Prognosis and prognostic factors in rosacea. In: Marks R, Plewig G (eds) Acne and related disorders. Dunitz, London, pp 331–333

Leyden JJ, Thew AM, Kligman AM (1974) Steroid rosacea. Arch Dermatol 110:619–622

Marks R (1989) Rosacea: hopeless hypotheses, marvellous myths, and dermal disorganization. In: Marks R, Plewig G (eds) Acne and related disorders. Dunitz, London, pp 293–299

Marks R, Wilson Jones E (1969) Disseminated rosacea. Br J Dermatol 81:16–28

Massa MC, Su WPD (1982) Pyoderma faciale: a clinical study of twenty-nine patients. J Am Acad Dermatol 6:84–91

Meschig R, Melnik B, Plewig G (1989) Ophthalmological complications of rosacea. In: Marks R, Plewig G (eds) Acne and related disorders. Dunitz, London, pp 321–325

O'Leary PA, Kierland RR (1940) Pyoderma faciale. Arch Dermatol Syph 41:451–462

Persi A, Rebora A, Burton JL, Lynfield YL (1985) Metronidazole in the treatment of rosacea. Arch Dermatol 121:307–308

Plewig G, Nikolowski J, Wolff HH (1982) Action of isotretinoin in acne, rosacea and gramnegative folliculitis. J Am Acad Dermatol 6:766–785

Plewig G, Braun-Falco O, Klövekorn W, Luderschmidt C (1986) Isotretinoin zur örtlichen Behandlung von Akne und Rosazea sowie tierexperimentelle Untersuchungen mit Isotretinoin und Arotinoid. Hautarzt 37:138–141

Plewig G, Jansen T, Kligman AM (1992) Pyoderma faciale – A review and report of 20 additional cases: is it rosacea? Arch Dermatol 128 (in Press)

Powell FC, Corbally N, Powell D (1989) Substance P levels in rosacea. In: Marks R, Plewig G (eds) Acne and related disorders. Dunitz, London, pp 307–310

Ramelet AA, Perroulaz G (1988) Rosacée: étude histopathologique de 75 cas. Ann Dermatol Venereol 115:801–806

Rebora A (1987) Rosacea. J Invest Dermatol (Suppl) 88:56–60

Rödder O, Plewig G (1989) Rhinophyma and rosacea: combined treatment with isotretinoin and dermabrasion. In: Marks R, Plewig G (eds) Acne and related disorders. Dunitz, London, pp 335–338

Rolleston JP (1933) A note on the early history of rosacea. Proc R Soc Lond 26:327–329

Rosen T, Stone MS (1987) Acne rosacea in blacks. J Am Acad Dermatol 17:70–73

Schmidt JB, Gebhard W, Raff M, Spona J (1984) 13-cis-retinoic acid in rosacea. Clinical and laboratory findings. Acta Derm Venereol (Stockh) 64:15–21

Sobye P (1950) Aetiology and pathogenesis of rosacea. Acta Derm Venereol (Stockh) 30:137–158

Turjanmaa K, Reunala T (1987) Isotretinoin treatment of rosacea. Acta Derm Venereol (Stockh) 67:89–91

Wilkin JK (1981) Oral thermal-induced flushing in erythematotelangiectatic rosacea. J Invest Dermatol 76:15–18

Wilkin JK (1983) Rosacea. A review. Int J Dermatol 22:393–400

Portrait of Rosacea

Rosacea has well-defined clinical characteristics with central facial redness and a copper-like hue which the French term *couperose*, circumoral and submental palor, small erythematous papules, some tipped with a yellowish pustule, and slight scaling. This woman knew she was a flusher–blusher, turning dark red after hot drinks, alcoholic beverages, and embarresments. This is stage II rosacea with many small papules on a red background. It responds well to oral tetracyclines or topical metronidazole.

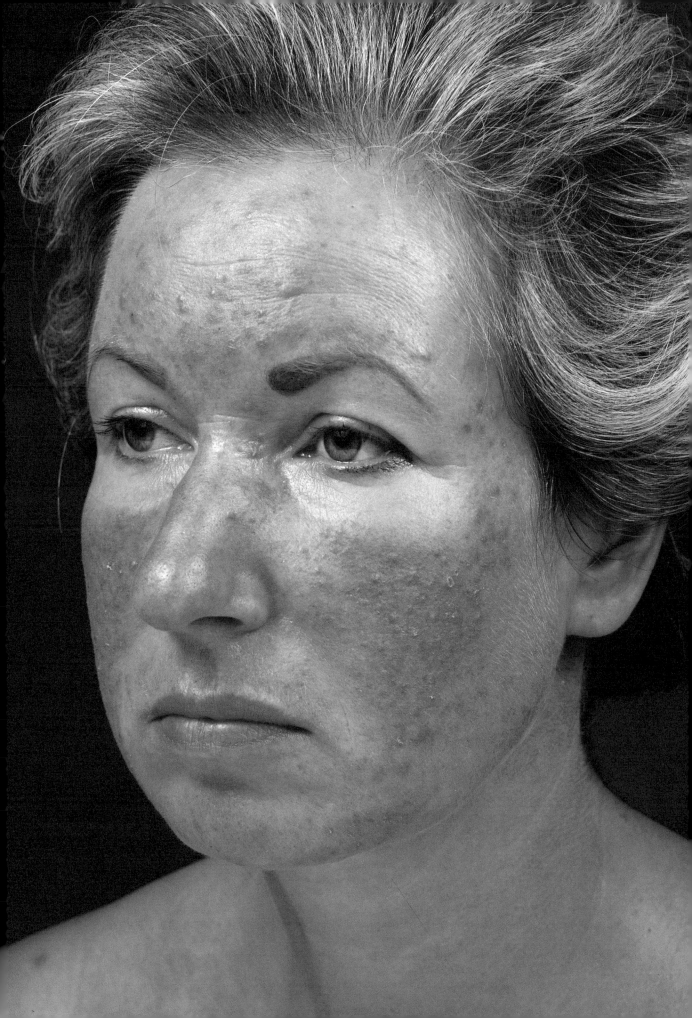

Rosacea

Rosacea evolves in well-defined stages.

Above

Left   Rosacea, stage I. This man is a flusher–blusher, showing the characteristic copper red hue. He has many fine telangiectasias and occasional papules on the nose and chin

Right   Rosacea, stage II. Papules and pustules in a centrofacial distribution on a background of copper red erythema accompanied by telangiectasias are diagnostic

Below

Left   Rosacea, stage II. All the typical signs of the disease can be found on the face of this young man

Right   Rosacea, stage III. Diffusely inflamed skin, confluent papules, and deep-seated painful nodules bespeak an unusually severe disease

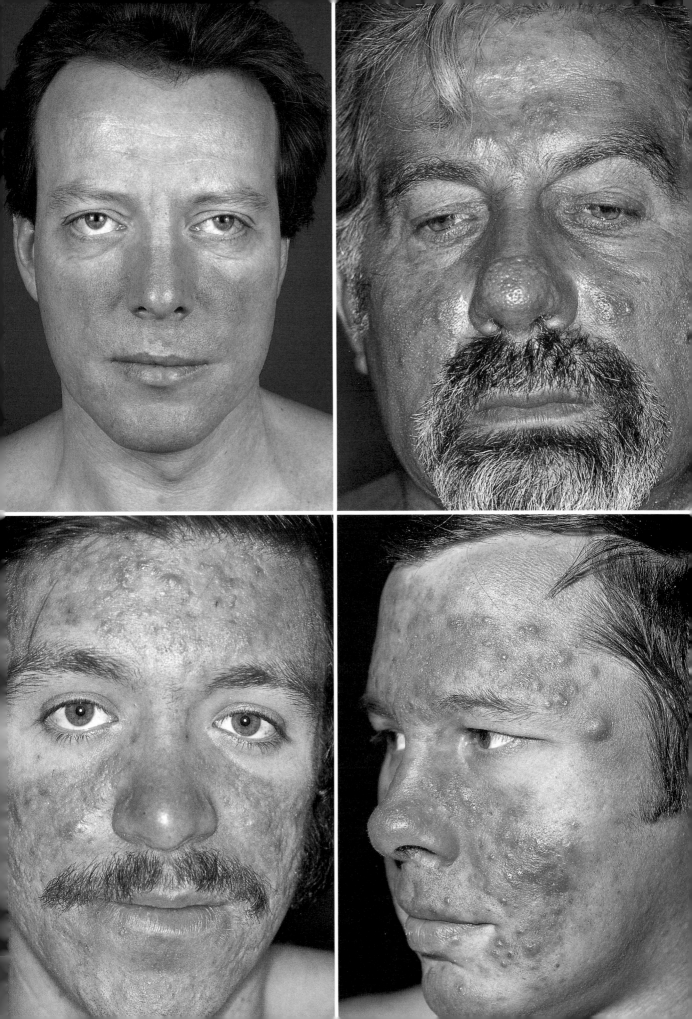

Rosacea: Extrafacial Locations

Although rosacea characteristically attacks the central face, other locations may be involved more frequently than appreciated because of failure to search.

Above   The central lesions are typical. What is unusual in this case are the densely aggregated papules on the forehead and bald scalp. The disease cleared with topical metronidazole.

Below   Severe rosacea, stage III, has deformed the face of this man (*left*). A patch of confluent deep papules and nodules on the chest is also part of the disease (*right*). Sometimes extrafacial rosacea is not suspected because blushing may be the only facial sign

Above: Courtesy of Professor Eckehard Haneke, Wuppertal, FRG

Haneke E (1986) Klinik und Therapie der Rosazea. In: Macher E, Knop J, Czarnetzki BM (eds) Jahrbuch der Dermatologie 1986. Regensberg and Biermann, Münster, pp 151–164

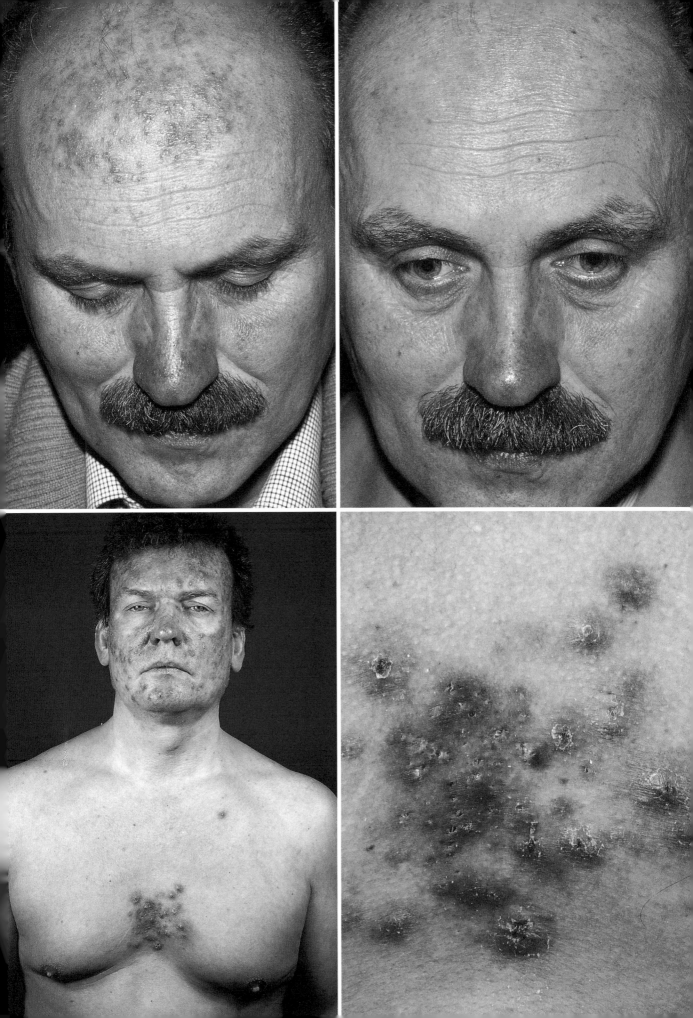

The Many Faces of Rosacea

Above

Left   Diffuse sebaceous gland hyperplasia, persistent erythema, telangiectasias, patches of edema, and irregular outcroppings of papulopustules are the features of rosacea in this man

Right   This is a complicated case with lumpy growths alongside the nose and on the cheeks, nonpitting edema, coarse facial pores, blepharitis, and edema on the forehead. The indurated growths are actually phymas

Below

Left   Decades of rosacea have left pitiful remnants on this man's face, e.g., diffuse and nodular sebaceous gland hyperplasia, coarse facial contures, telangiectases, a pebbly rugh surface, and prominent pores

Right   Rhinophyma is the ultimate, grotesque disfigurement of rosacea. The face is totally malformed. There is no truth to the vulgar belief that rhinophyma is caused by love of alcoholic drinks

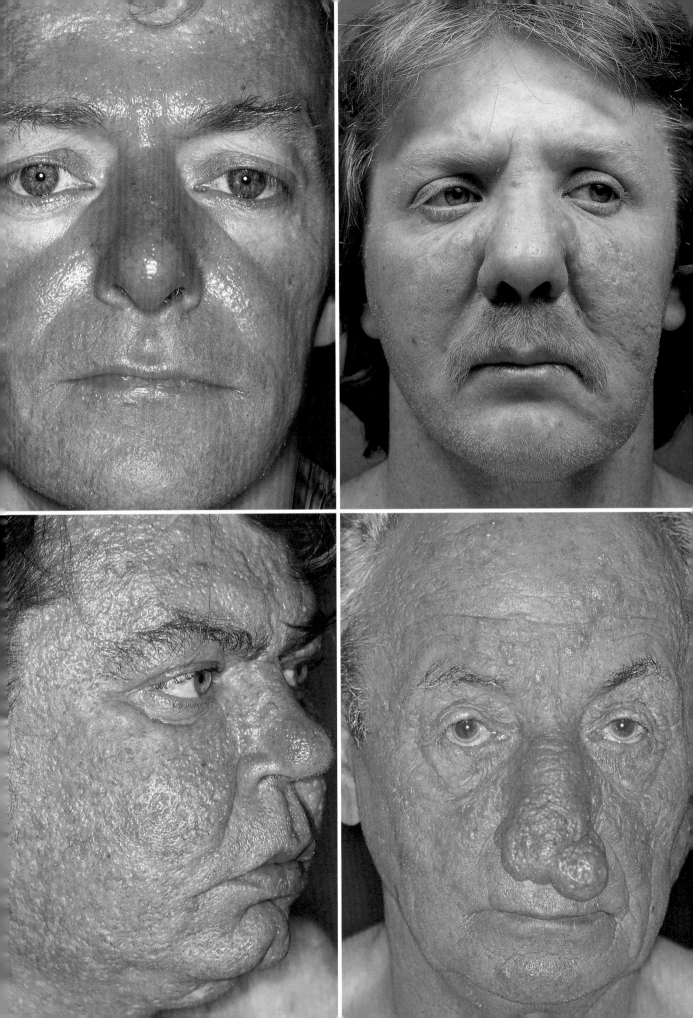

Exuberant Growths of Rosacea

Hyperplasia of various tissue components is typically seen in rosacea.

Above   Sebaceous gland hyperplasia. Circumscribed sebaceous gland hyperplasias are common in the face of the elderly. In particular, these dimpled growths are found in patients with rosacea. Many large sebaceous acini drain through sebaceous ducts and finally into one common infundibulum. The central pore is the equivalent of the dimple seen clinically

Below   Rhinophyma

Left   Cavernous follicular epithelium filled with loose corneocytes which do not form a compact comedo like in acne. Intrafollicular abscess, the equivalent of a pustule, and perifollicular infiltrate, extensive collagen hyperplasia, ectatic vessels, and interstitial edema are seen

Right   Many features of rosacea can be recognized in this specimen of rhinophyma: ectatic venules and lymphatics, edema, diffuse sebaceous gland hyperplasia, and perivascular and periadnexal infiltrate

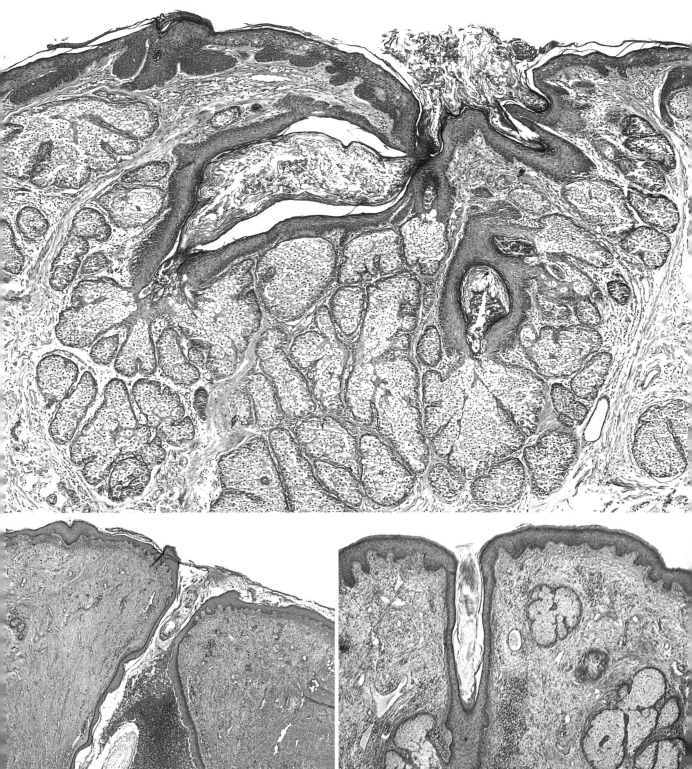
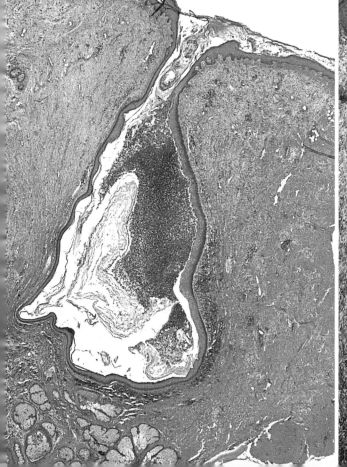
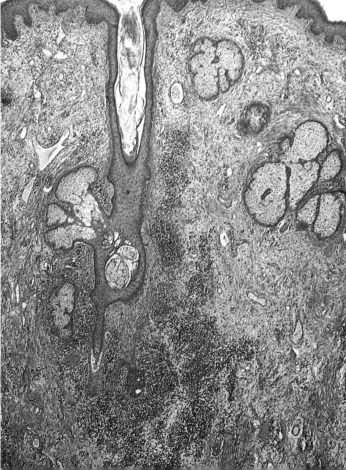

Rosacea and Rhinophyma

The bulging outgrowth of the nose, like all other phyma variants of the face, display quite typical features.

Above   Excessive overgrowth of connective tissue in sworled patterns produces the matrix of a phyma. Sebaceous glands, diffusely enlarged, cavernous sebaceous follicles filled with debris, wide and tortuous blood vessels, ectatic lymphatics, edema, and foci of a lymphohistiocytic infiltrate are complementary features

Below   Rosacea often has a peculiar edematous component to it. The collagen bundles are spread out, partly fine and thin, giving no good support for blood and lymph vessels, hence their ectasias. Occasionally one can find multinucleated giant cells and granulomatous niduses, not featured here

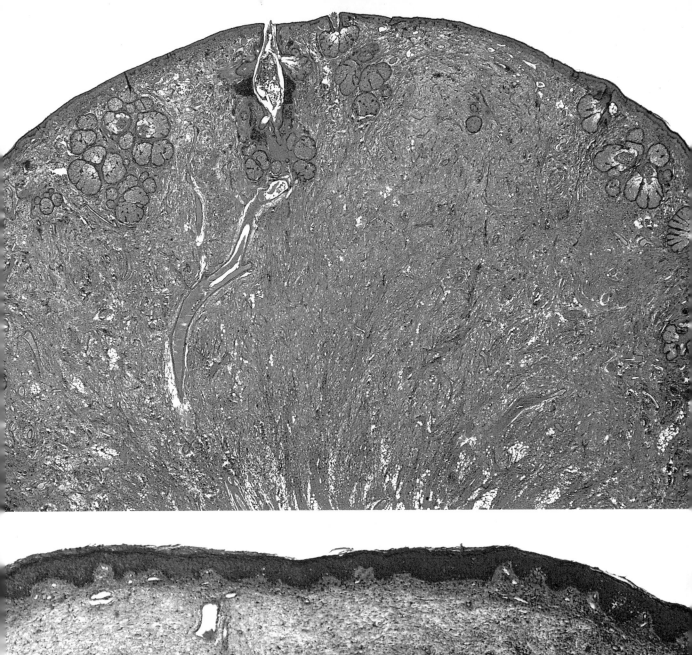
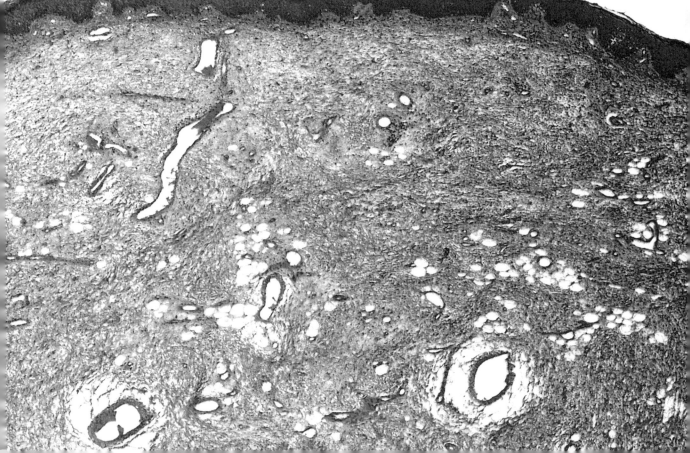

Rosacea and Red Eyes

A recognized but often overlooked complication of rosacea is inflammation of the eye. Indeed, this may be the heralding expression of the disease, masking the diagnosis until the face becomes involved. One clue is given by history. These are always flushers and blushers. Tetracyclines are effective, often in low doses, and may prevent severely afflicted patients from becoming blind.

Above

Left and The left eye was severely involved in this woman. Conjunctival injection,
right   photophobia, blepharitis, and corneal opacities were present, along with typical rosacea of the face. Oral minocycline immediately controlled all her lesions. Recurrence of ophthalmic rosacea is common, necessitating a maintained dosing schedule

Middle

Left and Chronic blepharitis, edema, and conjunctivitis create the typical red eyes.
right   Rosacea lesions on the face lead to the right diagnosis

Below

Left   Edema of eyelids, conjunctival injection, and blepharitis are the chief components of ophthalmic rosacea which knows no age limit

Right   Here facial rosacea is not severe but conjunctivitis and blepharitis are noteworthy

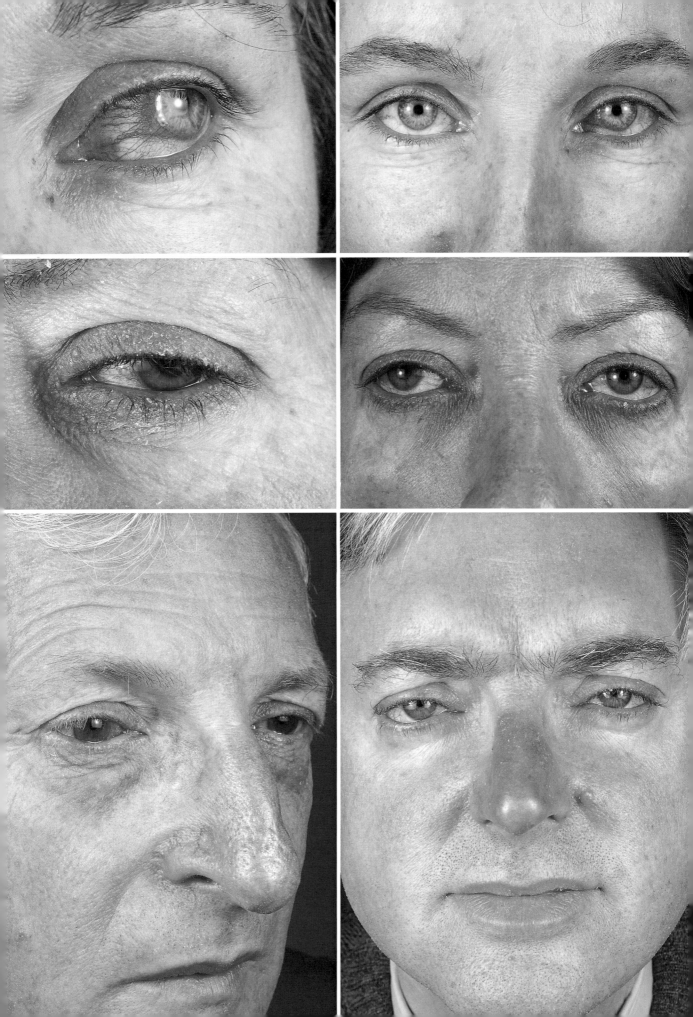

Persistent Edema in Rosacea

Uncommonly, patients with rosacea develop hard persistent edema, which is extremely distressing. A similar event occurs in acne. The origin of the edema is a puzzle. It calls for a variety of differential diagnoses, and is often not recognized as part of the rosacea spectrum.

Above

Left　Rosacea, stage II, in a young adult, who has a disfiguring nonpitting edema on the saddle of the nose, the glabella, and the maxillary region

Right　The forehead, both upper and lower eyelids, temples, and parts of the cheeks are swollen and edematous. Typical rosacea papules and pustules are present on the forehead and bald scalp

Below　Both men originally presented with stage II rosacea and persistent edema on forehead, upper, and lower eyelids. The rosacea cleared completely with low-dose isotretinoin, but not the edema. Despite full-dose isotretinoin therapy for 6 months there was only slight improvement
a

Above right: Courtesy of Professor Eckehard Haneke, Wuppertal, FRG

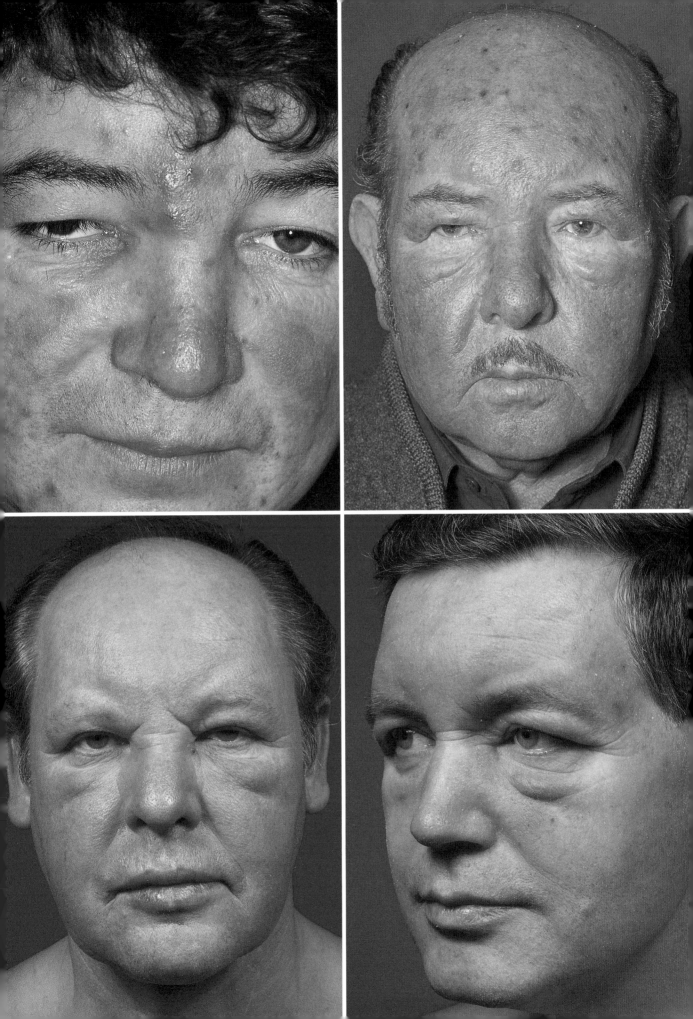

The Spectrum of Rosacea

Rosacea can take many forms, not unlike acne. Four variants are presented here.

Above

Left   Lupoid rosacea, with brown-red epitheloid infiltrates on diascopy covered the face of this young man for more than a year. Treatment is with orally given minocycline, or even better isotretinoin

Right   Steroid rosacea is the pitiful outcome of unnecessary topical corticoisteroid treatment. Fierce red, telangiectatic facial skin, studded with many tiny papules and papulopustules, accompanied by itching, make this man feel and look uncomfortable

Below

Left   Iodide-aggravated rosacea. Diagnostic procedures with iodide-containing radiopaques made the persistent low-grade rosacea in this woman explode into a conglobate-like stage within days

Right   Gram-negative rosacea is a difficult diagnosis. What are the clues? Seborrhea of unusual intensity, a male patient, papules and pustules fanning around mouth and nose, and failure to respond to conventional therapy with topical and oral antibiotics otherwise effective in this disease should alert one to search for gram-negatives. *Klebsiella* and *Escherichia coli* were recovered repeatedly in high numbers from the lesion. Treatment of choice is with isotretinoin, which cured the condition without a relapse. Parts of the nose and cheeks are covered by remnants from topical therapy

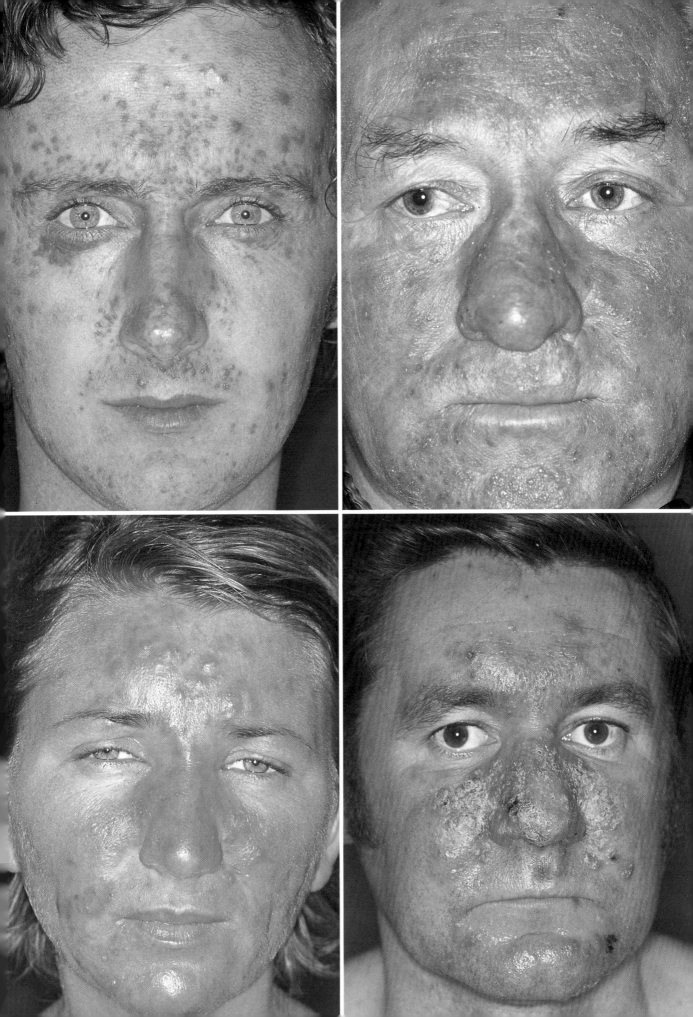

Horrendous Rosacea: Rosacea Conglobata and Rosacea Fulminans

Severe rosacea can be mutilating and devastating. Rosacea thus ferocious is rare in women.

Above   Rosacea conglobata. Conglobate hemorrhagic nodules in an unusual asymmetric pattern slowly developed over months, qualifying as a case of rosacea conglobata. More typical papules and pustules are scattered over the face. There were no lesions elsewhere

Below   Rosacea fulminans

Left   Rosacea fulminans, the counterpart to acne fulminans, suddenly appeared in the face of this young lady. Within a few weeks the face was overwhelmed by succulent hemorrhagic plaques, topped off by pustules, particularly on the chin

Right   Treatment with oral corticosteroids and isotretinoin brought about nearly complete resolution in 2 months. She was simultaneously thrilled and cured

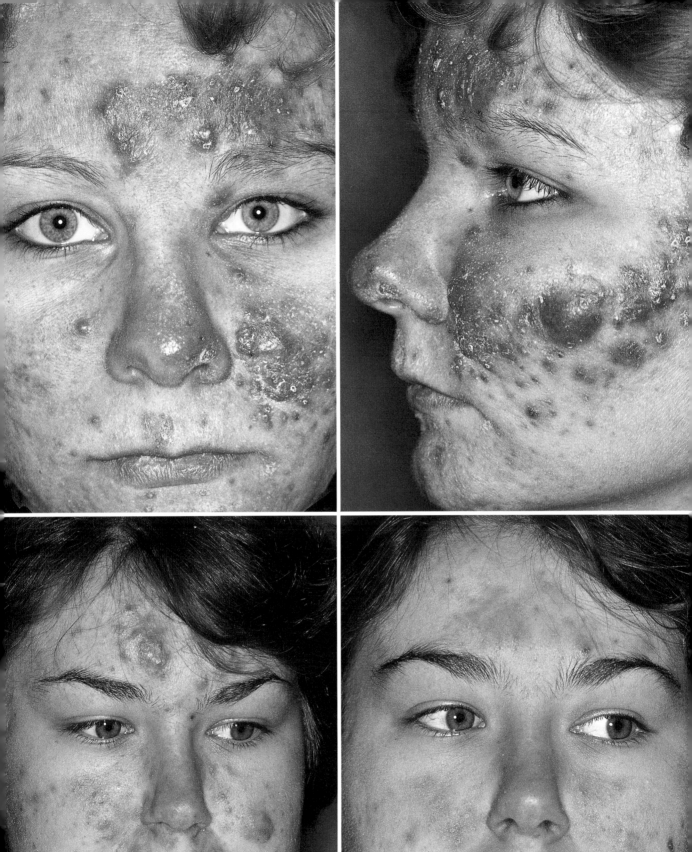

Ferocious Rosacea at Its Worst

Only two differential diagnoses are permitted: Rosacea conglobata or rosacea fulminans. The latter diagnosis is correct: a young woman with a history of flushing and blushing, fulminating onset a few weeks ago, no previous history of acne, confinement to the face, with maximal expression of confluent abscesses in the midline of the face. Seborrhea is typical. The rest of her body skin is smooth. Optimal treatment consists of oral contraceptives (antiandrogen type), isotretinoin (provided all precautions with this drug are met), and oral and topical corticosteroids. The results obtained with this all-round strategy (not shown here) are beyond words.

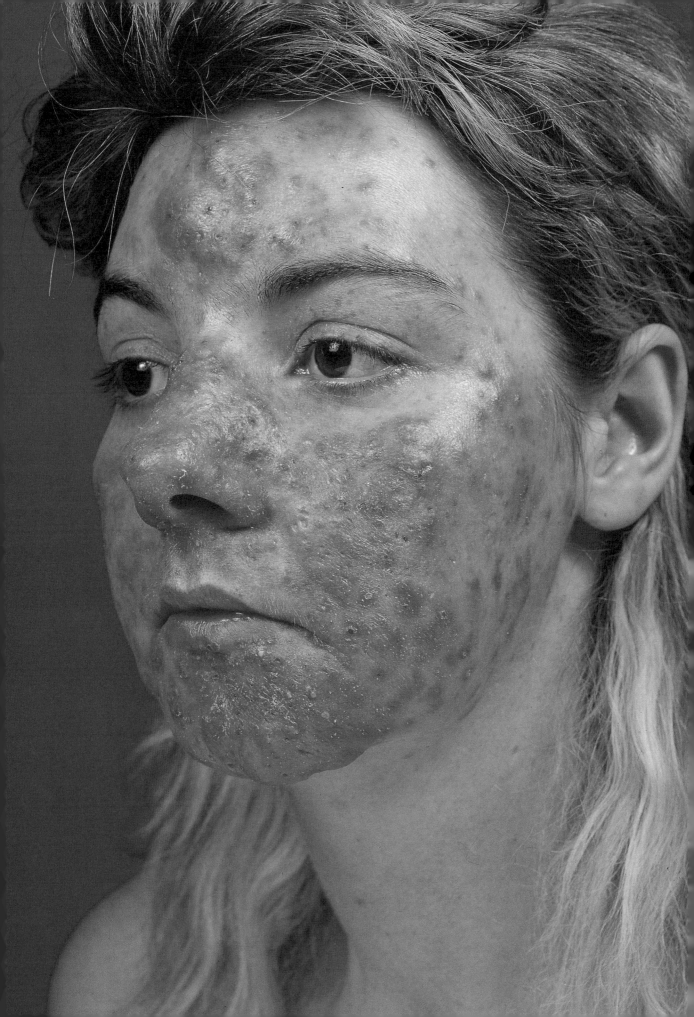

Rosacea Fulminans

This reckless attack of rosacea, afflicting only adult women, is the worst expression of this disease. The appearance is pitiful. All variants are displayed in this plate. Happily rosacea fulminans can be treated successfully with no recurrence.

Above

Left Incipient confluent lesions on the chin which were followed a few days later by further facial lesions

Right Boggy abscesses on the chin and early confluent abscesses in the nasolabial fold

Below

Left Chin, cheeks, and forehead satellites disfigure this young woman

Right One of the worst expressions of the disease

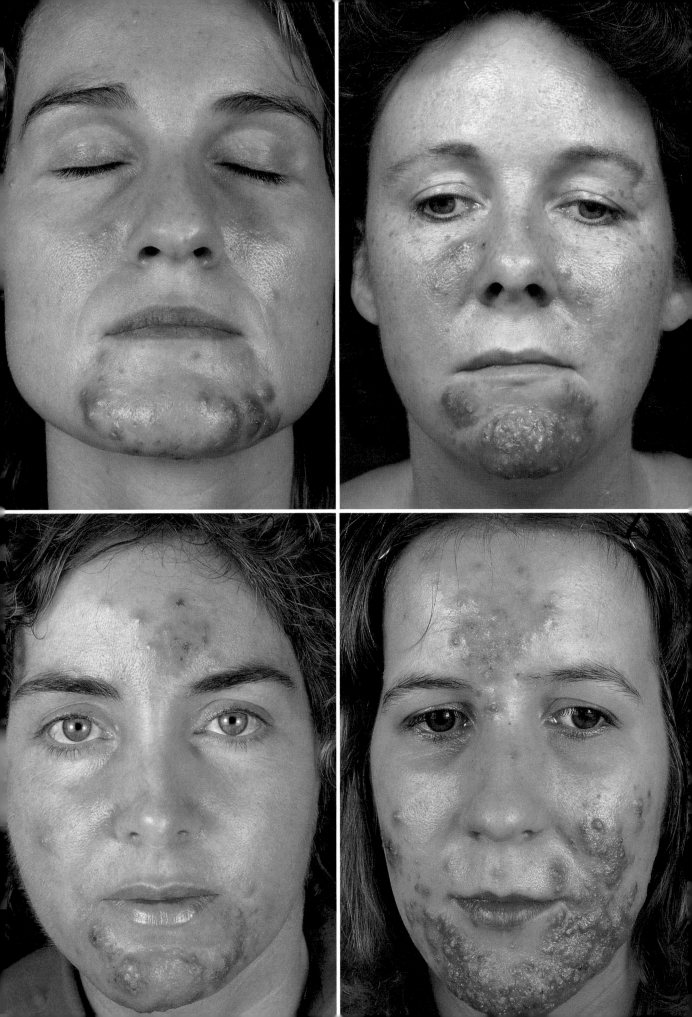

Pyoderma Faciale Is Rosacea Fulminans

It is astonishing that only a few biopsies of this strange disease have been reported in the literature. Histopathology from old lesions often informs us of unspecific secondary events. This plate shows early changes, about 72 h old, in a 25-year-old woman with rosacea fulminans.

Above

Left   The overview shows telangiectasias in the upper dermis and dense perivascular infiltrates in the middle and deep dermis, spilling over into the lobules of the subcutaneous fat

Right   Higher magnification reveals changes seen in rosacea: telangiectasias of veins and venules, ectatic lymphatics, edema, and a mixture of lymphocytes. There are also eosinophils, a few granulocytes in a perivascular pattern intermingled with a few epitheloid granulomas, and hypercellularity of the collagen

Below   The clinically telltale sign of hemorrhagic nodules is explained by considerable erythrocyte extravasation seen in the center. Telangiectasias, edema, nidusis of epitheloid granulomas, and scattered diffuse lymphohistiocytic infiltrate complete the picture

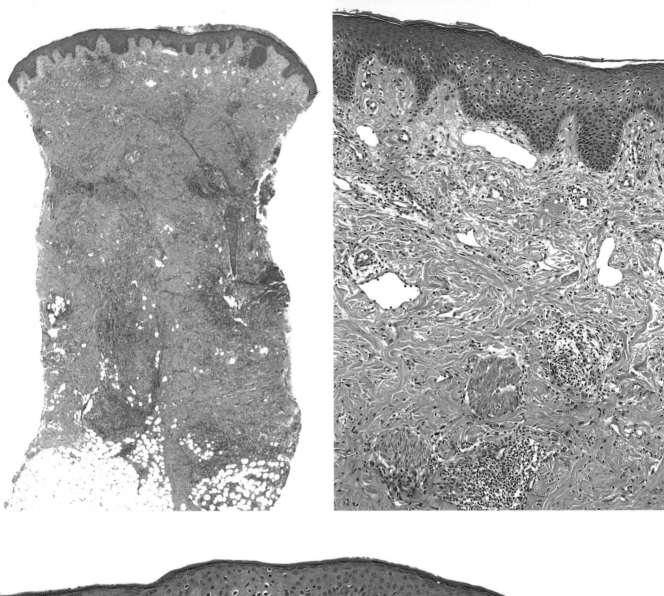
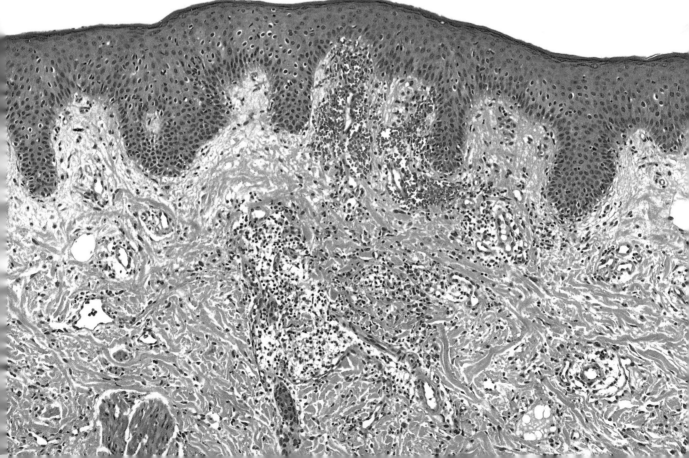

Rosacea Fulminans

It is still unknown why women are so fulminantly attacked by this disease, which curiously locates exclusively in the face and neck region. Suppuration and drainage plague the patients.

Above

Left   The findings are very varied, including small epitheloid granulomas, multinucleated giant cells of the Langhans type, lymphocytes, and extravasated erythrocytes. Granulocytes are sparse, and leukocytoclasia is absent

Right   The dense infiltrate distends deep down into the lower dermis with mixed lymphocytes, histiocytes, and a few eosinophils

Below   The inflammation spills over into the subcutaneous fat. Lobular panniculitis is present, with concomitant septal involvement

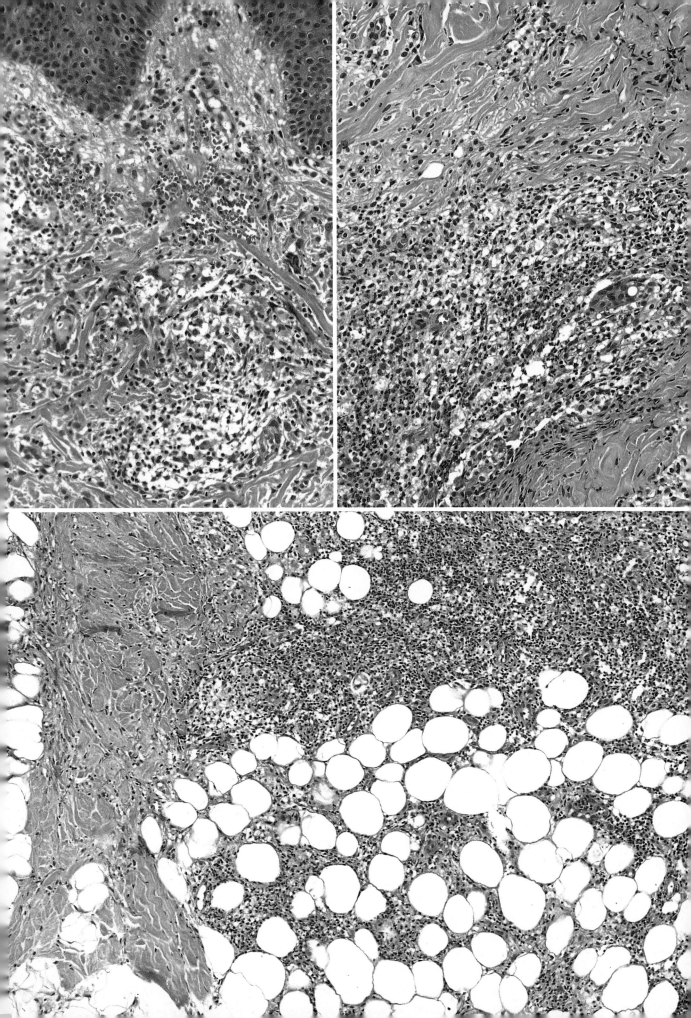

Rosacea Is an Eminently Treatable Disease

Above   Rosacea conglobata with edematous patches of the nose and cheeks (*left*) responded handsomely to oral isotretinoin within 12 weeks (*right*)

Below   Sadness speaks from these pictures. Rosacea can be aggressive and mutilating. When this severe (*left*), it requires immediate therapeutic action with isotretinoin. Isotretinoin given for 8 weeks (*right*) eliminated most of the inflammation

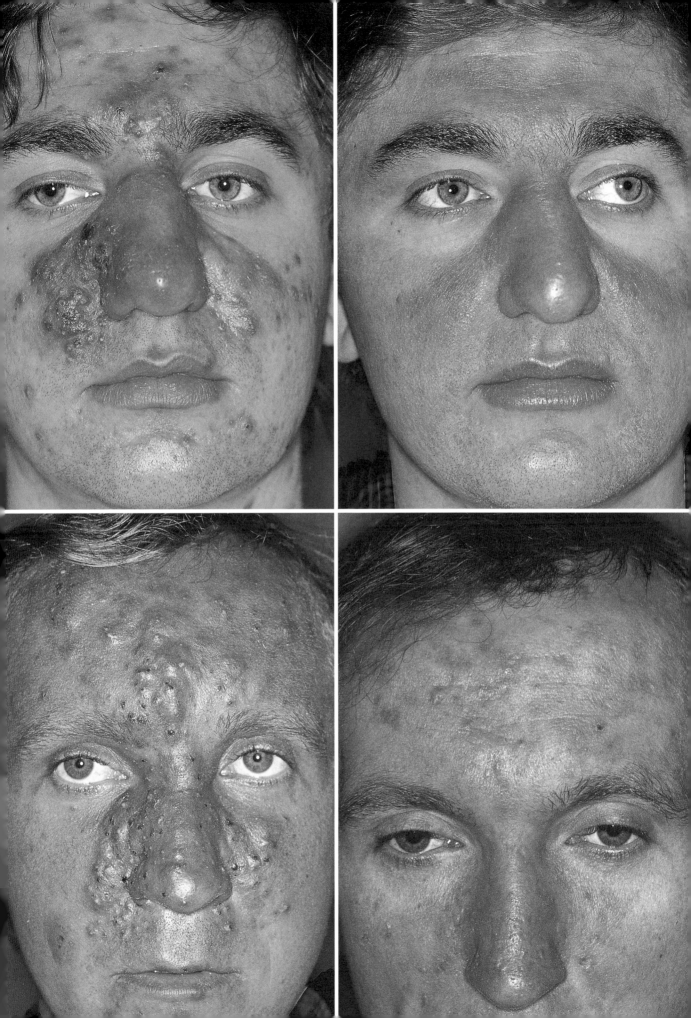

Rosacea Can Be Greatly Improved by Isotretinoin

Isotretinoin can be the choice of treatment in severe, recalcitrant rosacea. The biopsies are from the same patient of symmetrical areas from the forehead.

Above   Facial biopsy of a patient with a long-standing history of rosacea. The telltate features of the disease are mild acanthosis, slight spongiosis, marked ectatic veins and lymphatics, edema, and perivascular and periadnexal infiltrate of lymphocytes, with occasional granulocytes. The sebaceous acini of vellus and sebaceous follicles are very large

Below   8 weeks of isotretinoin have completely changed the view: sebaceous acini are gone except for one nidus in a vellus follicle (*center*). The infiltrate has been reduced by more than 80%. Ectatic vessels have become fewer and smaller in diameter, and the collagen is no longer separated by edema. Finally, there is no more spongiosis of epidermis and follicular epithelium

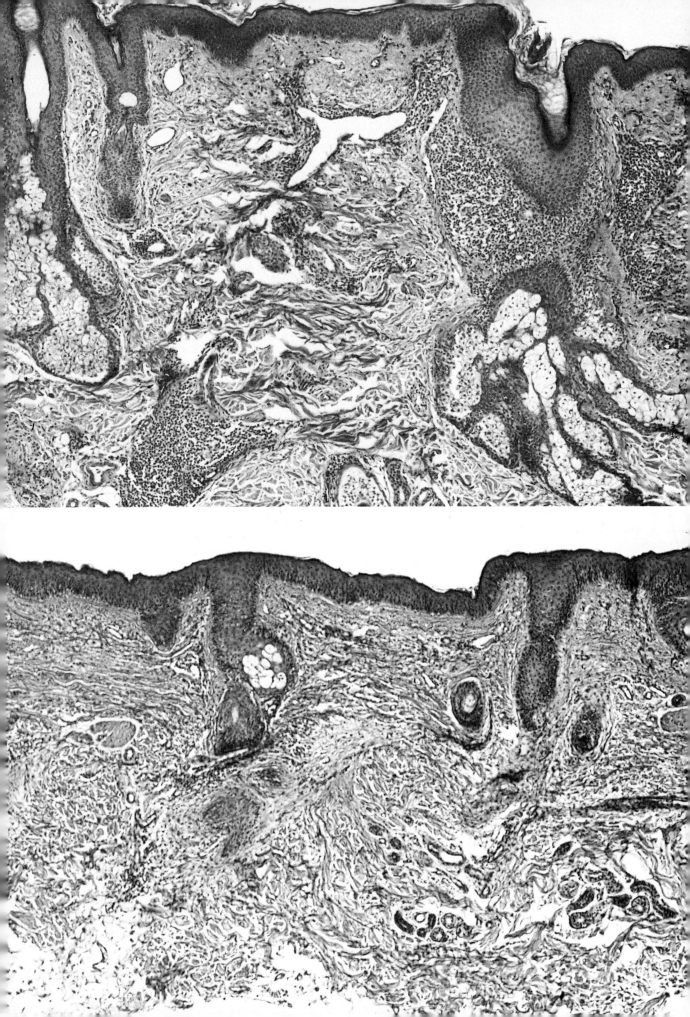

OTHER ACNE-LIKE DISORDERS

Perioral Dermatitis

Earlier synonyms for perioral dermatitis were light-sensitive seborrheid (Frumes and Lewis 1957) and rosacea-like dermatitis (Steigleder and Strempel 1968). The disease has made its way slowly around the world, starting in the United States and Western Europe, and then appearing in many other countries. It was common two decades ago; the prevalence has decreased substantially. Women are mainly affected, with rare instances in men. The peak age is between 20 and 30 years. The early reports offered a perplexing variety of putative causes including fluorinated toothpastes, mouthwashes, citrus fruits, soaps, handkerchieves, the beard of consorts, intestinal malabsorption, infection by *Candida* species or fusiform spirillae, hormones and oral contraceptives, and provocation by sun exposure. Others consider perioral dermatitis to be an abortive form of rosacea or a rosacea-like seborrheic dermatitis. We do not share any of these views.

We recognize two etiological agents, and there may be others. At the outset we must concede that some cases are inexplicable, perhaps manifestations of another disorder which mimics genuine perioral dermatitis. Facial cosmetics nowadays seem to be the number one culprit. Almost every woman with perioral dermatitis has a positive history of intensive use of cosmetics. These include a wide gamut of skin care products, especially moisturizers. Which ingredient is responsible is still a matter of debate, e.g., isopropyl myristate has been mentioned many times. Thorough questioning is necessary. Often a mix of factors are operative – excessive soap washing, use of abrasives and astringents. Many of these patients say that they have sensitive skin. The offending agents are likely to be irritants rather than possessing acneigenic activity. Proof of chemical causation comes from total abstinence, followed in 2–3 months by slow clearing. There is no doubt that topical corticosteroids were the most frequent cause of perioral dermatitis when the disease made its debut. The reasons for their (ab)use were mostly minor facial problems. Women came to believe that this miracle drug would take care of any imperfection. Perioral dermatitis has been experimentally induced by topical corticosteroids. When steroids are the cause, the lesions tend to spread beyond the classic perioral territory.

The clinical pattern is unmistakable. The disease is usually symmetrically distributed around the border and corners of the mouth, sometimes extending to the nasolabial folds and the cheeks, rarely to the lower eyelids. The typical location is perioral only. Comedones are notably absent. Initially there is only patchy redness on which tiny pustules are superimposed. As the disease progresses numerous papules or papulovesicles, 1–2 mm in diameter, develop on a diffusely reddened background. These have mainly a follicular location. Sparing of a narrow pale zone around the lips is a pathognomic feature explainable by the paucity of follicles in this special site.

The lesions are often accompanied by a feeling of tightness, moderate burning or stinging, dryness, and occasionally pruritus. Mild scaling is usually detectable on close examination. These symptoms suggest an external contactant. Quite typical is unpredictable waxing and waning, even from day to day. Aggravating factors include excessive washing with harsh soaps as well as exposure to sunlight. Rubbing and fingering the affected area add a traumatic factor. Thus, many factors may converge to trigger the disease which grinds on for many months even years.

The minimum requirement for a definitive diagnosis is papulopustules on an erythematous background in the perioral region. Otherwise almost any facial eruption can be dumped into the waste basket of perioral dermatitis.

Lupoid perioral dermatitis is a rare variant. Dense aggregations of somewhat larger red-brownish papules and papulosquamous lesions display a lupoid papule on diascopy. This form is most often due to topical application of corticosteroids.

Histopathologically perioral dermatitis is easily distinguished from acne. One always sees diffuse lymphohistiocytic perivascular infiltrations, edema, and spongiosis of the interfollicular epidermis and the follicular epithelium as well. Focal parakeratosis is always present. Perifollicular lymphocytic infiltrates are abundant. Microcomedones are absent. The smaller blood vessels are dilated and often engorged with red blood cells. The picture is that of a diffuse dermatitis which also involves the follicles. The latter are more numerous around the mouth and chin than elsewhere on the face, partially explaining the localization. *Demodex folliculorum* mites can sometimes be demonstrated but are incidental. However, in the granulomatous variant *Demodex* mites are considered a contributing etiologic agent.

Differential Diagnosis

This includes a wide range of facial dermatoses, especially rosacea and its variants, steroid acne, acne venenata (acne cosmetica), and seborrheic dermatitis.

Lupoid perioral dermatitis requires differentiation from lupoid rosacea and lupus miliaris disseminatus faciei, which by some is considered as a lupoid variant of rosacea or perioral dermatitis, by others as a true form of skin tuberculosis. We prefer the former classification.

Treatment

Dermatologists have varying opinions regarding the best treatment. Our approach is as follows:

Insist on total abandonment of all cosmetics: soaps, detergents, moisturizers, abrasives, adstringents, day or night creams, antiwrinkle creams (even in the periocular region as they will spread to the entire face), skin conditioners, rouges, etc. Wash with warm water only, using the fingers. This null therapy is hard for some patients. Tell them that exacerbations are to be expected, and that it may take many weeks to abate. After clearing cosmetics can be reintroduced, one at a time. Long-standing severe disease improves much faster with a full course of antibiotics. We prefer the lipophilic tetracyclines like minocycline or doxycycline. The dose is 50 mg twice a day for 3–4 weeks, rarely longer. The disease slowly regresses when exogenous insults are stopped. We strongly advocate oral antibiotics for destressed women who have had the disease for a long time.

The rare lupoid variant requires systemic treatment in every case. If there is no response to a full dose of tetracyclines, one may have to resort to isotretinoin. We have found that quite low doses are effective, usually 5 mg as a single daily dose for about 3 months. Even 2.5 mg/day is helpful. Precautions must be taken for women of childbearing potential (p. 635). Topical metronidazole twice daily is worth a try, but the results are inconsistent. Occasionally topical erythromycin is helpful.

Frumess GM, Lewis HM (1957) Light-sensitive seborrheid. Arch Dermatol 75:245–248

Marghescu S (1988) Lupoide Form der Rosazea-artigen Dermatitis. Hautarzt 39:382–383

Marks R (1976) Common facial dermatoses. Wright, Bristol, pp 25–31

Mihan R, Ayres S (1964) Perioral dermatitis. Arch Dermatol 89:803–805

Rufli T, Mumcuoglu Y, Cajacob A, Büchner S (1981) Demodex folliculorum: Zur Ätiopatho-genese und Therapie der Rosazea und der perio-ralen Dermatitis. Dermatologica 162:12–26

Steigleder GK, Strempel A (1968) Rosaceaartige Dermatitis des Gesichts. "Periorale Dermatitis." Hautarzt 19:492–494

Stieler W, Senff H, Kuhlwein A, Jänner M (1988) Lupus miliaris disseminatus faciei. Differential-diagnose und Pathogenese. Aktuel Dermatol 14:4–6

Wilkinson DS, Kirton V, Wilkinson JD (1979) Pe-rioral dermatitis: a 12-year review. Br J Dermatol 101:245–257

The Role of *Demodex*

The human integument provides a favorable substrate for the growth of bacteria, certain yeasts, and, in relation to the current topic, even mites. Most of these commensals live with us, and flourish and nourish themselves in our hair follicles, but curiously not within eccrine or apocrine sweat glands and their acrosyringa. Our skin may be likened to a botanical and zoological garden, supporting a diversity of species.

Mites of the species *Demodex folliculorum* and *Demodex brevis* prosper in the deep, large sebaceous follicles. It is rare to find a person in whom *Demodex* cannot be demonstrated after vigorous examination. *Demodex* is absent in children and surprisingly sparse in adolescents and young adults, even in oily persons. *Demodex* has an aversion for acne lesions, and is never found in comedones. Over the next three to four decades their numbers increase. The prevalence approximates 100% in older adults. However, it should be emphasized that the population density is low. To locate a few mites takes a lot of effort.

Demodex folliculorum are closely associated with sebaceous glands. They utilize sebum as nourishment. Their feeding grounds are, therefore, the spacious canals of the sebaceous follicles and sebaceous ducts. The best site to search for mites is the face. The nose, cheeks, forehead, temples, and chin are favorite locations, along with the balding scalp and neck.

Oily skin with large pores houses more *Demodex folliculorum* mites than asteatotic skin. On the cheeks and nose of some aged persons, hordes of *Demodex folliculorum* may infest the large sebaceous follicles. Not every follicle bears mites. Colonization is uneven, for unknown reasons.

Demodex folliculorum mites are mostly found head-down as if moving against the stream of sebum. Usually a whole family of mites dwells in the canal and ducts, comprising as many as 20 mites including parent and daughter generations.

Dermatologists have not been able to reach agreement concerning the pathogenetic potential of the mites. Most consider them to be merely passengers which can practically always be found in normal adult skin or coincidentally in diseased skin. It is important to emphasize that an etiologic role for mites can be proposed only when the follicles are crowded with them, a situation not unlike that of many bacteria which are harmless until the population becomes excessive.

Demodex Folliculitis

We must call attention to the fact that the role of *Demodex* as a cause of facial eruptions is controversial. We perhaps belong to the minority as we recognize a pathogenic role for this normal inhabitant.

Others who share our opinion have called this condition demodicidosis, an explicit term. Demodicidosis as a disease of follicles was first mentioned by Ayres and Ayres some 30 years ago. This seminal work is always mentioned in textbooks, but the majority of dermatologists have not been persuaded and believe they have never seen an incontestable case. This is in contrast to the ophthalmologists who recognize demodectic blepharitis. The clinical picture is typical, albeit subtle. Most of the patients are 50–70 years of age, males and females alike. The impression has been gained that women have a special predisposition, especially those who make heavy use at moisturizers, although there is no evidence for this. It may be that women have a keener interest in healthy skin. The clinical picture is not dramatic and often consists of a roughed surface from accumulation of scales in the infundibulum of sebaceous follicles. The finger may detect horny spines protruding from the orifices. Follicular papules, and papulopustules may be present to varying degrees. Thus, the central sign is a folliculitis, but this may often be sub-clinical, requiring biopsy for histologic confirmation. Proper diagnosis rests on demonstration of large numbers of mites and clearing after proper treatment. The course, if not diagnosed, is protracted over months and years.

Histopathology

There is spongiosis of the epithelia of sebaceous and vellus follicles containing a multitude of mites, including adults, larvae, and eggs. An especially vulnerable point is the thin epithelial lining where the sebaceous ducts merge with the infrainfundibulum. Breaks in the follicular epithelium occur, with spilling out of follicular debris. Small perifollicular abscesses may be present in early lesions.

Signs of diffuse chronic inflammation are always present. Displaced mites act as foreign bodies; their chitin bodies are seen in foreign body granulomas. It is noteworthy that perifollicular infiltrates occur only in those follicles in which mites are abundant.

Demodex Mites and Acne

Demodex can be disregarded as a potentially harmful intruder. Mites are absent or found in very low numbers. In the many hundreds of biopsies of lesional and clinically healthy skin from acne patients studied histologically, we have only occasionally demonstrated folliculitis possibly due to colonization by *Demodex folliculorum*. We have never seen mites in acne comedones or in papulopustules. *Demodex* dislikes the young and shows no partiality toward acne patients.

Demodex folliculorum Mites and Rosacea

Many dermatologists deny a role for *Demodex* in the pathogenesis of rosacea. In most cases, the association is merely coincidental. Since rosacea is a common disease of unknown origin it was convenient in the past to incriminate *Demodex*. Nowadays, hardly anyone blames mites. We believe, however, that mites may aggravate the disease and should be looked for in unusual patterns of rosacea, especially in patients who do not respond to conventional therapy or in steroid rosacea. Sometimes an asymmetrical distribution on one cheek is a clue. However, one particular lesion occurs in occasional rosacea patients which is undoubtedly due to *Demodex*. This is granulomatous rosacea with persistent, deep nodules. Biopsies show a foreign body granuloma with the chitinous remains of a mite in the center.

Demodex Folliculorum Blepharitis

Demodectic mites can cause inflammatory folliculitis of the eyelashes (blepharitis), a condition known to ophthalmologists. Many of the patients have seborrheic dermatitis with eyelid involvement, others have blepharitis associated with rosacea. The diagnosis can only be established by showing that the follicles are crowded with mites.

Demodex Infections in Veterinary Medicine

Demodectic mange in dogs, rodents, and cattle among many other animals is a bona fide follicular disorder, which may become extensive enough to destroy health, even the life of the animal.

How to Find the Mites

There is a noninvasive procedure for demonstrating *Demodex*. The fastest way, with small inconvenience to the patient, is the skin surface biopsy technique employing quick-setting polymers (cyanoacrylates), popularly known as crazy glue. A number of inexpensive brands are available. Place a small drop of the polymer directly on the skin and press down a glass slide so that the glue spreads into a thin film approximately 1 cm in diameter. The film hardens in 30–60 s, and then the glass can gently be peeled off the skin. Attached to the slide are a sheet of the outermost stratum corneum layers, many vellus hairs, and the follicular filaments from sebaceous follicles. Apply a drop of immersion oil onto the stratum corneum sheet, then use a cover glass, press down

gently to spread the oil, and view under a microscope. If mites are present they cling to the tops of vellus hairs and follicular filaments. Their movements, particularly of their short stubby legs on each side of the body, help to identify them. Again it is only when the mites are numerous that any pathogenic role can be considered. The polymers should not be used on eyelids or too close to the eyes. Squeezing out follicular filaments between fingers or with comedo extractors, or taking scrapings of pustules and papulopustules is another, though not an elegant, way to locate *Demodex folliculorum* mites; the yields are low. A biopsy is rarely indicated. However, when mites are abundant in cyanoacrylate specimens, a histologic diagnosis of demodectic folliculitis can be made. Accidental findings of mites in histologic specimens obtained for other reasons (excision of nevi, basal cell carcinomas, actinic keratoses, etc.) is well known to dermatopathologists.

Treatment

Mites call for eradication only when there is a clear relationship to infestation and disease.

Topical. A variety of antiparasitic compounds can be used, including benzoyl benzoate, lindane (γ-hexachlorocyclohexane), malathion, allethrin, crotamiton, and topical metronidazole. Most of these are registered for the treatment of scabies, and can be used in exactly the same way. The recently introduced pyrethrin formulation Elimite does not seem to work. We prefer applications to the entire face on two consecutive days, with a second treatment 1 week later. Metronidazole is used topically for the treatment of rosacea. A 0.75% gel (MetroGel) is commercially available in the USA. Proprietary formulations contain 1.0%–2.0% metronidazole in a cream base. We have seen good results in some patients, though formal proof of its success is lacking.

Systemic. Only metronidazole, as in the treatment of trichomoniasis, may be effective. There is no formal study available attesting its efficacy.

Aylesworth R, Vance JC (1982) Demodex folliculorum and Demodex brevis in cutaneous biopsies. J Am Acad Dermatol 7:583–589

Ayres SI, Ayres SIII (1961) Demodectic eruptions (demodicidosis) in the human. 30 years' experience with 2 commonly unrecognized entities: Pityriasis folliculorum (demodex) and acne rosacea (demodex type). Arch Dermatol 83:816–827

Bardach HG, Raff M, Poitschek C (1981) Nosologische Stellung der Demodicidosis beim Menschen. Hautarzt 32:512–518

Desch C, Nutting WB (1972) Demodex folliculorum (Simon) and D. brevis akbulatova of man: redescription and reevaluation. J Parasitol 58:169–177

Grosshans EM, Kremer M, Maleville J (1974) Demodex folliculorum und die Histogenese der granulomatösen Rosacea. Hautarzt 25:166–177

Landthaler M, Kleber R, Hohenleutner U (1988) Zum Krankheitsbild der Demodex-Follikulitis (Demodikose). Aktuel Dermatol 14:344–346

Lindmaier A, Jurecka W, Lindemayr H (1987) Demodicidosis mimicking granulomatous rosacea and transient acantholytic dermatosis (Grover's disease). Dermatologica 175:200–204

Mumcuoglu Y, Rufli T (1983) Dermatologische Entomologie. Humanmedizinisch bedeutende Milben und Insekten in Mitteleuropa. Beiträge zur Dermatologie 9. Perimed, Erlangen

Pajarre R, Peura R (1977) Scanning electron microscopy of Demodex brevis (folliculorum). Acta Derm Venereol (Stockh) 57:529–531

Purcell SM, Hayes TJ, Dixon SL (1986) Pustular folliculitis associated with Demodex folliculorum. J Am Acad Dermatol 15:1159–1162

Wätzig V, Zollmann C (1987) Demodikose – eine rosazeaartige Dermatose. Dermatol Monatsschr 173:158–162

Demodex and the Skin

Demodex folliculorum mites are commonly seen in elderly subjects. They dislike the acne-age.

Above

Left   Demodicosis is a disease sui generis. It mimics rosacea, is often unilateral as in this man, and does not respond to standard rosacea regimens. Proof of the disease rests on the demonstration of the mites in large quantities

Right   Several mites crowd this acroinfundibulum. Characteristic are spongiosis and perifollicular lymphohistiocytic infiltrate (*top*). With the cyanoacrylate skin surface biopsy a family of *Demodex folliculorum* mites together with debris of the follicular filament can be lifted up. The mites are always in a head-down portion. Unstained specimen, covered with immersion oil

Below

Left   Cyanoacrylate specimen from the cheek. One follicle is filled with approximately ten hairs (trichostasis spinulosa), the other one contains three *Demodex folliculorum* mites

Right   The mites feed on sebaceous lipids. Some mites are found deep in the glands; one is in the sebaceous duct, head down

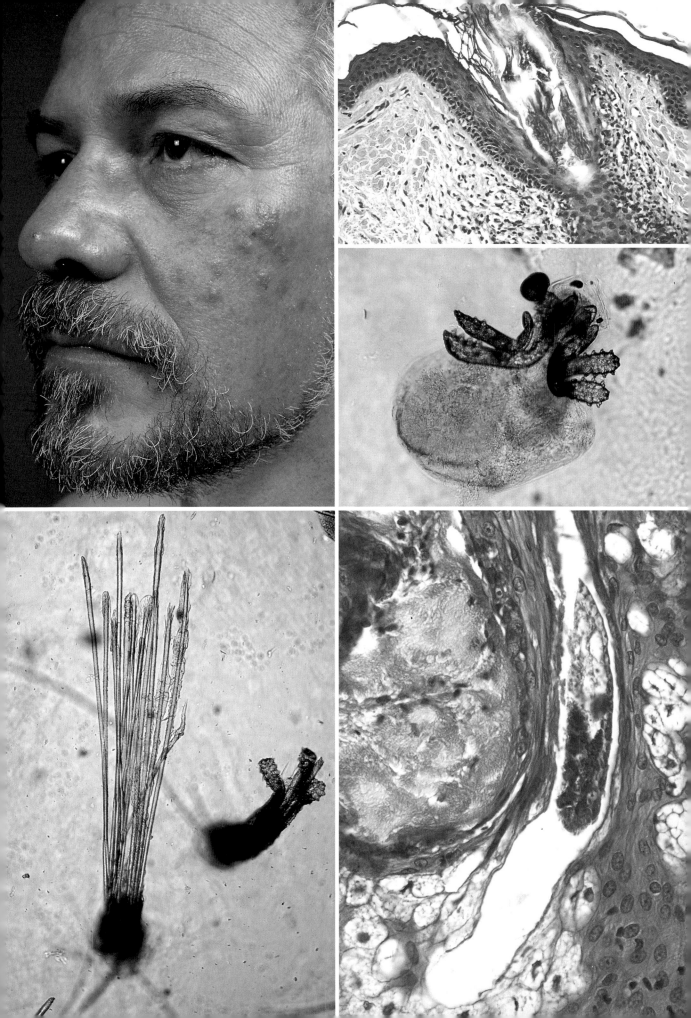

Gram-Negative Folliculitis

Gram-negative folliculitis was first reported in 1968 in a group of patients with longstanding therapy-resistant acne vulgaris. Since then the entity has been carefully studied, its clinical variants have been described in detail, and happily, effective therapy can now be offered. Rosacea patients, too, can suffer from this complication, and there is a poorly described scalp-folliculitis in another group of patients. The diagnosis is frequently missed and usually greatly delayed. Yet it can be suspected on purely clinical grounds. Proof comes from demonstration of gram-negative microorganisms on culture. The disease is actually more common than originally believed. There are reports of cohorts of 20–80 patients from different institutions.

A typical history of patients with gram-negative folliculitis reads as follows:

- Patients suffer from long-standing acne, rosacea, scalp folliculitis, or pyodermas (folliculitis).
- Oral or topical antibiotics, mostly tetracyclines, provide rapid improvement, followed by a swift recurrence once the drug is stopped.
- Readministration of the antibiotic is effective, but sooner or later it fails to provide adequate clearing of the pustules.
- Other antibiotics are prescribed, often in increasing doses. They are sometimes helpful at first, but are ineffective in the long run. Often sulfonamides are tried as well, than ampicillin, cephalosporins, macrolids (erythromycin, josamycin). All of them finally fail.

- Remission rates become shorter and shorter, a vicious cycle is evident. Exacerbation occurs days after the last antibiotic dose. In the worst case nothing helps any more.
- The clinical picture is quite typical. Most patients are men 18–30 years of age; few women have been reported so far.
- Oiliness, often an extremely slimy condition of the entire face, scalp, and neck is prominent and distressing.
- Numerous yellow fresh pustules, often on an erythematous base, are located in the central region of the face, on the upper and lower lips, chin, nasolabial folds, and cheeks. They seem to fan out from the nose and mouth. In other patients the skin between the pustules is diffusely inflamed.
- The pustules are short-lived, break open within 24–48 h, but new ones crop up over night.
- No comedo is clinically visible within the pustule, as is almost always the case in pustules of acne vulgaris.
- In some patients large inflammatory nodules and abscesses develop.
- Itching of the afflicted skin is typical.
- Gram-negative pustules also occur on the scalp, which is likewise very oily. Rarely pustules are also found on the chest (mostly in very hairy men).
- Histopathology reveals a typical folliculitis with granulocytes within the follicular canal and a granulocytic perfollicular abscess. There is no comedonal kernel.

Bacteriology reveals a wide range of gram-negative bacteria: *Escherichia coli, Enterobacter aerogenes, Klebsiella pneumoniae, Klebsiella oxytoca, Proteus mirabilis, Citrobacter freundii, Acinetobacter calcoaceticus, Serratia,* and *Salmonella panama.* Quantitative cultures before, during, and after appropriate therapy are recommended, not only from the pustules and the slimy facial skin surface but also from the anterior nares or even the throat. Between 10^4–10^6 colony forming units (CFUs) can be isolated before therapy from the facial skin surface, but none following adequate treatment.

Sometimes two or even three different gram-negative organisms, e.g., *Escherichia coli, Proteus mirabilis,* and *Klebsiella* may be recovered from one patient. Two types of gram-negative folliculitis are distinguished, types I and II. Type I is by far the most common with small juicy pustules around nose and mouth and is caused by one of the above-mentioned bacteria (not *Proteus mirabilis*). Type II is characterized by more deep-seated nodules and pustules, and is caused by a more virulent organism, *Proteus mirabilis.*

Problems often arise in establishing a correct microbiological diagnosis. Mostly technical problems account for this: inadequate sampling, dried out swabs, long delay between culturing the pustules and arrival of the specimen in the laboratory, etc. All this can be overcome with appropriate cooporation between dermatologists and microbiologists.

Pathogenesis is related to an ecological imbalance in the microbial flora of skin surface or mucous membranes. This usually originates from long-term antibiotics in the treatment of acne. The gram-positive resident organisms are suppressed, leaving a niche for gram-negatives to occupy the void. This is the typical background; however, gram-negative organisms may insinuate themselves into the microflora in the absence of oral antibiotics, especially in long-standing inflammatory acne.

One report describes multiple immunologic changes in a group of 41 patients, e.g., immunoglobulins M, G, A, and E, complement (total, C3, C4), α_1-antitrypsin, negative responses to recall antigens, lymphopenia, and low numbers of T cells. This is an interesting lead which deserves a serious follow-up.

How common is gram-negative folliculitis? This is hard to say since very few well controlled microbiological studies have been performed. In Philadelphia, the prevalence was estimated to be about 5% in acne patients. The German experience suggests 2%. Dermatology services in army medical centers now recognize the importance of this very troublesome and persistant disease.

Treatment

Antimicrobial therapy directed against gram-negative bacteria temporally produces improvement, but rarely a cure. The eradication of gram-negative organisms from the nasopharyngeal niches, where the organisms first take hold, is difficult. Inconsistent results have been obtained with intranasal applications of antibiotics highly effective against gram-negatives. Today the treatment of choice is isotretinoin. Since the first report in 1981 this has been confirmed in multiple centers. The drug is given orally as a single medicament. The dose is between 0.5 and 1.5 mg/kg body weight per day, usually for 20 weeks, with a range of 16–24 weeks. The overall results are rewarding. More than 90% of patients can be completely cleared.

Isotretinoin does not possess antibacterial properties, and therefore the elimina-

Mean counts of bacteria recovered from the foreheads of 12 patients with gram-negative folliculitis during (*above*) and after (*below*) treatment with isotretinoin. (From Neubert et al. 1986)

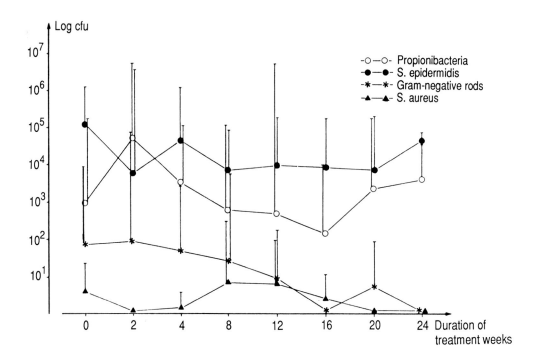

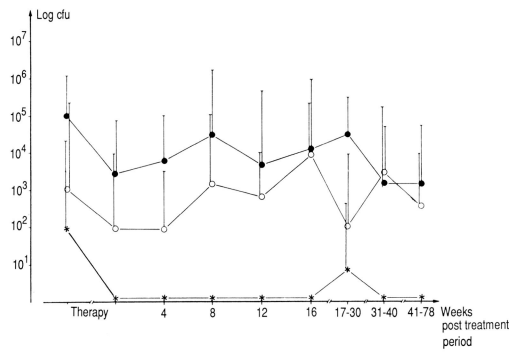

tion of gram-negative bacteria occurs in a different way. The mode of action is indirect. Gram-negative organisms are "wet germs" and normally require abundant moisture for survival. Isotretinoin dries out the skin, taking away this essential factor for the survival of these bacteria. This also happens in the mucous membranes but not to the same degree. Once the ecological niche has been established the normal skin and nasal flora will remain in balance.

Staphylococcus aureus colonization during isotretinoin treatment is more frequent than commonly appreciated. In our study, this organism was isolated from facial skin in 3 out of 12 patients before and in 10 of 12 patients during treatment, reaching its maximum density and incidence at weeks 8–12. In most patients *Staphylococcus aureus* disappears several weeks after cessation of the drug. The slight inflammatory reaction of the anterior nares and of the facial skin surface may exude enough serum to promote the implantation of *Staphylococcus aureus*. The routine application of antibiotic ointments to the anterior nares was recommended to reduce or inhibit colonization of *Staphylococcus aureus*, but it also failed and therefore is not encouraged any more.

Occasionally *Staphylococcus aureus* pyodermas develop in patients with acne, rosacea, or gram-negative folliculitis who are being treated with isotretinoin. Impetigo contagiosa or even deep abscesses (cellulitis) may also become a serious problem. If this occurs the retinoid must be withdrawn and appropriate systemic antibiotic treatment installed.

Blankenship ML (1984) Gram-negative folliculitis. Follow-up observations in 20 patients. Arch Dermatol 120:1301–1303

Fulton JE, McGinley K, Leyden J, Marples R (1968) Gram-negative folliculitis in acne vulgaris. Arch Dermatol 98:349–353

James WD, Leyden JJ (1985) Treatment of gram-negative folliculitis with isotretinoin: positive clinical and microbiologic response. J Am Acad Dermatol 12:319–324

Leyden JJ, McGinley KJ, Mills OH (1979) Pseudomonas aeruginosa. Gram-negative folliculitis. Arch Dermatol 115:1203–1204

Neubert U (1983) Immunabweichungen bei sogenannter gramnegativer Folliculitis. Hautarzt 34 (Suppl 6):277–278

Neubert U, Plewig G, Ruhfus A (1986) Treatment of gram-negative folliculitis with isotretinoin. Arch Dermatol Res 278:307–313

Plewig G, Braun-Falco O (1974) Gramnegative Folliculitis. Hautarzt 25:541–546

Plewig G, Nikolowski J, Wolff HH (1982) Action of isotretinoin in acne rosacea and gram-negative folliculitis. J Am Acad Dermatol 6:766–785

Simjee S, Sahm DF, Soltani K, Morello JA (1986) Organisms associated with gram-negative folliculitis: in vitro growth in the presence of isotretinoin. Arch Dermatol Res 278:314–316

Weissmann A, Wagner A, Plewig G (1981) Reduction of bacterial skin flora during oral treatment of severe acne with 13-*cis*-retinoic acid. Arch Dermatol Res 270:179–183

Gram-Negative Folliculitis

Though often mistaken for ordinary acne vulgaris, gram-negative folliculitis is a disease in which a variety of gram-negative organisms incite a folliculitis of sebaceous follicles. Extreme oiliness and male predominance are typical. The pyoderma is mostly confined to the face, but aberrant spread to scalp and chest occurs at times, affecting terminal hair follicles in the latter two locations.

Above

Left   Type I gram-negative folliculitis is caused by *Pseudomonas aeruginosa* (*pyocyaneus*) with deep-seated, broad, succulent, highly inflamed, and painful nodules, sometimes topped by pustules

Right   The much more common type II gram-negative folliculitis is caused by a variety of gram-negatives. Often two or three different species can be recovered. Face and neck are afflicted

Below   A typical example of type I gram-negative folliculitis with pustules fanning out around nose and mouth

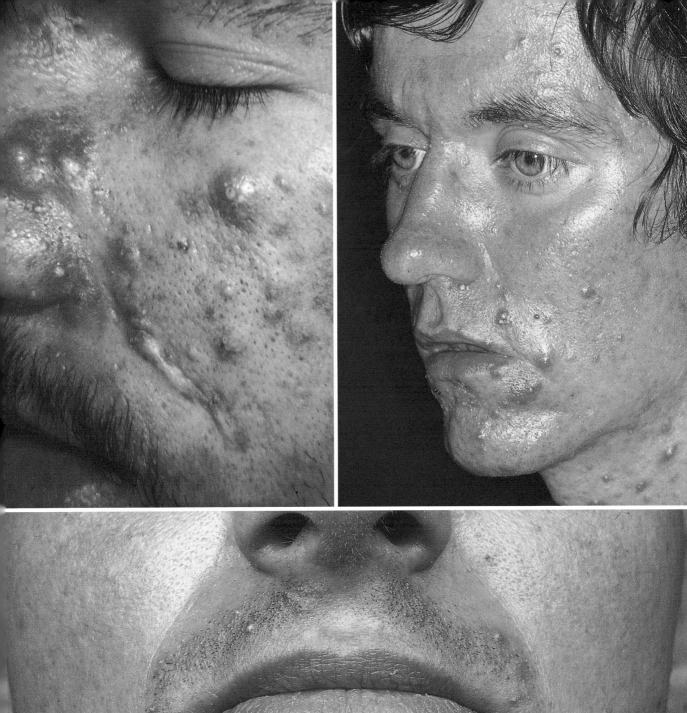
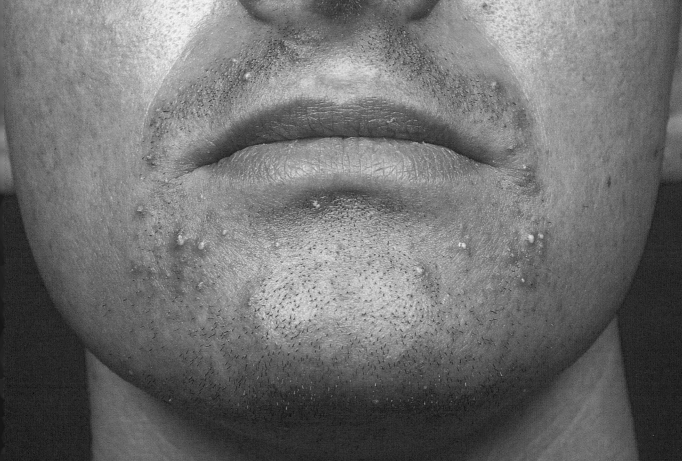

Gram-Negative Folliculitis

This disease often poses diagnostic problems. It is a great mimic. It is the fate of these patients to rotate through doctors offices till one is found who makes the correct diagnosis.

Above

Left   A male patient + seborrhea + pustules and papules particularly around the nose and mouth + no comedones + unresponsiveness to standard acne management = gram-negative folliculitis. The causative gram-negative organisms were cultured from pustules and the anterior nares

Right   Oral tretinoin has cleared all the lesions. The formerly extremly oily skin is dry; all pustules and papules have been eliminated. It is the best drug for this disease

Below   Gram-negative folliculitis rarely occurs off the face and would not be correctly diagnosed exept for the typical presentations on the face. The latter is always affected. In this 55-year-old man the extrafacial locations were the hairy chest and itchy pustules on the scalp

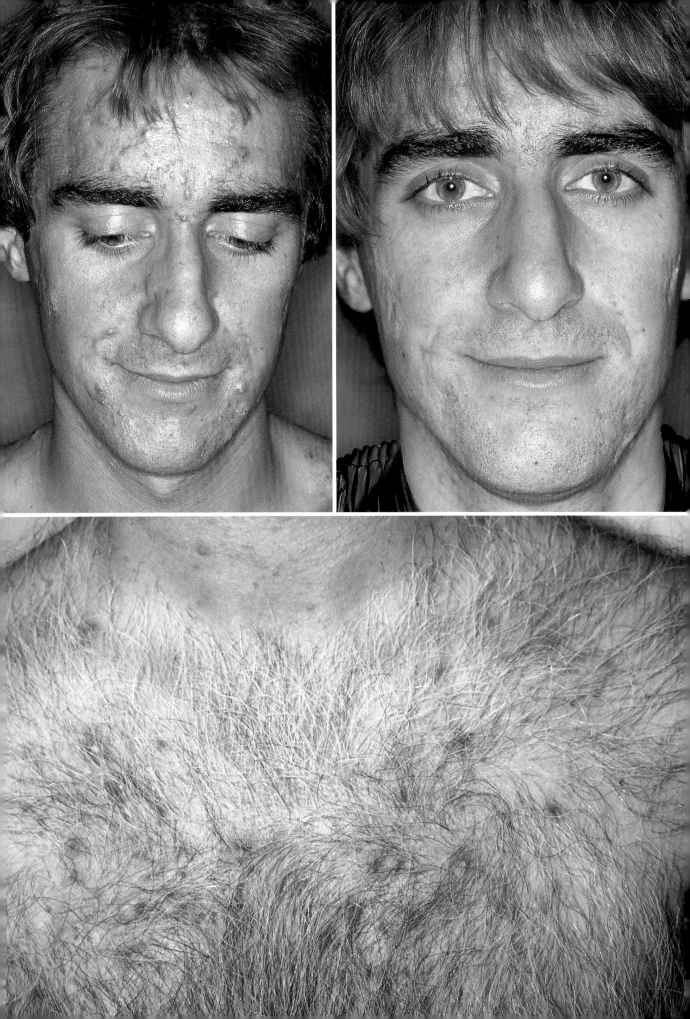

Pyodermas Mimicking Acne

Because acne vulgaris is so common, many lookalikes are misdiagnosed as acne.

Above　Scattered follicular papulopustules on the face, chest, and back suggest acne in this patient. However, there were no comedones and the lesions were only a few months old. Coagulase-positive staphylococci were isolated repeatedly (follicular impetigo). He responded quickly and permanently to oral antibiotics

Below　This young woman thought that the mild acne which she had had since adolescence had now turned vicious, with recurrent bouts of tender hot nodules. In fact the lesions were typical suppurating furuncles (boils) from which *Staphylococcus aureus* was recovered. A short course of full-dose oral antibiotics should be followed by maintenance therapy for those all too frequent patients who have recurrences. She had other signs of acne like comedones, papules, and scars

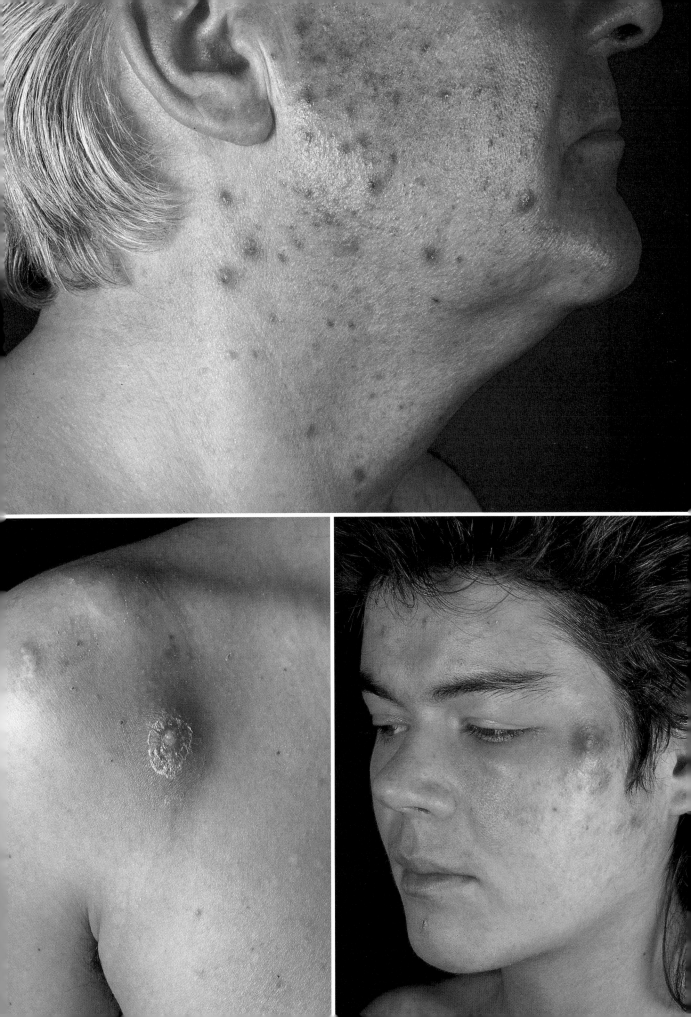

Staphylococcal Impetigo Presenting in an Acneiform Pattern

The referral diagnosis in this young man was acne. Some years ago he did go through some mild facial acne.

Above   The distribution pattern is acne-like in a V-shaped area of the chest

Below   Follicle-bound papules and pustules were seen on close-up examination. The eruption was itchy. *Staphylococcus aureus* could be isolated. The pyoderma was quickly wiped out with oral antibiotics

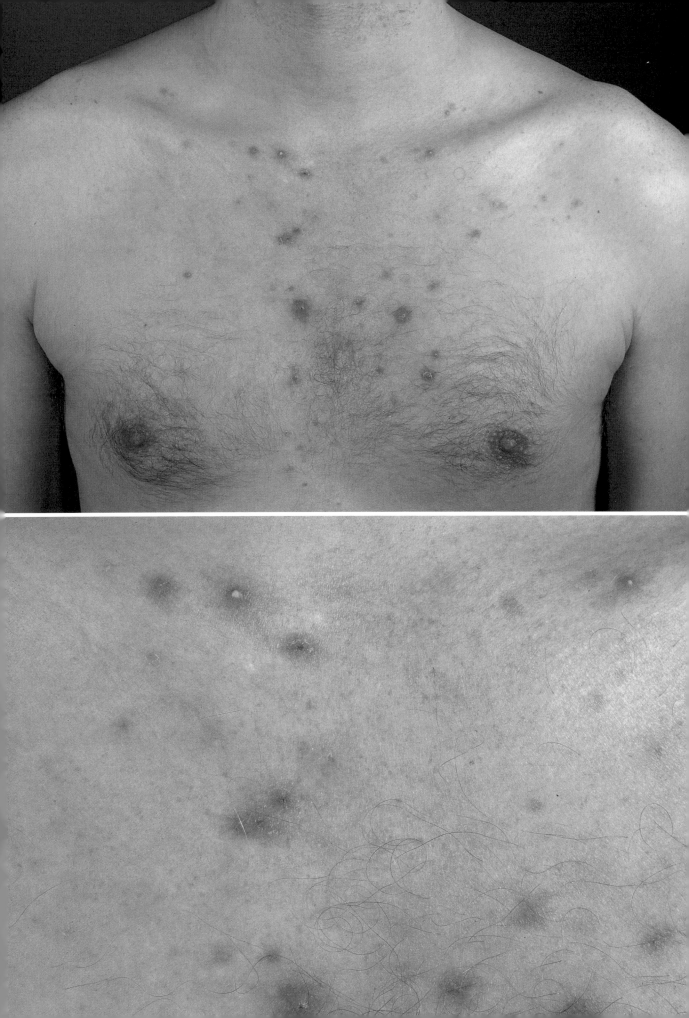

Acne Necrotica (Necrotizing Lymphocytic Folliculitis)

Historical Background

Acne necrotica is a mysterious disorder, unknown to many dermatologists, and usually unmentioned in recent texts. We acknowledge its existence despite its rarity. It has been called acne frontalis, acne varioliformis, acne pilaris, and acne necrotica. We suggest the term necrotizing lymphocytic folliculitis as used by others. Acne necrotica is actually a misnomer. The condition is not a variant of acne and bears only a superficial resemblance to an acneiform eruption.

Etiology

Ignorance prevails. Infection is routinely mentioned, but proof of bacterial, fungal, or viral invasion is lacking. Drugs, foodstuff, and allergies do not seem to play a role. Mechanical factors such as rubbing and scratching only aggravate the condition and are not the cause.

Clinical Features

The patients are mostly women past the acne age, from early until late adulthood. The main location is the face, with a peculiar distribution along the hairline, but also the scalp, the nape of the neck, rarely on the nose, cheeks, or extrafacial regions like the chest and back. Most notable is the chronicity, waxing and waning for many decades. Minor expressions are hardly recognized as such. Severer outbreaks cause considerable diagnostic problems. Descriptions in the older literature designate the scalp as the area of predilection. We recognize that follicular pustules on the scalp may be the sole expression.

The initial lesion is an umbilicated follicular papule, often very juicy, turning soon into a pustule, leaving hemorrhagic crusts and finally varioliform scars. The resemblance to smallpox or chickenpox explains its old name, acne varioliformis. Sometimes hundreds of lesions coexist with considerable inflammatory erythema in between. Small crusts develop within days leaving depressed scars.

Histopathology

Early lesions are characterized by perifollicular lymphocyte infiltrates, accompanied by lymphocytic spongiosis of the follicular epithelium. Soon necrosis of the follicular epithelium occurs, engulfing the infrainfundibulum, sebaceous ducts, and sebaceous glands. Foreign body granulomas may be seen. Necrosis of the epidermis may also occur. Hemorrhage is a prominent component, as is widespread necrosis of the corium. Neutrophils are usually lacking or come at a later stage. Fibrosis is evident finally.

Differential Diagnosis

Awareness of this bizarre disease is a prerequisite for an accurate diagnosis.

Gram-negative folliculitis may be considered but has distinctive features. So-called acnitis (lupus miliaris disseminatus faciei) is an altogether different process and its listing in the differential diagnosis is an act of desperation. Eosinophilic pustular folliculitis of Ofuji, eczema herpeticatum of the scalp and hairline, and pustular erosive dermatosis of the scalp might be at least tentatively considered.

Treatment

Treatment is unrewarding. Topical benzoyl peroxide, tretinoin, disinfectants and antibiotics are ineffective. Topical corticosteroids are inconsistently helpful. Oral tetracyclines and erythromycin are marginally beneficial. Systemic corticosteroids cool down the inflammation but are not curative. Isotretinoin has been tried in individual patients with varying results.

Baum J (1910) Ein Fall von sogenannter Acne urticata (Urticaria necroticans). In: Neisser A, Jacobi E (eds) Ikonographia Dermatologica. Atlas seltener, neuer und diagnostisch unklarer Hautkrankheiten. Urban and Schwarzenberg, Berlin, pp 5–8

Cunliffe WJ (1989) Acne. Martin Dunitz, London, pp 64–65

Gans O, Steigleder GK (1955) Histologie der Hautkrankheiten. Die Gewebsveränderungen in der kranken Haut unter Berücksichtigung ihrer Entstehung und ihres Ablaufs. Springer, Berlin Heidelberg New York, pp 376–378

Jacyk WK (1988) Pustular ulcerative dermatosis of the scalp. Br J Dermatol 118:441–444

Kossard S, Collins A, McCrossin I (1987) Necrotizing lymphocytic folliculitis: the early lesion of acne necrotica (varioliformis). J Am Acad Dermatol 16:1007–1014

Milde P, Goert G, Plewig G (1992) Acne necrotica. Hautarzt 43 (in press)

Pye RJ, Peachey RDG, Burton JL (1979) Erosive pustular dermatosis of the scalp. Br J Dermatol 100:559–566

Rook A, Dawber R (1982) Diseases of the hair and scalp. Blackwell, Oxford, pp 475–477

Acne Necrotica

Despite its name, this disorder has nothing to do with acne. It is also called necrotizing lymphocytic folliculitis. There is much uncertainty among dermatologists regarding nosology and therapy. Misdiagnosis is almost the rule.

Above

Left   Late stage of the disease with crusted and excoriated papules on the forehead and cheeks and along the hairline. The hairy scalp was spared

Right   Typical distribution pattern along the hairline, neck, and nape, with widespread involvement of the hairy scalp

Below   Close-up of the right and left side of the neck. Fresh, partly umbilicated papulopustules, many on an inflammatory background, resemble viral infections or drug eruptions. The disease perpetuated for several months. Scarring on the cheeks is a result of previous acne, a confounding factor

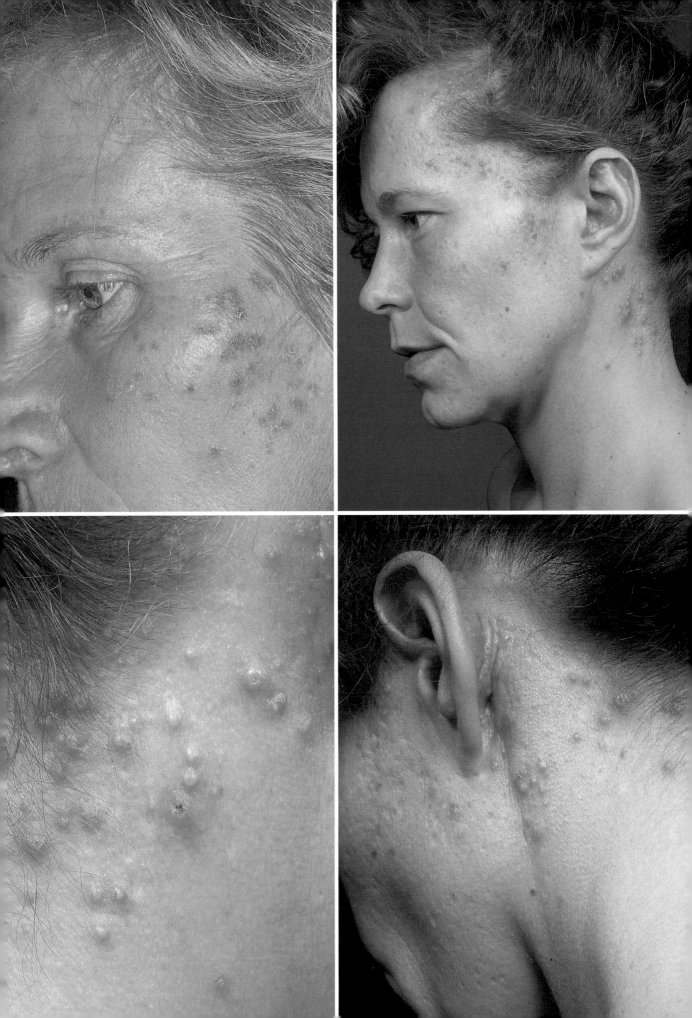

Acne Necrotica

The clinical features were shown on the previous plate; here the histopathology from this patient is presented.

Above   A wedge-shaped central necrosis, totally obscuring the original follicle prevails. A parakeratotic cap sits on top of a fibrinoid necrosis. The lymphocytic infiltrate is dense, stretching out bilaterally to cause prominent spongiosis of epidermis and neighboring follicles. Only resident flora can be cultured from such lesions

Below   Step sections through the block reveal another follicle afflicted in the same way. Here the remnants of the epithelium can be seen on the upper right side. Notably absent are comedones, *Demodex folliculorum*, viral particles (culture and electron microscopy), and leukocytoclasia

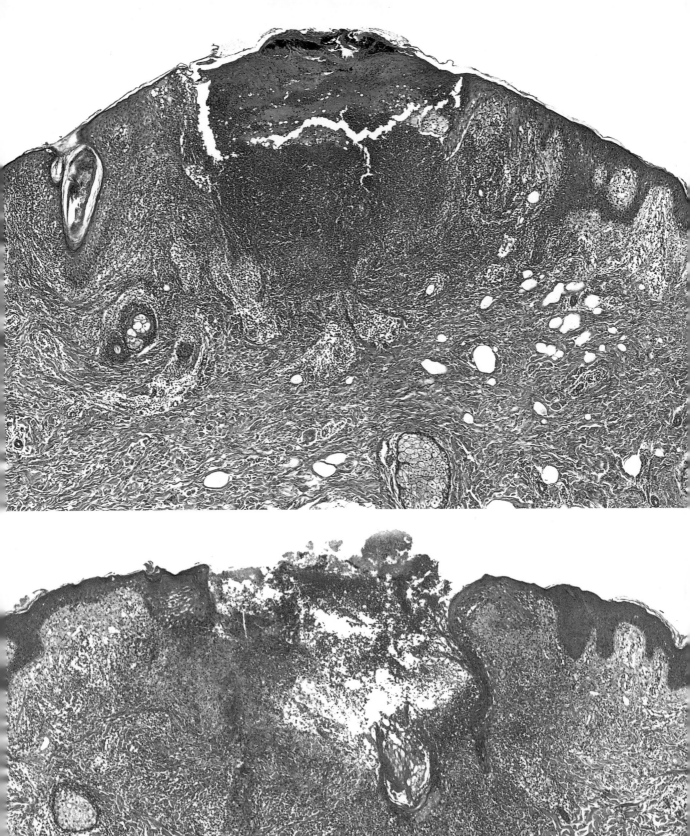

Sebaceous Gland Hyperplasia

The acini of sebaceous follicles sometimes become so large as to result in prominent papules. This is not due to androgen stimulation since this is not a phenomenon of puberty or early adulthood. Instead, these growths are found mainly on the photodamaged faces of the elderly. The novice easily confuses hyperplastic sebaceous glands with large, closed comedones.

Circumscribed Sebaceous Gland Hyperplasia

This is a common facial condition, usually found in elderly men, but also in women. Sometimes it occurs in adults, but only if the skin shows actinic damage. The old term senile sebaceous gland hyperplasia is disrespectful and should be avoided. Single or multiple lesions, as many as 100, are mainly located on the forehead, less often on the cheeks and nose. They are dome-shaped, slightly raised papules of yellowish hue, 2–4 mm in size. The surface may be lobulated. Often a central umbilical depression is present, sometimes with a comedo-like kernel. Curiously, visible sebum droplets are not discharged. Small telangiectasias may shine through the lesions.

The histopathology is characteristic. Large sebaceous acini drain into a common dilated follicular infundibulum. Compacted corneocytes form a comedo-like kernel, but do not attain the size of a genuine comedo. The spacious apical portion of the follicular infundibulum corresponds to the umbilical depression seen clinically. These lesions are not at all static as commonly supposed. Some growths regress completely with new ones springing up in the vicinity. Sebaceous glands have a known propensity to undergo remodelling. They have no malignant potential.

Differential diagnosis centers around closed comedones in older acne or rosacea patients. An early basal cell carcinoma may pose a problem. Sebaceous adenomas are clinically and histologically different.

Diffuse Sebaceous Gland Hyperplasia

This is a completely different picture which occurs mainly in young adults of either sex. This may run in families. Plaque-like or diffuse thickening of the face with wide open pores gives the surface an orange-peel appearance. Sometimes the neck, upper chest, and upper back may be involved. On the neck and trunk the huge sebaceous glands are often arranged in a bead-like pattern, mimicking erythrosis interfollicularis colli. A marked seborrhea is present. These patients look extremely oily, in contrast to those with the circumscribed variant. Surprisingly, these diffuse hyperplasias are not associated with any of the typical lesions of acne: comedones and inflammatory lesions are lacking.

The etiology of these enormous and widespread hyperplasias is unknown. Histopathologically, the individual lesions resemble those of circumscribed sebaceous gland hyperplasia. Huge sebaceous lobules drain into a common follicular canal.

Sebaceous Gland Hyperplasia in Rosacea and Rhinophyma

A diffuse thickening of facial skin, particularly of the nose, forehead, and cheeks, is associated with rosacea. This is typical of advanced rhinophyma. The patients have a leonine appearance, with coarse features and deep facial furrows. Prominent dilated facial pores are typical. The overall appearance suggests facial myxedema. Seborrhea, even in advanced age, is usually present. The worst cases occur in men. Histologically, one finds diffuse sebaceous gland hyperplasias, always accompanied by fibroplasia, telangiectasias, dilated lymph vessels, and lymphocytic infiltrates.

Odd Variants of Sebaceous Gland Hyperplasia

Giant Sebaceous Gland Hyperplasia. Instead of small papules, nodules up to 5 mm in size develop on the forehead and cheeks. One does not dare to make this diagnosis clinically, but rather has to suspect solitary tumors like basal cell carcinomas, metastatic cancers, and various adnexal tumors. Histopathology reveals confluent large sebaceous acini. The tumors are benign. Excision is indicated for cosmetic purposes.

Though not relevant for the differential diagnoses of acne, two rare sebaceous gland malformations occuring outside the acne-prone areas of the body are listed here. Both conditions often cause diagnostic problems.

Areolar Sebaceous Gland Hyperplasia. Confluent thickening of the areola mammae of both breasts. Histologically only sebaceous gland hyperplasia is found.

Fordyce Granules or Fordyce Spots. Circumscribed sebaceous hyperplasias of the vermilion border of the lip or oral mucosa, sometimes also on the genital mucous membranes, are not uncommon. The yellowish or whitish lesions are 1–3 mm in diameter, often aggregated into plaques, and completely asymptomatic. The sebaceous glands are not associated with a hair follicle. Otherwise they resemble circumscribed sebaceous gland hyperplasias. Fordyce spots contain lipids similar to those found in sebaceous glands of the skin.

Treatment

Large circumscribed sebaceous gland hyperplasias may be excised, preferentially with a small punch. They may also be ablated by laser or even by light electrocoagulation, followed by extrusion with pressure.

The only satisfactory ideal treatment for all other sebaceous gland hyperplasias is isotretinoin. This drug causes drastic shrinkage of the sebaceous glands, greatly improving appearance. Low doses of 0.05–0.2 mg/kg body weight daily for a few months are sufficient. Higher doses of 0.5–1.0 mg/kg shorten the treatment, often to 8 weeks. It should be made clear that recurrences are common after stopping treatment, hence one is obliged to find a maintenance dose. This may be as low as 2.5 mg daily or 10–20 mg once weekly. For women of childbearing age warnings concerning teratogenicity apply.

Burton CS, Sawchuk WS (1985) Premature sebaceous gland hyperplasia: successful treatment with isotretinoin. J Am Acad Dermatol 12:182–184

Czarnecki DB, Dorevitch AP (1986) Giant senile sebaceous hyperplasia. Arch Dermatol 122:1101

De Villez RL, Roberts LC (1982) Premature sebaceous gland hyperplasia. J Am Acad Dermatol 6:933–935

Dupré A, Bonafe JL, Lamon P (1983) Functional familial sebaceous hyperplasia of the face and premature sebaceous gland hyperplasia: a new and unique entity? J Am Acad Dermatol 9:768–769

Kaufmann R, Vranes M, Landes E (1987) Diffuse (präsenile) Talgdrüsenhyperplasie, eine neue Entität? Erfolgreiche Behandlung mit 13-cis-Retinsäure. Hautarzt 38:31–35

Keining E, Braun-Falco O (1953) Diffuse Talgdrüsenhyperplasie der Gesichtshaut in Analogie zum Bild des Rhinophyms. Dermatol Wochenschr 127:463–471

Luderschmidt C, Plewig G (1978) Circumscribed sebaceous gland hyperplasia: autoradiographic and histoplanimetric studies. J Invest Dermatol 70:207–209

Trichostasis Spinulosa

This is a skin change occurring mostly in elderly subjects that superficially shows some resemblance to open comedones. The black follicular plugs, especially common on the nose and cheeks, remind one automatically of blackheads. The pore of almost every sebaceous follicle is distended by a slightly pigmented, yellowish-brown to black elevated plug. No inflammation stems from these lesions. The matter is firmly rooted and cannot be easily delivered by pressure. The lesions always remain small and do not attain the size of true open comedones. Most of the patients are older, far beyond the acne age, though trichostasis spinulosa can occur after puberty and in early adulthood when acne vulgaris is still active. Therefore, this is an important differential diagnosis.

Histopathology

Vertical, or much better horizontal sections demonstrate the material that accounts for the plugs. Infundibula of sebaceous follicles are symmetrically round and distended with increased layers of loose corneocytes. The characteristic finding is a phenomenal aggregation of tiny vellus hairs, between a few and up to 50 or even 100. They are neatly arranged like a bouquet of flowers.

The hairs are easily lifted by a cyanoacrylate skin surface biopsy. A drop of magic glue is placed on a glass slide, which is gently pressed to the ala nasi or cheeks, waiting 60 s for complete polymerization. Peeling the hardened glue off the skin yields a sheet of follicular filaments. Cover with immersion oil and view through the microscope with low power. Fascicles of parallel hairs, all in the telogen phase and of the same size and quality, are visible. All hairs come from one and the same pilary unit.

In an acne comedo the hairs are less numerous, trapped in a solid mass, and coiled up in odd patterns.

Treatment

Topically applied tretinoin as in comedonal acne is quite helpful. Trichostasis spinulosa on the nose responds less well to this drug. Mechanical expulsion by comedo extractors or cyanoacrylate may then be indicated. A commercial kit for facial treatment with the powerful glue is available (Exolift, Cosmex Ltd., Great Neck, NY 11021, USA).

Braun-Falco O, Vakilzadeh F (1967) Trichostasis spinulosa. Hautarzt 18:501–504

Ladany E (1954) Trichostasis spinulosa. J Invest Dermatol 23:33–41

Goldschmidt H, Hojyo-Tomoka MT, Kligman AM (1975) Trichostasis spinulosa. Eine häufige follikuläre Altersveränderung der Gesichtshaut. Hautarzt 26:299–303

Mills OH, Kligman AM (1973) Topically applied tretinoin in the treatment of trichostasis spinulosa. Arch Dermatol 108:378–380

Trichostasis Spinulosa

Above   Looking at these black follicular plugs, which are especially common on the nose, one automatically thinks of blackheads. But the resemblance to open comedones is quite superficial. Viewing with a handlens reveals multiple hair tips. Here, the pore of every sebaceous follicle is thickened by a pigmented, slightly elevated plug, which is firmly anchored and cannot be expressed with the fingers. These hair bundles never become inflamed

Below

Left   Horizontal section of facial skin showing trichostasis spinulosa clinically. The follicles are hyperkeratotic, but the revealing finding is a phenomenal aggregation of tiny vellus hairs, in this case about 50 and 20, respectively. The hairs are trapped in a horny capsule

Right   An oil immersion mount of a plug removed by the cyanoacrylate technique shows a fascicle of parallel hairs, all of the same size. In a comedo, the hairs are less numerous, and being trapped in a solid mass are coiled up in odd patterns

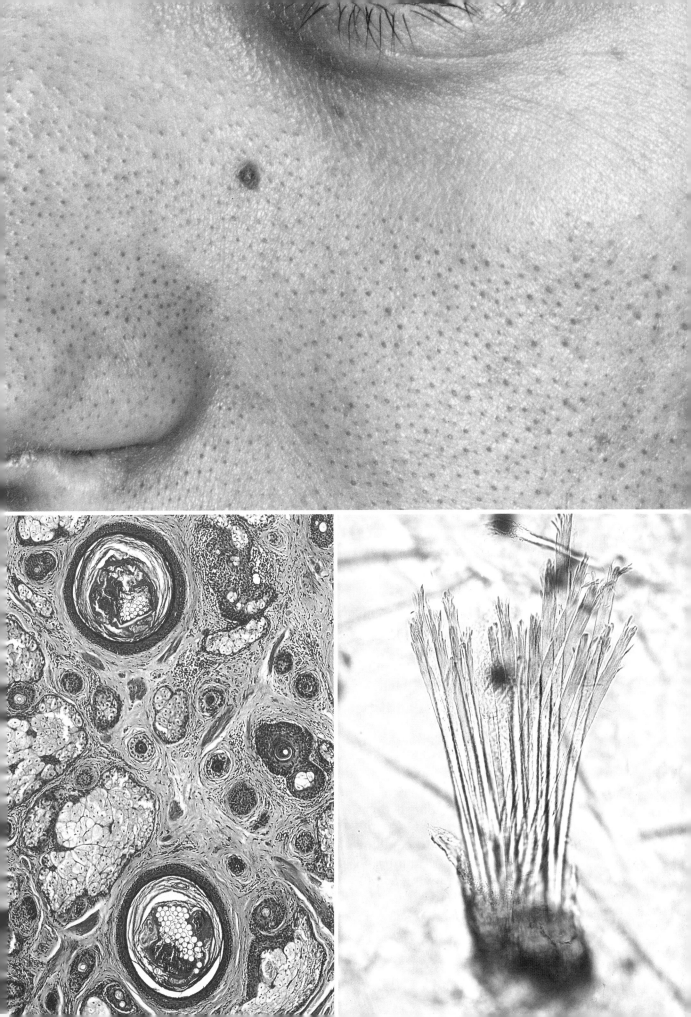

Steatocystoma Multiplex

These small tumors deserve mention because they may be mistaken for closed comedones or, when inflamed, for acne conglobata. They are neither a member of the acne family, nor an acneiform eruption.

Genetics

Pedigree analysis of many families indicates an autosomal dominant inheritance. Usually these androgen-dependent cystic tumors do not become clinically evident before puberty.

Clinical Findings

Sites of predilection are the V-shaped areas of chest and back, the axillae, and less often the face. The distribution is usually symmetrical. Cysts develop at puberty, although rudimentary elements are present earlier, awaiting hormonal stimulation. The cysts are mostly 3–10 mm in diameter, increasing slowly in size. They are rather uniformly spread over the chest and back. The individual lesions are small, raised, dome-shaped nodules. The smaller ones are detectable only after the skin is stretched. The color is that of the skin, at times with a slight bluish tinge. On palpation one feels firm, fixed structures in the dermis. There is no pain and usually no inflammation. The number of cysts varies considerably, ranging from a few to many hundred. Rarely one encounters large disfiguring lesions of steatocystoma multiplex on the trunk and in the face.

Steatocystoma Multiplex Suppurativum

This inflammatory variant is usually misdiagnosed as acne conglobata. Cysts rupture, become inflamed, and develop tunneled scars as in acne conglobata or acne inversa, particularly in the armpits.

Steatocystoma Simplex

A nonheritable form of steatocystoma was described by Brownstein, who termed it solitary steatocystoma. The solitary cysts are identical with those of the multiple form.

Histopathology

Steatocystoma is a cyst whose thin wall has the characteristics of the keratinocytes which line the sebaceous ducts with absence of keratohyalin granules. Sebaceous lobules of varying size are always found, sometimes only clusters of individual sebocytes. The wall of the cyst is wavy and crenulated. Invaginations and outpouchings are artifacts of histologic processing when the contents of the cyst are lost. These irregularities are not seen in frozen sections. Step sections through an entire cyst always reveal an epithelial cord or duct which connects the cyst with the overlying epidermis. It is the abortive remnant of the infundibulum of the normal sebaceous follicle. One vellus hair follicle is associated with each cyst. Often dozens of hairs lie freely within the cystic cavity. Bacteria are notably absent. The contents are sterile. Biochemical analysis shows high concentrations of triglycerides, but very little free fatty acids. In comedones, the latter are products of lipases, produced by *Propionibacterium acnes*. The absence of fatty acids may explain the lack of inflammation. Injection of living *Propionibacterium acnes* into the cyst induces rupture and the development of an inflamed nodule resembling acne conglobata. In steatocystoma multiplex suppurativum mechanical factors rather than bacterial colonization are blamed for the inflammatory development.

Differential Diagnosis

The most important differential diagnoses, which can be settled only by histopathology, are eruptive hydrocystomas and vellus hair cysts. Usually these are smaller. Other considerations are eccrine tumors, osteoma cutis, acne with unusual location of closed comedones, closed comedo-like scars, and acne inversa.

Treatment

This is usually not necessary, as the lesions are mainly a cosmetic nuisance. Anecdotal reports mention beneficial results of orally given isotretinoin, but any benefit can only be temporary. Surgical excision of large unsightly lesions is sometimes indicated.

Berendes U (1972) Zur Genetik multipler Hauttumoren. I. Multiple Lipome und Steatocystoma multiplex. Arch Dermatol Forsch 242:361–371

Brownstein MH (1982) Steatocystoma simplex. A solitary steatocystoma. Arch Dermatol 118:409–411

Gollhausen R, Besenhard HM, Ruzicka T (1988) Steatocystoma multiplex conglobatum. Hautarzt 39:177–179

Holmes R, Black MM (1980) Steatocystoma multiplex with unusually prominent cysts on the face. Br J Dermatol 102:711–713

Jamieson WA (1873) Case of numerous cutaneous cysts scattered over the body. Edinburgh Med J 19:223–225

Krähenbühl A, Eichmann A, Pfaltz M (1991) CO_2 laser therapy for steatocystoma multiplex. Dermatologica 183:294–296

Magid ML, Wentzell JM, Roenigk HH (1990) Multiple cystic lesions. Steatocystoma multiplex. Arch Dermatol 126:101–104

Moritz DL, Silverman RA (1988) Steatocystoma multiplex treated with isotretinoin: a delayed response. Cutis 42:437–439

Nishimura M, Kohda H, Urabe A (1986) Steatocystoma multiplex. A facial papular variant. Arch Dermatol 122:205–207

Plewig G, Wolff HH, Braun-Falco O (1982) Steatocystoma multiplex: anatomic reevaluation, electron microscopy, and autoradiography. Arch Dermatol Res 272:363–380

Rosen BL, Brodkin RH (1986) Isotretinoin in the treatment of steatocystoma multiplex: a possible adverse reaction. Cutis 37:115–120

Statham BN, Cunliffe WJ (1984) The treatment of steatocystoma multiplex suppurativum with isotretinoin. Br J Dermatol 111:246

Steatocystoma Multiplex

Usually the inconspicuous, small, skin-colored cysts pose no diagnostic problems; if located in the face they do, however.

Above

Left   The armpit is a choice location to look for steatocystoma multiplex. Sometimes the cysts become inflamed and may even mimic acne conglobata, a condition called steatocystoma multiplex conglobatum

Right   The chest over the sternum is another typical location. The cysts are best seen when the skin is folded or streched between two fingers. The close up of a single cyst features the characteristic bluish tinge. There is no pore, and pressure does not release any contents. The cysts are tightly sealed, the contents sterile

Below   The cyst has collapsed, as the contents (cellular debris, sebum, hairs) have fallen out during histologic preparation. The cyst wall is crenulated, and contains many sebaceous acini. In the center a small portion of the solid epithelial cord (→) connecting the cyst with the overlying epidermis is seen

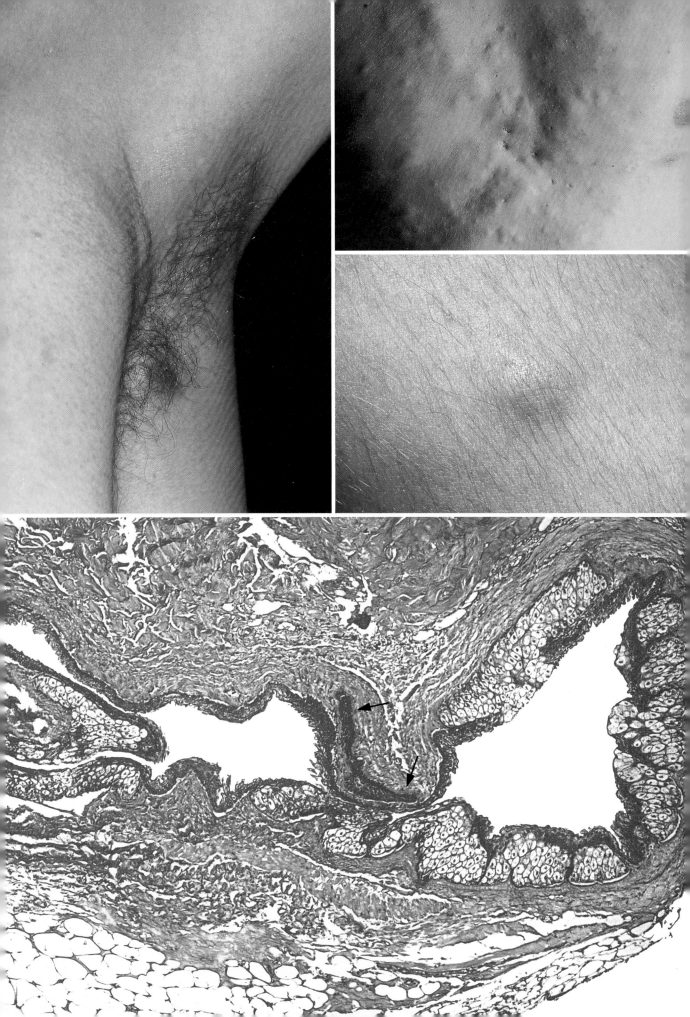

Steatocystoma Multiplex

Above These large, horn-filled cysts develop from nevoid malformations of sebaceous follicles. The epithelial lining derives from transformed sebaceous ducts. A tiny pilary unit produces vellus hairs which are shed into the cavity. Rudimentary sebaceous lobules are variably found around the periphery. The cyst is connected to the original infundibulum by a meandering thin cord. Thus the cyst is completely sealed off, the contents sterile

Below Semithin sections through the cyst showing multiple sections of vellus hairs floating in a matrix of loose horn and sebum. Semithin section, methylene blue

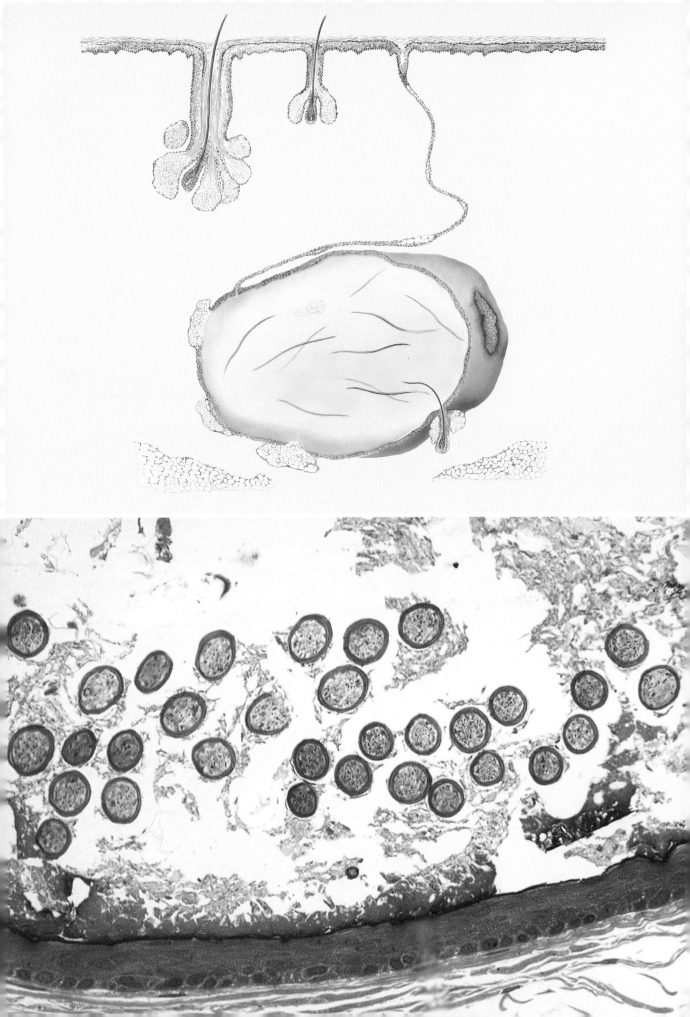

Eruptive Vellus Hair Cysts

This is not a real challenge for the acneologist but still an important differential diagnosis when crops of papules erupt. Surprisingly, this disorder was recently rediscovered after its first description some 80 years ago.

Clinical Findings

Patients present with many scattered papules, which they often say came up suddenly, hence the term "eruptive." This is unlikely. The same holds for eruptive syringomas, which in fact develop slowly. The papules have a cystic appearance, particularly when the skin is stretched. The color is that of the skin, at times intermingled with a bluish tinge. On palpation they are firm and solid but not painful. There is no visible punctum, nor any other sign that points to a follicular origin. Sites of predilection are the chest, abdomen, flank, upper back, and sometimes the face. The number varies from a few to several hundred. Very little is known about their final fate. Probably they are quite stationary and do not regress with time. Inflammatory reactions are rare.

Genetics

Familial cases and autosomal dominant inheritance have been reported in both sexes.

Histopathology

The lesions are thin-walled cysts whose epithelial lining has no stratum granulosum. No sebaceous glands are connected to the cyst wall as in steatocystoma multiplex. A solitary tiny vellus follicle is associated with the cyst. Many, sometimes dozens of shedded telogen hairs are trapped in the cavity. Pericystic fibrosis is sometimes seen.

Differential Diagnosis

At first glance steatocystoma multiplex comes quickly to mind and in fact may be almost indistinguishable clinically. Even histologically they share common features and sometimes seem to coexist. Some authors suggest that both are related cystic nevoid malformations. When acne persists with numerous closed comedones a false diagnosis is not unusual. Scars and other signs of acne vulgaris will generally keep one from making this eror.

Treatment

This is not necessary and almost impossible. Laser vaporization has been tried and is of uncertain value. Excision of course is effective but the trade-off of a scar for a cyst is dubious. Topical tretinoin is futile, even when aggressively used. A diagnostic biopsy of one or more cysts at least enables a correct classification.

Esterly NB, Fretzin DF, Pinkus H (1977) Eruptive vellus hair cysts. Arch Dermatol 113:500–503

Fisher DA (1981) Retinoic acid in the treatment of eruptive vellus hair cysts. J Am Acad Dermatol 5:221

Huerter CJ, Wheeland RG (1987) Multiple eruptive vellus hair cysts treated with carbon dioxide laser vaporization. J Dermatol Surg Oncol 13:260–263

Lee S, Kim JG, Kang JS (1984) Eruptive vellus hair cysts. Arch Dermatol 120:1191–1195

Mayron R, Grimwood RE (1988) Familial occurrence of eruptive vellus hair cysts. Pediatr Dermatol 5:94–96

Sánchez-Yus E, Aguilar-Martínez A, Cristóbal-Gil MC, Urbina-González F, Guerra-Rodríguez P (1988) Eruptive vellus hair cyst and steatocystoma multiplex: two related conditions? J Cutan Pathol 15:40–42

Sanchez Yus E, Requena L (1990) Eruptive vellus hair cysts and steatocystoma multiplex. Am J Dermatopathol 12:536–537

Sexton M, Murdock DK (1989) Eruptive vellus hair cysts. A follicular cyst of the sebaceous duct (sometimes). Am J Dermatopathol 11:364–368

Stiefler RE, Bergfeld WF (1980) Eruptive vellus hair cysts – an inherited disorder. J Am Acad Dermatol 3:425–429

Dilated Pore

Mostly solitary, sometimes with two or more lesions in one patient, dilated pores on the face of adults resemble large open comedones. However, its wide funnel-shaped opening and a pigmented cylinder of horny cells situated deeply in the crater help to differentiate this from a comedo. Men are more often affected than women. The facial skin always bears signs of solar elastosis. They mainly occur on the cheeks, less often elsewhere. Inflammation never occurs. Firm pressure yields an elongated comedo-like structure. A new horny impaction forms in several months.

The dilated pore, in our view, is neither a solitary trichoepithelioma nor an inverted seborrheic keratosis but a benign follicular malformation *sui generis*.

Histopathology

The histopathology is quite typical and diagnostic. The epithelial lining, in contrast to acne comedones, is hyperplastic with sprouts and outpouchings of a nevoid character. The whole lesion is asymmetrical and can extend with various cavities deep into the dermis. Hyperpigmentation along the basal cell layer throughout the lesion is also a typical feature. One pilary unit, often producing a fine silky hair, may be found on serial sections.

Treatment

Excision is the only way to permanently eliminate the pore.

Klövekorn G, Klövekorn W, Plewig, Pinkus H (1983) Riesenpore und Haarscheidenakanthom. Klinische und histologische Diagnose. Hautarzt 34:209–216

Winer LH (1954) The dilated pore, a trichoepithelioma. J Invest Dermatol 23:181–188

Dilated Pore

The dilated pore, first described by Winer, is a relatively common though often not diagnosed benign adnexal tumor. It occurs mostly often on the face of elderly adults with solar damage of the skin.

Above

Left   Solitary dilated pore on the forehead which looks like an open comedo. Indeed, a firm pigment-tipped cylinder of compact corneocytes can be squeezed out. A new blackhead-like structure reforms in a couple of months

Right   Close-up of a dilated pore almost indistinguishable from an open comedo

Below   Three-dimensional reconstruction of dilated pore. Three types are distinguished histologically: hair follicle, balloon, and multichambered type

Left   Hair-follicle type, reaching deep into the dermis. Acanthosis, papillomatosis, and one pilary portion at the bottom are typical

Right   Ballon type. A cavernous lesion with pronounced papillomatosis and a compact retention of corneocytes with apical melanin pigmentation

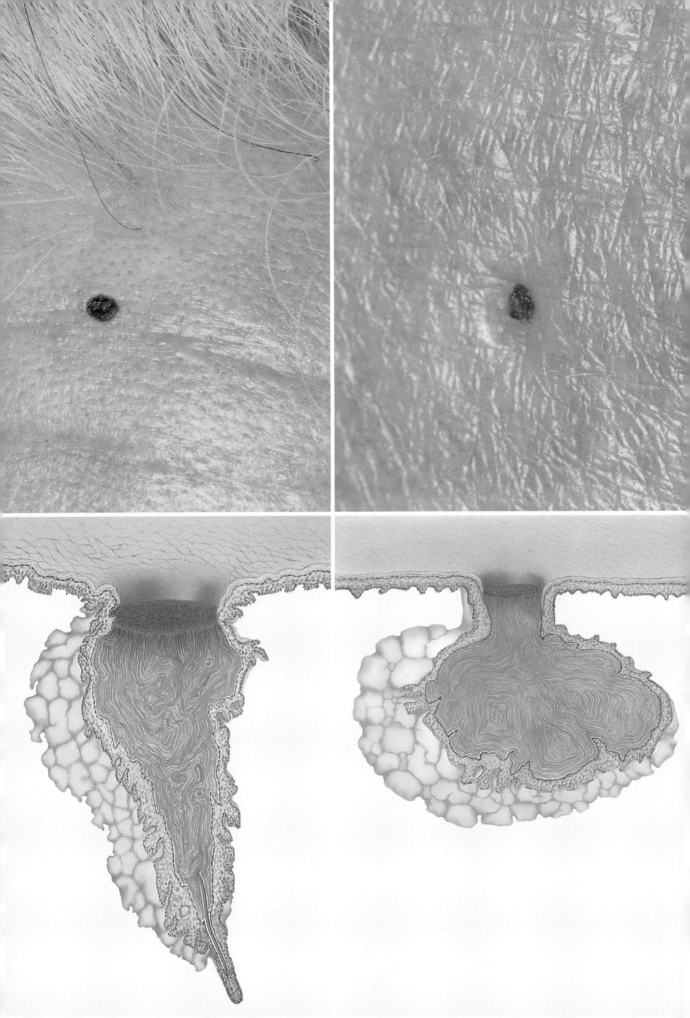

Pilar Sheath Acanthoma

This trough-like lesion, mostly occurring on the upper lip or chin in women, is not a real diagnostic challenge in acne patients. It does not occur in youngsters and is therefore rarely confused with acne. Elastotic skin is always a feature, reflecting actinic damage, the terrain in which the lesion develops. It can be mistaken for giant comedones, solar comedones, or even a scar. Pilar sheath acanthomas like dilated pores are easily diagnosed after one becomes familiar with their occurrence. The leading feature is a depressed trough-like opening, reminiscent of a shallow scar. Comedo-like impactions are sometimes visible. Inflammation is absent.

Histopathology

Restless nevoid epithelium with sprouts and islands compose this asymmetrical lesion, associated with a fine or coarse terminal hair. Melanin pigmentation along its base, with melanin deposits throughout the entire corneocyte layers, is quite typical.

Treatment

Surgical removal is the only effective therapy.

Mehregan AH, Brownstein MH (1978) Pilar sheath acanthoma. Arch Dermatol 114:1495–1497

Klövekorn G, Klövekorn W, Plewig G, Pinkus H (1983) Riesenpore und Haarscheidenakanthom. Klinische und histologische Diagnose. Hautarzt 34:209–216

Dilated Pore and Pilar Sheath Acanthoma

Two lesions mimic comedones in acne or in solar-damaged skin. Both of them are benign nevoid malformations of sebaceous follicles, occurring only in adult or elderly persons with actinic damage of the skin.

Above　　Pilar sheath acanthoma. A trough-like lesion, depressed, with hyperplastic irregular growth of keratinizing epithelium. Corneocytes are produced, but not as tightly compacted as in comedones in acne vulgaris. Most lesions are on the upper lip, as was this one. There is no perilesional fibrosis. It is not a secondary comedo or a scar

Below

Left　　Dilated pore. The solitary dilated pore on the face of adults looks like an open comedo. Indeed, a firm, pigment-tipped cylinder of horn can be squeezed out. A new blackhead reforms in a month or so. This is but one of many different follicular lesions in which comedo-like impactions form. The histopathology, however, is quite different. Here the epithelial lining, instead of being thinned out, is in fact hyperplastic with nevoid-like changes

Right　　A scarred follicle. This is not a giant pore, but a scarred follicle of an acne patient. Fifty days prior to the biopsy a comedo was squeezed out. The inflammatory reaction was not visible clinically. It distorted the follicle, which now has crazy patterns of acanthosis and papillomatosis. Sebaceous acini survived, as did the pilary unit. Note the tell-tate perifollicular fibrosis

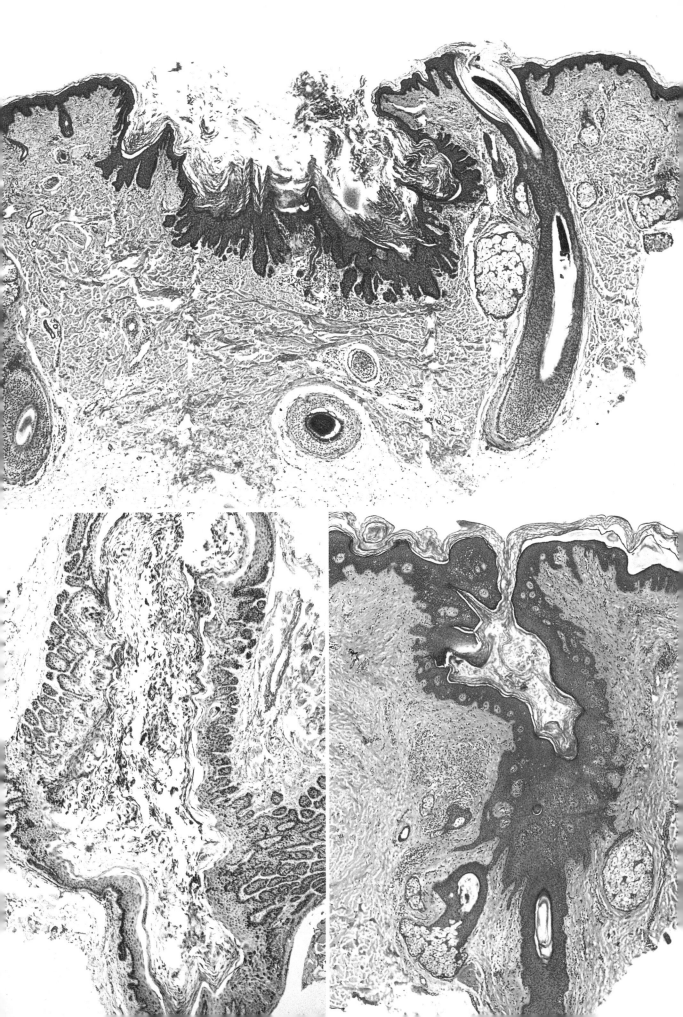

Omphalolith: The Ugly Nabelstein

Clinical Findings

Omphaloliths (*omphalos*, Greek = navel; *lithos*, Greek = stone) are curious lesions which have nothing to do with acne. They have the appearence of great blackheads. Synonyms are umbilical bolus, inspissated umbilical bolus, or navel stone. Persons with an exceptionally deep, invaginated navel are prone to retain corneocytes in the depths. Over years these become compressed into a compact hard bolus, a kind of pseudo-comedo. The opening is wide. The color is brown or black, corresponding to the skin type of the patient. The pigment is melanin, not dirt or lipid; the same accounts for the color of blackheads (open comedones). Inflammation is usually absent. The bolus is firmly rooted and surprisingly difficult to remove. It commonly takes years for the omphalolith to reform after being dislodged.

According to folklore, these curious lesions have magic powers, and are often valued as talismans (good luck charms). Some persons refuse to have them removed. In a museum in Delphi, Greece, one can admire a monstrous *Nabelstein*. The Hellenes considered Delphi the center – the navel – of the world, where the cosmic elements sky, earth, and hell came together. Similarly there was an umbilicus urbae Romanae at the Forum Romanum. In eastern cultures Buddha is sometimes decorated with a navel stone.

Differential Diagnosis

Malignant melanoma is often the first but incorrect diagnosis. Sometimes a chronic irritation (omphalitis) may lead to retention of cellular debris, often associated with a foul odor. Some authors have seen an analogy to cholesteatomas of the ear, and consequently called it cholesteatoma of the umbilicus (Nabelcholesteatom), or *corps étranger* (*étranger*, French = stranger). Invaginated scars with a deep recessus sometimes form similar solid impactions, also with a brown-black surface.

Treatment

The bearer will let you know if he wants the omphalolith to be removed. Forceful use of a forceps is sufficient to lift the bolus out of its deep hole.

Ehring F (1979) Der Nabelstein. Hautarzt 30:494–496

Fishman HC (1971) The inspissated umbilical bolus. Arch Dermatol 103:221–222

Longuet M (1875) Corps étranger de la cicatrice ombilicale. Bull Soc Anat Paris 10:367–368

Keratosis Pilaris

Occasionally keratosis pilaris causes diagnostic problems, particularly when it occurs concomitantly with acne on the lateral aspects of the upper arms. It is insufficiently recognized that keratosis pilaris frequently accompanies acne when looked for. It may simply be a marker for a tendency toward follicular hyperkeratosis in acne patients. The etiopathogenesis is still unknown. Though unproven, androgen stimulation is considered to be of importance. Some believe it to be associated with an atopic diathesis.

The condition generally starts before puberty when acne lesions are small or absent. Keratosis pilaris represents the diathesis to develop horny spines in terminal hair follicles. The chief locations are the lateral and dorsal sides of the upper arms, followed by rarer sites, e.g., thighs, cheeks, trunk, and scalp. The spectrum ranges from the mild expression of a fine sandpaper-like grainy appearance to grossly visible comedo-like impactions. Generally it is noninflammatory, but perifollicular inflammation with redness and tenderness rarely result in punctuate scars.

Keratotic follicles are a feature of several syndromes. It may appear in the lateral portions of the eyebrows (Hertoghe's sign). Another distressing, rare disorder is ulerythema ophryogenes of the cheeks (red apple cheeks). The spectrum encompasses scarring alopecia on thighs, back, and arms with punctate, reddish, follicular openings. Histopathology reveals a wide range of findings. The coarse though short hair shaft penetrates the follicular epithelium and leads to foreign body granulomas and scarring. Follicular units sometimes take a bizarre shape.

Therapy is only symptomatic with topical application of diluted tretinoin (0.025%), urea (5%–10%), or combinations of urea with NaCl (5% each). These treatments are helpful but not curative. After the skin becomes smooth, once or twice weekly applications are sufficient to prevent recurrence of the horny impactions.

Adam BS, Altmeyer P (1989) The histology of keratosis rubra pilaris compared with acne vulgaris. In: Marks R, Plewig G (eds) Acne and related disorders. Dunitz, London, pp 379–386

Barth JH, Wojnarowska F, Dawber RPR (1989) Is keratosis pilaris another androgen-dependent dermatosis? In: Marks R, Plewig G (eds) Acne and related disorders. Dunitz, London, pp 377–378

Pseudofolliculitis of the Beard

This disease, also called pili recurvati, has a wide spectrum of expressions which may mimic acne lesions to a certain extent. Afflicted persons have stiff, curved hairs. Most of them are adult Blacks, but minor examples also occur on the necks of Whites.

The tips of strongly curved stiff hairs penetrate the skin just before they exit through the follicular orifice. The hair pushes through the follicular epithelium and penetrates the dermis. Alternatively, the tip may emerge from the follicle and then soon reenter the nearby skin. Each tip provokes an inflammatory foreign body reaction (ingrown hairs), creating perifollicular papules. There are no comedones. Bacterial infections play no part. The condition eventually leaves criss-cross scars in Blacks with heavy beards. Sites of predilection are cheeks, chin, submental area, and lateral sides of the neck. The disease exists only in men who shave regularly. Razor blades create sharp tips on the strongly curved hairs. Close shaving with the skin stretched leads to retraction of the tip below the surface of the orifice. The shortened hair can then penetrate the infundibular epithelium.

Not shaving is curative. The hair forms an enlarging loop and the tip soon springs out of the skin. Of course, not everyone wants a beard. Less frequent and less close shaving is helpful, especially if electric shavers replace blades. We have also shown that electrolysis is curative, though this process is lengthy and costly. Topical tretinoin is helpful and may be alternated with a moderate strength steroid for a short while. Steroids rapidly produce atrophy on the face; this event may be prevented by concomitant use of tretinoin.

Alexander AM (1974) Pseudofolliculitis diathesis. Arch Dermatol 109:729–730

Alexander AM (1981) Evaluation of a foil-guarded shaver in the management of pseudofolliculitis barbae. Cutis 27:534–542

Kligman AM, Mills OH Jr (1973) Pseudofolliculitis of the beard and topically applied tretinoin. Arch Dermatol 107:551–552

Strauss JS, Kligman AM (1956) Pseudofolliculitis of the beard. Arch Dermatol 74:533–542

Acne-like Disorders

A surprising array of disorders have a resemblance to acne; the expert is usually not fooled.

Above   Pseudofolliculitis barbae (synonymous with pili recurvati) is a common problem in persons with stiff, curly hair of the beard. It is, therefore, very common in Blacks. The sharpened hair tips dig themselves back into the skin, causing foreign body granulomas

Left   Close-up of stiff hairs in a patient with folliculitis barbae

Right   There are longstanding papules, hypertrophic scars, and crisscross depressed scars in this person who has been suffering from pseudofolliculitis barbae for many years

Below

Left   Pseudofolliculitis not only occurs in the beard area, but in other hairy sites, like chest, abdomen, thighs, or buttocks. This man suffers from a pseudofolliculitis diathesis. Itching is frequent, leading to scratching, excoriations, and unsightly hyperpigmentation

Right   Pringle's disease with red angiofibromas in the centrofacial region of the face may be mistaken for acne. Characteristically, the angiofibromas are located in the center of the face and there are no comedones. Also there is no scarring. Other signs would include hypopigmented macules and angiofibromas on the gum, finger, or toe nails (Koehnen tumors). Dermabrasion or laser treatment offer excellent therapeutic results in this condition

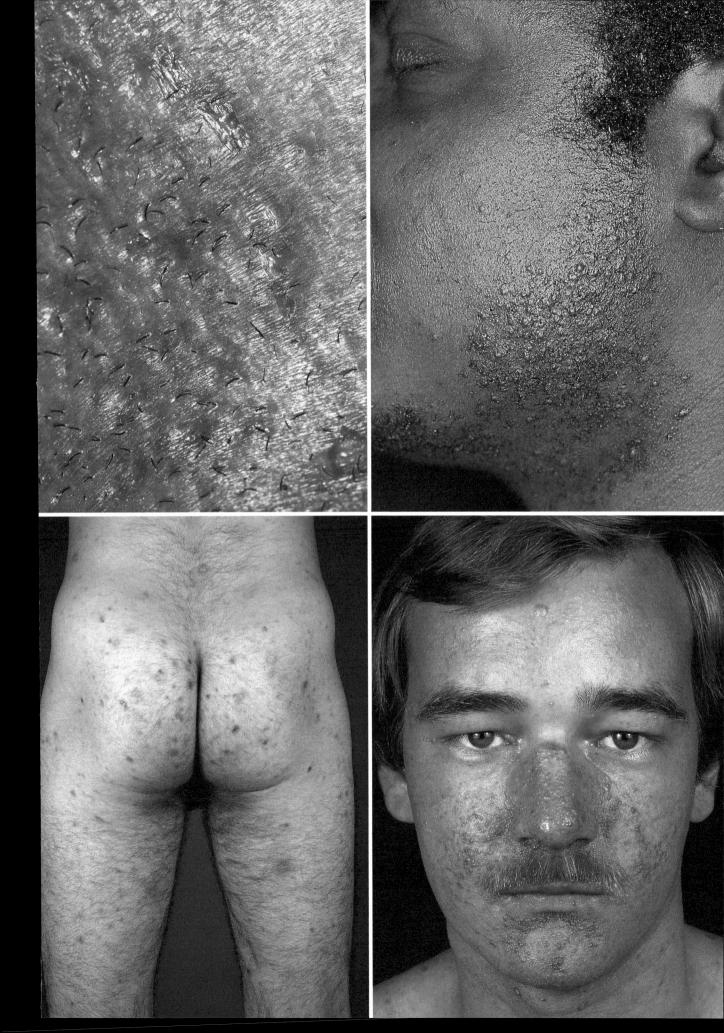

Osteoma Cutis and Pigmented Osteoma Cutis

Clinical Findings

Osteoma cutis (osteosis cutis, osteosis cutis multiplex) is a more common complication in acne than the less than 50 publications suggest. It is usually subclinical, showing up on X-ray examination in as many as 5%–10% of patients with persistent inflammatory acne. When (rarely) clinically apparent, ectopic bone formation can present baffling diagnostic problems. Osteoma cutis occurs as small, skin-colored, dome-shaped papules, 1–2 mm in diameter. Usually they are numerous, sometimes up to several hundred. They do not progess or regress, being permanent. Osteoma cutis favors the face but sometimes develops on the neck and on the chest. The nodules are rock-hard, painless, and noninflamed. Osteoma cutis is most often an unusual idiopathic response to a preexisting inflammatory acne lesion. The serum levels of calcium, phosphate, and parathyroid hormone are normal.

Facial osteomas sometimes acquire a bluish hue: pigmented osteoma cutis. Questioning reveals past therapy with tetracyclines, which form a complex with phosphate. Dozens to hundreds of small, blue, tattoo-like, pigmented macules or papules are dispersed over the face. When removed they look brownish; under UV-A radiation (Wood's light) they show the characteristic yellow fluorescence.

This is also the explanation for the disfiguring, crumbly teeth in young children taking tetracyclines, or in infants whose mothers were given tetracycline in early pregnancy.

Histopathology

The presence of well-defined round foci of typical bone in the mid-dermis is pathognomonic. Osteomas may contain blood vessels and fat cells. There is no fibrosis in primary osteomas, but scarring fibrosis in secondary ones.

Treatment

The only approach is surgical in desperate patients. Each lesion can be removed by a punch biopsy, with a replacement punch from the postauricular region. Alternatively, the contents can be expelled through a tiny incision.

Basler RSW, Watters JH, Taylor WB (1977) Calcifying acne lesions. Int J Dermatol 16:755–758

Burgdorf W, Nasemann T (1977) Cutaneous osteomas: a clinical and histopathological review. Arch Dermatol Res 260:121–135

Goldminz D, Greenberg R (1991) Multiple miliary osteoma cutis. J Am Acad Dermatol 24:878–881

Moritz DL, Elewski B (1991) Pigmented postacne osteoma cutis in a patient treated with minocycline: report and review of the literature. J Am Acad Dermatol 24:851–853

Wagner G, Lubach D, Jänner M, Mensing H (1987) Osteosis cutis multiplex. Aktuel Dermatol 13:60–62

Walter JF, Macknet KD (1979) Pigmentation of osteoma cutis caused by tetracycline. Arch Dermatol 115:1087–1088

Calcinosis and Osteoma Cutis: Refuse from Inflammatory Acne

Severe inflammatory acne always ends with scarring, either clinically or histologically. Buried beneath the skin surface within scar tissue are sometimes miraculous calcified or osseous objects. These hard corpuscular elements are rarely diagnosed clinically, but are more often seen in histologic sections, or sometimes when X-ray pictures are taken for other reasons. So far calcinosis and osteoma cutis have mainly been described in facial skin. This may be coincidental, as other body regions such as back or chest should be affected in the same way.

Calcification can be observed in many conditions unrelated to acne. Most commonly it is reported in trichoepitheliomas and basal cell carcinomas. A few reports mention calcification in acne-bearing skin. In osteoma cutis, nodular bone formations of small size are laid down in the tissue. Patients receiving tetracycline therapy, mostly minocycline, rarely develop pigmented osteoma cutis.

Above

Left   Calcinosis cutis from scarred face of an acne patient. The calcified nodule at the left is situated in a dermis which is diffusely infiltrated with inflammatory and multinuclear giant cells

Right   Osteoma cutis. Beneath sebaceous gland and follucular structures, the upper portion of an osteoma cutis is shown. The patient had acne in the past

Middle   X-ray picture taken from the patient shown above left. Multiple niduses of calcified tissue show up as opacities in the cheek

Below   Pigmented osteomata cutis

Left   The multiple bluish pigmentations in the face of this lady are all pigmented osteomas. She received tetracycline orally. As known from previous tragedies in prepubertal children, new bone formation combined with tetracycline causes disturbing pigmentation

Right   The surgically removed osteomas are brownish

Bottom   When viewed with a Wood's light, the osteomas fluoresce yellow

Courtesy of Joseph F. Walter, La Jolla, USA

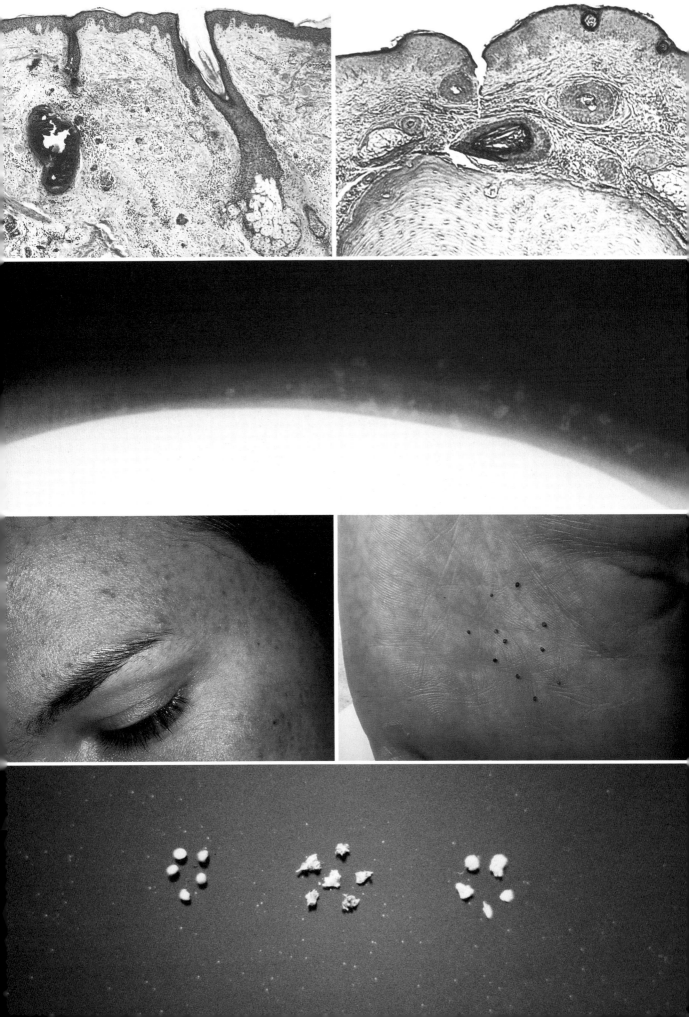

Bones in the Skin

Osteoma cutis means "bone in the skin." Osteomas arise in different ways, often without any explanation.

Above   Multiple, closed, comedo-like, skin-colored, flat, hard papules are difficult to diagnose clinically. Histologically these show bone formation

Below

Left   Histologically the small osteomas seem to float in a slightly inflamed elastotic skin from the face of an elderly man. These are probably postinflammatory osteomas

Right   A single osteoma from the man shown above. There is no inflammation and no fibrosis

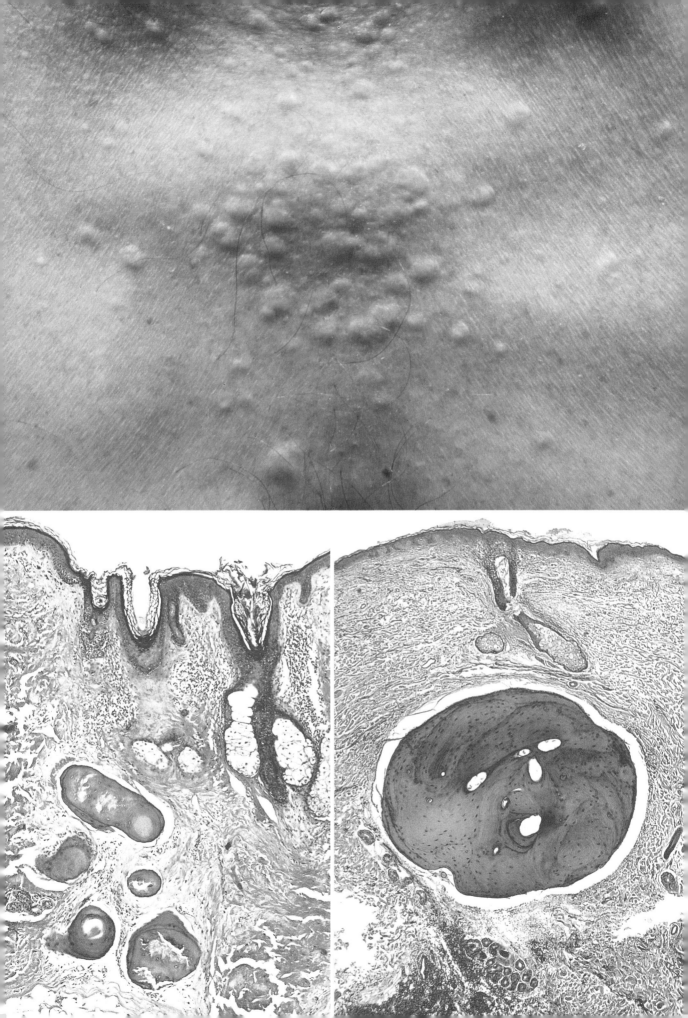

Minocycline-Induced Hyperpigmentation

Curious discoloration can occur occasionally from minocycline therapy of acne, rarely from other tetracyclines. Minocycline chelates to iron or calcium, and may then be oxidized to a colored quinone. A discrete or an intensive blue discoloration, resembling the color of coaldust tattoos in miners, is usually limited to scars on the face, mainly on the cheeks and temples. Pigmentation is often symmetrical. Another form is mottled hyperpigmentation unrelated to injury or scars. Finally there may occur a muddy-skin syndrome with generalized diffuse brown or gray discoloration.

Afflicted patients have a history of long-term treatment with minocycline hydrochloride, usually for many months or even years. Sun exposure seems to be contributory, since the hyperpigmentation is mostly limited to facial skin. However, it is also seen on the chest, back, or legs. Annoyingly, the blue color persists for years. The patients are highly embarrassed.

Brown–black pigment granules are deposited in the dermis, particularly around perivascular lymphohistiocytic infiltrates. Pigment deposition is most intensive in scarred tissue. Comedones and papulopustules are not pigmented.

Electron microscopy shows iron-containing electron-dense particles, probably hemosiderin, in histiocytes and macrophages, either surrounded by membranes or free within the cytoplasm. There is no resemblance to melanin. Electron probe microanalysis or energy-dispersive X-ray analysis have revealed that these particles contain iron and lesser amounts of calcium and sulfur.

In our experience, isotretinoin 0.5–1.0 mg/kg body weight daily given orally for several months clears the hyperpigmentation almost completely. The mechanism of action seems to be the anti-inflammatory property of the retinoid with removal of the chelate.

Basler RSW (1985) Minocycline-related hyperpigmentation. Arch Dermatol 121:606–608

Bridges AJ, Graziano F, Calhoun W, Reizner GT (1990) Hyperpigmentation, neutrophilic alveolitis, and erythema nodosum resulting from minocycline. J Am Acad Dermatol 22:959–962

Fenske NA, Millns J (1980) Cutaneous pigmentation due to minocycline hydrochloride. J Am Acad Dermatol 3:308–310

Gordon G, Sparano BM, Iatropoulos MJ (1985) Hyperpigmentation of the skin associated with minocycline therapy. Arch Dermatol 121:618–623

McGrae JD, Zelickson AS (1980) Skin pigmentation secondary to minocycline therapy. Arch Dermatol 116:1262–1265

Ridgway HA, Sonnex TS, Kennedy CTC, Millard PR, Henderson WJ, Gold SC (1982) Hyperpigmentation association with oral minocycline. Br J Dermatol 107:95–102

Sato S, Murphy GF, Bernhard JD, Mihm MC Jr, Fitzpatrick TB (1981) Ultrastructural and X-ray microanalytical observations of minocycline-related hyperpigmentation of the skin. J Invest Dermatol 77:264–271

Serwatka LM (1988) Minocycline-associated cutaneous pigmentation. J Assoc Milit Dermatol 14:10–12

Simons JJ, Morales A (1980) Minocycline and generalized cutaneous pigmentation. J Am Acad Dermatol 3:244–247

White SW, Besanceney C (1983) Systemic pigmentation from tetracycline and minocycline therapy. Arch Dermatol 119:1–2

Minocycline-Induced Hyperpigmentation

A troublesome though rare complication of oral minocycline therapy is a slate-blue persistent pigmentation. This occurs in scars, calcified tissue, and inflammatory foci. This young man's inflammatory acne responded well to minocycline. Unfortunately, tatto-like bluish discolorations appeared and persisted for more than a year prior to his seeking medical attention. Oral isotretinoin (0.5 mg/kg body weight per day) cleared the hyperpigmentation completely and permanently. The mode of action is probably related to the anti-inflammatory component, enabling removal of the macrophages which contain the pigment. Similar good results have been obtained in other patients.

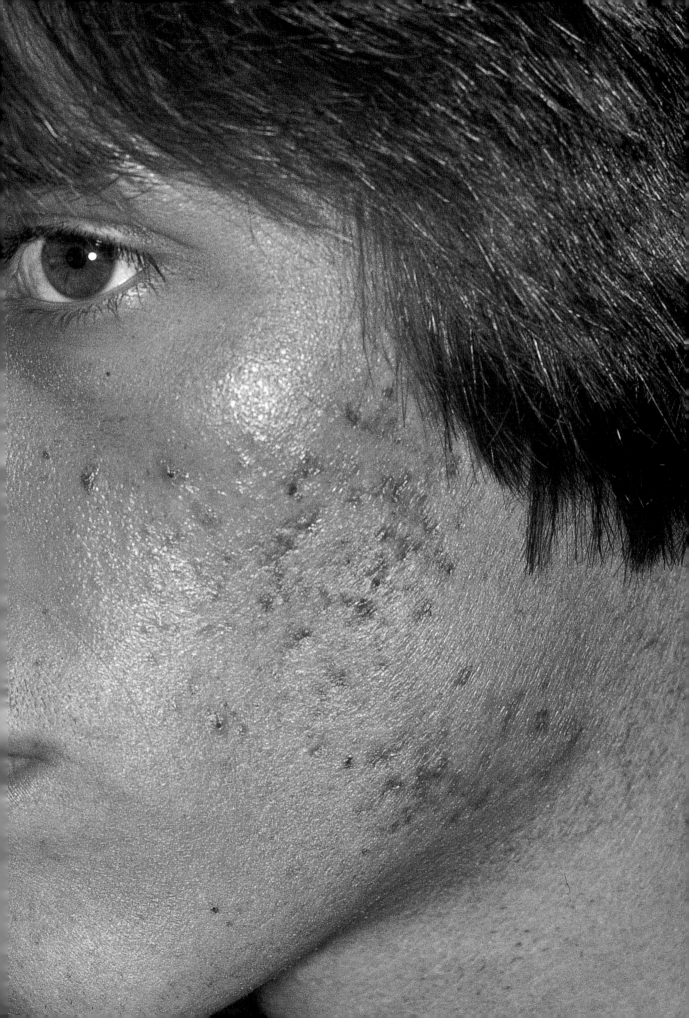

Histology of Minocycline-Induced Hyperpigmentation

Above   In this semithin section, macrophages containing conspicuous dark pigment granules have clustered around small vessels in which comma-shaped erythrocytes can be seen. This granular material accounts for the bluish discoloration seen clinically. (Electron microscopy, × 1240)

Below   Higher magnification with the electron microscope discloses the variably shaped pigment granules packed into the cytoplasm of a macrophage. (Electron microscopy, × 34000)

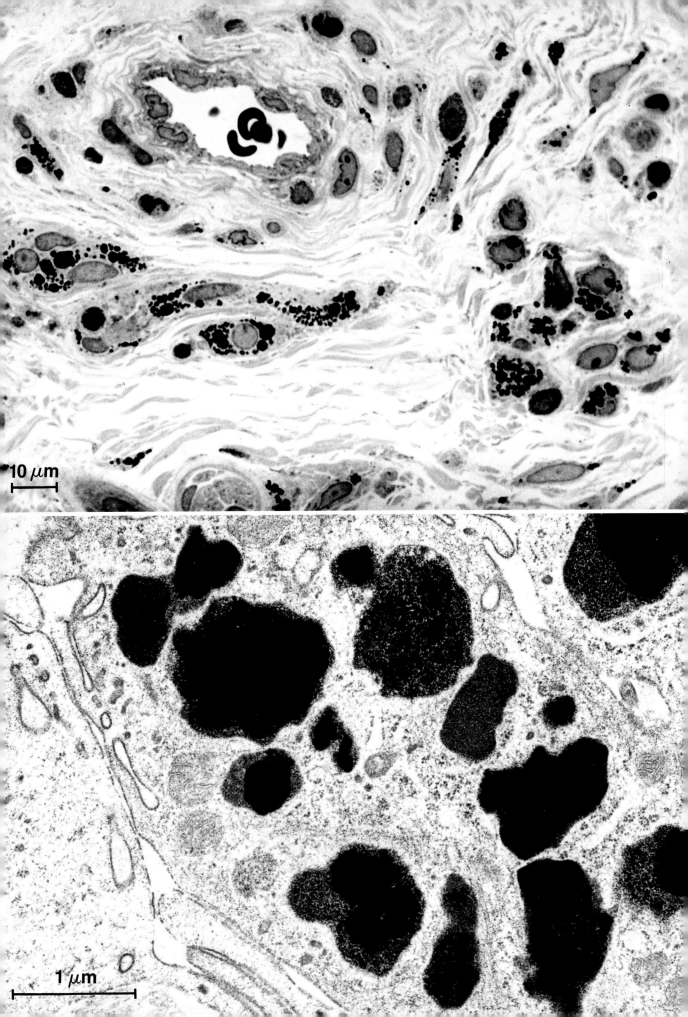

Differential Diagnosis of Closed Comedones

Above   Closed comedones. The forehead of this lady is studded with hundreds of closed comedones. "Whiteheads" is a very descriptive term. The camera provides enough magnification to see the tiny openings of the comedones

Below

Left   Colloid milia. The numerous whitish papules look like comedones. They are colloid milia, biopsy proven. Clinical considerations were milia, contact acne, steroid acne, eruptive vellus hair cysts, trichodiscomas, trichofolliculomas, etc.

Right   Milia. Many dome-shaped waxy papules on the cheek and the eyes were diagnosed as milia, sustained by a biopsy

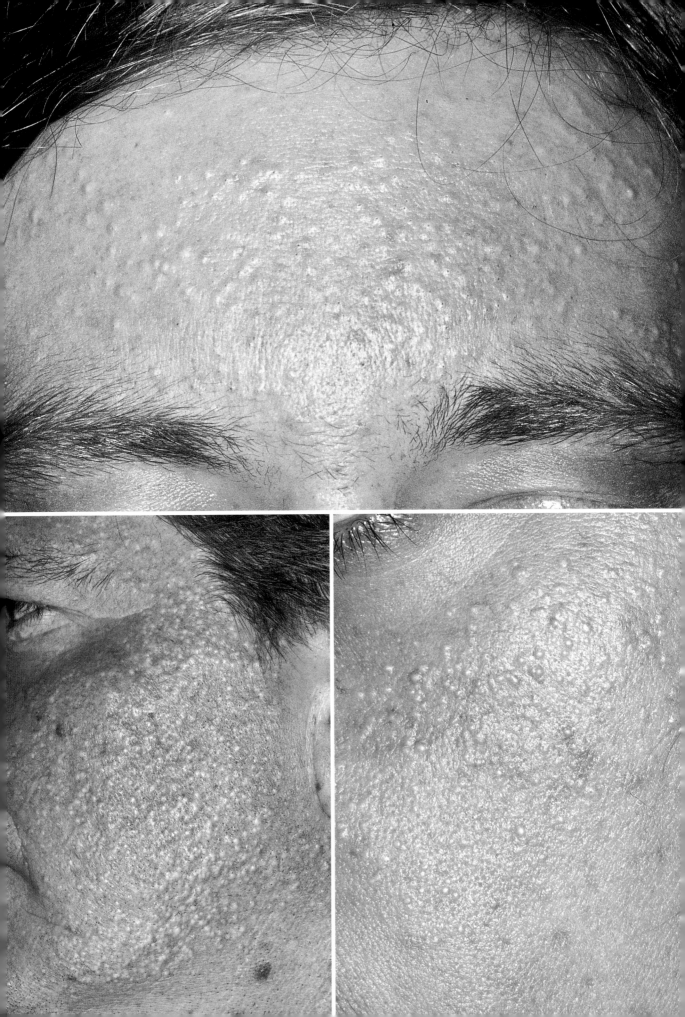

Epidermal Cysts

Epidermal cysts sometimes resemble giant comedones. They should be prophylactically excised to prevent spontaneous rupture and abscesses.

Above

Left   A huge epidermal cyst on the chest with a wide opening. The pigment is melanin

Right An old epidermal cyst with a spatulous central opening and a wide perforation to its lower left portion

Below The histopathology of epidermal cysts is quite characteristic, with a cyst wall, sometimes melanin pigment in its basal cell layer, a stratum granulosum, and corneocytes arranged in a wickerwork fashion

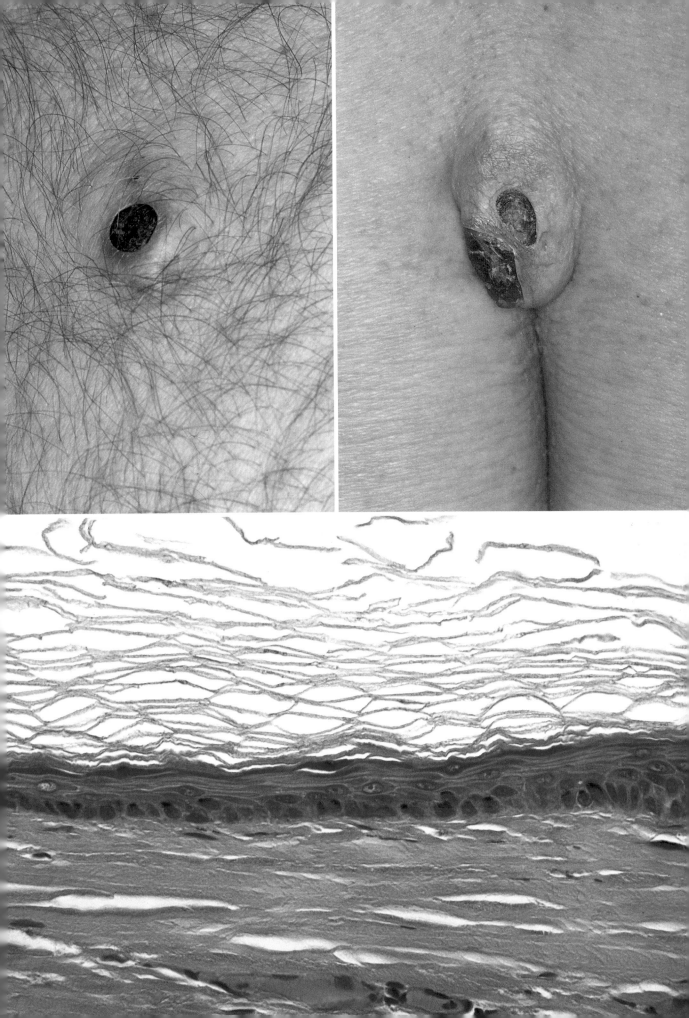

Trichilemmal and Epidermal Cysts

Cysts are part of the spectrum of lesions in acne. Epidermal cysts, trichilemmal cysts, eruptive vellus hair cysts, and steatocystoma multiplex are differential diagnoses.

Above   Trichilemmal cysts (atheromas, wens) are almost exclusively located on the hairy scalp, often several of them

Left   Three trichilemmal cysts of varying size are on the forehead and hairy scalp of this man

Right   The histopathology is quite typical. The overview gives an impression of the cast in relation to the normal hair infundibulum in its neighborhood. The cyst wall has pale-staining trichilemmal cells with a crenulated border towards the lumen. The stratum granulosum is typically absent

Below   Most epidermal cysts are on the face, trunk, and extremities and spare the hairy scalp. The scrotum is a site of predilection for epidermal cysts, originating from the terminal follicles

Left   More than two dozen cysts on the scrotum are cosmetically disturbing

Right   Epidermal cysts of the scrotum have a peculiar tendency towards calcification. The cyst presented here is completely calcified, with roughly 80% of the epithelial lining still present. Van Kossa stain

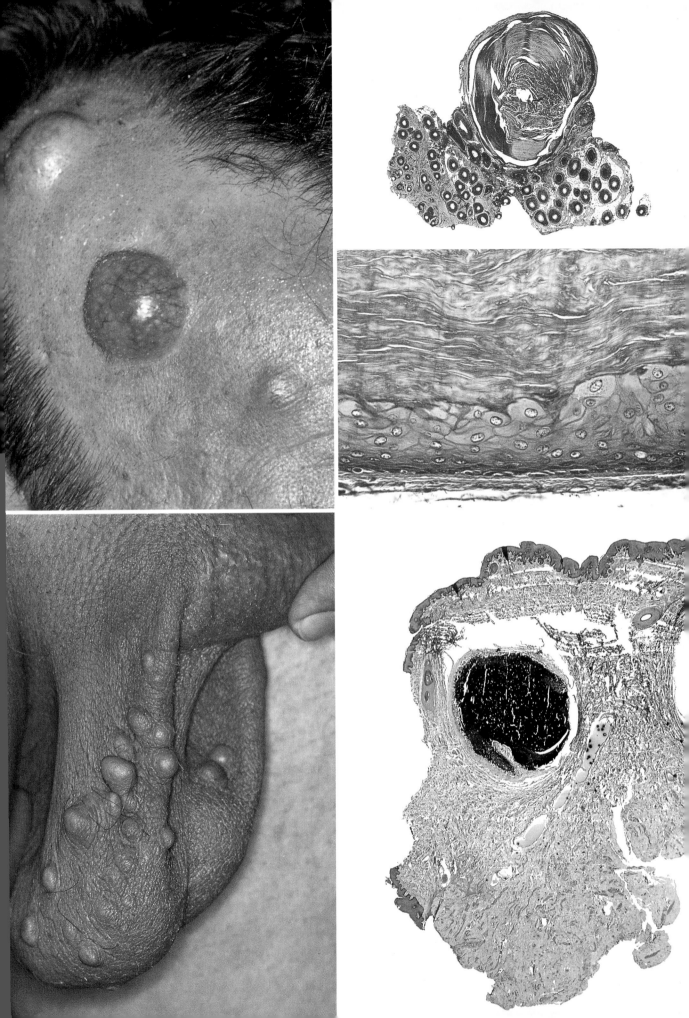

THERAPY

History of Therapy: Past, Present, and Future

Today dermatologists rightly feel confident when it comes to the treatment of acne. Topical and systemic drugs are now available which are highly effective in controlling the disease, even curing it. These impressive therapeutic resources are recent. Older physicians still remember the times when actually very little was available. They mainly dispensed enthusiasm and hope, along with drugs which were only marginally useful and sometimes harmful. We will briefly review the history of therapy because it illustrates how difficult it is to establish the safety and efficacy of drugs. It also reminds us to maintain a healthy scepticism regarding some of our current approaches which may also turn out to be passing fads.

X-rays were discovered 1895 by Roentgen in Germany, but it was America which passionately welcomed this painless, invisible yet highly effective physical modality. As early as 1902, reports appeared praising its efficacy. There was no question then, or for that matter now, about its efficacy. No other drug matched its beneficial effects. X-rays for inflammatory acne were given until the late 1960s. Unfortunately, without dosimetry and without long-term follow-up, X-rays were delivered in excessive doses, replacing acne lesions by radiodermatitis. Malignant tumors mostly of the thyroid gland developed decades later. There is a safe way to administer X-rays, but newer treatments have consigned these to the history books. First sulfonamaides and then antibiotics came into medicine in the 1930s and 1940s. Typically many reports praised sulfonamides, which are so effective in infectious diseases. But acne is not an infection, and sulfonamides are not only ineffective but entail many adverse effects. When tetracyclines came on the scene, they represented the first class of antibiotics which were truly effective when administered orally. It is a surprising fact that tetracyclines are almost useless topically, but are still being prescribed by many physicians. Erythromycin and later clindamycin, on the other hand, are effective both topically and orally.

The era of double-blind, well-controlled studies has a strong method for weeding out useless drugs. Benzoyl peroxide was synthesized 90 years ago, but it took half a century to bring it onto the skin of acne patients. The early preparations were unstable and inelegant. Today's formulations are first-class preparations which are both esthetic and dependable.

Tretinoin was introduced as topical medication about 25 years ago. It has stood the test of time, and today it is one of the leading preparation for acne. Because of irritation, it made its way slowly into the therapeutic armamentarium, and even today many physicians do not know how to use it effectively.

Hormonal treatment arose in the wake of oral contraceptives. This was followed by various hormonal combinations designed specifically for inflammatory acne in women. Antiandrogens played a key

Historical overview of the introduction of acne treatments and their registration in the United States and the Federal Republic of Germany

First Description of Use in Acne	US Registration	FRG Registration
1902 X-Rays		
~1930 Benzoyl peroxide, topical		
1954 Tetracycline, oral		
	1960 Benzoyl peroxide, topical	
1961 Tretinoin, topical		
1961 Cyproterone acetate, oral		
	1963 Tetracycline	
1965 Benzoyl peroxide, topical		
1969 Minocycline, oral		
	1971 Minocycline, oral	
1972 Clindamycin, topical	1972 Tretinoin, topical	1972 Minocycline, oral
		1973 Tretinoin, topical
		1973 Cyproterone acetate, oral
		1974 Tetracycline, topical
1974 Erythromycin, topical		1974 Benzoyl peroxide, topical
	1975 Erythromycin, topical	
1976 Tetracycline, topical		
		1977 Cyproterone acetate plus ethinyl estradiol, oral
		1977 Erythromycin, topical
1979 Isotretinoin, oral		
	1980 Tetracycline, topical	
	1980 Clindamycin, topical	
1982 Isotretinoin, topical	1982 Isotretinoin, oral	
1983 Azelaic acid, topical	1983 Erythromycin, topical	1983 Clindamycin, topical
		1984 Isotretinoin, oral
		1991 Azelaic acid, topical

role in this approach, with cyproterone acetate being the classical antiandrogen, along with its derivative, chlormadinone acetate. Spironolactone, an antiandrogen and aldosterone antagonist, is not approved for acne, but is also useful in the hands of experts for the control of resistant acne in women. No antiandrogen has been shown to be effective when topically applied. A breakthrough can be expected in less than a decade if partial successes in pharmaceutical achievements continue.

Possibly the most astounding drug found for the treatment of the most severe forms of acne is isotretinoin. It marks a real milestone in the history of our discipline. At the beginning, following published results of permanent cures in acne conglobata, this met with disbelief. The negative aspect of this "miracle" drug is its teratogenicity.

The most recent development is azelaic acid. Like new neighbors, it is viewed sceptically by some and hailed enthusiastically by others. It has shown activity, but only time will show its correct position.

Other refinements of therapy also need honorable mention: cryotherapy, dermabrasion, lasers, chemical peels, silicone and collagen injections, and at least half a dozen others which are the secret possessions of master clinicians. Ultraviolet radiation, popular in the past, can only be condemned.

Ad Hoc Committee Report (1975) Systemic antibiotics for treatment of acne vulgaris: efficacy and safety. Arch Dermatol 111:1630–1636

Baer RL, Witten VH (1960) Acne vulgaris: remarks on recent advances in knowledgement and management. Year Book of Dermatology. Year Book Medical, Chicago, pp 7–32

Becker FT, Fredricks MG (1955) Evaluation of antibiotics in the control of pustular acne vulgaris. Arch Dermatol 72:157–163

King WC, Forbes M (1955) Clinical trial of orally administered tetracycline in the management of acne vulgaris. Antibiotics Annual 1954–1955. Medical Encyclopedia, New York, pp 570–573

Loevenhart AS (1905) Benzoylsuperoxid, ein neues therapeutisches Agens. Therap Monatshefte 19:426–428

Pace W (1965) A benzoyl peroxide-sulfur cream for acne vulgaris. Can Med Assoc J 93:252–254

Peck GL, Olsen TG, Yoder FW, Strauss JS, Downing DT, Pandya M, Butkus D, Arnaud-Battandier J (1979) Prolonged remissions of cystic and conglobate acne with 13-*cis*-retinoic acid. N Engl J Med 300:329–333

Pusey WA (1902) Acne and sycosis treated by exposure to Roentgen rays. J Cutan Dis 20:204–210

Sulzberger MB, Witten VH, Steagall RW (1960) Treatment of acne vulgaris: use of systemic antibiotics and sulfonamides. JAMA 173:1911–1918

Treatment: General Statements

Acne is a malicious disease of adolescence. It strikes at a time when the impact of every lesion is momentous, when an emotional scratch may deepen into a life-long scar. Acne is a very serious disease in a society in which consciousness of cosmetic comeliness has been raised to a narcissistic obsession.

The list of therapy formerly thought to be effective is long, ranging from the silly to the preposterous. Medications were often offensive, and the victims urged to adopt the life style of monks. Healthy youngsters invariably defaulted. The doctor and patient then galloped around an ever-quickening vicious circle of crime and punishment. Worse still: many treatments were harmful. The record is sobering.

All this has changed. We know a good deal more about the nature of the disease and the informed physician rarely sees a patient he cannot help. The usual goal is to keep the flame low until the fire goes out spontaneously, and especially to control the conflagrations that leave scars. Cure is possible, even in the most serious cases.

A powerful collection of folkloristic beliefs has singled out the acne patient for special scorns, torments, and punishments. Numerous fictions regarding causation circulate among acne patients and indeed have too much currency among physicians. It is important to deal openly with the patients' beliefs and fears. A frank, emphatic approach distinguishes the doctors who obtain the best results.

Far too many physicians still think of acne as a curse that has to be endured and which responds to treatment uncertainly and unimpressively. Nondermatologists especially like to enjoy the old saw that patients with skin diseases never get well and never die. This view constrains physicians to follow outdated Hippocratic teachings of waiting for time to do its work. In view of the powerful remedies now in our instrumentarium, it is an execrable offense against suffering youngsters to treat acne passively and pessimistically. Acne is an eminently treatable disease. To bring these outcasts back into the bright light of society is satisfying.

The most serious forms require an attack with multiple drugs. The results are often impressive.

Diet

Except for starvation, which is nearly curative, diet rarely if ever plays an etiologic role. Severe calorific restriction results in about a 40% decrease in sebum production, enough to be beneficial. Semistarvation will, however, never be popular among teenagers, even if it is curative. Throughout history, foods have been reviled or favored in accordance with whether they were thought to be beneficial or harmful. Belief in the therapeutic benefit of diets flourish when little is known about causation and when medical practitioners can do little to change the course of the disease. Not long ago, for example, diets were manipulated to combat tuberculosis. The opposite situation has prevailed in acne. No special diet is prescribed, but some foods are proscribed with holy furor. The list of forbidden foods has one remarkable feature: All of the blacklisted items are delicious and delectable to the palate. Among these are chocolate, nuts, candy, soft drinks, shellfish, cheeses, and other tempting delights. No one inveighs against such mundane comestibles as rice and potatoes or exotic ones like artichokes and salsify.

Whether foods adversely influence acne in any way has been a matter of great scientific interest, which also affects the daily pleasure of living. We performed a study in which acne patients ingested a special bar of chocolate each day which contained ten times the quantity of cocoa butter in usual bars. Nothing happened! The great majority of them stayed the same, a few improved, and some got worse. Many patients hold on to such beliefs, incriminating this food or that. In our view they are victims of systematic brainwashing by those who are older, but not wiser. The conviction that delicous foods are bad for acne is so entrenched that physicians too issue injunctions against the delectables loved by adolescents, despite objective evidence to the contrary.

Management of acne in the past was by and large punitive. Possibly because adolescents have vigorous sexual drives and have trouble controlling their surging passions, society through parents and physicians invents measures to keep these imminent sinners in check. Denying pleasures in eating was one such measure, reinforcing the Calvinistic idea that pimples were a punishment for bad thoughts.

Reports that high carbohydrate and high fat intake increase sebum production or alter its composition have no validity whatever; the opposite has also been reported. The sebaceous glands are not an excretory pathway for ingested lipids. The lipids in serum do not pass into the sebaceous gland. The latter synthesizes all its components from simple carbon fragments such as glucose. The sebaceous lipids do not in any way resemble blood lipids. The glands have a high degree of physiologic autonomy and neither the rate of synthesis nor the quality of the product is much influenced by the external or internal milieu. In contrast to popular beliefs, most skin functions, fortunately, are not changed by the diverse diets which mankind has elaborated. We exclude from this pronouncement diets which are grossly deficient in calories or essential components (vitamins, minerals, etc.). Conversely, it is possible to imagine extreme diets which could upset skin homeostasis by damaging general health.

Unlike foods, certain drugs or their metabolites *can* end up in sebum. Some circulating substances will diffuse across the basement membranes of sebaceous glands to be transported to the exterior when the cells die and are shed (holocrine excretion). Tetracyclines, a benefical drug, and iodides, an acne excitant, are examples of substances that reach the surface in this way. We have no special dietary instructions for acne patients. We tell them that they can eat anything they want in moderate quantity. "Eat sensibly" contains all the advice one needs to know. In summary, dietary regimens do not influence the course of the disease. This should be clearly stated to the patient.

Finally, on rare occasions we have seen patients who actually do get worse after eating a forbidden food. This usually happens within a day or less after the "sin" is committed. Careful observation will usually establish the real cause, namely the fingers. Anxiety and tension lead the patient to pick, squeeze, and excoriate existing small lesions, hence provoking an inflammatory lesion.

Emerson GW, Strauss JS (1972) Acne and acne care. A trend survey. Arch Dermatol 105:407–411

Fulton JE, Plewig G, Kligman AM (1969) Effect of chocolate on acne vulgaris. J Am Med Assoc 210:2071–2074

Harrell BL, Rudolph AH (1976) Kelp diet: a cause of acneiform eruption. Arch Dermatol 112:560

Plewig G, Strzeminski YA (1985) Jod und Hauterkrankungen. Dtsch Med Wochenschr 110:1266–1269

Pochi PE, Downing DT, Strauss JS (1970) Sebaceous gland response in man to prolonged total caloric deprivation. J Invest Dermatol 55:303–309

Cleanliness

Because of oiliness, acne patients tend to wash frequently. Quite a few are in fact fanatics, scrubbing themselves with soap and water as often as eight to ten times daily. It is not hard to discern the source of this compulsive washing. Since ancient times skin diseases have been regarded as retribution for sinful thoughts and acts. Acne patients, burdened by the distempers of adolescence, already feel dirty. Their self-image is that of the leper, unclean and unacceptable. A healthy balance should be struck. Again, the physician should bring these common feelings within the light of consciousness.

There is no evidence that lack of washing worsens acne nor that frequent cleaning is helpful. The great unwashed are no more susceptible than the compulsive cleaner; the latter may enjoy his obsessive lathering, but he is not aiding his skin. The most frenetic washing removes only surface lipids, a process that is virtually complete in about 30 s. The lipid in the follicular reservoirs is not influenced, and it is in these deeper recesses that lipids create pathology. The spill-over on the surface is solely of cosmetic concern. After sebum has passed through the orifice it does not matter whether it is removed or not.

Anxiety about germs is often combined with tremendous concern about cleanliness. Hence, many acne patients, who listen avidly to television commercials, seek bacteriostatic soaps. These may contain agents such as hexachlorophene, tricarbanilides, and chlorinated salicylanilides. Repeated lathering with such soaps may reduce the surface flora, but has no effect on the real culprit, *Propionibacterium acnes*. The anaerobes continue to proliferate in their follicular sanctuaries. Bacteriostatic soaps and detergents are not indicated in acne. Although they generally do no harm, they can be irritating. We advise our patients to use whatever soap or detergents they like with no emphasis on such aspects as pH, mildness, natural, or synthetic. We emphasize moderation, twice daily is sufficient, using warm water and only the fingers. Scrubbing with rough cloths is aggravating.

Excessive oiliness of the face is easily removed by the use of adsorbent papers, e.g., Kleenex professional wipes. Patting the face several times with these tissues during the day reduces the appearance of oiliness. Several cosmetic houses produce good sebum-absorbant wipes which can be carried in the purse and do not require prior removal of make-up.

Scalp Care

The acne literature nearly always states that good management requires careful attention to scalp hygiene. Acne patients often have oilier scalps than persons without acne; this motivates degreasing operations. What we have said about face washing holds here too. Neither meticulous scalp care nor steady neglect has any effect on acne: this is another myth enshrined by endless repetitions. Although it is often said that dandruff and seborrheic dermatitis are more prevalent in acne patients, our survey has shown only a modest increase. We do advise treatment for these conditions when they coexist, not because they adversely affect acne but simply to reduce further discomforts. Shampoos containing selenium disulfide and zinc pyrithione are very effective in both scalp disorders.

We advise acne patients to use shampoos they like. Thrice weekly shampooing is generally enough to overcome the feeling of greasiness. This is a matter of personal preference. Daily shampooing is not harmful, except for possible damage to the hair shaft. Hair styling likewise is immaterial. We have no evidence that wearing bangs over the forehead intensifies acne in that area. Patients often adopt that hair style to conceal lesions of the forehead. We see no harm in that.

External Contactants

Acneigenic substances have greater effects on patients with acne than persons without acne. These chemicals induce comedones more swiftly and more abundantly in skin which bears or has borne acne lesions. The physician should be on the alert for comedogenic environmentals. The most frequent sources are cosmetics, pomades, sunscreens, and various medicaments. It is important to inquire about cosmetics especially in older women with acne.

Emotions and Psychosomatic Factors

Every conceivable point of view has been expressed in the literature. Some consider acne a psychosomatic disease originating in the affective reactions of adolescence, a period of emotional stress. Any statement that can be made in support of this idea can be countered by another which denies it. For example, acne is thought to be commoner in schizophrenics (a disease notably affecting the acne age group). On the other hand, acne was found to be equally common in mentally retarded youngsters. The protagonists often recommended psychotherapy by qualified professionals. Of course the term "psychotherapy" is about as explicit as the term "drugs". The methods include psychoanalysis (revealing the unconscious), the techniques of behavioral psychology (deconditioning and reconditioning), psycholinguistics ("you think badly"), and superficial psychiatric counselling ("let's talk it over").

Perhaps most dermatologists, correctly in our point of view, regard acne as a somatopsychic disease, that is, emotional responses are secondary. It is inconceivable that an adolescent with acne severe enough to see a doctor would not be disturbed. A face full of papulopustules is not a confidence builder. The physician should be alert to the plight of patients who deny this. It is normal for acne patients to resent their disease, to feel angry and hostile, to feel unfairly picked upon, isolated, and depressed. Of course, these responses may be out of all proportion to the severity of the disease. It is important to discuss feelings and provide reassurance. There is a healthy way to live with disease and doctors must help acne victims to do this. Our feelings may be summarized as follows:

- Every acne patient experiences anxiety. Guilt, anger, and depression are variably intermingled.
- The physician should transmit in his own way that he knows about these feelings and does not regard them as unusual.

- The physician should indicate clearly that acne does not come from bad habits, bad living, or bad thoughts. The skin one inherits is the dominant factor; no one is responsible for his integumentary allotment.
- On the other hand, intense anxiety aggravates and perpetuates the disease. We take this to be self-evident, but the mechanisms are far from obvious. Just enough is known to permit speculations on neuroendocrine influences.
- Acne tends to get worse under great stress, not in everyone and not in the same person every time. One mechanism is clear: acne patients have a great deal of manual nervousness; they have trouble keeping their hands off their face. Girls have a heavier emotional investment in beauty and are more susceptible than boys to manual maneuvers that intensify facial lesions. These include all kinds of posturing, picking, rubbing, squeezing, pinching, holding the chin in the hands, indeed all the forces which we have enumerated under the category of acne mechanica.
- Asymmetric localization of lesions and bizarre forms of excoriations or scars, for example on one cheek or on the chin, suggest mechanical factors. Patients will frequently deny these facial assaults even while busily engaged in them.
- The physician must announce that these are kinds of tics which are unconsciously performed. Every effort should be made to raise them to consciousness and to bring this harmful behavior under control.
- Formal psychotherapy is not advised. With modern dermatologic treatment, the informed physician can accomplish a great deal more than the best psychiatrist in the land.
- On the other hand, it is fatuous to deny that some patients with serious adjustment problems may need psychotherapy. Psychotherapy should never replace skin therapy. We retain control over the rare patients we refer for psychiatric consultations.
- Psychotropic drugs which influence mood and anxiety are probably not sufficiently utilized. The prevalence of depressive states in acne is much higher than realized. Antidepressants are helpful adjuncts in selected cases. Tranquillizers have a place in getting patients over rought periods. Hypnotics should be given when sleeplessness becomes a strain on health. Psychotropic drugs are not routinely prescribed. We use them for short periods along with repeated counseling to support unusually troubled youngsters.
- Finally, the best form of psychotherapy is optimism. This is no longer unrealistic or self-deluding. Acne is a highly treatable disease, and the results are quite good in the great majority of patients. This should be cheerfully communicated to the new patient.

Koo JYM, Smith LL (1991) Psychologic aspects of acne. Pediatr Dermatol 8:185–188

Myhill JE, Leichtman SR, Burnett JW (1988) Self-esteem and social assertiveness in patients receiving isotretinoin treatment for cystic acne. Cutis 41:171–173

Rubinow DR, Peck GL, Squillace KM, Gantt GG (1987) Reduced anxiety and depression in cystic acne patients after successful treatment with oral isotretinoin. J Am Acad Dermatol 17:25–32

Van der Meeren HLM, Van der Schaar WW, Van den Hurk CMAM (1985) The psychological impact of severe acne. Cutis 7:84–86

Wu SF, Kinder BN, Trunnell TN, Fulton JE (1988) Role of anxiety and anger in acne patients: a relationship with the severity of the disorder. J Am Acad Dermatol 18:325–333

How to Approach Acne

Treatment can be aimed at various steps in the pathogenic sequence. In order of importance these are:

Preventing the Formation of Comedones. This is the central goal. Strictly speaking, this is not treatment but prophylaxis. The disease would not commence at all if horny impactions could be prevented. Topical tretinoin in children at risk will accomplish just that. It is valuable to intervene early when the first comedones appear, which may occur before obvious pubertal changes. Parents who suffered from severe acne should be told about this.

Removing Comedones. Mechanical extraction of comedones with a variety of comedo extractors, in combination with facial masks, wet towels or steam bath to soften the impacted acne is an accepted, sensible, and useful technique. Dermatologists often bring in specially trained beauticians and cosmeticians to perform this useful service which may be called the acne toilet. These physical extractions are only one component of the entire program which, of course, includes comedolytic drugs such as tretinoin. Skilful comedo extraction, especially nicking and expelling closed comedones, results in an immediate benefit which patients appreciate. Too few doctors provide this important service, relying exclusively on drugs.

Reduction of Sebum Production. The aim here is to reduce what is poetically called the "fuel of the acne flame". Minor reductions of 10%–20% are not substantial and do not clearly ameliorate the disease. At least a 30% decrease in sebum production is necessary to demonstrate clinical benefit. Two classes of drugs are available: Hormones and isotretinoin. Hormonal treatment in women with estrogens in combination with a progestin or antiandrogen (cyproterone acetate or chlormadinone acetate, available in many European countries, but not in the United States as oral contraceptives) is highly effective. An alternative is spironolactone; this is an experimental drug in acne, and should be combined with an effective contraceptive measure. Isotretinoin is unexcelled in its capacity to reduce sebum production. It has revolutionized acne treatment. Very special attention has to be paid to the use of this drug, which can lower sebum production of 80%–90%.

Preventing Rupture of Microcomedones or Mitigating the Ensuing Inflammatory Reaction. Oral antibiotics such as tetracyclines and erythromycin have these effects. Similar effects are seen after topical administration of tetracyclines, erythromycin, and clindamycin. An anti-inflammatory component is insufficiently appreciated.

Promoting the Resolution of Inflammatory Lesions. The tactic of extinguishing the fire is the least satisfactory but the easiest to accomplish. Any chemical or physical modality which enhances local blood flow will accelerate the regression of inflammatory lesions, probably by enhancing tissue clearance of mediators of inflammation or by accelerating the removal of toxic products. A papulopustule which would spontaneously dry up in about 14 days can be made to resorb in less than a week. The course of indurated papules and nodules is undoubtedly shortened by such modalities as freezing and chemical irritants which cause peeling. The past popularity of such agents as sulfur, sulfides, and resorcinol probably reflected this activity.

Improvement of Scars. Correction of scars is the provenience of the expert. Its importance psychologically cannot be over-emphasized. First, the disease should be brought under control by drugs. As soon as this is achieved, the physician is challenged to cope with the more difficult task. Some improvement is to be expected with time, as with any scar following trauma, accidents, or surgery, though deep scars may not improve with time. Cooperation with another colleague, highly skilled in dermatosurgical techniques, is warranted. The list of corrective techniques encompasses dermabrasion, excision, punch-graft elevation, collagen implant, silicon implant, autologous fat cell implants, intralesional injection of corticosteroids, marsupialization of cysts and draining sinuses, and possibly lasers.

Outdated Remedies. Practically all the venerated methods of treatment can be stuffed into this disposable rag-bag; freezing with solid carbon dioxide slush, ultraviolet radiation, innumerable irritants (e.g., resorcinol, sulfur, phenol, zinc sulfate, betanaphthol). None of these have much impact on preventing or unseating comedones. Salicylic acid is an exception, because it is moderately comedolytic.

Combination Treatment. Best results are achieved by artful combinations, using drugs which have different modes of action, for example, oral antibiotics and topical tretinoin. Many choices are available and provide the therapist with a wide repertoire of options. One should never become dependent on a single, fixed regimen.

Communication. Intimate talk between the patient and the physician is the heart of acne therapy. Minors are often accompanied by their mother, father, rarely both parents, other family members, and boy or girl friends. Listening to what the patient thinks, feels, and has already tried

and with what outcome helps to break the ice. The amount of time spent with each patient – first consultation or follow-ups – does not matter. It should be sufficient to make the patient feel that during his visit with the doctor, he is the center of the affair and gets all the attention he needs. Doctors in a hurry are poor acne therapists. Printed material such as before-and-after photographs of successfully treated patients is very helpful. Brochures by professional organisations like the American Academy of Dermatology provide readable information on all aspects of the disease. Patients greatly appreciate educational materials which they can read in private. Our anchor position is that acne can be effectively treated with a handful of drugs. The consecrated therapist will also supplement this physical modalities such as comedo extraction.

Selection of Therapy

The therapy selected depends on the type of disease. Our general approaches are listed in the following.

Comedonal Acne. Treatment is exclusively done with a topical comedolytic. The most effective agent is tretinoin. Salicylic acid is often satisfactory for mild cases. Azelaic acid is also worth a trial. Extraction of comedones, especially blackheads, is cosmetically gratifying, instantly improving appearance.

Papulopustular Acne. Treatment is commenced with a topical or an oral antibiotic and a topical comedolytic agent. Again tretinoin, benzoyl peroxide, and azelaic acid are used for the latter purpose. Benzoyl peroxide acts mostly as an antibacterial agent. Combination products are available, or single drugs can be used in an alternating way to achieve the same purpose. Topical combinations of tretinoin with an antibiotic, of benzoyl peroxide with erythromycin or an imidazole, are available. Maintenance therapy is often necessary for months or years. Severe cases of this type of acne may require hormonal treatment (in women), or even oral isotretinoin.

Acne Conglobata. Outstanding results, even cures, have been achieved with isotretinoin. This drug attacks all components of the disease process, e.g., sebum production, comedones, and inflammation. The great danger of this miracle drug is its teratogenicity. There are a number of other troublesome side effects which require scrupulous attention by the physician. This is not a drug to be prescribed lightly. It can be combined with a variety of other topical and oral drugs. Where isotretinoin is not indicated, wanted, or available, a multiple-therapy approach with a topical comedolytic (tretinoin), topical benzoyl peroxide (antibacterial action, and mild exfoliant), topical azelaic acid, topical antibiotics, oral antibiotics, intralesional corticosteroids, hormones, and possibly a sulfone, *dia*mino*di*phenyl*s*ulfone (DADPS, or DDS) are alternatives.

Severe Varieties of Acne. All severe varieties of acne call for highly skilled acne specialists. The important examples include acne fulminans, acne inversa, gram-negative folliculitis, acne tropicalis, masculinizing syndromes in women, androgen excess acne in men, and chloracne.

Coleman WP, Hanke CW, Alt TH, Askin S (eds) (1991) Cosmetic surgery of the skin. Principles and techniques. Decker, Philadelphia

Cunliffe WJ (1987) Evolution of a strategy for the treatment of acne. J Am Acad Dermatol 16:591–599

Cunliffe WJ, Stainton C, Forster RA (1983) Topical benzoyl peroxide increases sebum excretion rate in patients with acne. Br J Dermatol 109:577–579

Goldstein JA, Pochi PE (1981) Failure of benzoyl peroxide to decrease sebaceous gland secretion in acne. Dermatologica 162:287–291

Hogan DJ, To T, Wilson ER, Miller AB, Robson D, Holfeld K, Lane P (1991) A study of acne treatments as risk factors for skin cancer of the head and neck. Br J Dermatol 125:343–348

Kotler R (1992) Chemical rejuvenation of the face. Mosby Year Book, St. Louis, Missouri

Mills OH Jr, Kligman AM (1983) Drugs that are ineffective in the treatment of acne vulgaris. Br J Dermatol 108:371–374

Mills OH, Kligman AM (1972) Is sulphur helpful or harmful in acne vulgaris? Br J Dermatol 86:620–627

Orlow SJ, Kalman L, Watzki KL, Bolognia JL (1991) Skin and bones. II. J Am Acad Dermatol 25:447–462

Pepall LM, Cosgrove MP, Cunliffe WJ (1991) Ablation of whiteheads by cautery under topical anaesthesia. Br J Dermatol 125:256–259

Shaw JC (1991) Spironolactone in dermatologic therapy. J Am Acad Dermatol 24:236–243

Strauss JS, Goldman PH, Nacht S, Gans EH (1978) A reexamination of the potential comedogenicity of sulphur. Arch Dermatol 114:1340–1342

Appraisal of Efficacy

Philosophers tell us it is important to learn about history in order not to have to repeat it. The record shows that almost anything that has ever been used in acne has been found beneficial at one time or another. The same might be said about many diseases for which there was no effective therapy. The cynic might conclude that no drug is ineffective in acne. There is scarcely an instance right up to the present time of an author stating unequivocally that the drug he studied was useless. Why can't doctors recognize ineffective drugs, or harmful ones for that matter? It is a sensible maxim that if everything works, probably nothing does. There are several reasons why efficacy has been so hard to estimate. Acne is chronic. It lasts for years. During that time the disease fluctuates in severity. Even without treatment, the disease is better at some times than others. Moreover, the disease is pleomorphic with diverse types of lesions; no two patients ever seem alike. Patients like to think well of their physicians, and the latter are similarly biased towards their treatment. Hence, improvement is not likely to be regarded as spontaneous.

Emotions color acne and influence its expressions. Sometimes worsening is explicable by picking, rubbing, and excoriating the lesions during periods of stress. The mechanisms by which anxiety and stress intensify acne are conjectural. The doctor–patient experience in itself alters emotions, especially if the doctor dispenses his drugs with conviction. Youngsters of course are exceptionally impressionable. Psychic effects are nebulous and mysterious, but it would be foolhardy to deny them a role in this or any other disease, as the great physicians have always taught.

The impact of the personality of the physician may contribute to the surprisingly good results sometimes achieved by placebos. According to some double-blind studies, beneficial effects can be obtained in 50%–75% of cases. While we regard results of this magnitude as uncontrolled enthusiasm, 25% might be a reasonable figure. It is substantial nonetheless and obliges one to think that acne tends to get better when under the care of physician.

These complexities are mild, however, compared to the overriding difficulty of assessing the severity of the disease and recording in some reasonable, objective way its response to treatment. Few techniques for objectively demonstrating slow progress are available. This is not the case with acne conglobata when a dramatic regression of lesions occurs after isotretinoin. The doctor's office is a less suitable place to acquire this kind of expertise than a university clinic. Modern photography, including polarized light and ultraviolet radiation, is very useful when all elements are standardized. Counting lesions is tedious but necessary in controlled trials. Finally, intelligent dermatologists have sometimes used treatments with overall effects which were probably harmful. These are worth mentioning as a cautionary lesson for all of us.

● Injections of testosterone have been found to be helpful even though in women and in men androgens will increase sebum production and can precipitate acne conglobata or acne fulminans.

● Virtual cures have been claimed for the combination of ultraviolet radiation and crude coal tar. The latter is a potent acneigen; moreover, its capacity to induce comedones is enhanced by sunlight.

● Penicillin and various sulfonamides do not enter the follicular canal and cannot affect *Propionibacterium acnes*; nonetheless, excellent results have been secured in some reports.

● Topical antiacne medications contained, for decades, corticosteroids, ranging from hydrocortisone to dexamethasone. It took a long time to convince physicians, patients, and pharmaceutical companies that corticosteroids are actually acneigenic. Once hailed, they are now of course banned.

● Topical antibiotics were greatly overrated when they were first introduced. Many dermatologists still believe, quite erroneously, that topical antibiotics are as effective as the same drug orally. An example of an almost ineffective topical antibiotic is tetracycline. This was introduced by a major US company which utilized the options of "experts" to launch it after controlled trials. It is encouraging to report that this was a flop and has been withdrawn.

We try to adhere to the following guidelines: accurate classification is the first step. Everyone realizes that a chronic disease may have different expressions and that treatment has to be accordingly adjusted to the type and severity. The three basic types of acne (comedonal, papulopustular, and conglobata) should therefore not be thrown together. Without due concern for these considerations even effective agents may be made to appear ineffective. For example, oral antibiotics do not eliminate existing open and closed comedones. Cases dominated by open and closed comedones therefore do not respond.

Severity can be assessed by a global estimate, an overall impression of the density of lesions, or by counting the lesions. One can enumerate the various lesions on one side of the face (comedones, pustules, papules). Counting the lesions is not so simple as it sounds, and the variance is great. It is desirable for statistical purposes to have numerical data, but this method is not always reliable.

The duration of study is another variable that will upgrade the effectiveness of some treatments and downgrade others. For example, no drug is able to expel comedones in less than 6 weeks, whereas any peeling agent will reduce small inflammatory lesions within 10 days. Most cases of acne show a mixture of lesions. It requires a minimum period of 10 weeks to gain an idea of efficacy. Longer periods are desirable for studies of comparative effectiveness, 12 weeks at the least.

Despite these uncertainties there has been substantial progess. One can get along very well in all varieties of acne with three to four drugs. A huge inventory has shrunken to a small list.

Comedolytics, Exfoliants, Keratolytics, Antiseborrheics, Counterirritants

Since the time of the Babylonians, drying and peeling agents, hereafter called exfoliants, have been the mainstay of topical therapy. A motley melange of chemicals and concoctions have been placed in this grab bag. In all these years no serious efforts have been made to sort these out according to mode of action and relative efficacy. A kind of pharmacologic legitimacy has been achieved by applying titles which suggest specific chemical actions. The commonest designations are such heady terms as keratolytic and keratoplastic, despite the fact that the latter is practically without meaning (besides being obsolete) and the former is not generally applicable to these agents. Other high-impact words are reducing agents, oxidants, and antiseborrheics. The truth is that these terms are pure jargon whose value lies in the comforting selfdelusion that the therapist knows what he is accomplishing with his pharmacologic tools.

A critical look at exfoliants is in order. Whatever else they may or may not be, they are all primary irritants. They damage the superficial layers of skin and incite an inflammatory response. This stimulates mitosis, the epidermis becomes acanthotic, corneocyte production increases, the horny layer temporarily thickens and soon begins to show scaling. Erythema often accompanies these events as might be expected for irritants.

Exfoliants are usually described as having the capacity to bring about drying and peeling. We avoid such language because the connotations are quite misleading. Dryness is usually interpreted as a sign of decreased oiliness. While the skin indeed looks dry, measurements of sebum production do not reveal a decrease. Indeed, this may even increase as a nonspecific response to irritation. Scales soak up sebum, masking the true secretion. Appearances are very deceiving as regards oiliness. Merely sweating or wetting the surface will instantly make the face look a good deal oilier than it is. Decreased sweating, often induced by exfoliants, creates an illusion of less oiliness, especially if accompanied by scaling.

Likewise, it is fallacious to imagine that peeling reflects a keratolytic action. Exfoliants, as a rule, do not attack fibrous proteins (keratins). Hence they are not keratolytics. Nice as it would be, they do not dissolve comedones. True keratolytics such as sodium hydroxide or barium sulfide cannot be tolerated. Salicylic acid has very limited ability to disorganize keratin unless used in high concentrations.

We use the term comedolytic to designate agents that accelerate the loss or retard the formation of comedones. We have revived the term counterirritants for agents that promote the resorption of inflammatory lesions. These are mainly chemical irritants. It seems that any measure which stimulates blood flow shortens healing time moderately. A pustule, for example, heals in about 14 days, depending on its size. With counterirritants this may take half as long.

Comedolytic activity is assayed in an experimental rabbit ear model. Tretinoin (retinoic acid) is unsurpassed in its comedolytic activity. Benzoyl peroxide is barely active; in fact, most proprietary 5%–10% formulations are comedogenic. One of the old veterans, salicylic acid, is moderately comedolytic, the following are not: phenol, resorcinol, betanaphthol, sulfur, and sodium thiosulfate. Hence, only a few agents which cause peeling are in fact comedolytic. The probable explanation is that most of them affect only the epidermis and not the follicular infrainfundibulum.

As regards counterirritants there is little to choose among them at doses which produce equivalent degrees of inflammation. They all promote resorption of inflammatory lesions, though differing of course in esthetic qualities. The more intensive the inflammatory reaction, the swifter the response. Therefore, the more powerful irritants are more effective, although more difficult to handle. We do not recommend counterirritants; they are historical leftovers.

The Sulfur Affair

The difficulties of assessing the therapeutic value of exfoliants is vividly illustrated by the special case of sulfur. Sulfur was for a long time the most common ingredient in antiacne formulations. It is still present in many proprietary preparations, often in combination with benzoyl peroxide, resorcinol, and others. It has been esteemed by laymen and dermatologists alike. Sulfur suddenly was seen in a new light when it was found to be strongly comedogenic in the rabbit ear model. Applied under admittedly unphysiologic conditions for several weeks to the backs of volunteers, microscopic comedones were evoked. We have been able to show that known comedogens such as tars always induce comedones in the rabbit ear. Because of this parallelism we consider the results of the rabbit test to be realistic. Consequently, we have raised the question whether sulfur may be more harmful than helpful in acne. It should be added that it is elemental sulfur and not compounds of sulfur that are comedogenic.

Sulfides, sulfites, thioglycolates, thiols, cysteines or thioacetamides do not provoke comedones.

We think that sulfur may actually perpetuate acne by laying down crops of new comedones. If so, how did keen clinicians all over the world become persuaded of its therapeutic powers? The foregoing discussion unlocks this paradox. Sulfur is undeniably an effective counterirritant. We see sulfur as truly subversive in its effects. It potentiates the natural tendency of acne patients to form comedones. This is an insidious activity for it takes many months for a comedo to become visible. Therefore, such an effect would be very difficult to discern. On the other hand, the doctor and patient both focus on the irksome, conspicuous pustules and papules. They are pleased when these symptomatic lesions are resorbed so quickly, an effect which can be seen in a few days. Thus, while sulfur banishes inflammatory lesions, at the same time it incites the comedones from which these spring. The subversive activity of sulfur is hard to expose because it acts on two levels: one above the surface in which it is benign, and one below in which it is malicious. We see little justification for the continued use of sulfur, as better and less offensive exfoliants are now available.

Therapeutic Adjuncts

Above   The surgical armamentarium for comedo extraction. Comedo extractors can be used effectively to remove comedones. Therapists have a wide choice of models

Below   The so-called acne toilet is an ancient elegant way to get rid of visible open and closed comedones. Cosmeticians, ideally trained and supervised by a dermatologist, can achieve respectable results

Left   A pointed blade has been inserted into a closed comedo to enable extrusion of the contents by gentle pressure with a comedo extractor

Right   An open comedo has just been unrooted *lege artis*. Closed comedones are sometimes resistant to ordinary extraction procedures. A refined technique consists of the ablation by cautery under topical anesthesia. The anesthetic is EMLA cream (0.025% lidocaine and 0.025% prilocaine). EMLA stands for *e*utectic *m*ixture of *l*ocal *a*nesthetics. It is applied 1–3 h prior to cautery under occlusive dressing

Pepall LM, Cosgrove MP, Cunliffe WJ (1991) Ablation of whiteheads by cautery under topical anaesthesia. Br J Dermatol 125:256–259

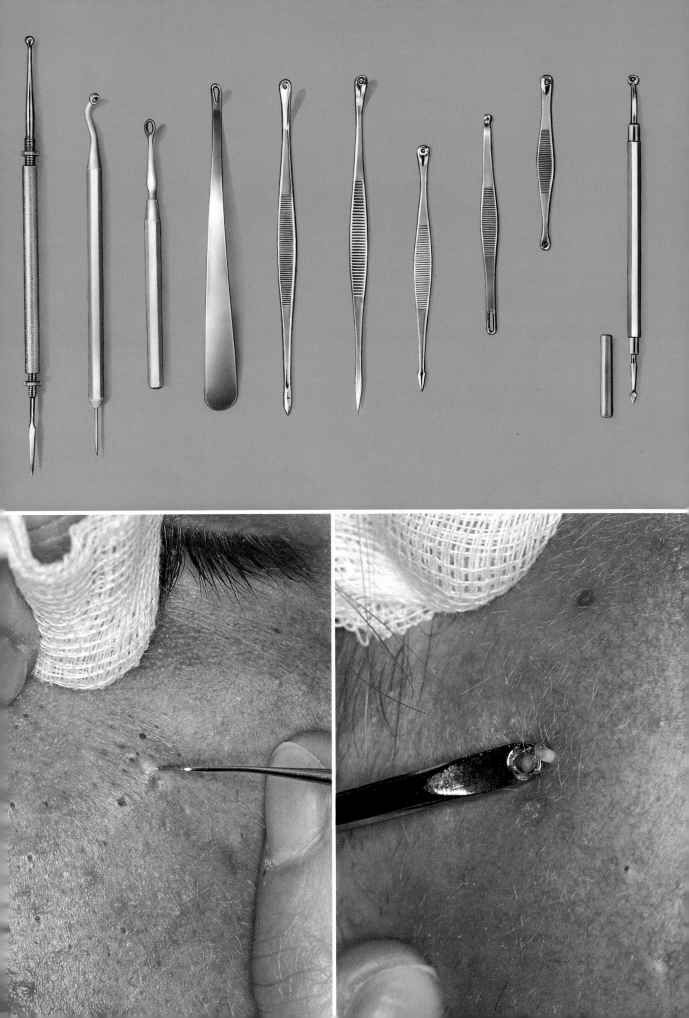

The Refinements of Comedo Extraction

Ideally the epithelium encapsulating comedones should be expelled along with the horny core, thereby obliterating the lesion permanently. Usually, the epithelial lining remains behind to continue a career of comedo-building.

Above   The epithelial lining remains in situ

Left   An open comedo immediately after extraction. The comedo has come out naked without any of its encapsulating epithelium. Loss of horn and bacterial lacunae during sectioning accounts for the large cavities. Open comedones can be much more readily extracted in toto than closed ones

Right   The collapsed follicle from which the comedo on the left has just been extracted. The epithelium is intact. Since it is no longer under pressure, it gets thrown into folds. In this case, most of the horny impaction has been extracted. By contrast closed comedones are more firmly anchored. Surprising quantities of horn may remain in the deeper portion

Below   The epithelial lining has prolapsed

Left   A large, mature comedo, full of bacterial cavities, has just been delivered by a comedo extractor. No stretch of the comedonal epithelium is connected with this kernel

Right   Biopsy immediately after extraction of the open comedo shown on the left. In this instance, the encapsulating epithelium has completely prolapsed through the orifice. The sebaceous acini remain in the dermis. In successful extractions, one can often see a tail of whitish, filmy material hanging from the base of the comedo. This is the everted epithelial capsule. Delivery of the capsule along with the horny core requires a spartan patient and a determined therapist. Most comedo extraction is too delicately performed, but too forcible extraction may cause scarring

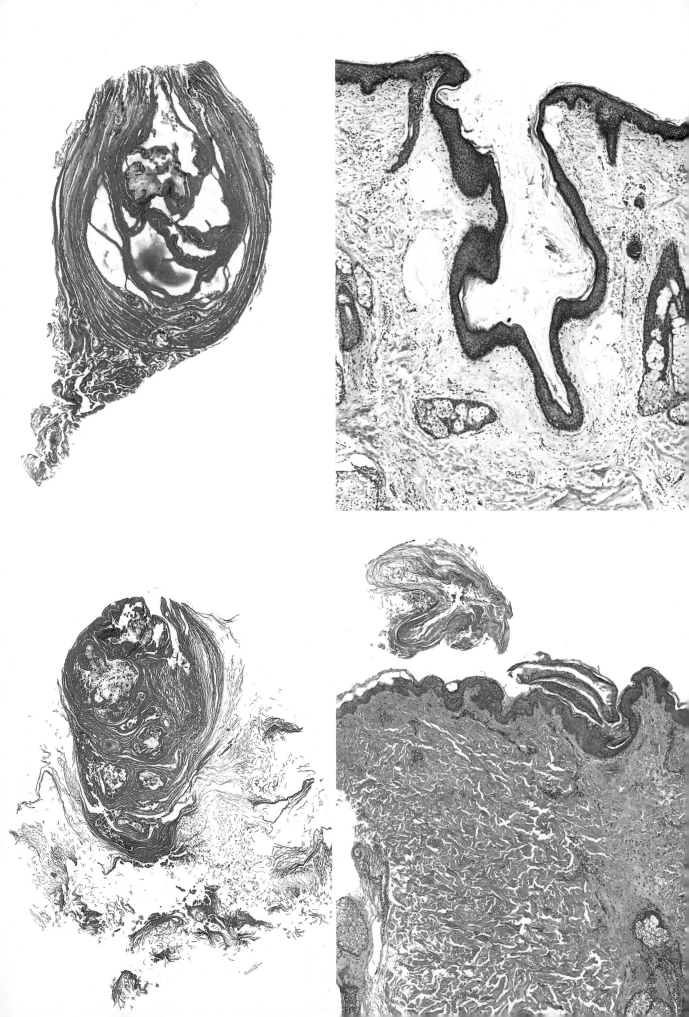

Comedo Extraction

Above

Left   The open comedo shown on the right was expressed, and the site biopsied 1 h later. A defect is visible where the comedo resided. Edema and perivascular lymphohistiocytic infiltrate remain as evidence of the injury. The epidermal wound will epithelialize very soon. A fine scar is possible, at least histologically

Right   The expelled comedo with the entire epithelium attached to it like a lasso

Below

Left   An open comedo was gently extracted, and the site biopsied immediately afterwards. The comedonal epithelium is thrown into folds and resembles a sebaceous follicle. It is surprising to find considerable quantities of corneocytes left in situ. There are two possiblities: a normal sebaceous follicle will be reconstituted, or a new comedo may form

Right   Two days previously an open comedo was extracted. Much of the comedo was evidently not delivered, a common happening even after careful comedo extraction

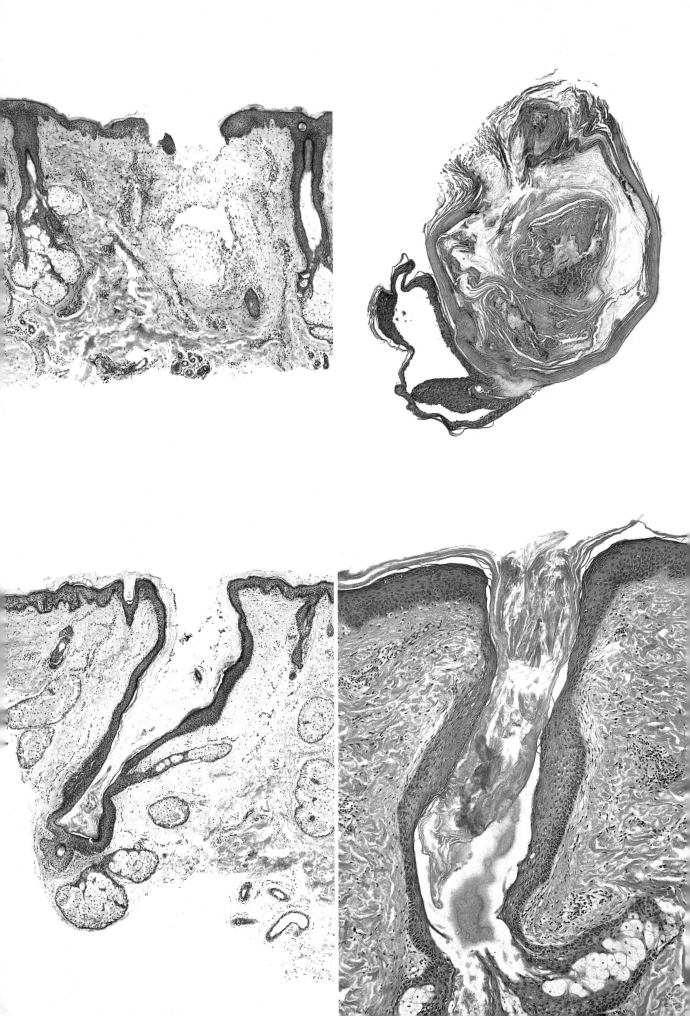

Comedo Extraction Is Often Incomplete, and Refilling Fast

Despite expertise in the manual extraction of open and closed comedones with comedo extractors, surprising quantities of the comedonal core are left behind. Also refilling is often very fast.

Above

Left   Biopsy 1 day after the comedo extraction. Although the inner core was successfully brought to the skin surface, the peripheral portion was not. The comedonal epithelium is intact except for a microscopic defect to the upper left with accumulation of granulocytes and lymphocytes. This comedo will definitely refill

Right   Considerable parts of this closed comedo were squeezed out 30 days ago. It must have caused inflammation, as can be appreciated from the parakeratotic and inflammatory debris in the center of the kernel, and the pericomedonal fibrosis

Below

Left   Open comedones are usually easier to extract than closed ones. This example is still in existence 15 days after comedo extraction, and is in the process of exactly repeating its previous life cycle. A comedonal core is being built up, and the sebaceous acini are intact, although small. Extensive pericomedonal scarring with hypercellular fibrosis shows that during the extraction the comedo epithelium ruptured

Right   If this open comedo had not been tattooed (one is to the left next to the vellus follicle, the right one outside this magnification), one would hardly believe that it was successfully extracted 28 days ago. It has completely refilled. Open and closed comedones refill fast. About three layers of corneocytes are produced in 2 days. Thus within 2–3 months a visible comedo reforms

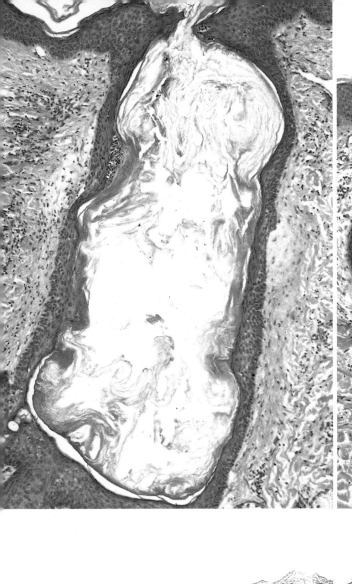
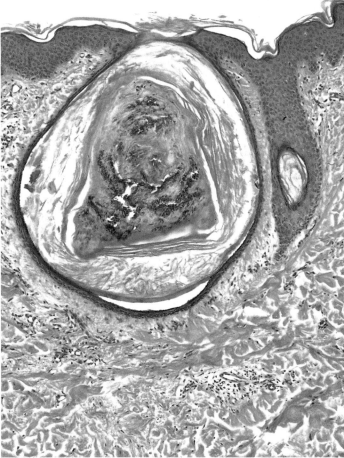
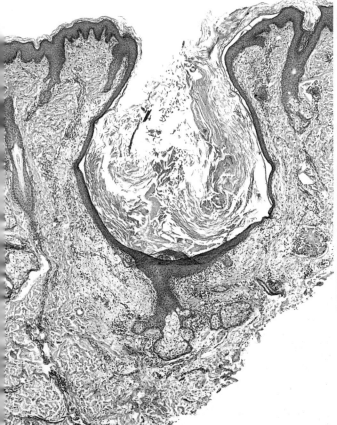
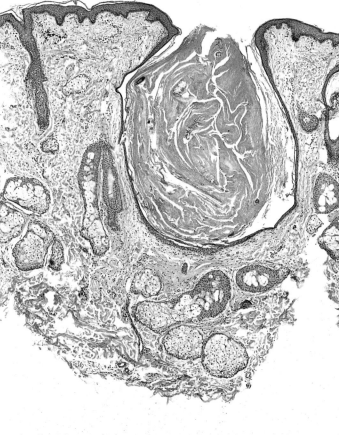

How Beneficial or Detrimental Is Comedo Extraction?

These figures illustrate the in situ reaction to properly performed comedo extraction.

Above

Left   An open comedo was extracted 24 h earlier. The comedonal epithelium has survived, although it is injured. It is acanthotic and engaged in wound repair. Considerable portions of the comedo kernel are still in place, now mixed with an granulocytic cell infiltrate. In essence this comedo will survive and leave a miniature scar

Right   This open comedo was extracted 24 h earlier. The upper part of the comedonal epithelium has survived, but this will not be enough to establish a new follicle or recurrent comedo. The lower portion of the comedonal epithelium has prolapsed. Localized hemorrhage and mixed granulocytic–lymphocytic infiltrate are typical sequels of comedo extraction. A fine scar will certainly remain

Below

Left   A closed comedo was not only expressed 24 days ago, but has been permanently laid to rest. The price is a scar, with many multinucleated giant cells, macrophages, and lymphocytes cleaning up the debris. smoldering inflammation will go on for weeks

Right   Three weeks previously a closed comedo was brought to the skin surface. No comedo has reformed, but the comedonal epithelium survived, transforming into an odd shaped follicle. In this section only its upper and lower pole are visible. The entire length of the epithelial structure is still surrounded by a dense infiltrate. Scarring fibrosis is a late consequence of this therapeutic maneuver

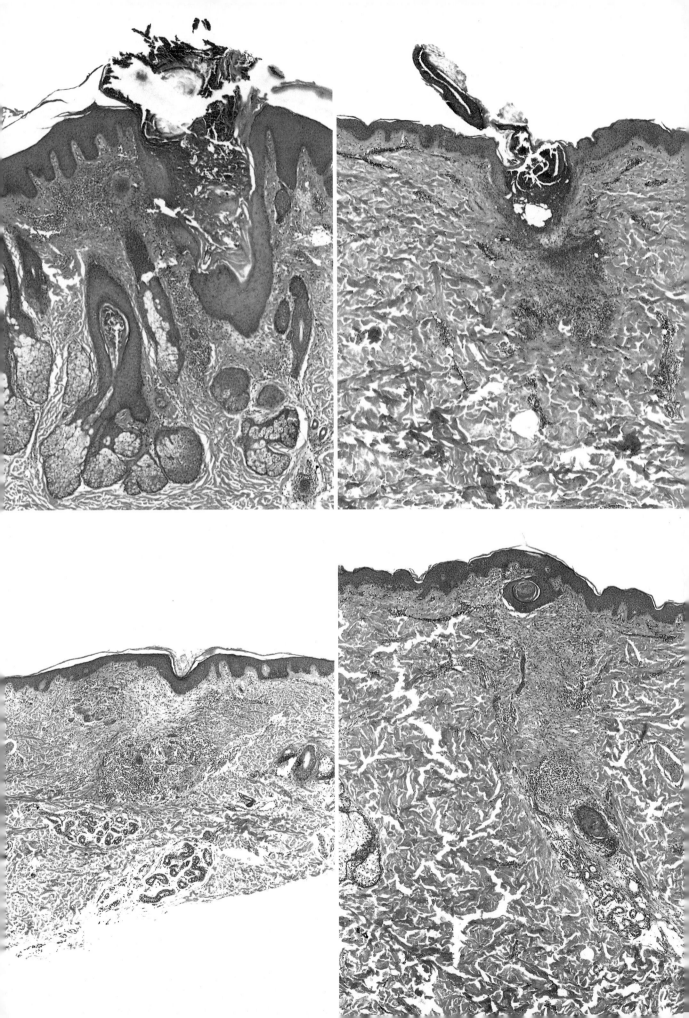

Sequels of Comedo Extraction

Removal of comedones is common practice, but the histologic events of this physical trauma are hardly studied. It is surprising how much inflammation and damage can result from this maneuver.

Above

Left   An open comedo was quite forcefully extracted, in a way that was painful to the patient. The same site was biopsied 24 h later. First of all, there is quite heavy inflammation where the comedonal epithelium was ruptured. Abscesses around and within the comedo almost amount to a papule. Hemorrhage is also present

Right   Thirty-five days previously a closed comedo was extracted. It has not reformed; instead a bizarre-shaped sebaceous follicle has formed, not producing coherent corneocytes. The tattoo to the right and left identifies the lesion

Below   A secondary comedo has formed 26 days after mechanical extraction of its kernel. The comedo is asymmetric and still full of dense horn. Pericomedonal fibrosis reveals that rupture of the epithelium and fibrosis followed the too forceful comedo extraction

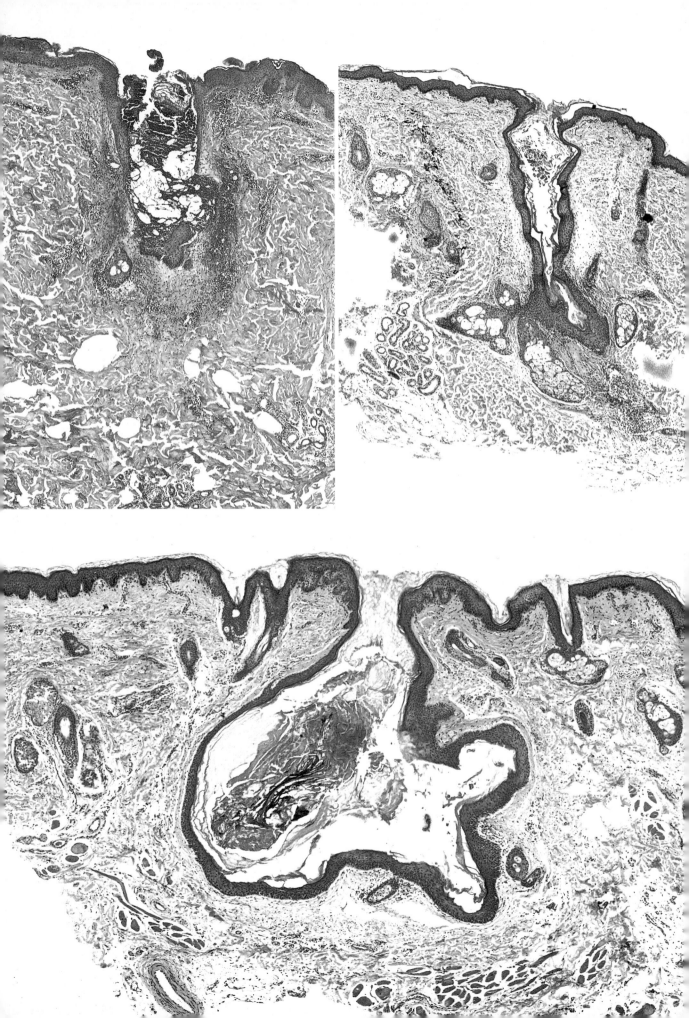

Complications Following Comedo Removal

The urge to remove comedones is understandable, but risky. Comedones are crushed between fingers too often, and their contents pushed into the dermis, thus inciting foreign body reactions.

Above This papulopustule was forcefully squeezed between the fingers 3 weeks prior to the biopsy. To encapsulate the abscess, the comedonal epithelium has to migrate far out. A chronic inflammation surrounds the lesion with lymphocytes, macrophages, and multinucleated giant cells

Below This open comedo was popped out using the fingers 2 months ago. The comedonal epithelium was simultaneously injured. Parakeratotic debris is indicative of the inflammation and repair. The comedonal epithelium is intact again. Wide spread, still inflamed fibrotic tissue indicates the extent of tissue damage

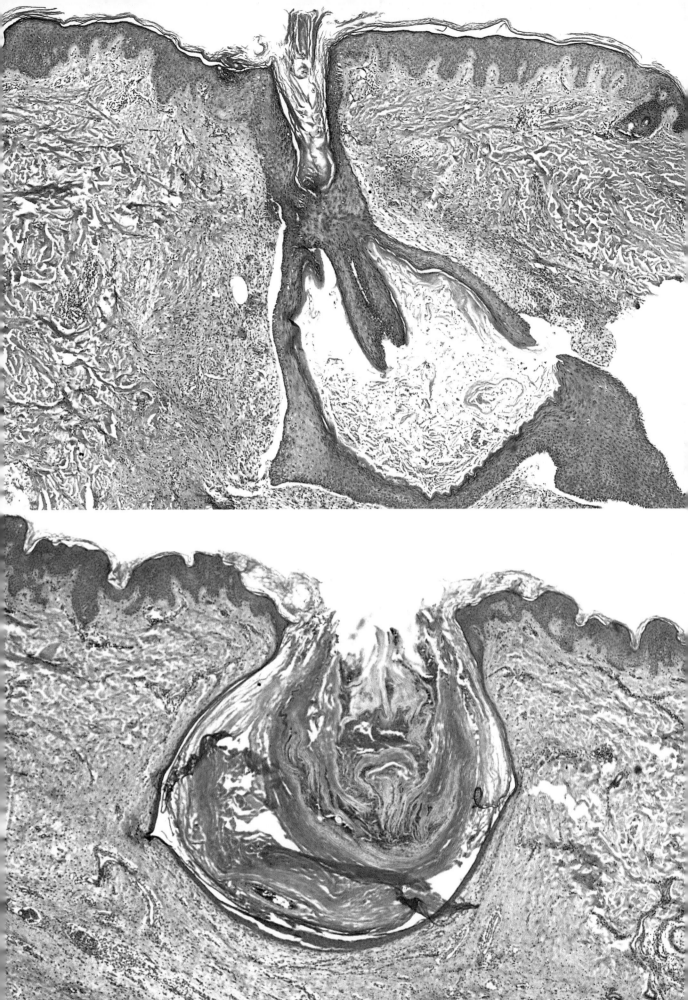

Tretinoin (*all-trans*-Retinoic Acid, Vitamin A Acid)

Historical Background

Vitamin A and its derivatives have been known for over 40 years to influence keratinization and epithelial differentiation. In 1962, Stüttgen in Düsseldorf and Beer in Basel independently demonstrated the efficacy of topical tretinoin (retinoic acid, vitamin A acid) in various neoplasms of the skin and chronic hyperkeratotic disorders, especially ichthyoses. They were not particularly impressed by the degree of benefit in acne vulgaris. In the late 1960s Kligman and his co-workers in Philadelphia were the first to show unequivocally that topical tretinoin was a very useful drug. Tretinoin did not become popular overnight. It took a decade before dermatologists finally became convinced that its beneficial effects were unique and predictable. Today it is the comedolytic prescription drug par excellence.

After that pioneering introduction, retinoid research took off like a rocket. The nuclear receptors of this family of hormones have been cloned, and include receptors for tretinoin, estrogen, progesterone, glucocorticoids, mineralocorticoids, thyroxin (T_3), and 1,25-dihydroxy vitamin D_3. Dermatologists, pharmacologists, toxicologists, oncologists, and immunologists have been caught up in retinoid investigation. Oral retinoids have revolutionized many fields of medicine. Next to corticosteroids and antibiotics, retinoids are the most interesting and important drugs to have appeared on the dermatologic scene.

Mode of Action

It will be sufficient here merely to mention those biologic effects which explain the efficacy of this drug in acne and acneiform disorders.

Comedolytic Effects. Tretinoin interferes with comedo formation by preventing corneocytes within the follicular canal from sticking together to form solid impactions. Thus the primary lesions are removed. No other drug matches the comedolytic action of tretinoin.

The drug inhibits synthesis of tonofilaments and promotes the detachment of desmosomes, thus lessening the attachment between keratinized cells. The result is premature shedding of epidermal corneocytes, leading to thinning of the horny layer. The mechanisms underlying enhanced dehiscence are poorly understood and may involve alterations of the intercellular lipids which are responsible for the cohesion of corneocytes. The fragile corneocytes thus fall apart soon after their formation. The prevention of comedo formation by tretinoin largely explains its prophylactic effect on the cause of the disease.

It cannot be too strongly emphasized that tretinoin is not simply a potent peeling agent. Ultrastructural studies and biochemical analysis show that the actions of the drug are specific and quite different from classical peeling agents such as resorcinol or phenol. In fact, the latter are not comedolytic.

Proliferation. Tretinoin increases mitotic activity of interfollicular and follicular epithelia and thus accelerates the turnover of keratinocytes. The rate of production of loose corneocytes is increased, as has been demonstrated with various autoradiographic techniques. This has two effects:

● Existing open comedones become loosened and expelled
● Closed comedones are more rapidly transformed into open ones followed by extrusion from the follicles

The follicular epithelium enclosing microcomedones as well as open and closed comedones becomes less sturdy and more permeable as a result of increased proliferative activity and the generation of a mucus-like substance which is deposited between keratinizing cells. This is accompanied by hyperplasia of the epithelium and intercellular edema. Toxic substances within follicles and comedones can leak out more easily, inciting rupture. The blow-up of inapparent comedones leads to their elimination. It is the detonation of these time bombs that accounts for the outcropping of pustules which sometimes occurs in the first weeks of treatment. Patients should be warned of this possibility, otherwise they will see this beneficial event as an unwelcome, disturbing side effect.

Tretinoin stimulates the formation of new blood vessels in the papillary dermis (angiogenesis) resulting in increased blood flow. The rosy hue of the skin of patients receiving tretinoin is in part due to this effect. The richly supplied skin heals faster, and toxic materials are cleared more quickly. It is well known that pretreatment of facial skin with tretinoin prior to dermabrasion and chemical peels promotes re-epithelialization and swifter healing, along with improvement of surface texture. Another useful effect is the gradual deposition of new collagen which

begins after several months of daily application. These various effects of tretinoin have been exploited in the treatment of photoaged skin in older people.

Counter Irritation. In our first reports we emphasized only the comedolytic action of this retinoid and understated its value in inflammatory acne. Subsequently impressive results were obtained with all inflammatory types of acne, including acne conglobata. Tretinoin stimulates blood flow and aids in the clearance of persistent papules and pustules. There is evidence that retinoids have anti-inflammatory activity and can lead to more rapid resolution of inflamed tissue, including granulomatous reactions. Contrary to our prior belief, tretinoin can be successfully and very effectively combined with other topical remedies. Combinations with antibiotics (erythromycin) and imidazoles are available, and concomitant or alternative application of benzoyl peroxide, topical antibiotics, sunscreens, and of course systemic drugs is en vogue today.

Miscellaneous

Tretinoin is not a contact sensitizer, and despite some controversy it is not photocarcinogenic. Twenty years of use have proved its safety in this respect. Patients may experience a sensation of burning when exposed to sunlight or even a mild sunburn while on tretinoin. This does not imply increased photosensitivity, but is easily explained by the thinned stratum corneum and a decreased shield of melanin within epithelial and stratum corneum cells.

Systemic toxicity is unlikely, since no more than 3%–4% of the applied dose is absorbed. This is important to know in view of the teratogenicity from oral tretinoin or its isomer isotretinoin. The effects of multiple and excessive topical applications of isotretinoin have not yielded measurable plasma concentrations of isotretinoin, tretinoin, or its major metabolite 4-oxy-isotretinoin. Hence there is no danger of teratogenicity, and the adverse effects of tretinoin are purely local.

Indications

The beneficial effects of tretinoin are most evident in comedonal acne. However, the drug can be used to advantage in all other forms of acne, particularly in combination with other drugs with different mode of action, e.g., antibiotics. It must be remembered that all expressions of acne begin with the microcomedo; hence, the comedolytic effect predicts clinical efficacy. All variants of contact acne due to external agents, e.g., acne cosmetica, pomade acne, oil acne, and chloracne, respond well. Tretinoin is very useful for prophylaxis after bringing inflammatory acne under control by systemic drugs such as isotretinoin. Application two to three times weekly is often sufficient as a maintenance dose to prevent relapse. All age groups can be treated, even infants.

Clinical Guidelines

Tretinoin is a potent drug and cannot be used in a casual way. It is exceedingly important to provide detailed instructions during the first consultation. The mode of action and the side effects should be carefully explained. Tolerance varies greatly, hence treatment must be individualized. Tretinoin is a powerful exfoliant and can cause tenderness, redness, and scaling with excessive use. Nonetheless we advocate aggressive therapy, guided by careful instructions. Benefits may be

secured more speedily in this way although some initial discomfort must be endured. Acne patients, especially those with severe disease, are usually a forbearing and cooperative lot if they trust the doctor.

At the start the patients are advised to apply the drug once nightly to the entire face from the hairline to the ear and laterally down to the jaw-line, including lips and nose, using just enough to provoke a modest flush or blush. This will be accompanied by a variable amount of stinging and burning. Smarting for a few minutes after application is common. After about 10 days, the patient will have learned how much to apply to produce mild scaling and slight redness. Pubertal children are more reactive than older adolescents. Fair-skinned, blue-eyed Northern Europeans, especially freckled, light-skinned Celts who sunburn easily and tan poorly, tend to react more strongly. For these and for anxious patients treatment should be at first every other day for about 2 weeks to allow the skin to accommodate. Thick-skinned, oily, pigmented, or Mediterranean skin types usually tolerate tretinoin very well, allowing one to start with higher concentrations. For those with sensitive skin, including flushers, blushers, and atopics, one must start with the lowest concentration and then slowly increased it. Tretinoin is more irritating in cold, dry, wintry weather. When prescribing a course of tretinoin, the following points should be borne in mind:

- Avoid the corners of the eyes and mouth; these areas are very easily irritated. Fissures at the mouth can be moderated by applying colorless lipstick several times a day or by frequently applying petrolatum.
- Stop all other local treatment. Inquire about cosmetic practices. Tretinoin intensifies the action of irritating chemicals. Severe reactions can develop this

way. It is surprising how often patients continue to use some other peeling or abrasive remedies unless explicitly told to cease. Combination therapy with antibiotics and benzoyl peroxide is recommended only after the patient has accommodated to tretinoin.

- Avoid excessive washing with soaps. The patient should wash no more than twice daily and washing should be gentle, with warm water, and fingers should be used rather than wash cloths. Soaps are irritants and are likely to be overused by acne patients obsessed with removing oil from the skin surface. Intensive use of soaps also make the skin more permeable by damaging the barrier. Inflammatory reactions arising in this way are sometimes blamed on tretinoin. Mild liquid soaps are available and are preferable to bar soaps for patients with sensitive skin.

- Do not apply tretinoin immediately after shaving. The package insert recommends waiting after washing before applying tretinoin. This is, however, not necessary and weakens compliance. We suggest that tretinoin be applied to the face after patting it dry. It spreads more easily on a damp surface. Prohibit toners, astringents, and pre- or aftershaves, which generally contain volatile solvents such as ethanol.

- Avoid direct and prolonged exposure to sunshine. Although tretinoin is not phototoxic and indeed does not appreciably increase the risk of a sunburn, sunlight, mainly through infrared radiation, induces painful sensations of smarting and burning. This is a transient phenomenon and disappears as tolerance develops. Sunscreens are always rcommended during the sunny season.

- In many patients an outcropping of pustules occurs within 2–4 weeks. It is important to inform the patients of this possibility. Pustulation is sometimes mistaken for bacterial infection. It represents in fact a blowing up of invisible microcomedones. Although the patient looks worse, this episode can be met with equanimity by the informed. The detonation of these occult lesions is a welcome event which arrests progression of the disease. Patients should be told that this is a favorable response. The pustules heal swiftly without scarring unless excoriated.

- Darkly pigmented individuals, including type IV Caucasians and Blacks, will sometimes experience some diffuse pigment lightening. This never amounts to more than slight hypopigmentation and is completely reversible. The very same effect is deliberately used in patients who want to get rid of mottled actinic hyperpigmentation, postinflammatory hyperpigmentation, melasma, and many other kinds of hyperpigmented lesions of the face. Tretinoin greatly shortens epidermal turnover. Keratinocytes do not remain in the basal region long enough to receive a full cargo of melanin from neighboring melanocytes. In Blacks, inflammatory lesions tend to leave hyperpigmented spots for a long time. These slowly bleach out after months of tretinoin use.

- Skin irritation generally occurs in the early stage of treatment. The skin invariably becomes hardened with continuous therapy. In the first weeks the skin may react strongly to a concentration which later will be completely innocuous. Generally inflammation reaches a peak within 4–6 weeks. Thereafter tretinoin treatment may be maintaincd with littlc or no visiblc rcaction. While we favor aggressive therapy to induce hardening, it must be emphasized that satisfactory therapeutic results can be secured without appreciable irritation.

- It has become clear that tretinoin cannot be used by all patients in the same way. Physicians do also not agree on the best way to use the drug. Irritant reactions are more common in winter, solutions are more irritating than creams, and of course, higher concentrations harsher than lower ones. Susceptibility of races and individuals varies greatly. Physicians practicing in cold climates encounter different problems from those in warm and moist climatic zones. Frequently patients who have experienced major side effects from excessive use of tretinoin prescribed by unknowledgeable doctors, abandon the drug and refuse to use it again. This can only happen when the effects of tretinoin are not properly explained. Manufacturers supply the drug in different vehicles and different concentrations to allow individualized treatment. In the USA there is only one manufacturer (Ortho Pharmaceuticals), whereas in other countries the market is more competitive. In Germany there are four pharmaceutical companies which provide tretinoin formulations. From 1992, the changing legislation of the Common European Market has allowed an even greater number of manufacturers. Presently the pharmaceutical forms include solutions (0.05% and 0.025%), creams (0.1%, 0.05%, and 0.025%), and gels (0.05% and 0.025%).
  Exact delivery from tubes to minimize over- or underapplication was recently made possible by a unit dispensing cap (Retin-A with Delcap). This allows the same dose to be applied each time from the metered cap.
- Swift improvement should not be promised. As a rule we urge patients not to judge the value of treatment until about after eight weeks. In Grade II–III comedonal acne or papulopustular acne, good to excellent results can be obtained in about 75% of cases within 3 months. A reduction in lesion count of more than 50% is considered good, and of more than 75% excellent. Of course some patients may not benefit at all, reject the drug vehemently, or are scared.
- Tretinoin should be used indefinitely as long as clinical activity is apparent. Relapse usually occurs within 6–10 weeks after stopping the drug. Complete withdrawal should be periodically tried in older patients in whom the signs of the disease have abated.
- Can tretinoin be used during pregnancy or nursing? Tretinoin falls into category C (key to the Food and Drug Administration's pregnancy categories). Category C means that a risk cannot be ruled out. Human studies are lacking. However, potential benefits may justify the theoretical risk. Also caution should be exercised when tretinoin is prescribed to a nursing mother. The threat of litigation has led many dermatologists in the USA to forswear tretinoin during pregnancy. We think the risk of teratogenicity is negligible to absent, but understand the decision to delay tretinoin during pregnancy and lactation.

Beer P (1962) Untersuchungen über die Wirkung der Vitamin-A-Säure. Dermatologica 124:192–195

Bernerd F, Ortonne JP, Bouclier M, Chatelus A, Hensby C (1991) The rhino mouse model: the effects of topically applied *all-trans* retinoic acid and CD271 on the fine structure of the epidermis and utricle wall of pseudocomedones. Arch Dermatol Res 283:100–107

Bollag W (1983) Vitamin A and retinoids: from nutrition to pharmacotherapy in dermatology and oncology. Lancet I:860–863

Cunliffe WJ, Miller AJ (eds) (1984) Retinoid therapy. A review of clinical and laboratory research. MTP Press, Lancaster

Fisher GJ, Esmann J, Griffiths CEM, Talwar HS, Duell EA, Hammerberg C, Elder JT, Karabin GD,

Nickoloff BJ, Cooper KD, Voorhees JJ (1991) Cellular, immunologic and biochemical characterization of topical retinoic acid – treated human skin. J Invest Dermatol 96:699–707

International Symposium Flims, Switzerland (1975) The therapeutic use of vitamin A acid. Acta Derm Venereol [Suppl 74] (Stockh) 55

Kligman AM, Fulton JE, Plewig G (1969) Topical vitamin A acid in acne vulgaris. Arch Dermatol 99:469–476

Korting HC, Braun-Falco O (1989) Efficacy and tolerability of combined topical treatment of acne vulgaris with tretinoin and erythromycin in general practice. Drugs Exp Clin Res 15:447–451

Lammer EJ, Chen DT, Hoar RM, Agnish ND, Benke PJ, Braun JT, Curry CJ, Fernhoff PM, Grix AW, Lott IT, Richard JM, Sun SC (1985) Retinoic acid embryopathy. N Engl J Med 313:837–841

Lehman PA, Malany AM (1989) Evidence for percutaneous absorption of isotretinoin from the photo-isomerization of topical tretinoin. J Invest Dermatol 93:595–599

MacKie RM (ed) (1988) Retinoids. Pergamon, Oxford

Orfanos CE, Braun-Falco O, Farber EM, Grupper C, Polano MK, Schuppli R (eds) (1981) Retinoids. Advances in basic research and therapy. Springer, Berlin Heidelberg New York

Plewig G, Braun-Falco O (1975) Kinetics of epidermis and adnexa following vitamin A acid in the human. Acta Derm Venereol [Suppl 74] (Stockh) 55:87–98

Saurat JH (ed) (1985) Retinoids: new trends in research and therapy. Karger, Basel

Schwartz E, Cruickshank FA, Mezick JA, Kligman LH (1991) Topical all-*trans* retinoic acid stimulates collagen synthesis in vivo. J Invest Dermatol 96:975–978

Stadler R, Roenigk H, Gollnick H, Peck GL, Vahlquist A (1987) Retinoids. Experimental and clinical results. Dermatologica [Suppl 1] 175:1–204

Stüttgen G (1962) Zur Lokalbehandlung der Keratosen mit Vitamin-A-Säure. Dermatologica 124:65–80

Willhite CC, Sharma RP, Allen PV, Berry DL (1990) Percutaneous retinoid absorption and embryotoxicity. J Invest Dermatol 95:523–529

An Excellent Therapeutic Result with Tretinoin

Above   This 13-year-old girl had numerous closed comedones and mildly inflamed papules

Below   Tretinoin solution 0.05% was applied twice daily. Clearing was complete in 2 months

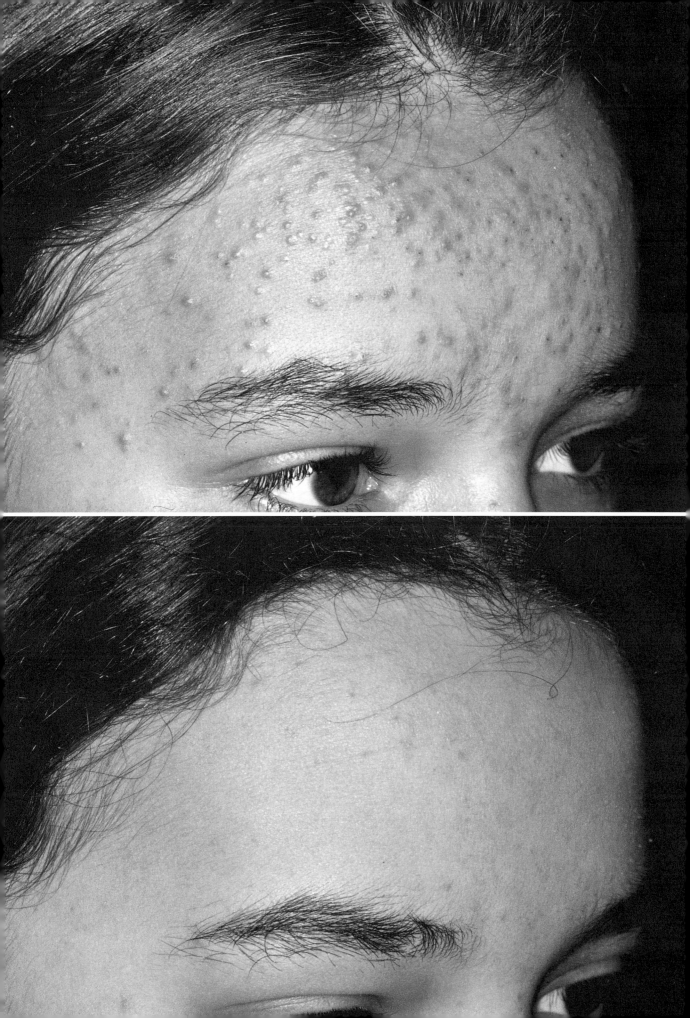

Acne Venenata: Successfully Treated with Tretinoin

Acne venenata (contact acne) is common in women, but also seen in men. Both illustrated cases came from inappropriate grooming habits.

Above   Prolonged use of a very popular moisturizing cream, applied daily for many months induced closed and open comedones. The woman was not aware of the causal relationship. Topical application of tretinoin removed all lesions. No maintenance therapy was required

Below   Another example of cosmetic-induced acne venenata. After shaving, this man preferred to use an aftershave cream on his face. Unfortunately it was comedogenic, and he acquired comedones all over his face. Tretinoin was highly effective

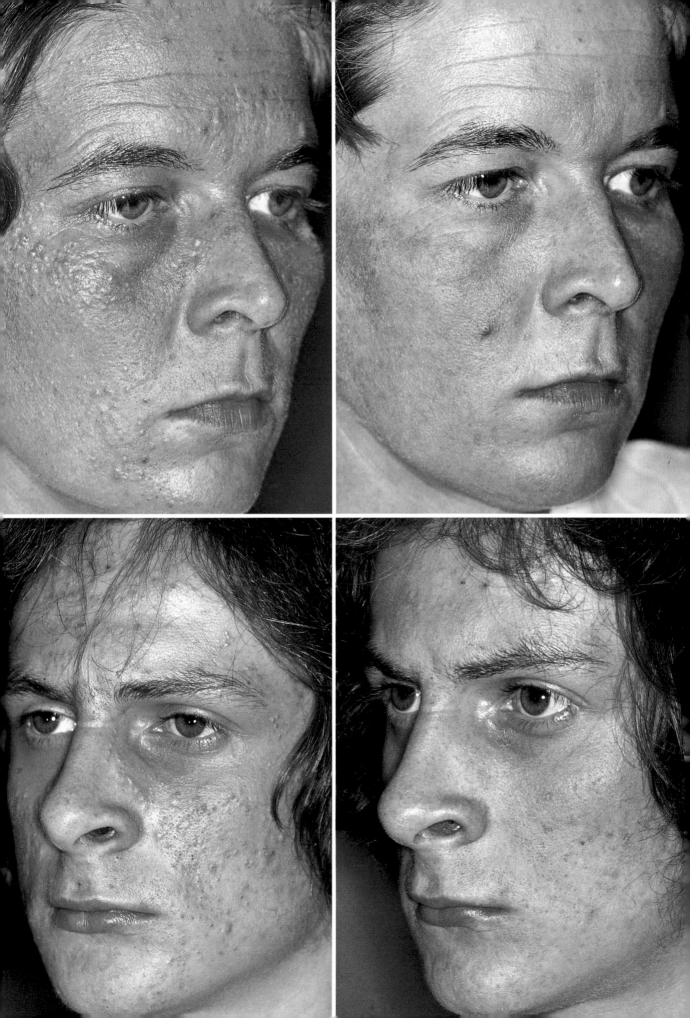

Proliferative Activity of Epidermis and Comedones and the Effects of Tretinoin

Autoradiographic techniques with tritiated thymidine incorporation provide an impression of proliferative activity. Normal untreated and normal tretinoin-treated skin of the upper back is compared with untreated comedonal and tetinoin-treated comedonal epithelium. All specimens are 45-min autoradiographs with tritiated thymidine, counterstained with hematoxilin.

Top Normal epidermis. Regular features with rete pegs and a few labeled cells in the basal cell layer. The labeling index is about 5%

Upper middle Tretinoin-stimulated epidermis. Marked acanthosis and papillomatosis, loss of granular layer, incoherent stratum corneum and a great many labeled cells, basal and suprabasal in location. 0.1% tetinoin for 2 days

Lower middle Wall of a closed comedo, untreated. The comedonal epithelium is stretched out with several labeled cells in this view. The labeling index of comedones is higher than of the adjacent epidermis, between 10%–15%

Bottom Wall of an open comedo, tretinoin stimulated. The comedo wall is acanthotic, has a pronounced granular layer and is labeled with many cells. This wall produces rapidly new corneocytes, which are loose and incoherent, leading to the sloughing of pre-existing comedones (comedolysis)

Plewig G (1991) Retinoide zur Kontrolle der Differenzierung von Epidermis und ihren Anhangsgebilden. Nova Acta Leopoldina 64:107–120

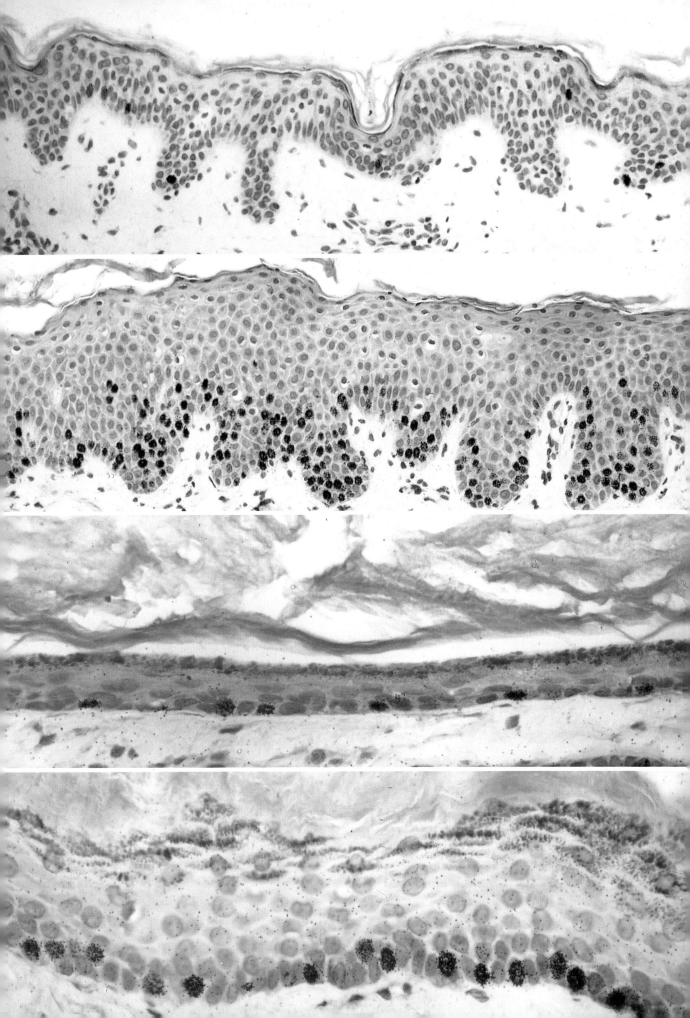

Topical Tretinoin Loosens Corneocytes

The most effective action of tretinoin is the uprooting of otherwise tightly anchored comedones, and the thinning of the stratum corneum, lining the infrainfundibulum of sebaceous follicles.

Above

Left   Normal skin to show the compact and tight cohesion of corneocytes, forming a sturdy wall, like bricks. The granular layer is on the left. (Electron microscopy, $\times 11\,500$)

Right   After tretinoin 0.05% for 11 weeks, intra- and intercellular lipid accumulates as a result of hyperproliferation. Corneocytes then begin to dehisce. (Electron microscopy, $\times 12\,800$)

Below

Left   After tretinoin 0.05% for 6 weeks, the lipid laden, swollen, flimsy corneocytes separate into a loose mass. (Electron microscopy, $\times 35\,000$)

Right   After tretinoin 0.05% for 6 weeks, odd-shaped, lipid-rich corneocytes replace the original, compact coherent stratum corneum. This is the distinctive ultrastructural image of the tretinoin effect. (Electron microscopy, $\times 13\,400$)

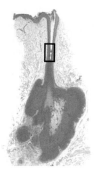

Courtesy of Professor Helmut H. Wolff, Lübeck, FRG

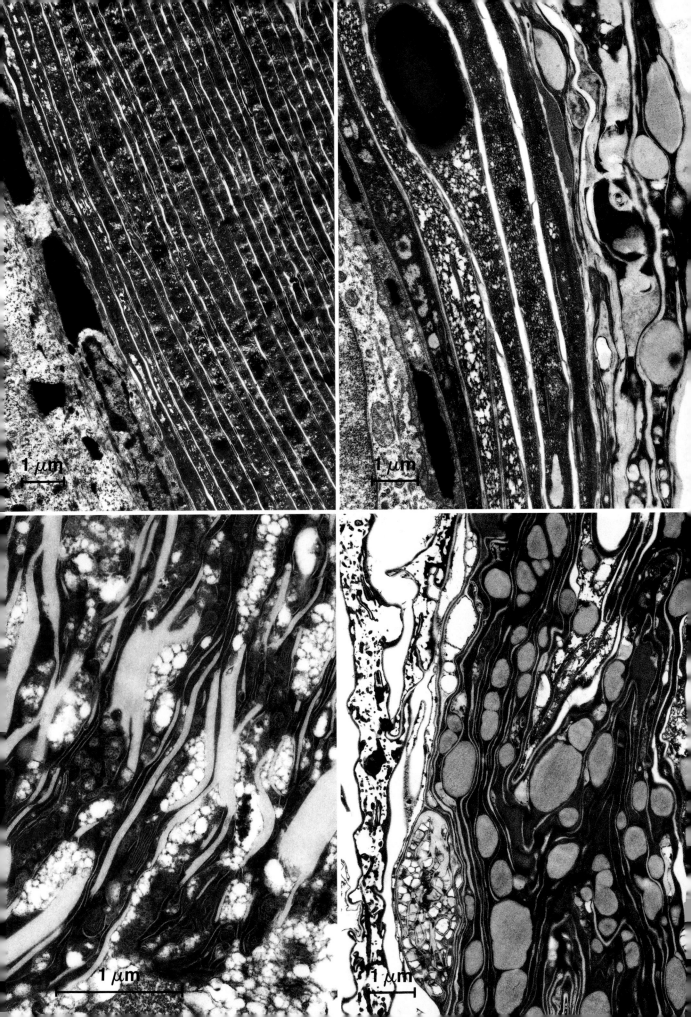

Benzoyl Peroxide

Benzoyl peroxide was synthesized by the chemist Loevenhard in 1905. There are many industrial uses, especially for bleaching fabrics and flour. The powerful antibacterial activity of peroxides has long been appreciated. It is this property which explains its use in acne. Benzoyl peroxide is available as an over-the-counter (OTC) drug in most industrialized countries. Ointments containing benzoyl peroxide and chlorhydroxyquinoline were marketed in 1930. These were messy and of questionable stability. To overcome this, benzoyl peroxide was subsequently distributed in a separate package to be mixed with the vehicle immediately before use. Benzoyl peroxide was registered for the treatment of acne in 1960 in the USA and in 1974 in Germany. It did not become popular until the late 1970s when much-improved products became available. Benzoyl peroxide is the leading OTC anti-acne topical and holds also an important position in office treatment.

Pharmacology

Benzoyl peroxide, $C_{14}H_{10}O_4$ is almost insoluble in water or ethanol, but soluble in ether, acetone, or chloroform. It degrades with increasing temperature, and is explosive above 60° C. It rapidly decomposes in the presence of light.

After application to the skin, benzoyl peroxide is rapidly metabolized to benzoic acid, a harmless chemical. Intensive use in humans has failed to demonstrate appreciable absorption. The drug is eminently safe. Its antimicrobial efficacy is noteworthy, with rapid destruction of gram-positive organisms and yeasts. These, of course, abundantly inhabit sebaceous follicles. *Propionibacterium acnes* is a prime target. In contrast to oral antibiotics the resident microflora does not become resistant to benzoyl peroxide; hence its efficacy does not decrease after years of use.

It is worth emphasizing that benzoyl peroxide depopulates *Propionibacterium acnes* much faster and to a greater extent than oral antibiotics. Negligible numbers are recoverable after 2 weeks. As a result the free fatty acids decrease swiftly.

Benzoyl peroxide stimulates epidermal mitosis, followed by acanthosis and hyperkeratosis, clinically evident as flaking. In contrast to tretinoin and salicylic acid, benzoyl peroxide is not comedolytic. In fact, some proprietary brands, especially those containing sulfur, are actually comedogenic. Were it not for this counteracting effect, benzoyl peroxide would be an incomparable drug for the treatment of most varieties of acne. Clinicans are generally not aware of the comedogenic handicap, but have learned to use it in combinations which offset this limitation, e.g., with comedolytic tretinoin.

Benzoyl peroxide is moderately irritating and often induces dryness and scaling. This peeling action is often mistaken for inhibition of sebaceous secretion. In fact the drug is not sebostatic despite earlier experimental reports and commercial claims. Currently, there is some worry concerning the extensive, uncontrolled use of this very popular drug. It has been found that benzoyl peroxide is a tumor promoter in the two-stage model of chemical carcinogenesis in hairless mice. Happily it does not promote carcinomas in mice irradiated with ultraviolet radiation. Thus, it is not photocarcinogenic and has been shown not to be mutagenic in various essays. There is much discussion among regulators whether tumor promotion occurs in humans. The record is clear. Extensive use for many decades is strong evidence that this drug is neither a carcinogen nor cocarcinogen. By this time, photocarcinogenicity would have become evident since the main usage is on the face.

How To Use Benzoyl Peroxide

The drug is indicated for mild to moderate papulopustular acne, but not for comedonal acne. It is available in a variety of concentrations: 2.5%, 3%, 5%, and 10% and in various formulations including emulsions, hydrogels, alcoholic gels, and creams to suit every preference. Fair-skinned persons who tend to have irritable skin, and very young or anxious patients should start with lower strength preparations, particularly on the face. For chest, shoulders, and back, higher concentrations are suitable. Emulsions are better tolerated than alcoholic gels. It should also be remembered that the skin is more readily irritated in winter. We have found that the suppression of *Propionibacterium acnes* is similar with 2.5%, 5%, or 10%, except that the action is a little slower. We prefer lower concentrations. They are less irritating and less comedogenic in the rabbit ear model. The

formulation has to be applied thinly to the entire affected area, e.g., total face, and not only onto the visible lesions, usually once daily to begin with. Some irritation with mild erythema, scaling, and itching frequently occurs within the first days or weeks, gradually subsiding. This is the well-known hardening effect. Twice daily applications are not warranted since maximal destruction of the follicular microflora can be achieved by a single daily dose. As always the treatment should be individualized to the needs of each patient.

Contact allergy to benzoyl peroxide is rare, although the drug is a troublesome allergen when used for the treatment of leg ulcers. Its rapid degradation on the facial skin probably accounts for the low incidence of contact sensitization. Still, physicians should be on the lookout for this unusual occurrence, which is easily mistaken for an exacerbation of the disease. Contact allergy on the face takes unusual forms. Patch testing provides proof. Pregnancy is not a contraindication. Patients should be warned that the drug bleaches hair, clothes, and bed linens.

Combination Therapy

It is highly desirable to combine benzoyl peroxide with other topical medications which have different modes of action. The best match is with tretinoin. This is an excellent choice when comedones are numerous along with inflammatory lesions. Tretinoin should be applied in the evening and benzoyl peroxide in the morning. Stubborn acne responds well to aggressive combination therapy. One must remember that both drugs are potential irritants; hence it is better to start with the lowest concentration of each. In patients judged to have sensitive skin it is wise to start with tretinoin alone, adding the peroxide after the skin has accommodated. Patients need to be counseled that acne does not disappear overnight.

Recently a combination of 2.5% benzoyl peroxide with 1% erythromycin (Benzamycin) was launched and has quickly gained a prominent position in the market place. *Propionibacterium acnes* is virtually extinguished and irritation is mild to absent. Theoretically, there is no rationale for adding erythromycin to an already highly effective antibacterial. Erythromycin might have other unrelated effects that account for the success of this combination drug.

Cartwright RA, Hughes BR, Cunliffe WJ (1988) Malignant melanoma, benzoyl peroxide and acne: a pilot epidemiological case-control investigation. Br J Dermatol 118:239–242

Cotterill JA (1980) Benzoyl peroxide. Acta Derm Venereol [Suppl 89] (Stockh) 60:57–63

Cunliffe WJ, Burke B (1982) Benzoyl peroxide: lack of sensitization. Acta Derm Venereol (Stockh) 62:458–459

Fulton JE, Farzad-Bakshandeh A, Bradley S (1974) Studies on the mechanism of action of topical benzoyl peroxide and vitamin A acid in acne vulgaris. J Cutan Pathol 1:191–200

Gloor M (1990) Benzoylperoxid in der dermatologischen Lokaltherapie. Zentralbl Hautkr 157:1010–1015

Harkaway KS, McGinley KJ, Foglia AN, Lee W-L, Fried F, Shalita AR, Leyden JJ (1992) Antibiotic resistance patterns in coagulase-negative Staphylococci after treatment with topical erythromycin, benzoyl peroxide, and combination therapy. Br J Dermatol 126:586–590

Iversen OH (1986) Carcinogenesis studies with benzoyl peroxide (Panoxyl gel 5%). J Invest Dermatol 86:442–448

Iversen OH (1988) Skin tumorigenesis and carcinogenesis studies with 7,12-dimethylbenz-[a]anthracene, ultraviolet light, benzoyl peroxide (Panoxyl gel 5%), and ointment gel. Carcinogenesis 9:803–809

Kligman AM, Leyden JJ, Stewart R (1977) New uses for benzoyl peroxide: a broad spectrum antimicrobial agent. Int J Dermatol 16:413–417

Leyden JJ, Kligman AM (1977) Contact sensitization to benzoyl peroxide. Contact Dermatitis 3:273–275

Loevenhart AS (1905) Benzoylsuperoxyd, ein neues therapeutisches Agens. Therapeut Monatshefte 19:426–428

Nacht S, Yeung D, Beasley JN, Anjo MD, Maibach HI (1981) Benzoyl peroxide: percutaneous penetration and metabolic disposition. J Am Acad Dermatol 4:31–37

Yeung D, Nacht S, Bucks D, Maibach HI (1983) Benzoyl peroxide: percutaneous penetration and metabolic circulation. II. Effect of concentration. J Am Acad Dermatol 9:920–924

Miscellaneous Exfoliants (Peeling Agents)

Acne is a capricious disease for which dozens of useless medications have been recommended in the past. Nevertheless, almost all purchasers of OTC anti-acne remedies judge them to be satisfactory. So-called peeling agents were very popular before the era of effective drugs. The efficacy of these remedies has never been proved; we now regard them as archaic. They lack comedolytic activity in humans and in the rabbit ear model and are merely irritants which provoke scaling, misinterpreted as a comedolytic effect: as scales absorb sebum this creates the illusion of sebum suppression by seemingly reducing oiliness. On the other hand, low-grade inflammation stimulates sebum production, and irritation produces hyperplasia of the sebaceous glands in humans and in hairless mice. Peeling sometimes hastens the regression of papulopustules helping to sustain a belief of efficacy.

Not only consumers, but even doctors have difficulties in identifying ineffective drugs. It takes an experienced professional to recognize harmful remedies in this multifaceted disease. We think that physicians often do not recognize treatments which are harmful. We advertise against the use of the following substances: phenol, resorcinol, β-naphthol, sulfur, zinc sulfate, and aluminium. We condemn out of hand the stinking medieval concoctions so familiar to earlier therapists: Vleminckx's solution and Kummerfeld's lotion. Now that effective topical drugs are available, there is no place for any of these pharmacologic assaults on the skin. Our antagonism includes peeling induced by physical agents such as liquid nitrogen and dry ice (cryotherapy).

We particularly inveigh against the use of sulfur. All preparations containing precipitated, particulate sulfur are actually comedogenic and will slowly induce more comedones, even though drying up papulopustules at the same time. Existing inflammatory lesions may benefit, but the disease is worsened in the long run. Sulfur drugs perpetuate the disease while creating the illusion of efficacy. We call attention to the adverse effects of combinations of sulfur with benzoyl peroxide. These are extremely comedogenic and have to be avoided at all cost.

Mills OH, Kligman AM (1972) Is sulphur helpful or harmful in acne vulgaris? Br J Dermatol 86:620–627

Strauss JS, Goldman PH, Nacht S, Gans EH (1978) A reexamination of the potential comedogenicity of sulfur. Arch Dermatol 114:1340–1342

Windhager K, Plewig G (1970) Wirkung von Schälmitteln (Resorchin, kristalliner Schwefel, Salicylsäure) auf Meerschweinchenepidermis. Arch Dermatol Res 259:187–198

Topical Antibiotics

Bacteriostatic treatment has a long history in acne. An extraordinary variety of bacteriostatical chemicals have been endorsed by the authorities and widely used. Among these are salicylic acid, sulfur, resorcinol, hexachlorophene, salicylanilides, bithionol, zinc pyrithione, carbanilides, a half-dozen quarternary ammonium salts, 8-hydroxy-quinoline, and many others that would fill this page. It is perhaps a sad commentary that none of these have appreciable antibacterial activity on facial skin, although some inhibit bacterial growth in vitro. This situation changes drastically with the introduction of topical antibiotics. These suppress *Propionibacterium acnes* in sebaceous follicles and are therefore clinically effective.

Three groups are currently used, namely tetracyclines, erythromycin, and clindamycin

Tetracyclines are bacteriostatic, mainly against gram-positive bacteria and act by inhibiting protein biosynthesis. Many strains of pathogenic *Staphylococcus* and *Streptococcus* have become resistant to tetracycline. Erythromycin has a similar spectrum of activity. The fear of development of resistant strains has led some countries to ban topical use, on the theory that this potentially life-saving drug would be ineffective when needed for serious infections.

Clindamycin, also a life-saving drug according to the WHO definition, is a broad-spectrum antibiotic, and it too has come under scrutiny by worried regulators. In our view these anxieties are unfounded and are merely theoretical objections. A list of selected products from the USA and German markets, their concentrations, vehicles, and trade names are provided in the table.

Recently, these have been formulated in combination with a variety of other anti-acne agents, mostly acting in a different way. For example, the inclusion of tretinoin confers comedolytic activity, supplementing antibacterial action. In most instances, the claim that the combination is more effective than either component alone has been substantiated by clinical trials.

Indication

All types of inflammatory acne, particularly milder grades, which do not require systemic antibiotic treatment are indicated.

Selection of Antibiotic

The selection of antibiotic is usually based on personal preferences, including particular brand names, vehicles, solutions, gels, ointments, patient acceptance, cost and of course efficacy. It would be a formidable task to establish with scientific rigor which of the available formulations are really superior.

Synopsis of single or fixed combinations of antimicrobial agents. A survey from the US (US) and German (G) market

Antibiotic	Percentage	Vehicle	Trade Name	Market
Tetracyclines				
Tetracycline hydro-chloride	3	Ointment	Imex	G
Meclocycline sulfo-salicylate	1	Cream	Meclan	US
Erythromycin	2	Solution	Erycette Pledges	US
	2	Gel	Erygel	US
	2	Solution	T-Stat Pads	US
	1	Solution	Aknefug El	G
	2	Solution	Aknemycin	G
	2	Ointment	Aknemycin 2000	G
	1, 68	Solution	Aknin-Winthrop	G
	2	Solution	Stiemycine	G
	1	Solution	Inderm	G
Clindamyin	1	Solution and Gel	Sobelin	G
			Akne Lösung	
			Cleocin T	US
Fixed Combinations				
Erythromycin and Benzoyl peroxide	3 5	Gel	Benzamycin	US
Erythromycin and Tretinoin	4 0.025	Gel	Clinesfar	G
Erythromycin and Zinc acetate	1.2 0.377	Solution	Zyneryt	G
Miconazole nitrate and Benzoyl peroxide	2 5	Cream	Acnidazol	G

Mode of Action

The mode of action is principally the same as for oral antibiotics. They act as bacteriostatic and bactericidal agents on coryneforme bacteria, notably *Propionibacterium acnes*, in sebaceous follicles and in microcomedones.

Bacterial Resistance

Bacterial resistance is of major concern, and is discussed elsewhere (p. 617).

Duration of Treatment

Efficacy

In our experience, topical antibiotics are less effective than their oral counterparts. Despite expectations to the contrary, the suppression of *Propionibacterium acnes* occurs slowly and is far from complete, even poor when compared to benzoyl peroxide. British dermatologists have a good reputation for looking soberly and critically at comparative efficacies. We call attention particularly to the thoughtful works of Eady et al. and Noble. Eady undertook the daunting task of critically analyzing data from 144 studies published between 1966 and 1989, and analysis considered nine criteria including overall trial design, clinical results, and methods of data analysis. The chief findings were not exactly reassuring:

- 33 trials had to be excluded because of major deficiencies in study design. Almost all of the remaining ones had serious technical shortcomings.
- Results of 15 double-blind placebo-controlled studies revealed that:
  – Tetracyclines were not effective, a credible result. These have no place in acne therapy. Clindamycin and erythromycin (1%–4% with or without the addition of zinc) were effective in inflammatory acne.
  – None of the antibiotics was more effective than benzoyl peroxide.
- A further 17 unpublished trials were reviewed from questionnaires. It was not clear why they were not published, except in one instance due to negative results.
- The overview showed that erythromycin and clindamycin were beneficial in inflammatory acne. It remains to be determined which types of acne respond best and how they compare to oral therapy.
  Eady's final message is: Journals should be more rigorous in refereeing drug trials in acne.

Side Effects

There are few side effects. Tetracyclines stain the skin yellow and fluoresce under UV-A radiation, e.g., at work places and in discos. They also smell bitter. Erythromycin is not a contact sensitizer and is not irritating. It is a trouble-free drug topically. Clindamycin also has a good safety record, except for rare instances of bloody diarrhea and colitis including pseudomembranaceous colitis, as happens more often with oral therapy. These signs reverse rapidly on stopping the drug. Local adverse effects from all these preparations include erythema, peeling, and burning, particularly around the eyes, attributable mainly to the vehicle. Phototoxicity has not been encountered.

Combination Therapy

Combinations are rational and are the forte of the dermatologist. Topical antibiotics are used along with tretinoin, benzoyl peroxide, hormones (oral contraceptives and antiandrogens), isotretinoin, azelaic acid, and so forth. There is not much point in giving the same antibiotic topically and orally at the same time. Fixed drug combinations with tretinoin, zinc acetate, benzoyl peroxide, or miconazole are currently available. This list will grow. Comparative studies must be done to determine the added value.

Eady EA, Holland KT, Cunliffe WJ (1982) Should topical antibiotics be used for the treatment of acne vulgaris? Br J Dermatol 107:235–246

Eady EA, Cove JH, Joanes DN, Cunliffe WJ (1990) Topical antibiotics for the treatment of acne vulgaris: a critical evaluation of the literature on their clinical benefit and comparative efficacy. J Dermatol Treat 1:215–226

Harkaway KS, McGinley KJ, Foglia AN, Lee W-L, Fried F, Shalita AR, Leyden JJ (1992) Antibiotic resistance patterns in coagulase-negative Staphylococci after treatment with topical erythromycin, benzoyl peroxide, and combination therapy. Br J Dermatol 126:586–590

Noble WC (1990) Topical and systemic antibiotics: is there a rationale? Semin Dermatol 9:250–254

Parry MF, Rha CK (1986) Pseudomembranous colitis caused by topical clindamycin phosphate. Arch Dermatol 122:583–584

Resh W, Stoughton RB (1976) Topically applied antibiotics in acne vulgaris. Clinical response and suppression of Corynebacterium acnes in open comedones. Arch Dermatol 112:182–184

Shalita AR, Smith EB, Bauer E (1984) Topical erythromycin v clindamycin therapy for acne. A multicenter, double-blind comparison. Arch Dermatol 120:351–355

Azelaic Acid

Historical Background

This is a newcomer in the antiacne repertoire. The Italian group of Nazzaro-Porro, Caprilli, and Passi reported in 1973 that the yeast *Pityrosporum* was able to oxidize unsaturated fatty acids to yield dicarboxylic acids. Diacids with a chain length from C_8 to C_{13} are competitive inhibitors of tyrosinase in vitro and might therefore affect melanin synthesis. In preliminary trials a 20% azelaic acid cream had a bleaching effect on hyperpigmented conditions such as toxic melanoderma, melasma, and lentigo maligna. It was coincidentally observed that acne also improved.

Chemistry and Toxicology

Azelaic acid is a naturally occurring, poorly water-insoluble, straight-chained, saturated dicarboxylic acid ($C_9H_{16}O_4$). Percutaneous absorption is slight (3.6%) and oral toxicity is negligible. A 20% cream applied topically to volunteers even three to four times daily for more than 1 year caused only slight initial erythema. The drug appears to be quite safe. Teratogenicity and fetal and neonatal toxicity has not been observed in laboratory animals.

$$HO-\overset{O}{\underset{}{C}}-CH_2-(CH_2)_5-CH_2-\overset{O}{\underset{}{C}}-OH$$

Trials in Acne

A 15% or 20% azelaic acid cream has been reported to be more effective than its vehicle in double-blind studies. European investigators consider it to be comparable in efficacy to topical and oral antibiotics. Side effects occur in about 10% of patients and include a transient redness, scaling, and burning. Irritation is probably due to acidity. Sebum production is not affected. At high concentrations the drug is bactericidal. Quantitative studies have shown a significant decrease in the density of *Propionibacterium acnes* and aerobic cocci after 4–8 weeks of daily treatment, with a corresponding reduction of free fatty acids. The degree of bacterial suppression is somewhat less than with benzoyl peroxide. Its effect on keratinization is not fully understood. Proponents claim the elimination of comedones in humans. We were not able to demonstrate a comedolytic effect on coal-tar-induced comedones in the rabbit ear.

Under in vitro conditions neither spontaneous resistant mutants nor phenotypic adaptation was detectable. In particular no azelaic acid resistant mutants of *Propionibacterium acnes* or *Staphylococcus epidermidis* developed. Azelaic acid is unrelated to antibiotics used in acne therapy which may cause resistance. Azelaic acid is now under intensive study in many countries. Its status is sub judice with varying opinions being exposed for and against. The drug was released in

1991 in several European countries (Skinoren) and will be available in 1993 in the USA.

Breathnach AS (1989) A new agent in the treatment of acne: history, metabolism and biochemistry. J Dermatol Treat [Suppl 1] 1:7–10

Cunliffe WJ, Holland KT (1989) Clinical and laboratory studies on treatment with 20% azelaic acid cream for acne. Acta Derm Venereol [Suppl 143] (Stockh) 69:31–34

Gollnick HPM (1992) Die C_9-Dicarbonsäure Azelainsäure als neue Substanz im Spektrum der Akne-Therapeutika. Dermatol Monatsschr 178:143–152

Gollnick H, Graupe K (1989) Azelaic acid for the treatment of acne: comparative trials. J Dermatol Treat [Suppl 1] 1:27–30

Holland KT, Bojar RA (1989) The effect of azelaic acid on cutaneous bacteria. J Dermatol Treat [Suppl 1] 1:17–19

Nazzaro-Porro M (1987) Azelaic acid. J Am Acad Dermatol 17:1033–1041

Passi S, Picardo M, Mingrone G, Breathnach AS, Nazzaro-Porro M (1989) Azelaic acid – biochemistry and metabolism. Acta Derm Venereol [Suppl 143] (Stockh) 69:8–13

Töpert M, Rach P, Siegmund F (1989) Pharmacology and toxicology of azelaic acid. Acta Derm Venereol [Suppl 143] (Stockh) 69:14–19

Azelaic Acid: A Newcomer

Topical azelaic acid was used as monotherapy in these patients. Comedonal and papulopustular acne seem to be the best indications. Improvement takes longer than with other topical regimes.

Above   Acne papulopustular before (*left*) and after 6 months (*right*) of 20% azelaic acid treatment

Below   The papulopustular acne (*left*) was successfully treated (*right*) with a 20% azelaic acid cream given for 12 weeks

Above: Courtesy of Professor Ole Fyrand, Oslo, Norway
Below: Courtesy of Ursula Schotte, M.D., Düsseldorf, FRG

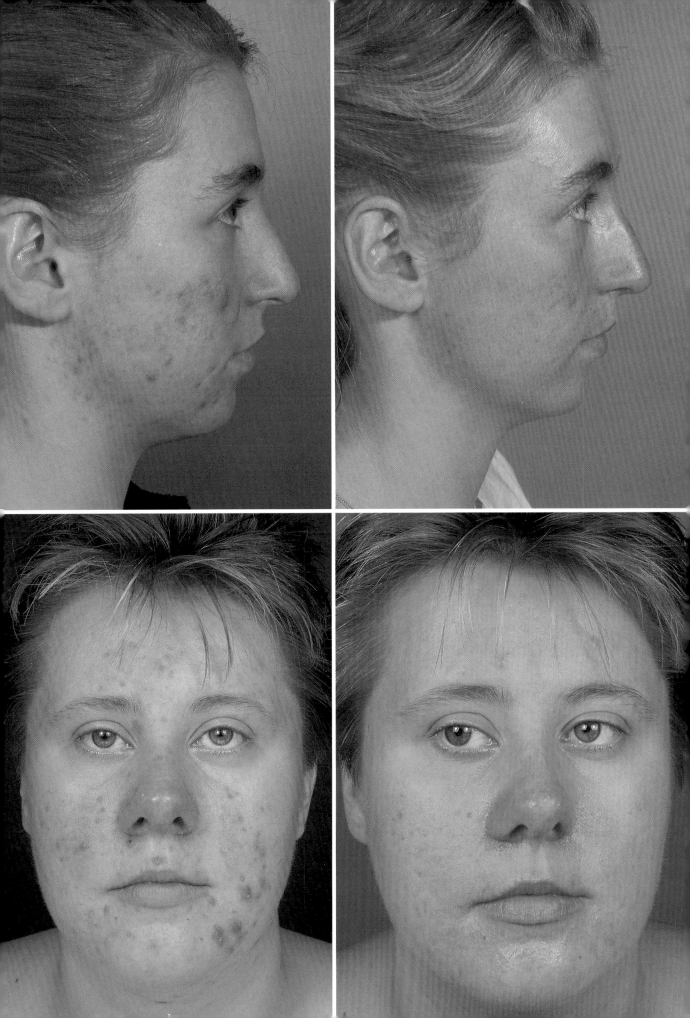

Antibiotics: Tetracyclines and Erythromycin

Starting with sulfonamides and penicillin each new antibiotic and chemotherapeutic drug has been enthusiastically welcomed as an effective acne treatment. This exemplifies the difficulties of therapeutic evaluations, for penicillin is ineffective and sulfonamides are hardly helpful. It is almost impossible to compare results from different investigators despite the efforts made to obtain objective data by controlled studies. The problems center around the following:

- Lack of uniform criteria for classifying and grading acne
- Biased selection of patients
- Variable standards for determining the degree of improvement
- Differences in the duration of treatment
- In large multicenter studies, the investigators vary greatly in experience and reliability
- Placebo effects
- Fluctuations in the natural course of the disease
- Concomitant topical therapy
- Influential variables that are not factored in, for example, season (summer versus winter) vacations, stress, and compliance

Caution dictates that we should not single out one antibiotic and declare it to be superior to the others. We here present a list of effective drugs and assume therapeutic equivalence until proved otherwise. It has been established beyond doubt that tetracyclines and erythromycin are valuable drugs in acne and have a long history of safe use. It is ironic, but highly instructive, that double-blind studies have sometimes found tetracyclines to be no better than the control. The placebo effect is substantial in this disease. The doctor's deportment and empathy contribute to the efficacy of all management programs. Acne is not an infectious disease, but antibiotics have a genuine role in treatment.

- *Propionibacterium acnes* is extremely susceptible in vitro to every antibiotic which is active against gram-positive organisms.
- Effective drugs without exception reduce the population of *Propionibacterium acnes* by 90% or more, accompanied by a decrease of about 50% in the proportion of free fatty acids in the surface lipids. At the same time follicular fluorescence under Wood's light disappears. These parameters can be used in healthy volunteers to screen and assess topical or systemic drugs. These measurements are more objective and more sensitive than clinical appraisals.

Fatty acids can be reduced without killing *Propionibacterium acnes*. One validated mechanism is inhibition of fat-splitting lipases by concentrations too low to inhibit bacterial growth. Tetracyclines inhibit bacterial lipases more effectively than erythromycin. Still, the two appear to be therapeutically equivalent. It has also been shown that concentrations of antibiotics which do not prevent the growth of *Propionibacterium acnes* can also suppress the synthesis of lipase in vitro. Perhaps the most dependable measure of monitoring antibiotic effects is the decrease of free fatty acids in the surface lipids, although follicular fluorescence is much simpler and surprisingly reliable. If the market place is any judge, clinicians prescribe tetracyclines far more frequently than erythromycin. Antibiotics, notably tetracyclines, but also sulfones have pharmacologic effects that are unrelated to bacterial inhibition. These posses a modest anti-inflammatory activity, mainly demonstrated by in vitro studies of neutrophil chemotaxis and macrophage functions. Accordingly these drugs are also effectively used in rosacea, perioral dermatitis, and pityriasis lichenoides, none of which is caused by bacteria.

Effective antibiotics have to be transported into the follicular canal, comedonal or papulopustular lesions, either via the sebaceous glands or the infundibular epithelium. The drugs enter the living cells, e.g., sebocytes or keratinocytes, and provided they are not metabolized, ride outwards with these finally being shed into the lumen of the follicular canal, sebaceous filament, or comedones. Penicillins G and V as well as sulfonamides do not possess this capacity. Thus, they are ineffective in vivo in contrast to having high antibacterial activity in vitro. Antibiotics do not directly affect open or closed comedones. They are not comedolytic. They are most effective in reducing inflammatory lesions, especially pustules. The beneficial effects take weeks to be perceived, probably by preventing the formation of new papulopustules. This is probably a result of inhibition of *Propionibacterium acnes* in preclinical lesions such as microcomedones. Rupture would thereby be forestalled by preventing accumulation of the multiple toxic products

synthesized by *Propionibacterium acnes*. Long-term use probably has a prophylactic action on the formation of comedones; surprisingly this has never been demonstrated. In any case, antibiotics have a multiplicity of effects in acne.

The porphyrins produced by *Propionibacterium acnes* provide another way of identifying effective antibiotics. Under Wood's light, emitting mainly long-wave UV-A, persons bearing high quantities of *Propionibacterium acnes*, usually those with oily skin and large facial pores, will show a punctate, orange–red follicular fluorescence, most evident in follicles of the nose. A high-intensity lamp must be used, which must first be "warmed up", the observer's eyes must become accommodated, and the examination room must be completely dark. The principle is similar to the detection of fluorescence in erythrasma. With effective antibiotics, virtual extinction of fluorescence occurs in about 1 month, well-correlated with a substantial reduction in *Propionibacterium acnes*. Incidentally, this is a convenient way of monitoring whether the patient is taking the drug.

The Management of Acne with Oral Antibiotics

A huge number of different antibiotics are now available. Only a few of this large family can be recommended. Since the drug will usually be given for long periods, toxicity must be low. The prevalence of side effects usually does not become known until a new drug has been used for years. Thus new drugs have to make their way slowly into the register of acceptability. Dermatologists have 40 years of experience with some of the older tetracyclines, the first of the broad-spectrum antibiotics. They are quite familiar with the risks and benefits. Tetracyclines are thus the premier antibiotics in acne. The ap-

Antibiotics	Unit dose (mg)	Daily dose (mg)
Tetracyclines		
Tetracycline hydrochloride	250, 500	500–1500
Oxytetracycline	250, 500	500–1500
Demeclocycline	150, 300	300–600
Doxycycline hyclate	50, 100, 200	50–100
Doxycycline monohydrate	100	100
Minocycline	50, 100	50–100
Macrolides		
Erythromycin	250, 333	500–1000
Erythromycin estolate	500	500–1500
Erythromycin ethylsuccinate	200, 400, 500	400–1500
Josamycin	500	500–1500

For more information the Physician's Desk Reference (PDR, 46th ed. 1992) or Rote Liste 1992 should be consulted.

propriate dosage derived from a vast clinical experience. This antibiotic is therefore the reference standard for all the others. It should be made perfectly clear that certain other antibiotics are doubtlessly therapeutically equivalent and may turn out to be at least as safe. Erythromycin, which has also been used extensively, is certainly one of those. Finally, geographical, historical, and educational aspects influence the selection of an antibiotic. Thus, the choice of antibiotics and the way they are used is somewhat different between the USA, the United Kingdom, and continental Europe.

As a matter of practicality only two groups of antibiotics will be discussed, tetracyclines and macrolides (Table). Lincomycin has not reached acceptability. We assume that these have parity at therapeutically equivalent doses. There is, however, no full consensus on what an equivalent dose is. Comparative efficacy is often estimated by measuring blood levels (concentration under the curve). This alone, while objective, may not be sufficient. Blood levels do not reveal much about concentrations in the target tissues. Lipophilic tetracyclines, like minocycline, have a better penetration into the lipid-rich domain of sebaceous follicles and microcomedones. Nonetheless, it is arguable whether minocycline is superior to doxycycline or tetracycline hydrochloride at "equivalent" dosage.

The newest development is the introduction of doxycycline monohydrate. It was shown that it is equally effective as minocycline, seems to have no central nervous system side-effects as may be encountered with minocycline, is virtually pH-neutral (pH 5–6) compared to doxycycline hyclate which is a highly acidic salt (pH 2–3), and can be taken with or without food. Happily the price is also substantially lower than that of its competitors doxycycline hyclate or minocycline. It remains to be seen how the dermatologic community accepts this newcomer.

The conventional dose for treating grampositive infections such as pyodermas is 1500 to 2000 mg of tetracycline hydrochloride per day, divided into three or four doses. In acne, the upper dose is actually 1500 mg, occasionally higher for acne conglobata. The starting dose for tetracycline hydrochloride or oxytetracycline is three doses of 500 mg per day (1500 mg), for demeclocycline hydrochloride 150 mg three times daily (450 mg), and for doxycycline hyclate or minocycline 50 mg twice daily (100 mg). For erythromycin ethylsuccinate, 500 mg thrice daily (1500 mg) is the recommended dose.

Guidelines for Antibiotic Therapy

Indications

The chief indications are moderate to severe papulopustular acne and acne conglobata. Age is not limiting, once permanent teeth are present. Antibiotics can be given without hesitation to boys or girls from the age 12 years and for long periods.

Selection

Tetracyclines are the most favored drugs. Tetracycline hydrochloride and oxytetracycline have a good record. Minocycline has recently gained much appreciation and is the leading antibiotic in acne. Doxycycline is similarly rising in popularity. Demeclocycline hydrochloride has fallen out of favor because of phototoxicity. Macrolides are less popular than tetracyclines, although erythromycin is certainly an acceptable alternative. None of the following can be recommended either because of lack of efficacy or considerations of safety: cephalosporines, aminoglycosides, chloramphenicol, clindamycin, sulfonamides, and gyrase inhibitors.

Dose

Physicians use different treatment strategies. Perhaps the most common approach is tetracycline hydrochloride or oxytetracycline, 500 mg three times daily for 1–2 months until there is marked improvement of inflammatory lesions. The drug is given on an empty stomach since food, especially milk products, reduces absorption. The drug is then tapered down to individual needs, usually 1000 mg daily. In many cases, a single dose of 500 mg daily is adequate.

The same rules hold for doxycycline and minocycline, starting with 50 mg bid and then 50 mg daily for maintenance. These drugs are much better absorbed and can be taken with meals. Advantages are also claimed for their lipophilia, enabling a higher concentration in target tissues.

Duration of Treatment

Again, there is no international consensus. Europeans use lower doses for shorter times than American dermatologists. Because of an excellent safety record, some prescribe it even for years. However, the status should be reviewed every 3 months. Patients often fall into a fixed routine and will even go to some lengths to obtain tetracyclines from friends and friendly pharmacists. Some patients have a pitiful record of needlessly taking antibiotics for years, even decades. It is not necessary for every pustule to be eliminated before stopping antibiotics. If a good response is not obtained in 3–6 months, pursue another avenue of treatment.

Laboratory Investigation

Happily the treatment of inflammatory acne with oral antibiotics is safe. There is no need to check white or red blood cells, liver or kidney enzymes, not even in patients on long-term treatment.

Side Effects

The side effects found depend on the drug. Unwanted side effects are uncommon and generally minor, and can be summarized as follows:

- Nausea, vomiting, and gastric distress are rare with tetracycline, but much more common with macrolides (erythromycin, josamycin). They are usually mild and transient.

- Phototoxicity is inherent to many tetracyclines. Demeclocycline is the major culprit and can cause severe phototoxic reactions on the face, lower arms, back of hands, lower legs and feet, including phototoxic onycholysis. In some sensitive fair-skinned persons, blistering reactions may be severe. Broad spectrum sunscreens absorbing well in the UV-A range should be used liberally. Doxycycline is far less phototoxic, while minocycline is borderline. Erythromycin is not a phototoxic drug.

- Allergic reactions are very rare. Tetracyclines sometimes cause acneiform eruptions with papules and pustules that can be easily mistaken for treatment failure. Fixed drug eruptions are uncommon.

- Superinfection come about as a result of ecologic imbalance. Susceptible resident organisms are repressed, creating voids which are then occupied by resistant organisms. Suppression of gram-positive organisms may pave the way for the entrance of gram-negative ones. Gram-negative folliculitis is the final outcome. Otherwise, changes in the composition of the microflora, especially acquired resistance to aerobic resident bacteria, are harmless and reverse completely after cessation of the drug.

- Quite commonly there is a substantial increase in the density of *Candida albicans* in the gut. Nevertheless, it is all to easy to blame bouts of diarrhea of proctitis on *Candida albicans*. Candida vaginitis is more common with broad-spectrum antibiotics, but the incidence has been exaggerated. Contraceptive pills also predispose to Candida vaginitis and so interpretation is often difficult. Candida vaginitis is less commonly reported than decades ago; the reason for this is unknown. Mucocutaneous candidiasis is a rare complication.

- Pigmentation may be affected. Tetracyclines cause discoloration and enamel defects of fetal dentition after the fourth month of gestation as well as in infants and children up to 8 years of age. Yellowish crumbly teeth were a life-long sequela; nowadays, this is rare. Minocycline can cause a slate-blue pigmentation, particularly in scars, which is not dose-related. It often but not always occurs in sun-exposed body sites, and is a puzzlement to the uninitiated. Osteomas in the skin also may become pigmented and shine bluish through the skin. Pigment deposition occurs also in the thyroid gland, bone marrow, and a number of other viscera. The pigment is a metabolite of minocycline often clustered in macrophages.

- Miscellaneous. High doses of tetracyclines may cause nephrogenic diabetes insipidus, hepatic toxicity, and increased intracranial pressure (pseudotumor cerebri). The latter is unusually frequent in combination with oral retinoids. Drug interaction, e.g., oral contraceptives, psychotropics, anticonvulsives, oral antidiabetics, must be carefully considered in the individual patient. Retinoids cannot be given concomitantly with tetracyclines because of severe toxic reactions including headache and gastrointestinal upsets. Some believe that tetracyclines render oral contraceptives ineffective, but this has not been proved.

Combination Therapy

Antibiotics alone only partially control inflammatory acne. Perhaps as many as 20% of cases respond feebly, even after higher doses. We never use antibiotics alone but always in combination with tretinoin. The therapeutic benefit of tetracycline plus tretinoin has been shown to be considerably better than either alone. This is understandable since these have entirely different modes of action. In addition, the increased vascularity caused by the tretinoin increases the tissue concentration of the antibiotic. It is well known that circulating drugs concentrate at sites of inflammation, owing to increased permeability of the blood vessels. This also holds for acne and can be directly perceived in patients on tetracyclines. When viewed under Wood's light, uninvolved skin does not show the typical yellow fluorescence of tetracycline. By contrast, inflammatory lesions fluoresce brightly. It has been erroneously concluded that antibiotics have no effect on comedones. It is true that existing ones, especially blackheads, are not expelled. After long-term use of 6 months or more, the comedo count decreases substantially indicating a prophylactic action on the formation of new comedones. We have demonstrated that *Propionibacterium acnes* synthesizes lipids which are strongly comedogenic. Keeping the population low will therefore deter the formation of comedones. Tretinoin alone is sufficient in comedonal acne. The combination becomes increasingly more useful with the severity of inflammation.

Bacterial Sensitivity

The determination of in vitro sensitivities is not warranted routinely. Aerobes quickly become resistant and are of no account anyway. Recent surveys have shown a disturbing increase in the percentage of *Propionibacterium acnes* isolations that are resistant to erythromycin and tetracycline, especially the former. This happens less frequently with the lipophilic tetracyclines. Antibiotic resistance has to be considered for those patients, who are no longer uncommon, who initially respond well but later do poorly with a return of papulopustules. Empirically, experienced clinicians know that switching to another antibiotic will again bring the disease under control. Lack of absorption could explain this, but has rarely been demonstrated. Moreover, one must ascertain whether the patient is taking the drug as directed. Noncompliance especially in teenagers is a real problem. In the case of tetracyclines, yellow fluorescence of the oral mucous membranes indicates compliance.

Long-Term Treatment

Patients on antibiotics for more than 12 weeks should be periodically re-evaluated, especially in regard to finding a maintenance dose. There is no doubt that many patients can be maintained on doses as low as 250 mg tetracycline daily, or 50 mg minocycline every other day, even though the blood levels are marginally antibacterial. This seems paradoxical and has intensified doubts concerning the pathogenic importance of *Propionibacterium acnes*. However, it is not necessary to eliminate *Propionibacterium acnes* to control the disease. Good therapeutic effects can be obtained with noninhibitory levels. We have shown that both fluorescence and free fatty acids can be greatly reduced even when there is no change in the density of *Propionibacterium acnes*. The reason is that low concentrations reduce the ability of *Propionibacterium acnes* to produce toxic metabolites such as chemotactic factors, which damage the follicular epithelium.

The ideal long-term goal is to stop oral antibiotics altogether and to rely exclusively on topical therapy. This is not always possible in severe cases. From time to time patients being controlled on low dosages should stop the drug. Exacerbations will generally occur within 3–4 weeks if the antibiotic was contributing to the therapeutic result. We think it wise to insist on revisits every 6–8 weeks, even for those who are doing well. The course of acne fluctuates upwards and downwards. The antibiotic dose should be adjusted accordingly. Stresses of various kinds, emotional or environmental may suddenly precipitate a recrudescence in a previously well-controlled case. This calls for a determination of the sensitivity of *Propionibacterium acnes* and exclusion of gram-negative folliculitis by bacterial cultures of the nose and adjacent skin lesions. There is no rationale for using combinations of oral antibiotics in acne. What about concomitant oral and topical antibiotics? Conventional microbiologists inveigh against this and offer good hypothetical reasonings. However, physicians are more influenced by practice than by theory. Many believe that these combinations are often highly effective. An example is the combination of an oral antibiotic with topical benzoyl peroxide, a powerful bactericidal drug against *Propionibacterium acnes*. Although we remain skeptical, we cannot in the absence of contrary evidence argue against such an approach. It must also be kept in mind that the possibility that topical antimicrobials may have actions beyond that of killing *Propionibacterium acnes*, for example, nonspecific anti-inflammatory effects.

Ad Hoc Committee Report (1975) Systemic antibiotics for treatment of acne vulgaris: efficacy and safety. Arch Dermatol 111:1630–1636

Baer RL, Leshaw SM, Shalita AR (1976) High-dose tetracycline therapy in severe acne. Arch Dermatol 112:479–481

Blank H, Cullen SI, Catalano PM (1968) Photosensitivity studies with demethylchlortetracycline and doxycycline. Arch Dermatol 97:1–2

Esterly NB, Furey NL, Flanagan LE (1978) The effect of antimicrobial agents on leucocyte chemotaxis. J Invest Dermatol 70:51–55

Frost P, Weinstein GD, Gomez EC (1972) Phototoxic potential of minocycline and doxycycline. Arch Dermatol 105:681–683

Hubbell CG, Hobbs ER, Rist T, White JW Jr (1982) Efficacy of minocycline compared with tetracycline in treatment of acne vulgaris. Arch Dermatol 118:989–992

Kurokawa J, Nishijima S, Asada Y (1988) The antibiotic susceptibility of Propionibacterium acnes: a 15-year bacteriological study and retrospective evaluation. J Dermatol 15:149–154

Leyden JJ, McGinley KJ, Kligman AM (1982) Tetracycline and minocycline treatment. Effects on skin-surface lipid levels and Propionibacterium acnes. Arch Dermatol 118:19–22

Noble WC (1990) Topical and systemic antibiotics: is there a rationale? Semin Dermatol 9:250–254

Olafsson JH, Gudgeirsson J, Eggertsdottir GE, Kristjansson F (1989) Doxycycline versus minocycline in the treatment of acne vulgaris: a double-blind study. J Derm Treat 1:15–19

Plewig G, Schöpf E (1975) Anti-inflammatory effects of antimicrobial agents: an in vivo study. J Invest Dermatol 65:532–536

Puhvel SM, Reisner RM (1972) Effect of antibiotics on the lipases of Corynebacterium acnes in vitro. Arch Dermatol 106:45–49

Simmons JJ, Morales A (1980) Minocycline and generalized cutaneous pigmentation. J Am Acad Dermatol 3:244–247

Antibiotic Resistance

Resistance generally arises by random mutation in which the antibiotic is only the selective but not the inducing agent. Three changes may occur with oral and/or topical antibiotic therapy:

617

- New organisms are selected out
- There is slow selection of chromosomally resistant variants
- Bacteria have acquired a resistance plasmid

These events and their potential clinical consequences have drawn much scientific attention. The relevant question here is: "Are acne patients on long-term antibiotics at increased risk of serious infections?"

In the hospital setting, superinfection with newly acquired bacteria is fairly common. There are counterparts in acne, for example, suppressing of gram-positive cocci and coryneforms by oral antibiotics may lead to their replacement by gram-negative ones. This is the explanation of gram-negative folliculitis, in which an ecologic niche is created by suppression of the dominant organisms.

The second event, the selection of resistant chromosomal variants, varies with the antibiotic and the organism. Rifampicin, which is not used in acne, but is used in, e.g., tuberculosis readily induces resistant strains during therapy; therefore combination treatment with other antibiotics is indicated. The selection of chromosomally resistant strains of *Propionibacterium acnes* will surely affect therapeutic efficacy. For instance, oral tetracycline reduces the minimal inhibitory concentration (MIC) by a factor of four to five. After erythromycin, there may be a hundred-fold increase. These considerations apply to patients on long-term antibiotics.

Understandably patients with resistant strains do not respond as well to standard therapy as controls with sensitive strains, or they escape completely. A word of caution is necessary, as a replacement of the previous flora is possible instead of the development of chromosomal resistance. This cannot be solved at present as there are no typing methods for *Propionibacteria*.

Eady et al. have suggested the possibility of a gene transfer to account for *Propionibacterium acnes* resistance. In their studies with oral erythromycin or topical clindamycin, acne patients developed an erythromycin- and lincosamide-resistant *Propionibacterium acnes* population. Once the antibiotics were stopped the original strains of *Propionibacterium acnes* were restored. The mechanism was identically due to methylation of the 23S ribosomal RNA.

The third mechanism involves the transfer of resistance by plasmids (plasmid aquisition). Gentamycin-resistant plasmids have been extensively investigated in *Staphylococcus aureus*. Similar tetracycline-resistant plasmids in coagulase-negative and coagulase-positive staphylococci have been demonstrated. Unfortunately erythromycin-resistant plasmids appeared in strains of *Corynebacterium diphtheriae*, and frequently plasmids may be found in coryneformes on normal human skin. Mupirocin, the latest topical antibiotic (not registered for acne treatment), has led to the selection of transmissible resistant plasmids to *Staphylococcus aureus*.

Information on bacterial resistance may also be encoded in the DNA of extrachromosomal plasmids. This genetic material may easily be transferred from a resistant to a sensitive strain. R (resistance) plasmids may contain multiple drug-resistance determinants.

Resistance to erythromycin is due to modification of bacterial ribosomes, either by mutation or by plasmids. Resistance as a result of chromosomal mutation is associated with an altered specific protein component (protein L4 or L12) of the 50S ribosomal subunit. This leads to a change of the conformation of the receptor site which is less favorable for erythromycin binding. A second mechanism which occurs especially in *Staphylococcus aureus* is plasmid-mediated and involves the demethylation of a specific adenine sequence of the 23S RNA of the 50S subunit by a plasmid-mediated ribosomal RNA methylase. The modified ribosomes are cross-resistant to macrolide antibiotics.

Bacterial resistance to tetracyclines is mostly based on decreased cell permeability which is mostly resistance (R) factor dependent. To attack the bacterial ribosome, the antibiotic has to pass the cell membrane to enter the cell. This happens readily in sensitive cells. In R factor-bearing tetracycline-resistant strains, the intracellular concentration is too low to inhibit protein synthesis.

It is important to appreciate that long-term tetracycline therapy induces multiple antibiotic-resistant organisms in patients and their relatives. Erythromycin does not do so. So far, the risks to acne patients and their relatives have been negligible. In conclusion, the main effect of the development of resistant strains in acne patients is loss of efficacy.

Adams SJ, Cunliffe WJ, Cooke EM (1985) Long-term antibiotic therapy for acne vulgaris: effects on the bowel flora of patients and their relatives. J Invest Dermatol 85:35–37

Cohen ML, Wong ES, Falkow S (1982) Common R-plasmids in Staphylococcus aureus and Staphylococcus epidermidis during a nosocomial Staphylococcus aureus outbreak. Antimicrob Agents Chemother 21:210–215

Cooksey RC, Baldwin JN (1985) Relatedness of tetracycline resistance plasmids among species of coagulase-negative staphylococci. Antimicrob Agents Chemother 27:234–238

Eady EA, Ross JI, Cove JH, Holland KT, Cunliffe WJ (1989) Macrolide – lincosamide – streptogramin B (MLS) resistance in cutaneous propionibacteria: definition of phenotypes. J Antimicrob Chemother 23:493–502

Eady EA, Cove JH, Holland KT, Cunliffe WJ (1989) Erythromycin resistant propionibacteria in antibiotic treated acne patients: association with therapeutic failure. Br J Dermatol 121:51–57

Eady EA, Holland KT, Cunliffe WJ (1982) Should topical antibiotics be used for the treatment of acne vulgaris? Br J Dermatol 107:235–246

Kerry Williams SM, Noble WC (1988) Plasmids in coryneform bacteria of human origin. J Appl Bacteriol 64:475–482

Leyden JJ, McGinley KJ, Cavalieri S, Webster GF, Mills OH, Kligman AM (1983) Propionibacterium acnes resistance to antibiotics in acne patients. J Am Acad Dermatol 8:41–45

Noble WC (1990) Topical and systemic antibiotics: is there a rationale? Semin Dermatol 9:250–254

Rahman M, Noble WC, Cookson B (1987) Mupirocin-resistant Staphylococcus aureus. Lancet 2:387–388

Richmond MH, Linton KB (1980) The use of tetracycline in the community and its possible relation to the excretion of tetracycline-resistant bacteria. J Antimicrob Chemother 6:33–41

Westh H, Jensen BL, Rosdahl VT, Prag J (1989) Development of erythromycin-resistance in Staphylococcus aureus as a consequence of high erythromycin consumption. J Hosp Infect 14:107–115

Severe Inflammatory Acne Often Responds Well to Therapy

The entire face of this 18-year-old boy was studded with succulent, deep-seated persistent papules and pustules. Tetracycline hydrochloride was given for 1 month, along with 0.05% tretinoin solution applied twice daily. The gratifying result shown below was secured in only 9 weeks. Topical tretinoin is used here, which is mistakenly regarded as having only comedolytic effect

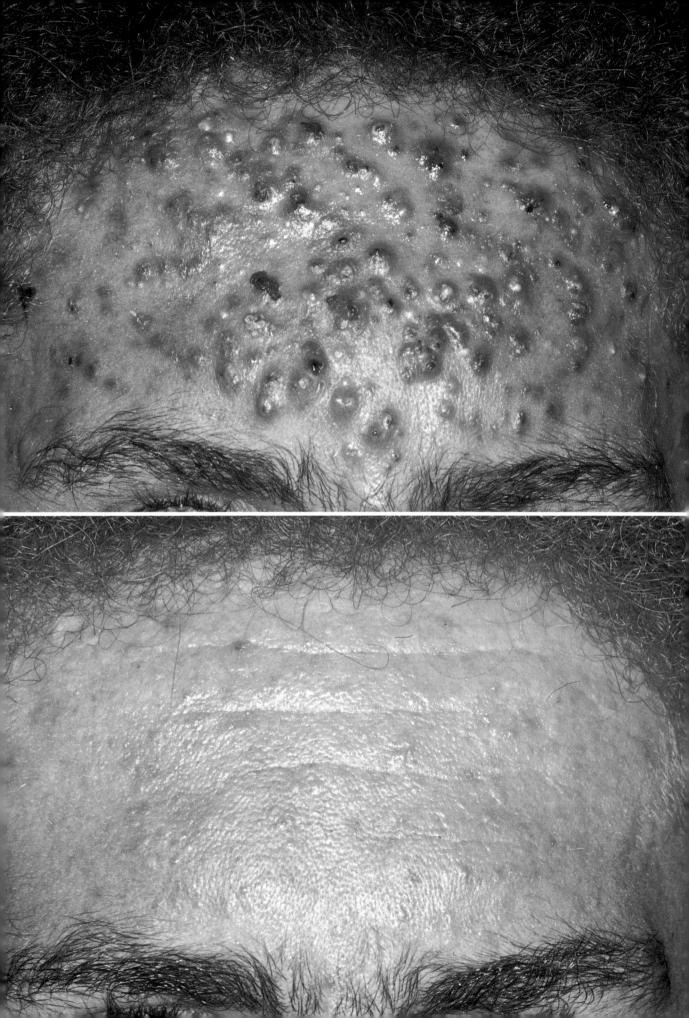

Treatment of Severe Inflammatory and Conglobate Acne

Prior to the marketing of isotretinoin, one had to adopt all kinds of strategies to help the afflicted patients.

Above   Severe inflammatory acne, papules, pustules, and widespread inflammation on a very seborrheic skin troubled this 16-year-old boy. The combination of tetracyclines given orally and benzoyl peroxide topically cleared most of the disease, except the seborrhea

Below   Acne conglobata on chest, neck, and back (not shown here) and sparing of the face are quite typical features of this acne variant. The therapeutic approach consisted of tetracycline 1.5 g/day, DADPS 100 mg/day, tretinoin, benzoyl peroxide topically, and lifting his spirits. Scars were left behind

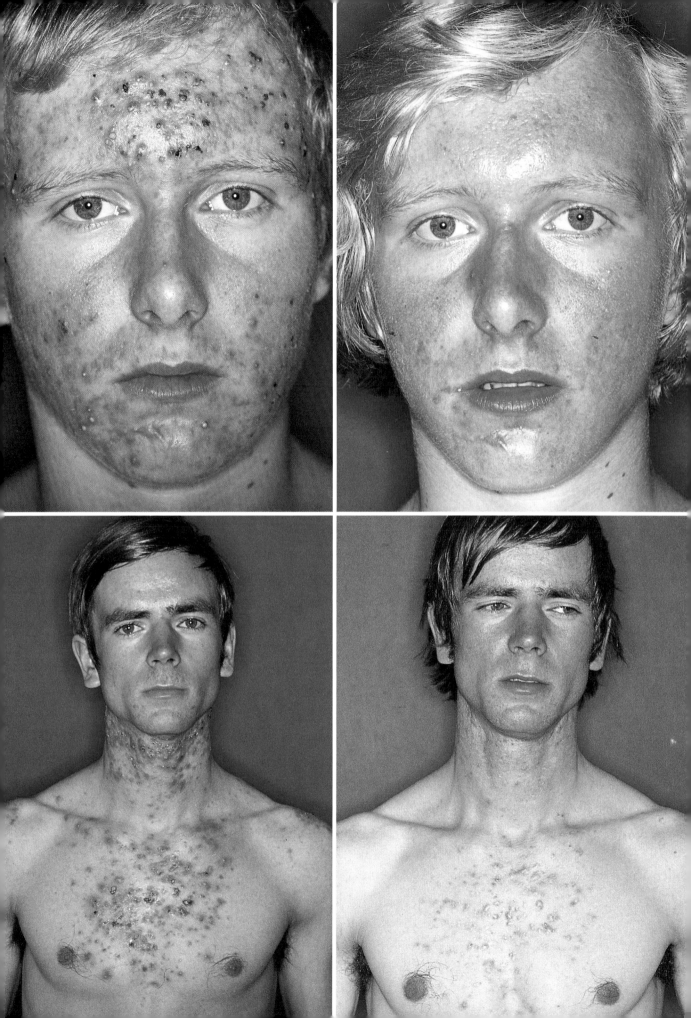

Isotretinoin (13-*cis*-Retinoic Acid)

Historical Note

While searching for retinoids with less severe side effects than tretinoin, Bollag (Hoffmann-La Roche, Switzerland) discovered and then synthesized isotretinoin (13-*cis*-retinoic acid) in 1971. As early as 1973 the drug was tried in psoriasis, but the results were not encouraging. However, by 1976 isotretinoin was found to be highly effective in the treatment of disorders of keratinization, particularly Darier's disease, lamellar ichthyosis, and pityriasis rubra pilaris. It happened that one patient who also had severe acne responded dramatically. Thus serendipity led to the discovery of a drug which is incomparable effective in acne conglobata. Credit must go to Peck and his colleagues from the National Institutes of Health who showed conclusively that isotretinoin could suppress and even cure severe inflammatory acne. Systematic studies regarding dosage, toxicity, and effects on sebum production were published in 1979 in the USA and in 1980 in Germany and Great Britain.

Pharmacology

The drug is rapidly absorbed after oral administration, producing peak levels of 180–460 ng/ml in 1–6 h (average 3.2 h) after a single dose of 80 mg. Its main metabolite is 4-oxo-isotretinoin. Isotretinoin is more than 99% bound to plasma albumin. Bioavailability is rather low, about 25%. Three binding proteins are identified:

Retinol-Binding Protein (RBP) acting specifically as a carrier for the transport of retinol from liver stores to the target tissue via the blood stream;

Cellular Retinol-Binding Protein (CRBP) which exists in the cytoplasm and is responsible for the intracellular transport; and

Cellular Retinoid Acid-Binding Protein (CRABP) which is responsible for the transport of retinoic acid, the main metabolite of retinol, and of isotretinoin.

The nuclear receptors for isotretinoin have been identified. Much of the drug is eliminated via biliary excretion with some enterohepatic recirculation. The terminal elimination half-life is much shorter than for etretinate and ranges from 10 to 20 h. There seems to be no deep compartment storage in fatty tissue, as is the case with etretinate. Absorption of isotretinoin is moderately enhanced by food. Accordingly, intake is recommended with or after the main meal of the day, or with some milk.

Toxicology

Therapeutic doses of isotretinoin invariably induce a variety of toxic effects which are specific expressions of the hypervitaminosis A syndrome. Hypervitaminosis A was well known to pioneers of the polar regions after having eaten polar bear liver: The symptoms included weight loss, fatigue, weakness, lethargy, dry skin, hair loss, and headaches. There is no antidote. The more frequently discussed problems center around:

Mutagenicity

No mutagenic effects have been seen in various systems such as Ames test, gene mutation test with hamster cells, and mouse micronucleus test. A dose-dependent increase in sister chromatid exchanges (SCE) was induced by isotretinoin in human diploid fibroblast cultures.

Carcinogenicity

There is no evidence of carcinogenicity in the human. On the contrary, retinoids have been shown to be effective against tumor promotion in many systems. Retinoids including isotretinoin are used for chemoprevention of various malignant tumors. This field is under intensive investigation worldwide.

Teratogenicity

All therapeutically useful retinoids, e.g., retinol, vitamin A palmitate, tretinoin (*all-trans*-retinoic acid), etretinate, and isotretinoin, are unequivocally embryotoxic and teratogenic when administered in sufficient doses at susceptible stages of pregnancy. The teratogenic dose varies from species to species. The threshold teratogenic dose for humans is not known. Federal agencies have laid firm restrictions on the sale and use of synthetic retinoids, including vitamin A. The latter is freely available over the counter, especially in health food stored and often in association with multivitamin preparations. Many food faddists take as many as 100000 IU of retinol daily. There is little doubt that such doses can cause congenital deformities. It should be remembered that teratogenicity is also possible from ingestion of products with high amounts of vitamin A by women of childbearing age, or from vitamin A supplementation specifically recommended for vitamin fortification during pregnancy. In the USA one can buy any quantity of retinol in health food stores. In Germany, specific warnings were recently placed by law on all packages.

Direct evidence of teratogenicity comes from laboratory studies with various animal species, and also from circumstantial evidence in women. This is not the case with topically applied tretinoin and isotretinoin, because the concentrations and amounts applied are too low.

The vitamin A malformation syndrome is manifested in the central nervous system (hydrocephalus, microcephalus), craniofacial skeleton (cleft palate), eye and ear defects (micropinna, absent ear canal), skeleton abnormalities (axial and at the extremities), and cardiovascular defects (septum defect, aorta anomalies, tetralogies).

Fertility

Isotretinoin poses no hazard to the male reproductive system. Teratogenicity cannot be transferred via the ejaculate or sperm to the woman, a question which is commonly asked. It is noteworthy that certain sperm aberrations were actually reversed in acne conglobata patients receiving isotretinoin. This was probably due to the elimination of severe inflammation and secondary effects on general health.

Indications

Indications vary from country to country. In the USA the specific indication is for severe, recalcitrant, nodular and inflammatory acne. Because of teratogenicity, regulators in the USA insist that isotretinoin should be reserved for patients with severe cystic acne who are unresponsive to conventional therapy, including systemic antibiotics. In Germany, the spectrum is broader including acne conglobata, severe inflammatory acne resistant to conventional drugs, acne fulminans, and acne inversa.

Despite the exhortations of the regulators, physicians have made up their own mind regarding the patients for whom they will prescribe isotretinoin. The sale of the drug is much greater than the narrow indications of the package inserts. This is as it should be, since doctors are in the best position to decide who should receive this "miracle" drug. Thus, isotretinoin has been effectively used in severe acne, rosacea, and pyodermas, e.g., gram-negative folliculitis, dissecting cellulitis of the scalp, and rosacea fulminans (pyoderma faciale). We even allow its use in persistent papulopustular acne which has responded poorly to conventional therapy. The manufacturer has prepared an elaborate educational program to reduce the risk of teratogenicity. The number of annual cases of congenital abnormalities has been decreasing steadily. Nonetheless, physicians are responsible for explaining the potential side effects of the drug.

Contraindications

Isotretinoin is contraindicated in pregnancy (category X by American standards) and in patients with paraben sensitivity, since paraben is used as a preservative in the gelatin capsule.

Mechanisms of Action

These are only partly understood. Certain pharmacologic effects have been established.

Sebum Suppression

One of the stunning properties is the decreased sebum production in every patient. The decrease is unequalled by any other drug (estrogen, estrogen-progestin combinations, or antiandrogens), of rapid onset within the first 2 weeks, and dose-dependent. Quantitative studies reveal a dose-dependent suppression of about 30% with 0.1 mg, 40% with 0.5 mg, and 70% with 1.0 mg per kilogram body weight/day, reaching almost 90% with the latter dose after 3 months of therapy. Histologic and electron-microscopic studies reveal an astonishing reduction of the population of sebocytes. The previously large cauliflower-like sebaceous acini regress to barely discernible miniature buds of nondifferentiated epithelial cells. Not surprisingly, qualitative analysis of the skin surface lipids reveals significant alterations. Owing to the cut-off of sebum, there is an increase in the amount of cholesterol, with a decrease in wax esters and squalenes. This reflects the pattern seen in childhood before androgens stimulate the sebaceous glands. What is left on the surface is mainly the contribution from epidermal lipids. Normally about 95% of the skin surface lipids are of sebaceous origin. Cholesterol values in excess of 10% are seen when sebum production falls to less then $0.4 \text{ mg}/10 \text{ cm}^2$ every 3 h (the normal value in untreated young men is 2.5 mg).

After discontinuation of therapy, sebum production begins to increase within 2–3 weeks and slowly returns to nearly nor-

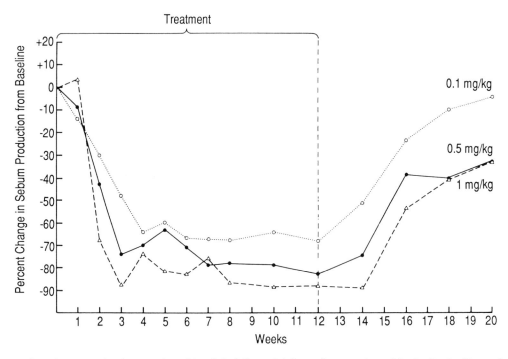

Changes in sebum production produced by 0.1, 0.5, and 1.0 mg/kg per day of isotretinoin (Reproduced from Farrell et al. 1980, with permission of the publisher and the authors)

mal levels by 10–12 months. In some patients sebum production never reaches its original value.

The clinical benefits of sebum suppression are particularly noteworthy. Even the worst cases of seborrhea improve; the skin looks and feels dry. Likewise seborrhea of the scalp, common in acne patients, completely vanishes. Instead of shampooing the greasy scalp and hair daily, shampooing is reduced to intervals of 3–7 days. The cessation of sebum production can become a severe problem in other body sites, e.g., trunk, flank, lower legs, or upper arms, as dry, scaling, asteatotic, itching skin develops, sometimes accompanied by patchy eczematous dermatitis. Another area of drying out is the conjunctiva bulbi, and dry eye symptoms develop. This is dealt with further below.

Comedolytic Effects

Unlike any other drug given orally, isotretinoin prevents the formation of new comedones, stopping the disease at its inception. The comedones are loosened and unrooted, literally popping out of the follicle; follicular filaments (follicular casts) and microcomedones are likewise eliminated. It is not unusual to observe finger-like protrusions of oil-soaked casts from prominent facial pores. The diameter of facial pores, which are wide and spacious in acne patients, is remarkably reduced to a third or a fifth of their original size.

Histologically one can readily appreciate the elimination of excess of corneocyte material retained in comedones, follicular filaments, and normal sebaceous follicles. The number of corneocyte layers in a normal sebaceous filament is about 30–60; with isotretinoin it is reduced to 10–15. Much less sebum is available for colonization by *Propionibacterium acnes*; no cavernous lacunae are maintained in the follicular filaments. The tiny vellus hair comes into close contact with the follicular eptihelium. The biochemical alterations that lead to the enhanced dehiscence of corneocytes are still unknown. Possible mechanisms are: (a) incomplete formation of attachment plaques and so-called corneosomes, analogous to desmosomes of the malpighian layers, and disturbance of tonofilaments inserting into these disk-like cellular-binding sites; and (b) alteration of intercellular lipids, the mortar-like domaine, which is responsible for the barrier function of the stratum corneum. Ceramides, sphingolipids, and other lipid classes, but also proteins and sugars may be modulated by the retinoid. There is evidence of reductions in the major lipid classes, especially ceramides and sphingolipids; these make up more than 50% of the intercellular lipids.

Anti-Inflammatory Action

The term "anti-inflammatory" is loosely used to describe the rather rapid resolution of inflammatory lesions: papules, pustules, persisting nodules, and inflammatory components of various scars all respond to isotretinoin. Long periods of remission are achieved. In vitro models have shown that serum from patients on isotretinoin inhibits chemotaxis of neutrophils. In vivo models in acne patients using the potassium iodide patch test support this observation. In the latter model, erythema, edema, papules, and pustules are significantly reduced. Further indirect evidence comes from the histologic studies of scars: the lingering macrophages, monocytes, and lymphocytes, always present around secondary comedones, papules, and almost all types of scars, are swept away.

Other inflammatory diseases like rosacea, perioral dermatitis, and particularly their lupoid variants, also respond very well to isotretinoin.

Effects on Bacteria

Isotretinoin is neither bactericidal nor bacteriostatic. Yet the high density of organisms in the sebaceous follicles of acne patients falls drastically. The removal of sebum on which *Propionibacterium acnes* depends for nutrition accounts for this. This is also the explanation for the great reduction, even elimination, of the mixed gram-negative organisms which are the principal pathogens in gram-negative folliculitis. No other therapy, not even antibiotics, is as effective as isotretinoin. Additionally, the elimination of horny material and the channels within comedones deprive these organisms of living space. Gram-negative folliculitis is a particularly good example. Curiously the colonization of *Staphylococcus aureus* is sometimes enhanced during isotretinoin treatment, leading clinically to boils and furunculoid lesions. Colonization starts in the nose, possibly a consequence of isotretinoin-induced rhinitis. One has to be aware of this complication. A short course of antibiotics quickly solves this problem. The prophylactic application of mupirocine ointment into the anterior nares is no longer recommended.

Immunomodulation

Few studies are available which address immunomodulation in animals or humans. Mostly other retinoids, but not isotretinoin, have been used but it may be assumed that isotretinoin exerts the same effects. There is mounting evidence that retinoids can modulate immune processes. They can inhibit the delayed hypersensitivity response when the drug is given in the sensitization phase. T-cell activation may contribute to the therapeutic effects by affecting the release of cytokines. However, retinoids have no effect on antibody formation. The action on the immune system is complex, with immunopotentiation occurring simultaneously. Many more studies are needed to resolve contradictory observations in the literature.

Side Effects

There are numerous side effects ranging from minor to major and from common to rare. The clinical spectrum is essentially that of hypervitaminosis A.
The following signs are frequent when the dose is 0.5 mg/kg body weight per day or more:

Cheilitis and Vestibulitis

The incidence of cheilitis or vestibulitis approaches almost 90% in patients treated with 0.5 mg isotretinoin or more per kilogram body weight per day. Accordingly bland emollients such as petrolatum and chapsticks are routinely recommended for every patient. Epistaxis occasionally is bothersome.

Asteatotic, Dry Skin

The face, lateral aspects of upper arms, wrist, lower legs, and flanks are commonly affected, particularly in the cold season with low humidity. Patients present with itching, scaling dermatitis of the craquelé or nummular-discoid type. Heavy moisturizers such as petrolatum or lanolin and water-in-oil creams are highly recommended.

Ophthalmologic Side Effects

Dry Eye Syndrome. Blepharoconjunctivitis in acne, particularly discomforting in rosacea, can be so severe as to require lowering the dose or stopping the treatment. The Meibomian glands and the glands of Zeiss provide lubrication of the tear film for the smooth movement of the eyelids across the conjunctiva bulbi. The trilamellar water–mucus–lipid film which is normally present is deprived of its lipid and mucus moiety. Patients who wear contact lenses are often very uncomfortable with a sandpaper-like foreign-body sensation in the eyes. Sometimes it is necessary to switch from contact lenses to glasses.

Decreased Night Vision. It is very rare for patients to suffer a decrease in night vision. Patients should be advised and cautioned when driving at night.

Corneal Opacities. It is also rare for patients to develop corneal opacities, and these are mostly seen in patients receiving high doses. After discontinuation these completely resolve.

Sticky Palms and Soles

Less than 5% of patients complain of a peculiar moist-like, sticky feeling of hands and feet. The thinned stratum corneum and an abnormal barrier, resulting in increased transepidermal water loss and other structural changes, such as increased carcinoembryonic antigen account for this phenomenon.

Friction Blisters

Heavy-duty work, sports (tennis, squash), and other manual activities may cause blistering with bulla formation on palms, fingers, and soles. Thinning of the horny layer is the cause.

Musculoskeletal Symptoms

In about 15% of patients, minor to major forms of arthralgia occur, which sometimes severe enough to require discontinuation of the drug. It mainly follows strenuous exercise, and intensive physical activity. Elevated values of creatine phosphokinase (CPK), particularly of the isoenzyme fraction MM (skeletal musculature) has been reported.

Hyperostoses and DISH

Fortunately hyperostoses are rare, and of minor clinical significance in acne patients, where dosage is comparatively low and treatment limited to a few months. However, it may be more prominent in patients with disorders of keratinization when much higher doses over extended periods are used. Disseminated Interstitial Skeletal Hyperostosis (DISH) occurs spontaneously in young persons, mainly affecting the anterior ligaments of the cervical and lumbar spine, the Achilles tendon, and the tibial tuberosity. Radiological examination discloses fine bony spicules on the vertebra, the small bones of the feet and hands, or the hips. Calcification of tendons and ligaments has also been reported. The alterations are usually asymptomatic, mainly reflecting the ability of modern image-analysis techniques to reveal subtle changes. In essence, it is not worrisome, and we do not have our patients X-rayed before and during therapy.

Pseudotumor Cerebri

The term pseudotumor cerebri refers to benign intracranial hypertension. It may be caused by a variety of drugs, including tetracyclines and vitamin A derivatives. Patients report symptoms such as headaches, impaired vision, blurred vision, "seeing yellow", emotional instability, paresthesia, and drowsiness. Often but not always, this is dose-dependent. The diagnosis is easily made by an ophthalmologist or neurologist. The drug must be discontinued; symptoms disappear spontaneously within a few days. In desperate cases, it is sometimes possible to start over again. Tetracyclines and isotretinoin must not be given together as pseudotumor cerebri is common with this combination.

Depression has been very rarely reported, but its relationship with the drug is problematic since a depressed affect in patients with severe acne is fairly frequent.

Skin Infections

Isotretinoin promotes colonization by *Staphylococcus aureus* in some patients, initially in the nasal antrum. Impetiginization should be looked for. The infection may present as impetigo contagiosa anywhere on the body as boils or furuncles, but mostly in the face with angular cheilitis. Other infections are impetiginized eczema, paronychia of the fingers or toes, meatal urethritis (mostly in men), scalp folliculitis, folliculitis barbae, and Bockhardt's folliculitis, particularly on arms and legs.

Hair Loss

Hair loss is a well-known side effect of retinoids and was earlier reported after high doses of retinol (vitamin A). This is especially seen with etretinate. Some clinicians think this occurs with oral isotretinoin, but the data are not conclusive. We have studied trichograms in a series of patients before and during isotretinoin therapy, and were unable to demonstrate telogen effluvium (loss of club hairs). Hair loss is mentioned in the package insert; hence some comments may be in order. Discoloration of hair, e.g., temporarily lightening of natural hair color has been reported.

Increased Sunburn

There is a good deal of confusion regarding sunburn. The stratum corneum gets thinner and loses some of its melanin protection due to increased turnover rates. This means a poorer shield against ultraviolet radiation. A sunscreen with a sun protection factor (SPF) of 15 or more, preferably protecting against UV-B and UV-A, is recommended for patients while they are outdoors during the sunny season.

Laboratory Abnormalities

Important changes in laboratory values occur which require a policy of routine monitoring.

Lipids

Approximately 25% of patients develop elevated plasma triglyceride levels, although these are rarely above 400 mg%. A mild to moderate increase of high-density lipoprotein (HDL) levels may occur. Much rarer are elevated cholesterol levels, overestimated in the past. All these lipid abnormalities are reversible once the drug is stopped. Known risk factors are familial hyperlipidemias, obesity, smoking, alcoholic beverages, diabetes mellitus, oral contraceptives, diets high in fat, and inactivity.

Hepatotoxicity

Mild to moderate elevation of liver enzyme activities occurs in about 15% of patients. This is usually asymptomatic and reverses quickly after discontinuation. Hepatitis has been reported, but the causative role of isotretinoin has not been proved.

Inflammatory Bowel Disease

There are rare reports of exacerbations of chronic colitis and regional ileitis in patients with prior histories of these afflictions.

Pyogenic Granuloma-like Lesions

Although only a cutaneous nuisance pyogenic granuloma-like lesions are a troublesome complaint, especially when misdiagnosed, as is usually the case. The mushroom-like granulation tissue is characteristically observed in patients with acne conglobata and acne fulminans. Single or multiple, bright-red, denuded, moist nodules spring up on the trunk, particularly the shoulder belt, upper back or chest, reaching dimensions of 1–2 cm in diameter, and 5–10 mm in elevation. They bleed quite easily and soil underwear and bed linens. They soon become covered with a thick black hemorrhagic crust. Unfortunately they heal with wide atrophic or hypertrophic scars. Not infrequently, impetiginization with *Staphylococcus aureus* is superimposed and unfortunately is not obvious clinically. Bacterial cultures should be performed. The same granulomatous lesions may develop spontaneously in patients with acne conglobata and acne fulminans without isotretinoin treatment.

The best approach consists of topical application of potent corticosteroids. We use clobetasole propionate several times daily for a few days. Excessive angiogenesis and collagen formation is arrested. Intradermal injections of triamcinolone acetonide is also effective. Cautery, curettage, silver nitrate sticks, and other painful intrusions are outdated.

Erythema Nodosum

Erythema nodosum is rare. It presents as painful nodular lesions on the shins, especially in men. Again, the acne fulminans patient is particularly prone. Bed rest, elevation of legs, occlusive dressings with potent corticosteroids, and, if necessary, oral corticosteroids calm down the vasculitis.

Practical Guidelines for Therapy

- Establish the correct diagnosis and type of severity of acne.
- Explain the drug, its modes of action, and the anticipitated side effects.
- Hand out a brochure provided by the manufacturer which lists all details patients should know about, including indications and contraindications. The physician assumes great responsibility in prescribing this potent drug. Take enough time to explain its benefits and risks.
- Minors should be accompanied by a parent or guardian. The drug must not be given without parental consent.
- Blood chemistry is performed before initiation of therapy and at control visits (*) at 2, 6, and 10 weeks, and thereafter if necessary: hemoglobin, erythrocytes, leukocytes, SGOT*, SGPT*, GGTP*, LDH, triglycerides*, cholesterol*, bilirubin; sedimentation rate, urine analysis.
- Remember the precautions of the detailed program for women of childbearing age (p. 635).
- Ask for patient's body weight to adjust dose.
- Discuss concomitant topical and systemic therapy. Patients should not take vitamin A supplementation to avoid additive toxic effects (hypervitaminosis A).
- Unmedicated emollients (basis ointments preferred) should be used to combat dry skin, lips, and nose. Hydrophobic "moisturizers" (petrolatum) are most effective, though greasy. Next best are water-in-oil emulsions (e.g., Eucerin cream, Moisturel cream). Sunscreens should be used when solar exposure is extensive.
- Hand over the prescription only if laboratory results are normal, and to women only after completion of a special check-up list.
- Explain possible flare-ups of acne; this is common in the first 2–4 weeks.
- Note that decreased tolerance to contact lenses may require switch to glasses.
- It is recommended that patients do not donate blood during therapy and for 1 month thereafter (theoretically transfer of a teratogenic blood level to a woman of childbearing potential is possible).
- Be cheerful! Most patients and parents are shocked after they have read the package insert with its long account of potential problems.

Dosage Forms

Isotretinoin was registered as Accutane in 1982 in the USA, and as Roaccutan in Europe, and since then in some 50 countries. In the USA the drug is available in capsules containing 10, 20, and 40 mg. In Germany 2.5, 10, and 20 mg capsules are also sold. Hoffmann–La Roche is the sole producer.

Dosage

The dose ranges from 0.1 to 2.0 mg/kg body weight daily for 15–20 weeks.

Isotretinoin should be divided into two daily doses if the dose is greater than 40 mg daily. Dosage is dependent on a number of variables. Moderately severe inflammatory acne generally responds well to 0.5 mg/kg body weight. We include persistent papulopustular acne as an indication for isotretinoin. A dose as low as 0.1 mg/kg body weight is surprisingly effective in many cases; however, resolution is slower and the relapse rate higher. Low dosage is recommended for very anxious patients, in cold, dry, wintery climates, or for those with Celtic skin type I, and is surprisingly well tolerated. Inexperienced or very cautious physicians are well advised to start with 0.5 mg/kg body weight, adjusting the dose according to the response.

Another tactic which seems promising in moderately severe inflammatory acne is to start with 0.1 mg/kg body weight and to maintain this for 5–6 months. High doses are associated with faster response, complete instead of incomplete clearing, and lower recurrence rates. The inevitable price is troublesome side effects.

Duration of Treatment

A course of 15–20 weeks is recommended by the manufacturer, and this was also the duration in early trials. Common practice and experience is teaching that longer periods, 24–32 weeks, are best to achieve complete healing in severe cases with deep nodules. As always treatment programs should be individualized. Some patients require less than 15 weeks, and others more than 32 weeks. It is a common observation that the disease continues to improve after discontinuation of the drug.

Relapse Rate

Recurrences, although milder than the original presentation, are fairly common, although less frequent when high doses are given. The relapse rate is indirectly proportional to the therapeutic dose. At 6 months after withdrawal of the drug, 95% of patients receiving 1.0 mg/kg body weight did not relapse, but 74% of the cohort receiving 0.2 mg did. This figure rises to about 50% with 0.1 mg/kg body weight.

Retreatment

It is sometimes necessary to undergo retreatment; this is entirely feasible. Usually one waits a few months before starting a second or even third course. Longer drug-free intervals are preferred by us. Severe relapse requires higher doses, and in rare cases adjunctive therapy such as adrenal suppression with dexamethasone.

Concomitant Therapy

Most patients are maintained on monotherapy; nothing else is needed. Prophylactic greasing of lips and vestibuli nasi is sufficient. Oral contraceptives in women enhance the therapeutic benefit. The addition of topical treatment is a doctor's choice, largely determined by his experience.

Concomitant Topical Therapy

Most patients do not require tretinoin. It must be used cautiously to avoid excessive irritation. Tretinoin is very worthwhile in patients with innumerable closed comedones, some of which are so tightly closed that prolonged isotretinoin fails.

Benzoyl peroxide and azelaic acid are rarely needed, and no formal studies are available.

Severe inflammatory acne conglobata, acne fulminans, as well as rosacea conglobata and rosacea fulminans (pyoderma faciale) all calm down much faster if potent topical corticosteroids are applied twice daily for 7–10 days. Edema, hemorrhage, crusting, and granulation tissue quickly respond to this additional anti-inflammatory regimen. Above all, scarring is minimized. With this short course, neither local nor systemic side effects have occurred. Corticosteroids must not be given alone to acne patients.

As regards antibiotics, topical tetracyclines, erythromycin, and clindamycin are sometimes added. We do not make use of this, but see no harm in it.

Concomitant Systemic Therapy

Tetracyclines are contraindicated, as they enhance the risk of pseudotumor cerebri as well as other complications, especially gastrointestinal complaints.

Erythromycin and other macrolids, e.g., josamycin, are not indicated. In one study, isotretinoin 0.5 mg/kg body weight daily was compared to a combined therapy with 1.0 g of erythromycin daily. The combination produced a more rapid rate of improvement though the final result was not superior. We do not recommend this combination.

We advocate the addition of corticosteroids for severe inflammatory acne conglobata, acne fulminans, as well as rosacea conglobata and rosacea fulminans. We start with the steroid, usually prednisolone 1.0–1.5 mg/kg body weight daily for about 1 week. The steroid is then tapered within 10–14 days after starting isotretinoin. Longer use in unusual cases of acne fulminans may be justified.

A combination of antiandrogens and oral contraceptives is most frequently used in women of childbearing age for the improvement of acne as well as to prevent pregnancy. Consult the gynecologist. Where available 2 mg cyproterone acetate in combination with 35 µg ethinylestradiol (Diane 35, Dianette) probably is the best alternative, as a speedy resolution of inflammatory lesions, and a particularly rapid sebum suppression is achieved.

As regards interactions with other drugs, the problem of drug interference is complex and many questions remain unsolved. As yet there are no clear guidelines. Drugs most commonly discussed in this context are anticonvulsives, oral antidiabetics, insulin, estrogens, progesteron, and antidepressants such as lithium. Before coming to any decision, consult the specialty physician, look into the ever-growing reports in the literature, and use the assistance of drug information networks, or the help of the manufacturer.

We have used isotretinoin effectively in patients on oral antidiabetics, insulin, anticonvulsives and in those bearing kidney transplants receiving azathioprine, cyclosporine A, and corticosteroids for immunosuppression. All tolerated isotretinoin, experienced no deleterious effects on their basic disease, and achieved clearing of their acne.

Precautions in Women of Childbearing Potential

Isotretinoin is a teratogen, like all retinoids including retinol itself. Unfortunately the teratogenic hazard was not sufficiently emphasized earlier. More fetal abnormalities were seen in the USA than in Europe. This has all changed. Exhaustive information is now provided by the manufacturer. It is well summarized in the advertisement: "Start right, or don't start." Much of the following information is directly taken from the manufacturers' educational brochures.

Contraindication and Warning

Major fetal abnormalities have been reported. Isotretinoin must not be used by women who are pregnant, who may become pregnant while undergoing therapy and 1 month thereafter, or who may not use reliable contraception for 1 month before treatment, during treatment, and 1 month after treatment.

If the dermatologist wishes to refer his patient to a consulting physician for contraceptive counseling, the manufacturer of isotretinoin will pay for the initial counseling and the serum pregnancy testing (in the USA only).

Treatment Rules

Women must have a sensitive urine or serum pregnancy test done to exclude pregnancy before taking isotretinoin. A prescription should not be filled in until a report of a negative pregnancy test has been obtained.

Do not start isotretinoin until the third day of the menstrual period. Effective contraceptive measures must be used 1 month before, during, and 1 month after cessation of isotretinoin.

Some countries, e.g., the USA, provide a special form to sign up for a confidential follow-up survey.

A special consent form, written in easily understandable language, is provided. The patient, parent, or guardian signs it. The prescribing dermatologist countersigns it. This record is kept by the physician.

Bershad S, Rubinstein A, Paterniti JR Jr, Le NA, Poliak SC, Heller B, Ginsberg HN, Fleischmajer R, Brown WV (1985) Changes in plasma lipids and lipoproteins during isotretinoin therapy for acne. N Engl J Med 313:981–985

Bigby M, Stern RS (1988) Adverse reactions to isotretinoin. J Am Acad Dermatol 18:543–552

Blumental G (1984) Paronychia and pyogenic granuloma-like lesions with isotretinoin. A report from the adverse drug reaction reporting system. J Am Acad Dermatol 10:677–678

Camisa C, Eisenstat B, Ragaz A, Weissmann G (1982) The effect of retinoids on neutrophil functions in vivo. J Am Acad Dermatol 6:620–629

Chivot M, Midoun H (1990) Isotretinoin and acne: a study of relapses. Dermatologica 180:240–243

Chytil F (1986) Retinoic acid: biochemistry and metabolism. J Am Acad Dermatol 15:741–747

Cunliffe WJ, Miller AJ (eds) (1984) Retinoid therapy. A review of clinical and laboratory research. MTP Press Limited, Lancaster

Dai WS, La Braico JM, Stern RS (1992) Epidemiology of isotretinoin exposure during pregnancy. J Am Acad Dermatol 26:599–606

David M, Hodak E, Lowe N (1988) Adverse effects of retinoids. Med Toxicol Adverse Drug Exp 3:273–288

Farrell LN, Strauss JS, Stranieri AM (1980) The treatment of severe cystic acne with 13-*cis*-retinoic acid. J Am Acad Dermatol 3:602–611

Gold JA, Shupack JL, Nemec MA (1989) Ocular side effects of the retinoids. Int J Dermatol 28:218–225

Hennes R, Mack A, Schell H, Vogt HJ (1984) 13-*cis*-retinoic acid in conglobata acne. A follow-up study of 14 trial centers. Arch Dermatol Res 276:209–215

James WD, Leyden JJ (1985) Treatment of gram-negative folliculitis with isotretinoin: positive clinical and microbiologic response. J Am Acad Dermatol 12:319–324

Kilcoyne RF, Cope R, Cunningham W, Nardella FA, Denman S, Franz TJ, Hanifin J (1986) Minimal spinal hyperostosis with low-dose isotretinoin therapy. Invest Radiol 21:41–44

Kiraly CL, Valkamo MH (1991) Renal transplantation and isotretinoin. Acta Derm Venereol (Stockh) 71:88

Lehucher Ceyrac D, Serfaty D, Lefrancq H (1992) Retinoids and contraception. Dermatology 184:161–170

Leyden JJ, McGinley KJ, Foglia AN (1986) Qualitative and quantitative changes in cutaneous bacteria associated with systemic isotretinoin therapy for acne conglobata. J Invest Dermatol 86:390–393

MacDonald Hull S, Cunliffe WJ (1989) The safety of isotretinoin in patients with acne and systemic diseases. J Dermatol Treat 1:35–37

MacKie RM (ed) (1988) Retinoids. Pergamon Oxford

Neubert U, Plewig G, Ruhfus A (1986) Treatment of gram-negative folliculitis with isotretinoin. Arch Dermatol Res 278:307–313

Oral retinoids. A workshop (1982) J Am Acad Dermatol 6:573–832

Orfanos CE, Braun-Falco O, Farber EM, Grupper C, Polano MK, Schuppli R (eds) (1981) Retinoids. Advances in basic research and therapy. Springer, Berlin

Peck GL, Olsen TG, Yoder FW, Strauss JS, Downing DT, Pandya M, Butkus D, Arnaud-Battandier J (1979) Prolonged remissions of cystic and conglobate acne with 13-cis-retinoic acid. N Engl J Med 300:329–333

Penneys NS, Taylor R, Hernandez D (1992) Etretinate increases carcinoembryonic antigen in palmar scrapings. J Am Acad Dermatol 26:940–2

Plewig G, Nikolowski J, Wolff HH (1982) Action of isotretinoin in acne, rosacea and gramnegative folliculitis. J Am Acad Dermatol 6:766–785

Plewig G, Wagner A (1981) Anti-inflammatory effects of 13-cis-retinoic acid. An in vivo study. Arch Dermatol Res 270:89–94

Rappaport EB, Knapp M (1989) Isotretinoin embryopathy – a continuing problem. J Clin Pharmacol 29:463–465

Robertson DB, Kubiak E, Gomez EC (1984) Excess granulation tissue responses associated with isotretinoin therapy. Br J Dermatol 111:689–694

Rollman O, Vahlquist A (1986) Oral isotretinoin (13-cis-retinoic acid) therapy in severe acne: drug and vitamin A concentrations in serum and skin. J Invest Dermatol 86:384–389

Saurat JH (ed) (1985) Retinoids: new trends in research and Therapy. Karger, Basel

Scheinman PL, Peck GL, Rubinow DR, Digiovanna JJ, Abangan DL, Ravin PD (1990) Acute depression from isotretinoin. J Am Acad Dermatol 22:1112–1114

Sporn MB, Roberts AB, Goodman DS (eds) (1984) The retinoids. Vols I and II. Academic Press, Orlando

Sporn MB, Roberts AB, Roche NS, Kagechika H, Shudo K (1986) Mechanism of action of retinoids. J Am Acad Dermatol 15:756–764

Strauss JS, Rapini RP, Shalita AR, Konecky E, Pochi PE, Comite H, Exner JH (1984) Isotretinoin therapy for acne: results of a multicenter dose-response study. J Am Acad Dermatol 10:490–496

Thomson EJ, Cordero JF (1989) The new teratogens: accutane and other vitamin A analogs. Am J Nurs 14:244–248

Tripp TB, Abele DC (1986) Creatine phosphokinase levels and isotretinoin therapy. J Am Acad Dermatol 14:130–132

Vogt HJ, Ewers R (1985) 13-cis-Retinsäure und Spermatogenese. Spermatologische und impulszytophotometrische Untersuchungen. Hautarzt 36:281–286

Weleber RG, Denman ST, Hanifin JM, Cunningham WJ (1986) Abnormal retinal function associated with isotretinoin therapy for acne. Arch Ophthalmol 104:831–837

Therapeutic Triumphs with Isotretinoin

The therapeutic outcome in these two young men is spectacular. Pictures like these should be shown to new patients with severe acne. They inspire hope and promote compliance.

Above Severe acne conglobata (*left*) was completely cleared by 12 months of isotretinoin (*right*) with no recurrences

Below Acne fulminans (*left*) struck this 13-year-old boy who also had ulcerating lesions on chest and back, accompanied by fever, leukocytosis, arthralgias, and erythema nodosum. Twelve weeks of isotretinoin (*right*) made him smile again

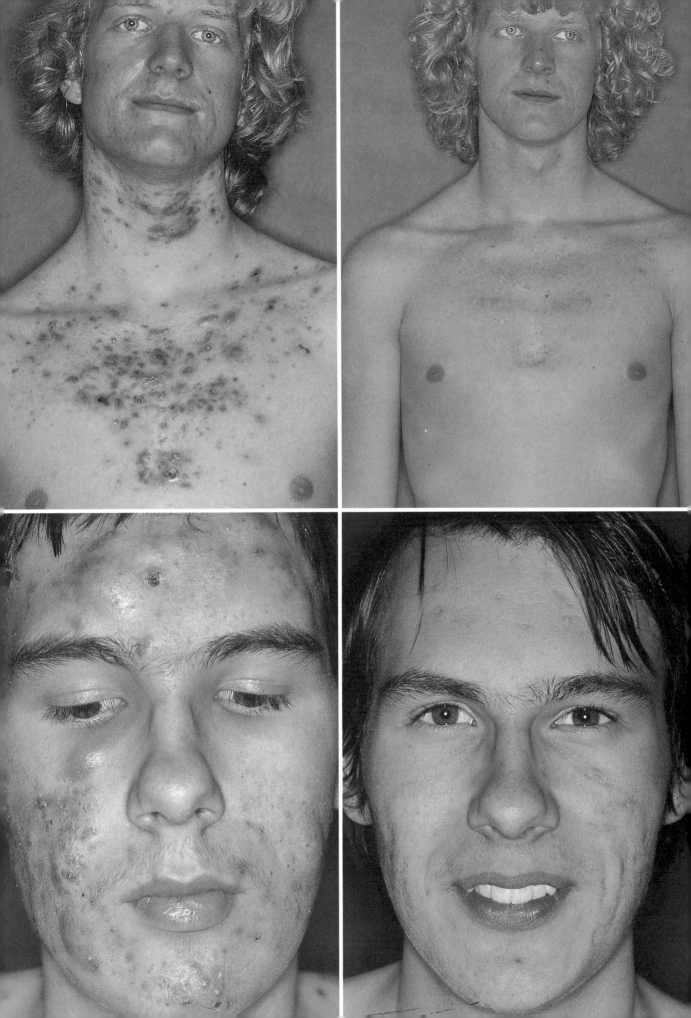

Isotretinoin Is the Miracle Drug in Acne Conglobata

Confluent, long-lasting nodules and abscesses are typical of acne conglobata. The patient suffered from widespread, fulminant acne conglobata (*above*). Closed comedones, papules, pustules, and confluent nodules, as shown here in the submandibular area and on the neck are usually very stubborn and complicated to treat. A 12-week course of 1.0 mg/kg body weight isotretinoin produced complete and permanent clearing (*below*).

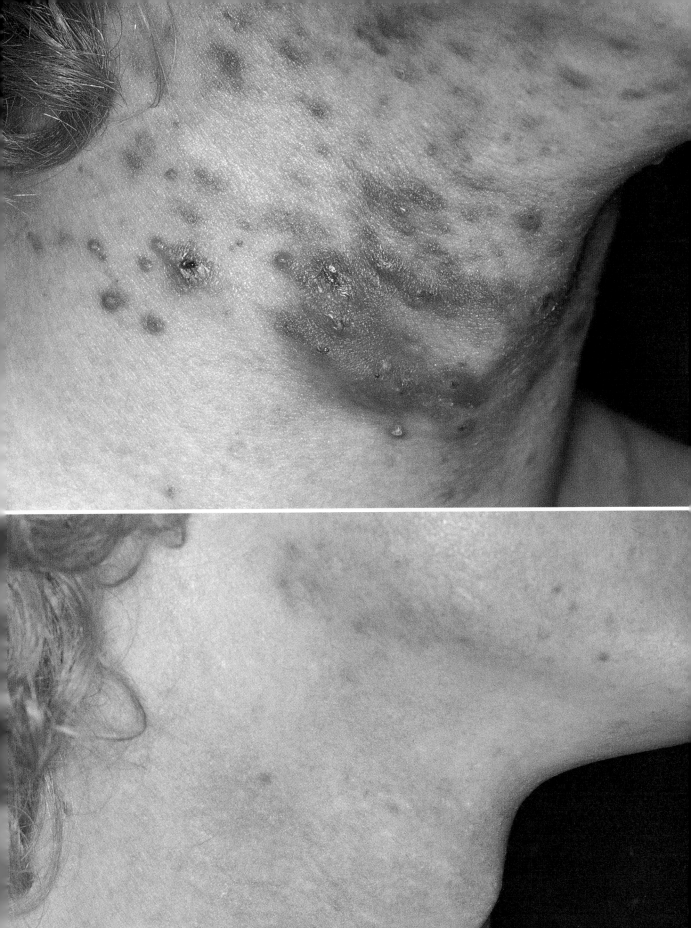

Isotretinoin Loosens and Expels Corneocytes

One of the miraculous effects of oral isotretinoin is that existing comedones are expelled and the formation of new ones inhibited. For orientation the hair shaft is always to the left.

Above

Left   Normal sebaceous follicle. About 15 layers of compact corneocytes fill the space between the hair and the follicular epithelium (Electron microscopy, × 4400)

Right   After isotretinoin 0.5 mg/kg for 3 weeks. Malformed, swollen corneocytes are detaching from each other and forming loose, disorganized masses. (Electron microscopy, × 4400)

Below

Left   Isotretinoin 0.5 mg/kg for 7 weeks has greatly reduced the number of corneocyte layers (Electron microscopy, × 4200)

Right   After isotretinoin 0.5 mg/kg for 12 weeks, only three to four corneocyte layers fill the narrow space between hair and epithelium. This thinning of the intrafollicular stratum corneum accounts for the smoother looking skin. Less horn in the follicular orifice creates the impression of shrinkage of the pores. The removal of follicular horny casts and microcomedones in acne-prone subjects certainly improve the complexion and cosmetic appearance. (Electron microscopy, × 6200)

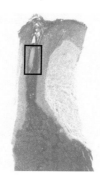

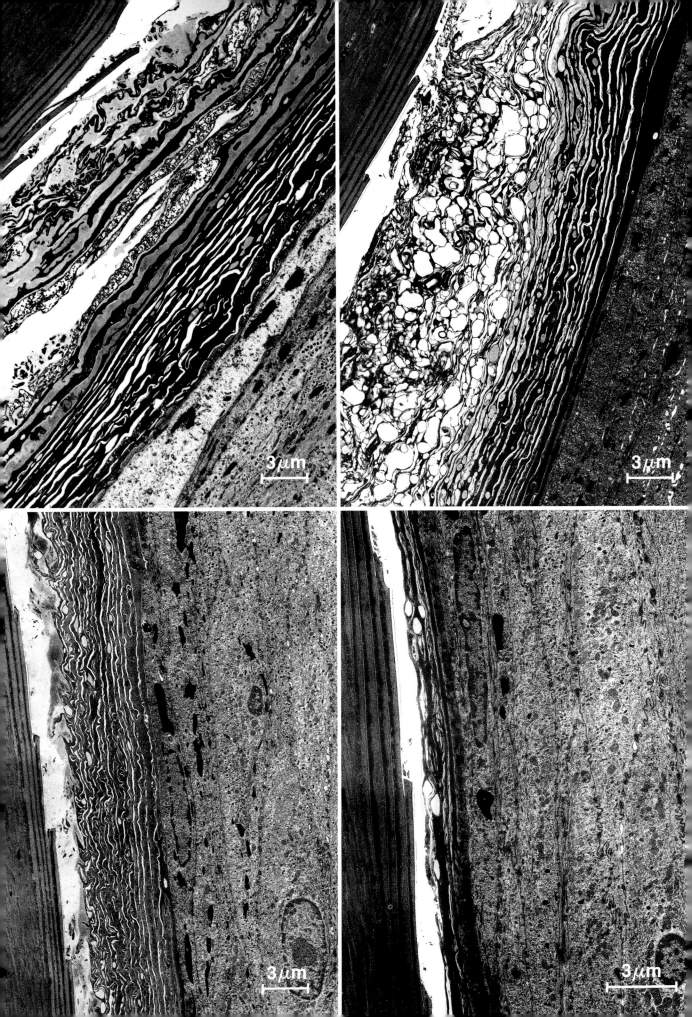

3 μm

3 μm

3 μm

3 μm

Isotretinoin Drastically Changes Cornification

Oral isotretinoin not only loosens the attachments between corneocytes but markedly alters their morphology. Transmission electron microscopy of the follicular epithelium of a comedo under isotretinoin therapy showing tightly bound layers of dense corneocytes adjacent to the granular layer. Further out the corneocytes are swollen with lipid droplets, have assumed bizarre shapes, and are separating from each other. Interference with cohesion leads to falling apart of the comedo (Electron microscopy, × 18400)

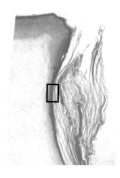

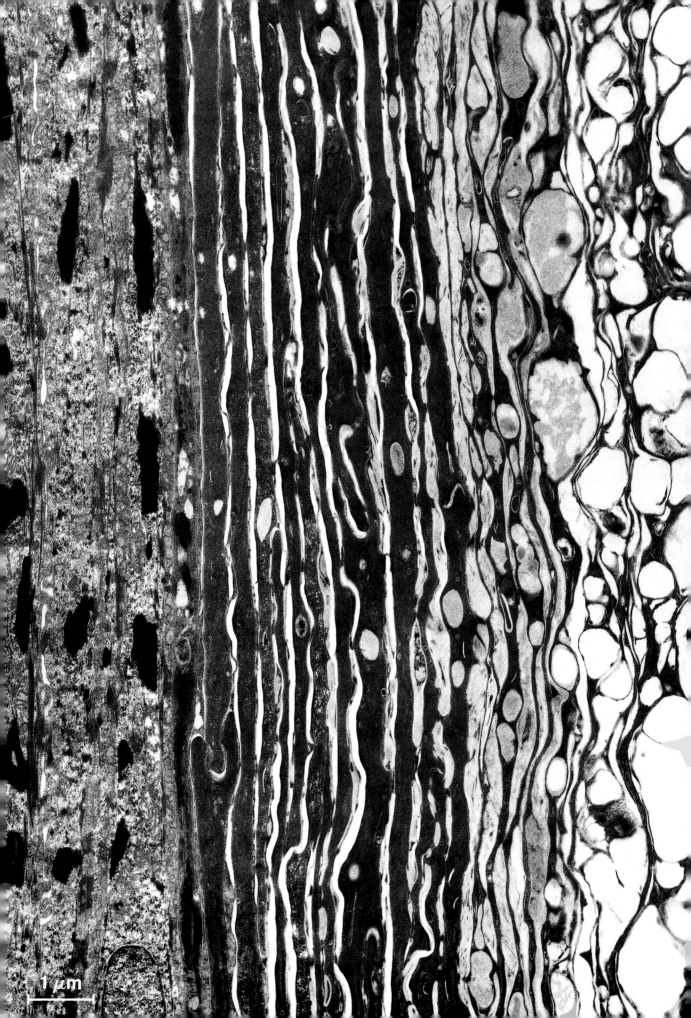

1 μm

The Miraculous Sebum Suppression of Isotretinoin

One of the most surprising actions of this retinoid is the virtual elimination of sebocytes. When these histologic sections were seen for the first time, one felt alarmed: is this permanent? Fortunately it is not. Glands re-establish weeks and months after discontinuation of the drug. It is surprising that the exact biochemical steps leading to this drought have not been described.

Above   Two facial biopsies from the same acne patient, 12 weeks apart

Left   Large sebaceous follicle with prominent sebaceous acini, one pilary unit, and a spatious follicular canal filled with cornecytes, bacteria, one hair and sebum. Before treatment. (Hematoxilin and eosin)

Right   Even serial sections through this follicle disclose nothing but a nude follicular canal with epithelium and the pilary unit. No sebaceous acini are left. Slight perifollicular fibrosis around the upper half of the follicle reveals where the sebaceous lobules were located once. Twelve weeks of oral isotretinoin completely cleared the severe acne as well. (Hematoxilin and eosin)

Below   Another example of sebum-suppressing with two facial biopsies from the same acne patient

Left   A beautiful architectural pattern of a sebaceous follicle with several sebaceous lobules draining into a cavernous follicular canal. (Before treatment. Semithin section, methylene blue)

Right   After only 2 weeks of oral isotretinoin the whole sebaceous follicle has converted into a wick-like structure, standing lonely in the dermis. The arrows point to the buds, which were once the sebaceous acini (→). The hair fits snugly into the follicular canal, with almost no corneocyte material left in between. Bacteria are absent. Isotretinoin often makes the skin surface look very smooth by reducing the spacious follicular pores to very narrow opening. (Semithin section, methylene blue)

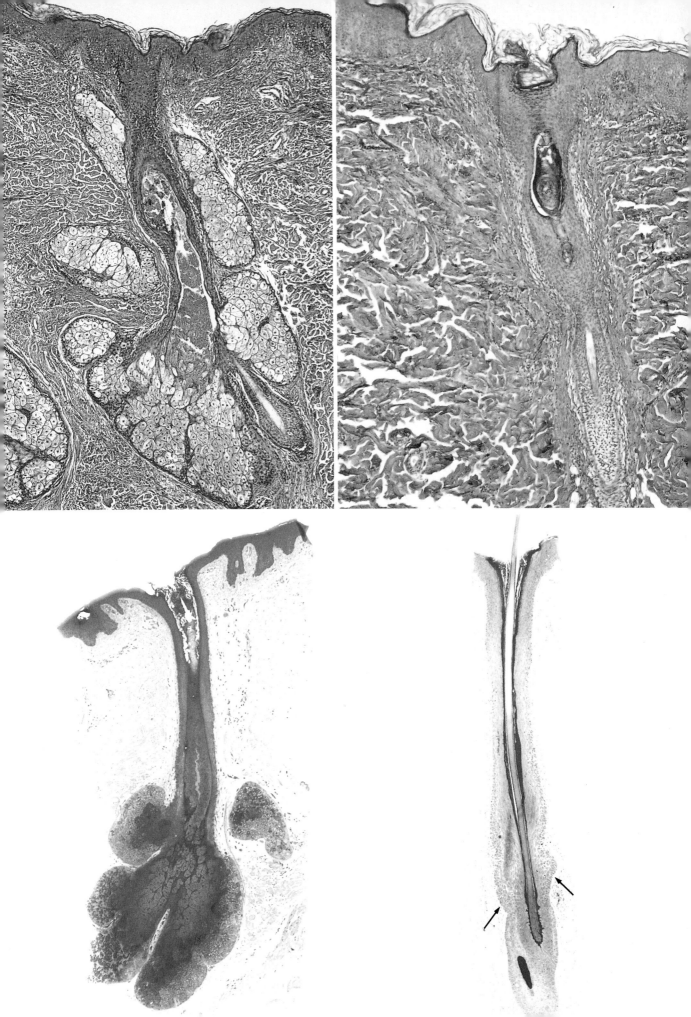

Isotretinoin Stops Sebum Production

Ultrastructurally isotretinoin switches sebum (lipid) production off completely. The semithin sections stained with methylene blue (*above*) are compared with electron microscopical views (*below*).

Above

Left   Part of a large sebaceous follicle with multilobular sebaceous acini. Lipid productions starts with small lipid inclusions at the periphery of the gland; larger droplets are seen with further maturation

Right   One week of 2.0 mg/kg body weight isotretinoin has arrested lipid production. The newly formed cells look undifferentiated. The old sebocytes have moved upward and outward and contain their original load of lipid droplets

Below

Left   Sebaceous acinus before treatment. All sebocytes produce lipid material. The basement membrane is at the bottom. (Electron microscopy, ×5200)

Right   The newly produced cells of this acinus have abruptly ceased to produce lipid. The basement membrane is below and not shown here. The two sebocytes on the top are loaded with lipid droplets, which were synthesized before treatment. (Electron microscopy, ×5200)

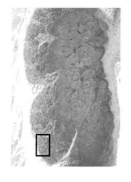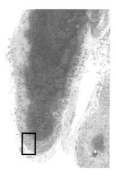

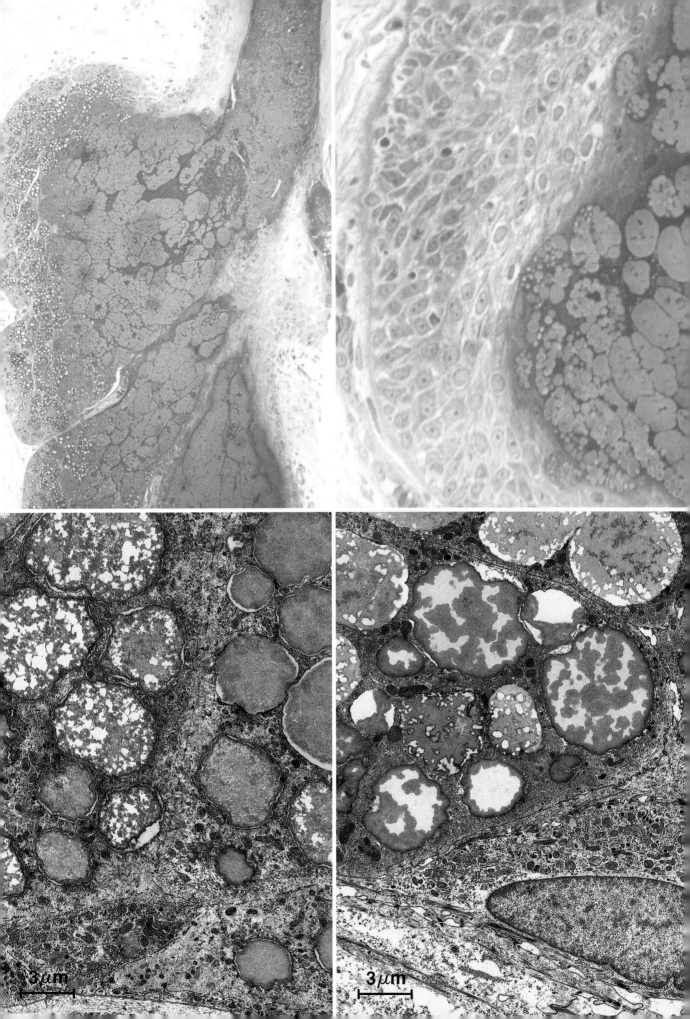

Isotretinoin: Cutaneous Side Effects

Above   Cheilitis with dry, fissured, tender lips and desquamation occurs in almost every patient, if the dose is 0.2 mg/kg or above. Greases like petrolatum and lanolin offer some relief

Below

Left   Paronychia is surprisingly frequent, an expression of the tendency of the drug to induce excess granulation tissue. One must also watch for superinfection with *Staphylcoccus aureus*

Right   Fragility of the skin, resulting in blisters and erosions, is a well-known side effect of full doses. Blunt trauma or friction causes intraepithelial and subepithelial separations

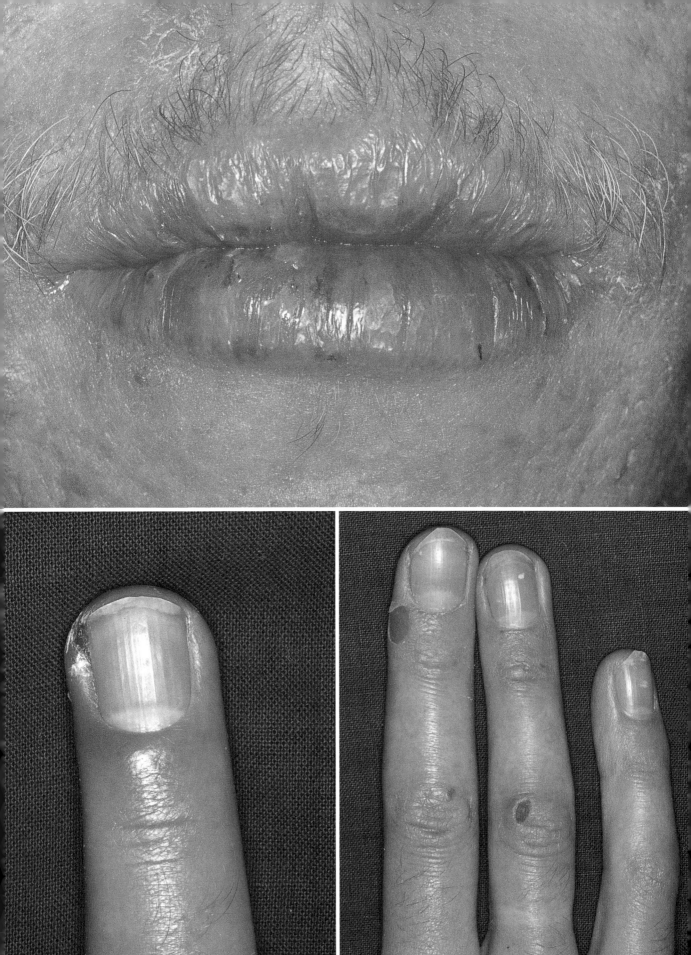

Pyoderma Superimposed on Acne

This young man with acne conglobata was responding very well to isotretinoin when suddenly there was a worsening of facial lesions. The skin of the cheeks and chin became infiltrated. Honey-colored, hemorrhagic crusts appeared. *Staphylococcus aureus* impetigenization and phlegmonous infection was suspected. Isotretinoin was discontinued. Bacterial swabs from the crusts and the nasal antrum yielded dense colonies of *Staphylococcus aureus*. Oral erythromycin cleared the superinfection within days. Impetigo contagiosa due to *Staphylococcus aureus* is not rare in isotretinoin-treated patients, but phlegmonous deep cellulitis is.

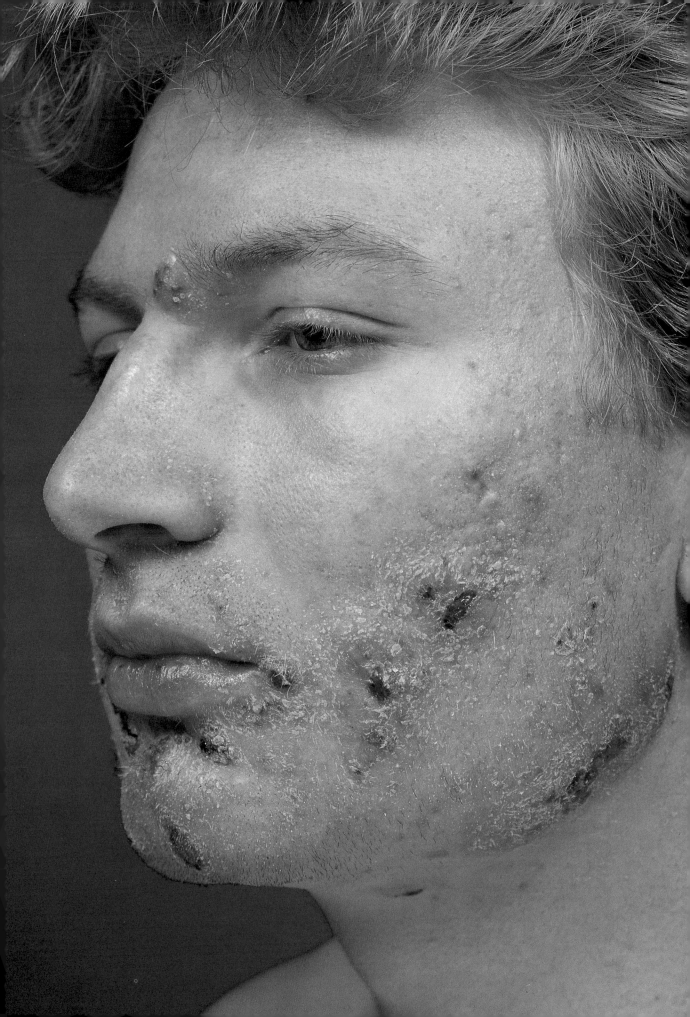

Vitamin A (Retinol)

Vitamin A is readily available anywhere around the corner: drug stores, supermarkets, health shops, pharmacies and, of course, all without a prescription. Many laymen think retinol has multiple benefits in promoting health. Vitamin A (retinol) was formerly extolled as a remedy for acne. It is still praised by some, and still used widely as a supplementary agent to other therapies. At least half a dozen multiple-combination drugs are registered alone in Germany for the treatment of acne, containing between 10000 and 50000 IU of retinol palmitate per dose, often in combination with other vitamins and assorted nutrients. Studies have shown that the amount of oral vitamin A that produces significant therapeutic effect is of the order of 300000–400000 IU units a day. This entails a definite risk of toxicity, including teratogenicity. The recommended daily dose to avoid vitamin A deficiencies is only 5000 IU.

The side effects are similar to those from other oral retinoids such as isotretinoin, namely, dry skin, cheilitis, puritus, transient skin eruptions, headache (increased intracranial pressure), nausea, hair loss, and elevation of serum lipids. Isotretinoin, a better tolerated drug, has literally thrown retinol onto the trash heap. In those countries where isotretinoin is not available, vitamin A is still widely prescribed, thankfully in doses usually not exceeding 100000 IU daily. Even when combined with other antiacne medicaments, it is doubtful that 50000 IU have any effect. We never use oral vitamin A, but always make sure to ask how much the patient may be taking, especially if isotretinoin is being contemplated. We inveigh against any dose over 10000 IU. Retinol is often given with vitamin E. Such a combination may be rationalized on theoretical grounds, but proof of efficacy is lacking.

Goodman DS (1979) Vitamin A and retinoids: recent advances. Introduction, background, and general overview. Fed Proc 38:2501–2503

Kligman AM, Leyden JJ, Mills O Jr (1981) Oral vitamin A (retinol) in acne vulgaris. In: Orfanos CE, Braun-Falco O, Farber EM, Grupper C, Polano MK, Schuppli R (eds) Retinoids. Advances in basic research and therapy. Springer, Berlin Heidelberg New York, pp 245–253

Muenter MD, Perry HO, Ludwig J (1971) Chronic vitamin A intoxication in adults. Am J Med 50:129–136

Rollman O, Vahlquist A (1985) Vitamin A in skin and serum – studies of acne vulgaris, atopic dermatitis, ichthyosis vulgaris and lichen planus. Br J Dermatol 113:405–413

Stüttgen G (1975) Oral vitamin A acid therapy. Acta Derm Venereol [Suppl] (Stockh) 74:174–179

Sulfonamides

Sulfonamides are rarely used in acne and only trimethoprim-sulfamethoxazole is presently advocated. There are two dosage forms containing a fixed combination of 80 mg trimethoprim with 400 mg sulfamethoxazole, or a double-strength combination containing 160 mg trimethoprim with 800 mg sulfamethoxazole. The latter is given twice daily.

The trimethoprim component inhibits bacteria dihydrofolate reductase; the sulfamethoxazole is a competitive inhibitor of *p*-aminobenzoic acid. The combination, therefore, has a synergistic effect on microbes. This formulation should not be casually prescribed and should be reserved for unusually subborn cases. Side effects are fairly common and may be quite serious. Allergic reactions take the forms of toxic epidermal necrolysis, erythema multiforme, and exfoliative erythroderma. We do not use sulfonamides and mention them here only for the sake of completeness. The risks seem disproportionate to the benefits.

Feingold DS, Wagner RF (1986) Antibacterial therapy. J Am Acad Dermatol 14:535–548

Cotterill JA, Cunliffe WJ, Forster RA, Williamson DM, Bulusu L (1971) A comparison of trimethoprim-sulphamethoxazole with oxytetracycline in acne vulgaris. Br J Dermatol 84:366–369

Sulfones (DADPS, DDS, Dapsone)

The sulfones have achieved eminence because of their ability to moderate all forms of leprosy, one of the world's most common and terrible infectious diseases. The antibacterial effects of sulfones have been appreciated for more than 50 years. Like sulfonamides, to which they are related, they inhibit the utilization of *p*-aminobenzoic acid by bacteria. In dermatology, however, sulfones have secured a place of distinction in a variety of nonbacterial diseases, e.g., dermatitis herpetiformis, pyoderma gangrenosum, subcorneal pustulosis, chronic pustular eruptions, and others, in which chronic inflammatory reactions are prominent. Acne is also added to this list. It was in an endemic area of leprosy that sulfones were first found to be valuable in inflammatory acne. This occurred in 1950 at about the same time the drug was found to be effective in dermatitis herpetiformis. All the sulfones are broken down in the gastrointestinal tract to diaminodiphenyl sulfone (DDS, dapsone). This is apparently the active form. The leprologists and the malarialogists have taught us that dapsone is not a drug for amateurs. The therapeutic index is narrow; effective dosage involves a substantial amount of toxicity. Studies of DDS in acne are curiously few in number.

Nevertheless, having treated many cases, we are convinced that DDS has real value in severe cases of acne. Its dangers, while real, have probably been overstressed. This is a powerful agent. Dapsone is reserved for serious, inflammatory acne, notably acne conglobata and its relatives (acne fulminans, tropical acne, etc.). Stubborn severe papulopustular acne is another indication. Comedonal and garden varieties of acne are off-limits for this drug.

DDS is rarely used alone. It is usually combined with an antibiotic and a comedolytic drug. We have observed questionable in vivo suppression of *Propionibacterium acnes*. Its mode of action thus differs from antibiotics. In some unknown way, DDS antagonizes the extensive flooding of the dermis with neutrophils, restraining abscess formation and tissue destruction. In this respect its action resembles that of corticosteroids. It thus belongs to that motley group of drugs which are designated crudely as "anti-inflammatory." Like the latter it has been shown to stabilize lysosomes. Despite a host of theories regarding its mode of action, we do not know how the drug works. Justification for its use rests on empirical grounds.

DDS is completely absorbed and accumulates in all body tissues. For this reason, leprologists usually give the drug two or three times weekly. Our approach is less cautions, for it is a rare that a patient will require the drug for more than 4 months. We use DDS as an "opener" to roll back the disease, withdrawing it as soon as that is accomplished. This usually takes about 3 months. We see the patient weekly for the first 2 weeks and every 2–4 weeks thereafter. The red blood count, or even better, measurement of methemoglobin, are the most useful laboratory tests. These are repeated every 2–4 weeks. Some anemia can be anticipated, usually the result of hemolysis of older red blood cells. Black and to a lesser extent Mediterranean patients require special monitoring for the existence of 6-glucose-phosphate-dehydrogenase deficiency. DDS induces severe hemolysis in such persons.

We begin with a daily dose of 100 mg. Mild gastrointestinal reactions may sometimes occur, but can usually be ignored. If reasonably tolerated for a week, the dose is increased to 150 or 200 mg daily and maintained at that level till the fire has been subdued. This goal can generally be reached in 4–5 months, especially in deep-seated nodulocystic acne. Sometimes it is difficult to reach the 200 mg dose until after several weeks. Cyanosis of the lips and nailbeds represent methemoglobinemia and is not an indication for lowering the dose in the absence of anemia. Treatment has to be individualized, for which hands-on experience is obligatory.

We have not encountered patients in which the drug had to be stopped altogether. Unresponsiveness to the quadruple regimen of DDS, an antibiotic, retinoic acid, and benzoyl peroxide lies outside our experience. Since DDS is reserved for only the most ferocious cases, appraisal of the risk–benefit ratio is not easy. We estimate that about in 50% excellent results are achieved. The disease can be calmed down to a socially acceptable level in most of the remainder. Occasionally, successful treatment is followed by recrudescence months or even a year or more later. We attack this event as if dealing with a fresh case, i.e., full doses of all drugs. The eventual goal is to maintain the patient on topical therapy alone. This can be achieved in about 60% within 6 months. The ideal patient behaves something like the following:

- First period: 2–3 months; 100–200 mg of DDS daily; full dose of an antibiotic, topical retinoic acid and benzoyl peroxide once to twice daily.
- Second period: 2–3 months; withdraw DDS, lower antibiotic stepwise to maintenance dose.
- Third period: indefinite; stop antibiotic; maintain by topical retinoic acid.

Side Effects

The list of side effects reads like a tale of horrors, not excluding deaths from agranulocytosis. DDS is an effective drug with risks to match. We take comfort in the fact that DDS has been used in many millions of people with health-destroying diseases, although in smaller doses. This has provided an unparalleled opportunity to uncover every conceivable type of adverse reaction. Properly monitored, DDS is a relatively safe drug in adolescents and young adults.

The most important adverse effects relate to the blood and chiefly take the form of hemolysis; leukopenia and agranulocytosis are rare. Methemoglobinemia is usually no more than an oddity but patients should be apprised of this possibility. Neuropathy is also feared, but is uncommon and usually reversible.

Nausea, vomiting, headache, and dizziness can be moderated by lowering the dose. These become a problem in about 10% of the patients. Skin reactions of all kinds have been noted, some allergic, most probably toxic. Exfoliative dermatitis is the worst of these.

Since the introduction of the wonder drug isotretinoin, we have not used DDS any more. We like to have it in reserve and have accorded it due space in this text. It is especially useful in countries or in situations where isotretinoin is not an option.

Barranco VP (1974) Inhibition of lysosomal enzymes by dapsone. Arch Dermatol 110:563–566

Kaminsky CA, Kaminsky AR De, Schicci C, Morini MV De (1974) Acne: treatment with di-aminodiphenylsulfone. Cutis 13:869–871

Bernstein JE, Lorincz AL (1981) Sulfonamides and sulfones in dermatologic therapy. Int J Dermatol 20:81–88

Lang PG Jr (1979) Sulfones and sulfonamides in dermatology today. J Am Acad Dermatol 1:479–492

Lorincz AL, Pearson RW (1962) Sulfapyridine and sulfone type drugs in dermatology. Arch Dermatol 85:42–56

Estrogens and Oral Contraceptives

The knowledge that estrogens suppress sebum secretion antedates the widespread use of oral contraceptives. Contraceptive pills are administered either as a combination of estrogen and a progestin, or sequentially with the progestin given along with the estrogen toward the end of the cycle: The progestin serves to normalize menstruation. The latter has no effect on sebum production. Indeed some progestins actually stimulate sebum output. These are sometimes called androgen-dominant contraceptives. The oral contraceptive is simply a convenient way of administering estrogen to acne patients.

The estrogenic component is either ethinyl estradiol or mestranol. The oral contraceptives that are most effective in acne contain 50 µg of ethinyl estradiol, an amount sufficient to suppress sebum secretion moderately in the majority of women. Recently, manufacturers of oral contraceptives have created a mini-pill, containing much less estrogen, to avoid coronary and peripheral thrombosis. The mini-pill is almost useless in acne.

Of course, contraceptive pills are used exclusively by women. Feminization is unavoidable in men with any dose capable of suppressing sebum production; indeed, higher doses are required to achieve sebum suppression. Estrogens should be reserved for women or teenagers (who are at least 16 years old) with rather severe acne and who have responded poorly to conventional therapy. Severe seborrhea, persistent inflammatory lesions, and scarring encourage one to try hormonal therapy. Estrogens are not the drug of first choice in severe acne. Estrogen therapy should be augmented by topical medication such as tretinoin (first choice), or antimicrobials (antibiotics or benzoyl peroxide). In severe cases, oral antibiotics are added. When isotretinoin is given to women of childbearing potential, effective contraception is mandatory (see p. 635). We favor oral contraceptives, but personal preferences should be explored. Candidates for oral isotretinoin are referred to a gynecologist for adequate counseling of side effects, complete physical and gynecological examination, and follow-up check-ups approximately every 6 months. The ability of estrogens to suppress sebum production should make these an excellent therapeutic choice. Moreover, there should be little worry about a drug that millions of women use daily. Unfortunately this is not the case. Estrogens are far from ideal and in fact have limited applications for special situations. First of all improvement is slow, taking about five cycles for substantial improvement. It generally takes a couple of cycles until sebum production begins to decrease. The reduction is usually not more than 20%–30%, and rarely up to 50%. Some women respond little or not at all. Responsive women become aware of decreased oiliness after three to four cycles. The effect of estrogens is mainly prophylactic by inhibiting the formation of comedones. Existing inflammatory lesions including papulopustules are mainly not affected. Improvement is slight or absent in about one-third of patients, a rather high failure rate about which patients should be informed. In these patients we do not advocate switching to a more potent contraceptive or doubling the dose. Rather we select another therapeutic approach. A disturbing event in a fair number of patients is an inexplicable flare of papulopustules during the first few cycles. An outcropping of many new inflammatory lesions can be alarming. Patients should be informed of this possibility and assured of its transient nature.

While contraceptives eventually lower the circulating level of androgens by inhibition of pituitary gonadotrophins, sometimes the reverse, namely an androgen-stimulating effect, seems to occur. There have been even cases of hirsutism in women receiving substantial doses of oral contraceptives. This unusual side effect is probably due to the progestin component, certain of which are weak androgens. Dermatologists have learned to avoid androgenic progestins. One should also mention that there exists a pathway for the metabolic conversion of estrogens to androgens.

Another curious limitation is estrogen escape. Patients whose acne has been brought under good control will sometimes begin to worsen after a year or two. First sebum secretion increases, then a few cycles later the disease exacerbates. Such cases are by no means rare.

Women are quite familiar with a variety of unpleasant side effects. These are quite annoying even though they are transient or episodic, and include nausea, fluid retention with weight gain, and breast tenderness. Intermenstrual spotting can sometimes happen; if frank bleeding occurs, a gynecologist should be consulted.

The most worrisome side effect of estrogen therapy is the definitely increased risk of thrombosis in the central nervous system or the periphery. A careful family history of vascular diseases should be obtained. Women with Sneddon's syndrome and anticardiolipin antibodies (livedo reticularis, which is synonymous with livedo racemosa in the European terminology) are particular at risk. There is often a family history of miscarriages. Additional risk factors are smoking, obesity, and alcohol consumption. Estrogen therapy frequently provokes melasma, at least in 30% of women. If one accepts multiple, small, pigmented lesions as expressions of melasma, the prevalence may exceed 50%. Melanin hyperpigmentation is intensified by ultraviolet radiation, and sometimes by cosmetics and fragrances. Sunscreens should be used daily in the sunny season.

Finally a very common event is a mild papulopustular eruption when the oral contraceptive is discontinued. It may last for months, and the skin may become even oilier than before. The cause of this rebound phenomenon is unknown.

Without question, serious acne in women can sometimes be considered a hyperandrogenic syndrome. The literature is contradictory and confusing, owing to technical difficulties in essaying androgens accurately. The endocrine status of most women is normal. Many studies have established that free and bound testosterone, follicle-stimulating hormone (FSH), luteinizing-hormone (LH), and prolactin are normal.

An endocrinologic work-up would be reasonable when there is evidence of masculinisation, hirsutism, hair loss of the androgenetic type, menstrual abnormalities, etc. Furthermore therapy-resistant acne belongs in this category. Polycystic ovaries are overdiagnosed. This subject is a rather complex and not fully sorted out, even by expert endocrinologists.

Darley CR, Kirby JD, Besser GM, Munro DD, Edwards CRW, Rees LH (1982) Circulating testosterone, sex hormone binding globulin and prolactin in women with late onset or persistent acne vulgaris. Br J Dermatol 106:517–522

Fanta D (1980) Hormone therapy of acne. Clinical and experimental principles. Springer, Vienna New York, pp 4–12

Hammerstein J (1980) Possibilities and limits of endocrine therapy. In: Hammerstein J, Lachnit-Fixson U, Neumann F, Plewig G (eds): Androgenization in women – acne, seborrhea, androgenic alopecia and hirsutism. Excerpta Medica, Amsterdam, pp 221–238

Lookingbill DP, Horton R, Demens LM, Egan N, Marks JG Jr, Santen RJC (1985) Tissue production of androgens in women with acne. J Am Acad Dermatol 12:481–487

Lucky AW, McGuire J, Rosenfield RL, Lucky PA, Rich BH (1983) Plasma androgens in women with acne vulgaris. J Invest Dermatol 81:70–74

Pochi E (1983) Hormone therapy of acne. Dermatol Clin 1:377–384

Wishart JM (1991) An open study of Triphasil and Diane 50 in the treatment of acne. Australas J Dermatol 32:51–54

Antiandrogens and Aldosterone Antagonists

Sebum is the fuel of the acne flame. It is not only comedogenic in its own right but provides the substrate for the growth of *Propionibacterium acnes.* Any drug that reduces sebum secretion by 30% or more will have a therapeutic beneficial effect.

Hormone Treatment of Acne

Several options exist for the hormonal treatment of acne:
- Estrogen (ovarian androgen suppression)
- Glucocorticoid (adrenal androgen suppression)
- Estrogen plus glucocorticoid (ovarian plus adrenal androgen suppression)
- Cyproterone acetate plus estrogen
- Chlormadinone acetate plus estrogen
- Megestrol acetate plus estrogen
- Spironolactone (aldosterone antagonist)

Here we shall discuss only cyproterone acetate, chlormadinone acetate, megestrol acetate, and spironolactone.
Antiandrogens for the treatment of acne which have been available in Germany for almost 20 years, have become available only quite recently in Great Britain and other European countries, but are not available in the USA. They offer an excellent alternative in certain difficult cases. Many clinical trials have proved that none of the antiandrogens are topically effective, probably because of poor absorption. Antiandrogens are an important therapeutic resource for the expert.

These drugs inhibit the action of androgens on androgen-dependent tissues, e.g., prostate, seminal vessels, and, of course, sebaceous ducts and sebocytes. They prevent the target from responding to the chemical stimulus. Dihydrotestosterone (DHT), the active metabolite of testosterone, has a high affinity for cytoplasmic androgen receptors in target cells. The necessary conversion of testosterone to DHT within the cell is catalyzed by the enzyme 5-*a*-reductase. Antiandrogens generally act by competitive inhibition by binding of DHT to androgen receptors. The receptor translocation is prevented, and the nuclear concentration of free DHT reduced. Antiandrogens block like a wrong key in the keyhole.

Cyproterone Acetate

Cyproterone acetate was discovered accidentally when researchers were looking for an orally effective progesterone. To their surprise they observed complete feminization of male rat fetuses. Cyproterone acetate was the most potent of hundreds of compounds evaluated. Some chemically related steroids, e.g., chlormadinone acetate and megestrol acetate, also display antiandrogenic effects. The only other potent nonsteroidal antiandrogen is glutamide and its hydroxylated metabolite. In contrast to the steroidal antiandrogens, the latter is not being used for acne treatment.

Cyproterone acetate was originally marketed in 1978 as a combination contraceptive containing 2 mg cyproterone acetate and 50 µg of ethinyl estradiol (Diane). The estrogen content has recently been reduced. The commercial product now contains 2 mg cyproterone acetate and only 35 µg ethinyl estradiol (Diane-35, Dianette). A package contains 21 pills, and the first pill is taken on the first day of menstruation. Since no drug is given for the last 7 days, withdrawal is followed by bleeding. In stubborn cases, the estrogen can be supplemented with extra amounts of cyproterone acetate ranging from 5 to 100 mg per day for 10 days. High-dose therapy was developed by the gynecologist Hammerstein and has come to be known as the reverse sequential schedule.

Cyproterone acetate in combination with an estrogen is restricted to women only; in men it would lead to feminization. Full information and consent, especially in minors, is mandatory. We reserve it for the following: extreme seborrhea in acne patients, therapy-resistant papulopustular acne, and refractory acne conglobata. Each patient should be seen by a gynecologist who will carry out the following requirements: exclusion of pregnancy, complete physical and gynecological examination, explanation of the action of the drug, side effects, and the appropriate response to bleeding. Follow-up examination every 6 months is encouraged.

By the second or third cycle, oiliness is generally reduced, but only by 25%–35%. Fewer inflammatory lesions develop, and the formation of comedones slows down. Curiously some patients do not respond at all, neither with respect to sebum production nor with reduction of acne lesions.

Particular attention has to be paid to side effects which are very common. These include menstrual abnormalities, breast tenderness and enlargement, nausea and vomiting, fluid retention, leg edema, headache, and melasma. Coronary and peripheral thrombosis, although rare, is the most serious complication and is the main reason why some Federal Authorities are reluctant to approve the drug. Thromboembolic episodes are more likely in those who smoke, are sedentary, overweight, or have had previous arteriosclerotic disease. It should not be given to women who suffer from livedo reticularis (livedo racemosa in the European literature) associated with Sneddon syndrome (anticardiolipin antibodies).

The cyproterone acetate–ethinyl estradiol combination is an appropriate choice for the treatment of persistent inflammatory acne. At the same time it is an oral contraceptive. Accordingly it has an important place in preventing pregnancy in woman who are receiving isotretinoin for severe acne. The combination of isotretinoin with an antiandrogen exploits two different pharmacologic actions.

Duration of treatment varies, according to individual needs, and sometimes continues for years. The beneficial effect can be enhanced by concomitant use of tretinoin or benzoyl peroxide.

Chlormadinone Acetate and Megestrol Acetate

Chlormadinone acetate and megestrol acetate are chemically closely related steroidal antiandrogens. Both are weaker than cyproterone acetate, but have very similar modes of action, indications, and contraindications.

Again these are registered as an oral contraceptive in only a few countries, e.g., in Germany (Gestramestrol N, containing 2 mg chlormadinone acetate and 50 µg mestranol); this drug is also approved for the treatment of acne. Another drug is Menova (containing 2 mg chlormadinone acetate and 20 µg ethinyl estradiol) which is not registered for the treatment of acne).

Spironolactone

Aldosterone antagonists like spironolactone compete with mineral steroids for their receptors on tubular cells of the kidneys, preventing binding and thus inhibiting their action. They also act as an antiandrogen as they alter steroidogenesis by the adrenals and gonads. They also block target organ receptors for circulating androgens. The blood concentration and secretion of corticosteroids are not influenced. Spironolactone selectively destroys microsomal cytochrome P-450 in adrenals and testes leading to a subsequent decrease in the activities of cytochrome P-450-dependent enzymes, e.g., 17α-, 11β-, and 21-hydroxylases.

Spironolactone is registered for the treatment of primary or secondary hyperaldosteronism, edema, and ascites. Because of its antiandrogenic activity it is also used to treat therapy-resistant acne. However, it has not been approved for this disorder. Physicians are free to prescribe it, but should be aware of this. It is noteworthy that it is neither a contraceptive nor a component of any oral contraceptive. Spironolactone is more likely to be used in those countries where antiandrogens are not registered, e.g., the USA. The drug is to be used only by experts and mainly in cases which are resistant to conventional therapy.

Its mechanism of action is similar to that of cyproterone acetate. Spironolactone has been employed in some open clinical trials for the treatment of seborrhea, severe scarring acne, and so-called idiopathic hirsutism. These sometimes occur together and are a prime indication for this type of intervention. In acne its mode of action is to reduce sebum production. Obviously it cannot be given to men in whom it would reduce libido and induce feminization. Side effects are similar to cyproterone acetate, e.g., breast tenderness, headache, nausea, melasma, risk of thromboembolism, or amenorrhea. Aldosterone antagonists are contraindicated in patients with renal failure. In women of childbearing age, it must be combined with an oral contraceptive to avoid feminization of male fetuses.

The following guidelines are recommended (adapted from Shaw 1991). The drug is indicated in women with severe persistent inflammatory acne, particularly of the face, and in those with a history of premenstrual flares, adult onset acne, seborrhea, and hirsutism. Furthermore, it can be prescribed in the case of inadequate therapeutic response to other standard modalities, and where there are associated hormonal symptoms such as irregular menses and premenstrual weight gain. The drug is contraindicated in hypotensive patients. Determination of serum androgens before therapy is not mandatory but may be helpful in complex cases. Effective birth control measures are mandatory (oral contraceptives preferred). The physician should explain drug action and unwanted side effects to the patient.

Oral treatment begins with 1–2 mg/kg body weight per day (roughly 50–100 mg/day) as a single dose.

Monthly or bimonthly check of blood pressure should be performed, and potassium levels should be monitored. A red and white blood cell count is optional. Concomitant topical therapy, especially tretinoin, is encouraged. Oral antibiotics may augment efficacy in resistant cases.

In the case of clinical failure, the dose can be increased to 150–200 mg/day after 3 months. Lower dose in case of unwanted side-effects. Hirsutism usually requires higher doses and longer treatment.

Like topical antiandrogens spironolactone is topically ineffective.

Finally, some clinicians like to give 50 mg a day to control persistent but moderate pustular acne. It is worth noting that low-dose spironolactone can moderate the premenstrual tension syndrome, accompanied by reduction of premenstrual acne flares.

Fanta D (1980) Quantity and quality of sebum production. In: Fanta D: Hormone therapy of acne. Clinical and experimental principles. Springer, Wien, pp 4–12

Fanta D (1990) Cyproterone acetate in acne. J Dermatol Treat (Suppl 3) 1:19–22

Goodfellow A, Alaghband-Zadeh J, Carter G, Cream JJ, Holland S, Scully J, Wise P (1984) Oral spironolactone improves acne vulgaris and reduces sebum excretion. Br J Dermatol 111:209–214

Hammerstein J (1980) Possibilities and limits of endocrine therapy. In: Hammerstein J, Lachnit-Fixson U, Neumann F, Plewig G (eds) Androgenization in women – acne, seborrhea, androgenic alopecia and hirsutism. Excerpta Media, Amsterdam, pp 221–238

Lucky AW (1983) Endocrine aspects of acne. Pediatr Clin North Am 30:495–499

Lucky AW (1988) The paradox of androgens and balding: where are we now? J Invest Dermatol 91:99–100

Lucky AW (1985) Topical antiandrogens. What use in dermatology? Arch Dermatol 121:55–56

Lucky AW, McGuire J, Rosenfield RL, Lucky PA, Rich BH (1983) Plasma androgens in women with acne vulgaris. J Invest Dermatol 81:70–74

Lucky AW, Rosenfield RL, McGuire J, Rudy S, Helke J (1986) Adrenal androgen hyperresponsiveness to adrenocorticotropin on women with acne and/or hirsutism: adrenal enzyme defects and exaggerated adrenarche. J Clin Endocrinol Metab 62:840–848

Muhlemann MF, Carter GD, Cream JJ, Wise P (1986) Oral spironolactone: an effective treatment for acne vulgaris in women. Br J Dermatol 115:227–232

Pochi PE (1983) Hormonal therapy of acne. Dermatol Clin 1:377–384

Pocchi PE, Langcope C (1989) 5α-androstane-3α-, 17β-diol glucuronide blood levels and sebum secretion in acne and normal subjects. I: Marks R, Plewig G (eds) Acne and related disorders. Dunitz, London, pp 67–69

Redmond GP, Bergfeld WP (1990) Treatment of androgenic disorders in women: acne, hirsutism, and alopecia. Cleve Clin J Med 57:428–432

Redmond GP, Gidwani GP, Gupta MK, Bedocs NM, Parker R, Skibinski C, Bergfeld W (1990) Tratment of androgenic disorders with dexamethasone: dose-response relationship for suppression of dehydroepiandrosterone sulfate. J Am Acad Dermatol 22:91–93

Rich BH, Rosenfield RL, Lucky AW, Helke JC, Otto P (1981) Adrenarche: changing adrenal response to adrenocorticotropin. J Clin Endocrinol Metab 52:1129–1136

Rosenfeld RL, Rich BH, Lucky AW (1982) Adrenarche as a cause of benign pseudopuberty in boys. J Pediatr 101:1005–1009

Schindler AE (1987) Antiandrogen therapy for signs of androgenization: an overview. In: Schindler AE (ed) Antiandrogen-estrogen therapy for signs of androgenization. De Gruyter, Berlin, pp 15–20

Shaw JC (1991) Spironolactone in dermatologic therapy. J Am Acad Dermatol 24:236–243

Vexiau P, Husson C, Chivot M, Brerault JL, Fiet J, Julien R, Vilette JM, Hardy N, Cathelineau G (1990) Androgen excess in women with acne alone compared with women with acne and/or hirsutism. J Invest Dermatol 94:279–283

Persistent Inflammatory Acne in Adult Women

Therapy-resistant serious acne in women is not a rarity and requires aggressive treatment after ruling out endocrinologic abnormalities. Antiandrogens are appropriate, as are combinations with other drugs which suppress sebaceous secretion.

Above   Severe inflammatory scarring acne associated with marked seborrhea (*left*) responded very well within 6 months (*right*) to a course of oral cyproterone acetate (2 mg/day) in a fixed combination with 50 µg ethinyl estradiol. No other therapy was given

Below   Two women with refractory papular and nodular acne on the face and trunk. Hyperandrogenism was ruled out in both of them. There are a number of treatment options which are generally sucessful: (a) antiandrogens, e.g., cyproterone acetate or chlormadinone acetate, (b) spironolactone, or (c) oral isotretinoin. Combinations of these are quite effective

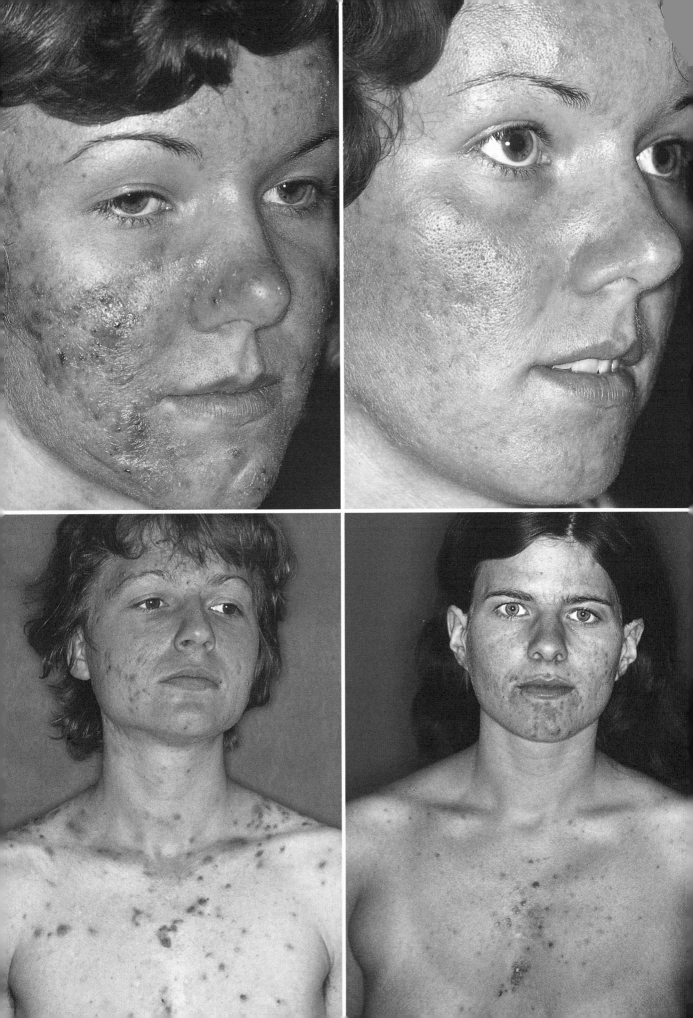

Spironolactone Treatment

Antiandrogens and the aldosterone antagonist spironolactone can provide excellent therapeutic results in selected cases. In this plate the achievements with spironolactone in a woman with persistent papular, nodular and scarring acne, associated with massive seborrhea are demonstrated before (*left*) and after (*right*) oral treatment with spironolactone for several months.

Courtesy of Peter Pochi, MD, Boston, USA

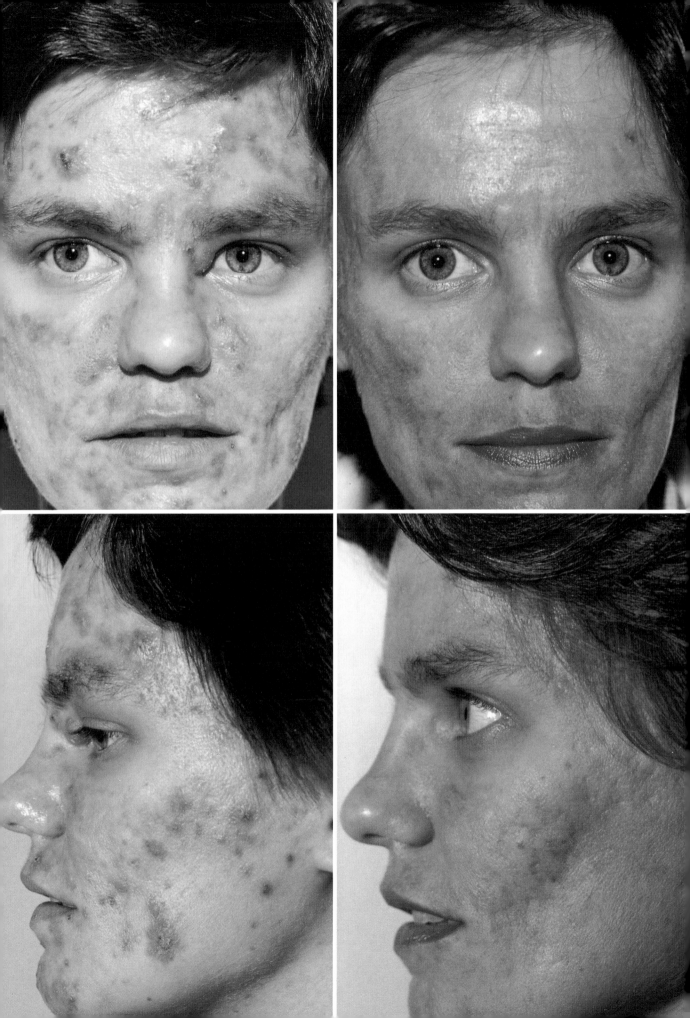

Corticosteroids

Topical and systemic corticosteroids are used sparingly in acne but have powerful effects in properly cases.

Topical

Clinicians quite logically sought to take advantage of the dramatic anti-inflammatory properties of topical steroids in the 1960s and 1970s to treat papulopustular and conglobate acne. With the introduction of high-potency topical steroids, enthusiasm grew rapidly. Indeed, the suppression of inflammatory lesions was dramatic and more prompt and more rapid than with any other treatment. Despite early warnings, it took an inordinately long time for physicians to discover that steroids are immediately beneficial only to be followed by a variety of serious delayed side effects. These can be devastating and include skin atrophy, flares of papulopustules (steroid acne), perioral dermatitis, a wild rebound dermatitis, and exacerbation of rosacea. Many were injured before physicians finally stopped prescribing topical steroids.

This unhappy history again highlights how difficult it is to recognize harmful drugs. There is, however, a place for this approach, but preferably in the hands of experts. Steroids may be very useful as an opening strategy for severe inflammatory acne, especially acne conglobata. High potency steroids applied to face, chest and back, twice daily for 7–10 days can rapidly cool down the fiery lesions. There can be no exceptions to this time limit otherwise one courts disaster. We prefer clobetasole-17-propionate or halobetasol propionate. This short course will convince patients with intractable disease that they have finally found the doctor who really knows how to bring acne under speedy control. Faster resolution means less scaring too. Oral drugs such as isotretinoin can augment efficacy.

Another justification for topical steroids is to treat the granuloma pyogenicum-like lesions that sometimes erupt after oral isotretinoin. Shortly after starting isotretinoin, dense outcroppings of vascularized, oozing, bleeding, fragile, red nodules are extremely alarming. In addition to soiling clothing and bedlinen, the lesions are extremely tender. Rather than withdrawing isotretinoin it is advisable to apply the steroid two or three times daily, covering each lesion with a band aid. The exuberant granulation tissue will resolve in about 2 weeks. A short course of oral corticosteroids is an equally effective alternative, especially when there are numerous angry lesions.

Systemic

Acne Conglobata. Corticosteroids are not the drugs of first choice in acne conglobata. There are, however, narrowly defined indications for the expert confronted with stubborn acne. The chief indication is raging acne conglobata and its variants. A short course of steroids will generally quench the fire immediately. We prescribe 60–80 mg prednisolone daily for 1 week, tapering off to discontinuation by 2 weeks. An alternative favored by some is a single intramuscular injection of 40 mg triamcinolone acetonide. These are solely opening maneuvers. The positive psychological impact of immediate benefit within a few days can relieve despair and generate hope. Exudative pustular and hemorrhagic lesions dry up, pain is reduced, and drainage to the clothing and bed sheets is eliminated. No harm can result in otherwise healthy subjects from one salvo of steroids. We always combine steroids with either isotretinoin as a first choice or oral antibiotics at full doses.

Acne Fulminans. Steroids are a conditio sine qua non in acne fulminans. There is no alternative for this terrible disease. We start with oral steroids a few days prior to isotretinoin, maintain it for 1 or 2 weeks, and then taper off in another week. For more details see p. 318.

Acne Tropicalis. Another disorder which warrants a short course of steroids is acne tropicalis, now exceedingly rare.

Androgen Excess in Women with Acne. Women with or without polycystic ovary disease (PCO) greatly benefit from low-dose corticosteroid treatment for adrenal androgen suppression. For details see p. 347.

Intralesional Injection

An effective tactic for suppressing large, long-lasting inflammatory nodules is intralesional injection of corticosteroids. Torpid nodules may last for months. The method is superior to any other therapy in promoting the resolution of inflammatory nodules in acne conglobata. Within a few days, hard, hot, and tender nodules soften, and become flat and quiescent by about a week. Reinjections may be necessary if the lesion reactivates, a fairly common occurrence.

Another lesion to be attacked this way is the draining sinus. This is the most relentless acne lesion, erupting unpredictably, like a volcano. The drug of choice for intralesional injection is a crystalline suspension of triamcinolone acetonide. Because of its insolubility the drug persists as a depot for months, achieving a local effect with less likelihood of adrenal suppression than with more soluble corticosteroids. There is no need to use the full-strength suspension of 10 mg/ml. The suspension is diluted with physiological saline or a local anesthetic to 2.5 mg/ml. We use 1% meaverine without adrenaline. A volume of about 0.5 ml is injected into the center of the nodule and not beneath it. Sometimes the nodule inflates like a balloon, indicating an optimal technique. The quantity injected into different nodules at one session should not exceed 10–20 mg in order to avoid systemic effects.

It may be necessary to repeat the injection one or more times at about 2-week intervals to achieve complete involution of large torpid nodules. Only inflammatory nodules, and not horn-filled cysts should be injected. Fluctuant lesions may first be aspirated with a wide-bore needle and a small syringe (2.5 ml or 5 ml) to achieve complete evacuation of the sometimes chambered nodule. Steroid atrophy at the injection site is not a problem. The patient has to understand, however, that these nodules, even without steroid injection, often heal with depressed scars due to the inflammatory destruction of the collagen bed which improve with time. Occasionally a nodule will reappear after months of quiescence. Reinjection is usually effective. Bacterial superinfection does not occur. Never incise nodules or draining sinues; this always induces a scar.

Histologic examination of nodules a few days after injection reveals a great mop-up of neutrophils. It is no wonder that nodules shrink so quickly when these enzyme-loaded cells are removed from the scene.

Certain areas of the face, particularly around the eye and nose must be approached with caution. Inadvertent injection of crystals into the vessels which drain into the cerebral vasculature or even more threatening, the central artery of the retina, can cause Hoigne's syndrome, with agitation, sweating, restlessness, hypotension, visual impairment, or even blindness.

Callen JP (1981) Intralesional corticosteroids. J Am Acad Dermatol 4:149–151

Levine RM, Rasmussen JE (1983) Intralesional corticosteroids in the treatment of nodulocystic acne. Arch Dermatol 119:480–481

Potter RA (1971) Intralesional triamcinolone and adrenal suppression in acne vulgaris. J Invest Dermatol 57:364–370

Zinc

The trace element zinc is an essential element for many physiologic reactions in man. It is part of the molecular structure of various enzymes, e.g., alcohol dehydrogenase, lactate dehydrogenase, several other dehydrogenases, and DNA polymerase. It is also involved in the synthesis and release of the retinol-binding protein (RBP), which is a specific transport protein. Its plasma levels reflect the amount of vitamin A available in the tissues. With a regular diet and no metabolic disturbances there is no need for supplement of zinc in our food.

Zinc works like a miracle in zinc deficiencies such as acrodermatitis enteropathica and those arising in a variety of other ways. Many laymen believe in the magical powers of zinc in multiple common disorders. The role of zinc in health food stores is big business. The struggles of our colleagues to prove efficacy in disorders like psoriasis, atopic dermatitis, hair loss, and leg ulcers had been unconvincing and often resulted in preposterous claims. With regard to acne, our position is strong and unequivocal.

It must be remembered that it takes a keen dermatologist to recognize ineffective drugs in acne. The zinc story is a splendid example of this mischief. In the late 1970s and early 1980s a series of publications touted the efficacy of zinc in acne. Zinc sulfate was administered in doses of 135–400 mg daily or 220 mg three times daily. There were studies comparing zinc to vitamin A (300 000 IU daily), or oxytetracycline up to 750 mg daily. Zinc was found to be more effective than the placebo and equivalent to the tetracyclines. In properly controlled double-blind studies, other authors failed to demonstrate any benefit from zinc over the placebo. Moreover, uncitrated zinc sulphate 220 mg three times daily, caused considerable gastrointestinal side effects with nausea, gastric erosions, and gastric ulcers, sometimes requiring surgical intervention. Zinc has no place in acne therapy.

Cunliffe WJ (1979) Unacceptable side-effects of oral zinc sulphate in the treatment of acne vulgaris. Br J Dermatol 101:363

Dreno B, Amblard P, Agache P, Sirot S, Litoux P (1989) Low doses of zinc gluconate for inflammatory acne. Acta Derm Venereol (Stockh) 69:541–543

Hillström L, Pettersson L, Hellbe L, Kjellin A, Leczinsky CG, Nordwall C (1977) Comparison of oral treatment with zinc sulphate and placebo in acne vulgaris. Br J Dermatol 97:681–684

Holland KT, Bojar RA, Conliffe WJ, Cutcliffe AG, Eady EA, Farooq L, Farrell AM, Gribbon EM, Taylor D (1992) The effect of zinc and erythromycin on the growth of erythromycin-resistant and erythromycin-sensitive isolates of *Propionibacterium acnes*: an in-vitro study. Br J Dermatol 126:505–509

Michaëlsson G, Juhlin L, Ljunghall K (1977) A double-blind study of the effect of zinc and oxytetracycline in acne vulgaris. Br J Dermatol 97:561–566

Michaëlsson G, Juhlin L, Vahlquist A (1977) Effects of oral zinc and vitamin A in acne. Arch Dermatol 113:31–36

Michaëlsson G, Vahlquist A, Juhlin L (1977) Serum zinc and retinol-binding protein in acne. Br J Dermatol 96:283–286

Moore R (1978) Bleeding gastric erosion (oral zinc sulphate). Br Med J I:754

Weismann K, Wadskov S, Sondergaard J (1977) Oral zinc sulphate therapy for acne vulgaris. Acta Derm Venereol (Stockh) 57:357–360

Ultraviolet Radiation

Everyone knows that acne improves in summer, especially after sunbathing. Patients are keen to reap the benefits of sunlight in hastening the resorption of papules and pustules. Faster clearing of inflammatory lesions can be experimentally demonstrated. Not so long ago artifical radiation with ultraviolet radiation was a standard treatment offered by dermatologists. Sunburning doses were given with weekly or biweekly exposures for many months. It turns out that the situation is far more complex. We shall argue that sunlight and ultraviolet is more harmful than helpful, actually perpetuating the disease and of course also inducing irreparable photodamage. Stated simply: ultraviolet itself is comedogenic! Solar comedones in photoaged skin are a great example of this baleful effect. Moreover, we have induced microcomedones on the backs of acne-prone subjects after many doses of ultraviolet radiation.

When we irradiated skin bearing many closed and open comedones with UV-B, they were not loosened and expelled, even with intense sunburning doses. In fact after 2 months of thrice weekly irradiations many comedones enlarged.

We have also shown in the rabbit ear model that ultraviolet radiation, in mild doses, consistently enhances the formation of comedones by a variety of comedogenic substances. We call this photocomedogenicity and have evidence of its existence in humans. Paradoxically, some sunscreens show photocomedogenicity,

usually because of a comedogenic component in the vehicle. There is striking resemblance to what happens when elemental sulfur is applied to acne-bearing skin. Existing inflammatory lesions dry up, but new crops of microcomedones are slowly induced. The paradox is that visible lesions regress but invisible ones (microcomedones) are laid down, assuring continuation of the disease. The reappearance of acne in the fall may have a quite different explanation than the absence of sunlight. Comedones, it will be recalled, take months to reach visibility. Summer lasts about 3 months, a suitable time period for the emergence of clinical comedones. Then, too, it is worth noting that about some acne patients actually get worse in the summer as has long been known. Sun exposure brings about several subjective and very pleasant side effects: A nice tan, the image of looking much better, and of feeling great. This doubtlessly lifts up the spirits of acne-ridden patients, but the overall effect is negative. We studied sebum secretion, its qualitative composition, the amount of free fatty acids and the density of *Propionibacterium acnes* in patients with a heavy sunlight exposure. None of these changed.

We condemn the treatment of acne by repeated exposures to ultraviolet radiation, both UV-B and UV-A. Physicians who stick to this archaic method do more harm than good. People have begun to understand that excessive sunbathing in youth produces premature aging in late adulthood. Acne patients are still likely to believe that sunlight is good for their acne. This is simply another of the myths that have a baleful effect on the course of the disease. Incidentally one of the reliable ways to induce crops of comedones on the upper back is psoralens and UV-A (PUVA) therapy, in which the patient takes 8-methoxypsoralen (a phototoxic drug) by mouth and is exposed to UV-A about 2 h later.

Mills OH, Kligman AM (1978) Ultraviolet phototherapy and photochemotherapy of acne vulgaris. Arch Dermatol 114:221–223

Mills OH, Porte M, Kligman AM (1978) Enhancement of comedogenic substances by ultraviolet radiation. Br J Dermatol 98:145–150

Saint-Leger D, Bague A, Cohen E, Chivot M (1986) A possible role for squalene in the pathogenesis of acne. I. In vitro study of squalene oxidation. Br J Dermatol 114:535–542

Sunshine Does Not Always Improve Acne but May Paradoxically Aggravate It

Many patients experience substantial improvement of inflammatory acne lesions. However, as many as 20% report that sunbathing worsens the disease. Intensive sun exposure may sharply aggravate severe acne. This man with acne conglobata certainly did not benefit from solar exposure sufficient to induce tanning.

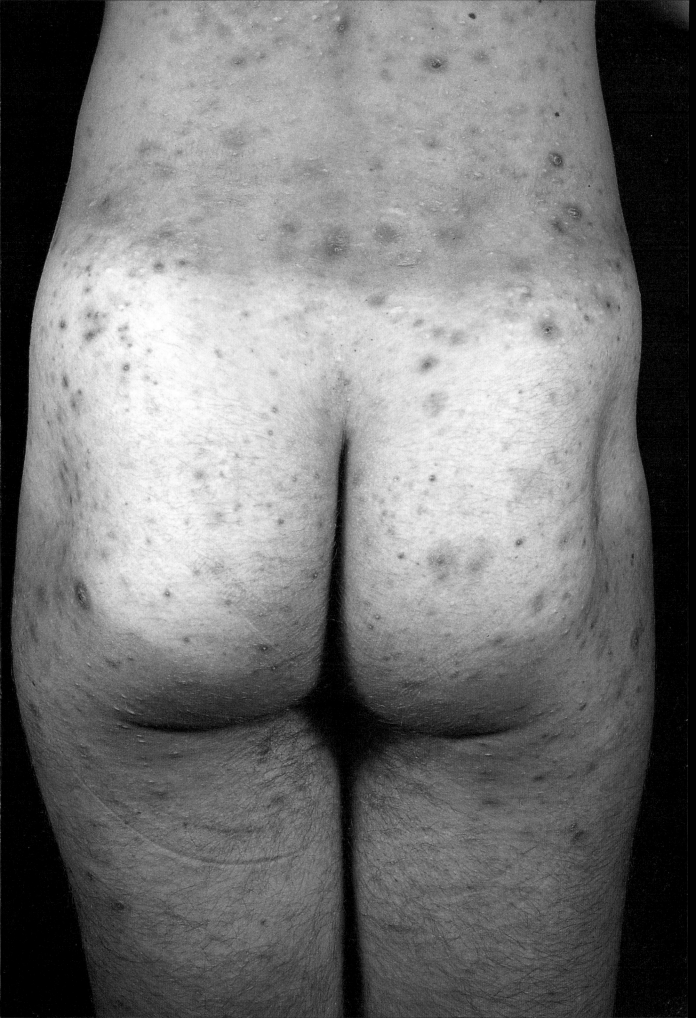

Cryotherapy

Before the age of really effective topical or systemic acne treatment modalities, cryotherapy was en vogue in the management of acne patients. The procedure involved swabbing the skin with a slush prepared with acetone and carbon dioxide. Freshly prepared in front of the patient, impressively supported by the noise of escaping carbon dioxide, the snow-like crystals were thinly applied to the affected area, mostly the face, just long enough to create an erythema. This was performed two to four times weekly, resulting in a superficial desquamation.

Volatile refrigerants such as ethyl chloride, dichlorotetrafluoroethane, and others were developed. Open systems spray the refrigerant directly onto the skin; closed systems use frozen metal pellets, disks, and various other tools held against the skin. The latter technique is quicker, cleaner, and more practical, though not necessarily better than spraying applications.

The beneficial effects of cryotherapy have been greatly overrated. Treatment of the whole face induced peeling, but did not release comedones. Spot cryotherapy was used to treat all inflammatory lesions like papules, pustules, and even tender persistent nodules. This is moderately helpful but is painful. The freezing effect is like a counterirritant, causing inflammatory lesions to disappear faster than without treatment. Open or closed comedones cannot be uprooted by this means.

The most severe side effects are hypo- or hyperpigmentation; cryotherapy is contraindicated in Blacks and Orientals. The amelioration of minor scars, mostly flat ones, was another indication for cryotherapy. In some patients the scars softened, but the effect was temporary. Cryotherapy belongs to the dark ages of acne therapy. We never use it.

Leyden JJ, Mills OH, Kligman AM (1974) Cryoprobe treatment of acne conglobata. Br J Dermatol 90:335–341

Colver GB, Dawber RPR (1989) Cryosurgery – the principles and simple practice. Clin Exp Dermatol 14:1–6

Abrasives

Abrasives consist of hard particles of aluminum oxide, plastics, or ground nutshells which, one gathers from the advertisements, are supposed to physically unroof or loosen the anchoring of comedones. Nothing like this happens. Open and closed comedones are too firmly rooted to be exfoliated in this way, no matter how frenetically one rubs. The overall effects are slight, certainly inferior to comedolytic agents such as tretinoin or salicyclic acid. Rubbing and scouring the face seems to satisfy some primitive instinct for automanipulation. Some rub their face so vigorously that superficial excoriations result. We deem abrasives to be potentially more harmful than helpful. Aggravation of existing lesions is fairly common, especially in conjunction with tretinoin or benzoyl peroxide. Abrasives are often compounded with other traditional peeling chemicals, increasing the chances for irritation. Surfactants are sometimes incorporated to aid washing. Abrasives are a holdover from a previous area when effective therapies did not exist. We do not use abrasives.

α-Hydroxy Acids: A Peeling Agent for Acne?

The α-hydroxy acids, lactic acid and glycolic acid among others, have been recommended for the removal of hyperkeratotic stratum corneum. These agents have been popularized by the writings of Van Scott in Philadelphia. Their mode of action is to loosen the adhesion between corneocytes, thereby promoting desquamation. They definitely thin down the excessively thick horny layer, smoothing ichthyotic skin. Lachydrin contains 12% ammonium lactate and has beneficial effects in xerotic skin.

Certain formulations of glycolic acid have received much publicity with regard to therapeutic benefits in acne. Theoretically, α-hydroxy acids could be comedolytic by loosening the binding of corneocytes making up the comedo.

However, we have studiously assessed these in regard to their ability to eliminate comedones induced in the rabbit ear by coal tars and have been unable to demonstrate any comedolytic effect, even at high concentrations in a variety of vehicles. No persuasive clinical studies have been published. We do not recommend these for acne. Besides, they can be quite irritating.

Van Scott EJ, Yu RJ (1989) Alpha hydroxy acids: procedures for use in clinical practice. Cutis 43:222–228

Van Scott EJ, Yu RJ (1984) Hyperkeratinization, corneocyte cohesion, and alpha hydroxy acids. J Am Acad Dermatol 11:867–879

Lasers

The magic tool of lasers, so effectively used in neurosurgery, gastrointestinal surgery, vascular surgery, and other ever increasing indications also has its place in dermatologic surgery, particularly in vascular nevi and vascular malformations. There seems to be a limited application in the treatment of acne scarring. Expectations, notably from patients and laymen, are very high. Controlled clinical studies are unfortunately very scarce.

Carbon Dioxide Laser

Laser abrasion of focal size is offered in the treatment of pitted acne scars. Either conventional continuous-wave carbon dioxide (CO_2) laser or superpulsed CO_2 lasers are used. The wavelength of the latter is 10660 nm. The average laser provides 5–25 W; the sports are small, between 1 and 5 mm; the delivery is continuous or with short pulses.

Not only depressed but also papular or nodular or even keloidal scars can be attacked in this way, i.e., vaporized. Local anesthesia, mostly with 1% meaverine or 1% lidocaine is necessary. The laser beam is passed once or repeatedly over the scarred skin. An eschar develops immediately. Postoperative care is minimal, if necessary at all with rinses, bland ointments, or antiseptics. The scab falls off within 1–3 weeks. Frequently several sessions are necessary. Treatment results are evaluated not only immediately after wound healing, but also 6–12 months thereafter.

The best results are obtained by experts in the field. Laser treatment requires intensive training like all other surgical modalities. Important factors among others are estimating the optimal laser depth intraoperatively, the extent of contouring, and minimal heat development during vaporization to reduce thermal damage to surrounding healthy tissue.

Dye Lasers

Too little critical information is yet available to recommend these laser types for the improvement of scars. Undisputedly they have their place in vascular lesions, birthmarks, and nevi. Rarely are these vascular elements of importance in acne scars. However, in rosacea, and particularly in rhinophyma, they are definitely indicated.

Argon Laser

The most widely used type of laser (wave length 488–514 nm) to treat vascular malformations, e.g., in rosacea and rhinophyma, is the argon laser. It is not suitable for correcting scars in acne.

Neodymium YAG Laser

The neodymium YAG (Nd: YAG) is a near-infrared laser (wavelength 1.064

nm). Usually this laser is used with a contact mode (mostly synthetic sapphire) and provides bloodless incisions. In the noncontact mode, coagulation is possible, which is a method to destroy scar tissue.

André P, Chavaudra J, Daima E, Guillaume JC, Avril MF (1990) Les lasers en dermatologie. Ann Dermatol Venereol 117:377–395

Brauner GJ, Schliftman A (1987) Laser surgery for children. J Dermatol Surg Oncol 13:178–186

Dover J, Arndt KA, Geronemus RG, Olbricht SM, Noe JM, Stern RS (eds) (1990) Illustrated cutaneous laser surgery: a practitioner's guide. Appleton & Lange, Norwalk

Garrett AB, Dufresne RG Jr, Ratz JL, Berlin AJ (1990) Carbon dioxide laser treatment of pitted acne scarring. J Dermatol Surg Oncol 16:737–740

Hobbs ER, Bailin PL, Wheeland RG, Ratz JL (1987) Superpulsed lasers: minimizing thermal damage with short duration, high irradiance pulses. J Dermatol Surg Oncol 13:955–964

Kantor GR, Ratz JL, Wheeland RG (1986) Treatment of acne keloidalis nuchae with carbon dioxide laser. J Am Acad Dermatol 14:263–267

Kantor GR, Wheeland RG, Bailin PL, Walker NPJ, Ratz JL (1985) Treatment of earlobe keloids with carbon dioxide laser excision: a report of 16 cases. J Dermatol Surg Oncol 11:1063–1067

Landthaler M, Haina D, Brunner R, Waidelich W, Braun-Falco O (1986) Neodymium-YAG laser therapy for vascular lesions. J Am Acad Dermatol 14:107–117

Nakagawa H, Tan OT, Parrish JA (1985) Ultrastructural changes in human skin exposure to a pulsed laser. J Invest Dermatol 84:396–400

Steiner R, Kaufmann R, Landthaler M, Braun-Falco O (eds) (1991) Lasers in dermatology. Springer, Berlin

Wheeland RG (1991) Lasers 1990. Adv Dermatol 6:125–142

X-Ray Therapy: A Historical Note

Four to five decades ago, the best dermatologists in university centers typically gave 100 R of superficial X-rays once weekly for 7–10 weeks. This reduced sebum production and very often produced a remarkable degree of clearing, especially in the worst cases such as acne conglobata. Except for isotretinoin probably no other single remedy is as effective as X-ray therapy. Improvement was rapid to the great delight of the patients. Seborrhea quickly disappeared, with an 80% reduction in sebum production after a total dose of 1.000 R. The authorities recommended one course, but patients with recurrences simply sought a new doctor. Radiodermatitis was the result, often not becoming visible for many years. Unfortunately safety precautions were not as stringent in earlier days as in later decades, causing an increased risk of malignant tumors of thyroid or parotid gland in patients irradiated 20–40 years earlier. Thirty-five percent of about 400 patients in one series developed malignant tumors, but none occurred in control subjects. All this is history now. With the advent of modern drugs, X-rays no longer have a place in the treatment of severe acne.

Braun-Falco O, Lukacs S, Goldschmidt H (1976) Dermatologic radiotherapy. Springer, Berlin Heidelberg New York, pp 34, 118, 132

Goldschmidt H (1975) Ionizing radiation therapy in dermatology. Current use in the United States and Canada. Arch Dermatol 111:1511–1517

Goldschmidt H, Panizzon RG (1991) Modern dermatologic radiation therapy. Springer, Berlin Heidelberg New York

Paloyan E, Lawrence AM (1978) Thyroid neoplasms after radiation therapy for adolescent acne vulgaris. Arch Dermatol 114:53–55

Preston-Martin S (1989) Prior x-ray therapy for acne related to tumors of the parotid gland. Arch Dermatol 125:921–924

Pusay WA (1902) Acne and sycosis treated by exposure to Roentgen rays. J Cutan Dis 20:204–210

Strauss JS, Kligman AM (1959) Effect of x-rays on sebaceous glands of the human face: radiation therapy of acne. J Invest Dermatol 33:347–356

Acne Surgery

Dermabrasion

Historical Note

The first comprehensive description of dermabrasion was by Kromayer in 1905, although this was not the first report on dermabrasion. Wire brush or diamond fraise heads introduced in the 1950s are still the instruments of choice, depending mostly on the operator's skills and preferences. We only use diamond fraises.

Indication

Almost every type of scar, except the deep ice-pick type, lends itself to dermabrasion, e.g., trough-like, shallow, linear, small papular, or nodular scars. Dermabrasion is limited to the face, elsewhere the procedure itself may leave a scar.

Contraindication

A tendency for spontaneous keloids, especially in youngsters, poses a hazard. In older subjects with a history of hypertrophic scars, the procedure may be justified. Most dermabraders tend to avoid dermabrasion in Blacks and Orientals because of the fear of persistent or permanent hypo- or hyperpigmentation. This outcome has probably been exaggerated by practitioners with limited experience in abrading deeply pigmented skin. Some cosmetic surgeons who are themselves black do not hesitate to abrade.

Technique

Long-term training with an expert in the field is the only way to learn the essentials of this art in order to avoid common pitfalls and to be prepared for unusual intra- or postoperative problems. One becomes skilled only after doing hundreds of dermabrasions. This is not the place to discuss techniques. In the early days, it was the custom to freeze the skin to a hard state, which simultaneously provided anesthesia. Volatile refrigerants were used, some achieving quite low temperatures, often leaving persistent hypopigmentation. While still used by those who know which cryorefrigerants to use and how to use them, there has been a growing tendency to abandon freezing altogether. Some physicians prefer full anesthesia, most use local anesthesia in stages. This may be accompanied by diazepam 1 h preoperatively, atropine intramuscularly and fentanyl intravenously prior to regional block anesthesia with a lidocaine and bupivacaine mixture (other caines work as well, e.g., meaverine). A supraorbital, infraorbital, and mental foramina block provides anesthesia for about 70% of the face.

Dermabrasion may provoke an extensive eruption of herpes simplex in the abraded areas. The diagnosis of herpes simplex

Patient	Physician
● Too high expectations with incomplete ablation of scars	● Infections through aerosolized blood and tissue particles
● Hyperpigmentation, including the borders of the abraded scars	● Hepatitis B
● Hypopigmentation	● Acquired immunodeficiency (HIV)
● Mottled pigmentation following sun exposure	● Law suits when the patients' expectations are not met or when complications occur
● Increased sun sensitivity with severe sunburns	
● Avoidance of sun exposure or artificial ultraviolet tanning postoperatively	
● Scarring from too deep dermabrasion	
● Milia	
● Herpes simplex	
● Pyodermas, mostly Staphylococcus aureus	
● Unphysiological skin appearance with loss of skin markings, fine facial natural lines and skin pores	

can be difficult in a moist, eroded, epidermis-free skin; the infection is heralded by unusual postoperative pain. The antiviral drug acyclovir is therefore routinely used if there is a history of recurrent herpetic infections. On the preoperative day, acyclovir is given three times 400 mg orally, then continued for the next 3–5 days. The diagnosis of postdermabrasion herpes requires instant administration of full doses of acyclovir.

There is evidence that tretinoin applied topically prior to dermabrasion enhances wound healing. Several studies on large cohorts support this practice. We advise at least a month of vigorous pretreatment. Others think that 2 weeks is sufficient. Re-epithelialization occurs in about half the time. Moreover, pretreatment markedly cuts down the development of milia and also yields a better cos-

metic result. It is advisable to institute daily use about 10 days after healing, starting with low concentrations. This improves the texture of abraded skin and results in uniform pigmentation.

Should dermabrasion be performed on patients receiving oral isotretinoin? There are unconfirmed reports of hypertrophic scarring in several patients treated in this way, but only time will tell. We personally have not witnessed it in our patients. The specter of litigation may be a deterrent.

Practices differ in regard to postdermabrasion dressings. The development of modern biosynthetic materials, especially hydrogels, has seemingly settled this question. Re-epithelialization is doubtlessly enhanced, postoperative pain reduced, and the patient comforted with less bulky dressings. We use these routinely. One has a choice of at least a half-dozen films, providing occlusion without sticking to the wound. There can be no fundamental objection to a second or even third dermabrasion in selected cases. Cautious physicians perform shallow dermabrasions, allowing them to assess the results before going on. This reduces complications.

Protection of the physician and assisting personnel in the operating theater includes careful handling and disinfection of surgical instruments, blood-splattered dressings, and the meticulous use of gloves, masks, goggles, and splatter guards.

This chapter should not end on a pessimistic note, as dermabrasion has been and still is an effective tool to improve acne scars. Whether chemical peels or dermabrasion give the best results will probably never be settled. Practically speaking, each dermatologist settles on one technique and perfects it over the years.

Alt TH (1987) Facial dermabrasion: advantages of the diamond fraise technique. J Dermatol Surg Oncol 13:618–624

Burke J (1956) Wire brush surgery. Thomas, Springfield

Dzubow LM (1985) Survey of refrigeration and surgical technics used for facial dermabrasion. J Am Acad Dermatol 13:287–292

Eaglestein WH, Davis SC, Mehle AL, Mertz PM (1988) Optimal use of an occlusive dressing to enhance healing. Effect of delayed application and early removal on wound healing. Arch Dermatol 124:392–395

Fulton JE Jr (1990) Modern dermabrasion techniques. Am J Cosm Surg 7:19–24

Hung VC, Lee JYY, Zitelli JA, Hebda PA (1989) Topical tretinoin and epithelial wound healing. Arch Dermatol 125:65–69

Kromayer E (1905) Rotationsinstrumente: ein neues technisches Verfahren in der dermatologischen Kleinchirurgie. Dermatol/Zeitschr/12:26–36

Mandy SH (1991) Advances in dermabrasion. Adv Dermatol 6:113–123

McCollough EG (1989) Dermabrasion and chemical peel: a guide for facial plastic surgeons. P. Royal Langsdon Thieme Med. Publ., New York

Orentreich N, Durr NP (1983) Rehabilitation of acne scarring. Dermatol Clin 1:405–413

Petres J (1977) Dermabrasion. In: Konz B, Burg G (eds) Dermatochirurgie in Klinik und Praxis. Springer, Berlin, pp 211–218

Roenigk HH Jr, Pinski JB, Robinson JK, Hanke CW (1985) Acne, retinoids, and dermabrasion. J Dermatol Surg Oncol 11:396–398

Rubenstein R, Roenigk HH Jr, Stegman SJ, Hanke CW (1986) Atypical keloids after dermabrasion of patients taking isotretinoin. J Am Acad Dermatol 15:280–285

Silverman AK, Laing KF, Swanson NA, Schaberg DR (1985) Activation of herpes simplex following dermabrasion. Report of a patient successfully treated with intravenous acyclovir and brief review of the literature. J Am Acad Dermatol 13:103–108

Weber PJ, Weber M, Dzubow LM (1989) Sedation for dermatologic surgery. J Am Acad Dermatol 20:815–826

Yarborough JM Jr (1987) Dermabrasive surgery. State of the art. Clin Dermatol 5:75–80

Dermabrasion

Shallow facial scars can be markedly improved by superficial mechanical abrasion, a technique now known for almost 90 years. In the hands of experts, it is a marvellous therapeutic adjunct.

Above Improvement of flat, shallow scars before (*left*) and after dermabrasion (*right*)

Below The dermabrasion equipment consists of a high-speed electrical motor (not shown here), the handle, and a wide choice of abrading tools. Diamon-studded steel heads of various sizes and shapes to deal with the geometry of facial contures are preferred by us. The hand piece has an attachment shield to prevent splashing of tissue and fluids

Above: Courtesy of John Yarborough, M.D., New Orleans, USA

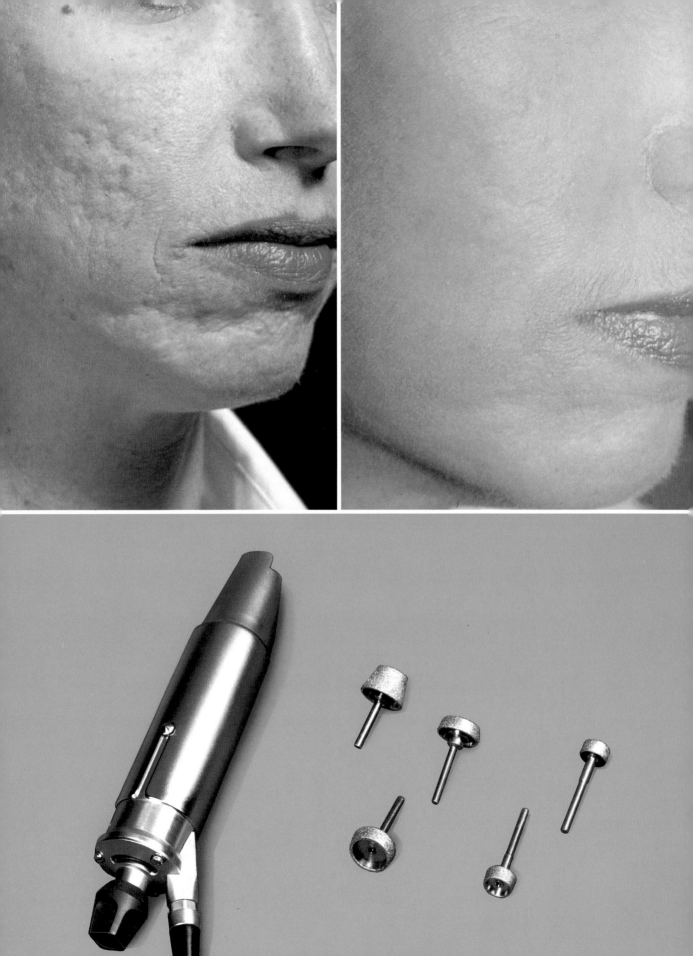

Excision

Some scars are not improved by dermabrasion, punch-graft elevation, punch-graft transplants, laser treatment, or collagen injections. In these cases other surgical techniques are indicated. This is particularly true for scars larger than 5 mm in diameter, odd-shaped irregular scars, wide trough-like scars, flat atrophic scars, keloidal scars, fistulated scars (fistulated or polyporous comedones), and occasionally the worst of all scars, the draining sinus.

Before grasping a scalpel, the physician should lay out very individualized treatment plans and discuss the pros and cons of every step. Acne patients, and in particular older women with residual acne scars, sometimes have unrealistic expectations. Explain the possibilities, make sure the patient understands what is planned and what is to be expected, mention every possible unwanted side effect; take preoperative photographs. It is often wise to treat one scar only and to wait for several months to see if the patient is pleased.

Excision, primary closure, rotation flaps, and many other technical approaches all depend on the anatomical situation of the patient and the skill of the physician. It is not appropriate to discuss these here. It is often possible to improve the result by light dermabrasion several weeks later. Draining sinuses need special care. Pre- or intraoperative delineation of the extent of the bizarre labyrinth is necessary. A visible scar following this more extensive surgery is inevitable. A final touch-up with collagen implants, laser, or dermabrasion is sometimes added. Excision surgery can be most rewarding, but also hopelessly disappointing. Circumspect predictions are in order.

Punch-Graft Elevation or Punch-Graft Transplant

Pitted scars (ice pick scars) are difficult to treat. Dermabrasion is too superficial, and collagen implants and silicone are only mildly helpful because of fibrosis. There are, however, effective surgical corrections.

Punch-Graft Elevation

Orentreich, a master of dermabrasion and hair transplantation, introduced the procedure of punch-graft elevation. With a punch slightly larger in diameter than the scar, a cylindrical incision is made in the surrounding skin, allow the central core to rise up like a cork from a bottle but still connected to the underlying tissue. The elevated tissue is kept in place by adhesive strips and is not sutured. Healing is rapid. Later the site may be dermabraded to blend in with the skin level. The end result is not predictable. Sometimes the cylinder retracts, leaving a circular depression, or healing may be uneven with fibrotic irregularities.

Punch-Graft Transplant

Johnson, a cosmetic surgeon in Philadelphia, devised the procedure of punch-graft transplant, which generally gives superior results to punch-graft elevation. The scar is first punch-excised, and the tissue discarded. Then punch-grafts 0.5–1.0 mm larger than the recipient site are obtained from the mastoid or back of the ear. In the bearded area the recipient punch must be parallel to the hairs to avoid ingrown hairs and sinus tracts. Ideally the donor graft fills the recipient hole firmly. The donor graft is secured by tissue glue (isobutyl cyanoacrylate, Ellman International) adhesive or strips (Steri-

Strips). The strips may be additionally fastened with surgical glue (e.g., Mastisol, Fermdale Laboratories). Larger grafts may be fixed with sutures running over the transplant, steel pins through the transplant, or by suturing the edges. Dozens of scars can be corrected at one setting. Experts do not hesitate to excise more than a hundred pitted scars if required. The published results are impressive. Physicians need to know that this is a viable option that offers great improvement of the badly scarred face.

Complications from punch-grafts include:
- Failure to take the graft
- Depressed grove at junction with normal skin
- Depressed graft, crocked graft
- Elevated graft despite dermabrasion
- Hypertrophic scar

- Pigmentary abnormalities from punches or dermabrasion
- Infection
- Excessive bleeding
- Problem sites are bearded areas in men, and areas lateral to the angles of the mouth

Johnson WC (1988) Treatment of pitted scars: punch-graft transplant technique. Am J Cosm Surg 5:73–77

Mancuso A, Farber GA (1991) The abraded punch graft for pitted facial scars. J Dermatol Surg Oncol 17:32–34

Orentreich N, Durr NP (1983) Rehabilitation of acne scarring. Dermatol Clin 1:405–413

Orentreich D, Orentreich N (1987) Acne scar revision update. Dermatol Clin 5:359–368

Solotoff SA (1986) Treatment for pitted acne scarring – postauricular punch grafts followed by dermabrasion. J Dermatol Surg Oncol 12:1079–1084

Punch-Graft Technique and Dermabrasion

Experts can achieve remarkable fine results when it comes to the correction of scars. Punch-graft technique and subsequent dermabrasion comprise a series of steps.

Above

Left Wide shallow trough-like scars without ongoing inflammation are a proper indication for this multiple-step technique

Right More than 75 scars were punched out on the left cheek alone; the tissue that is punched out is then discarded

Below

Left Graft punches from other donor sites were placed into the holes some weeks previously, and have now healed in well but remain bumpy with a cobblestone like surface. The prominent tissue is dermabraded

Right Excellent cosmetic result after healing of dermabraded skin

Below: Courtesy of Waine C. Johnson, M.D., Glenside, Pennsylvania, USA

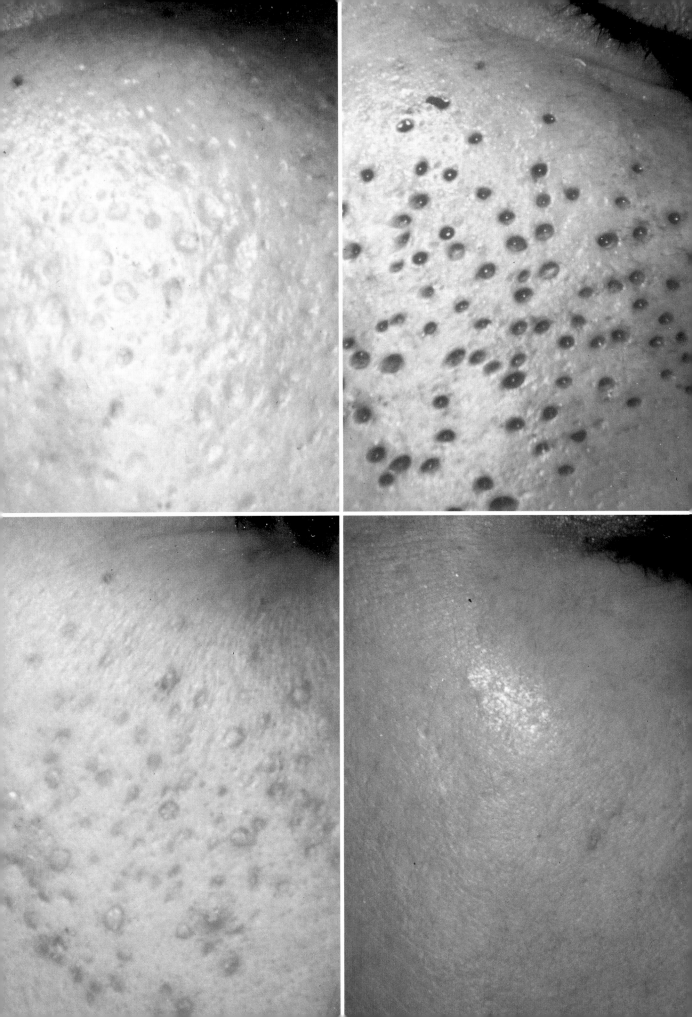

An artist's sketch to demonstrate the punch graft technique. A deep-seated scar is seen histologically and from above. The punch biopsy has removed the scar en bloc, and another punch biopsy has provided a healthy donor cylinder, slightly larger than the recipient hole. The donor graft is healed in with a fine scar (histologically) with perfect skin architecture following dermabrasion.

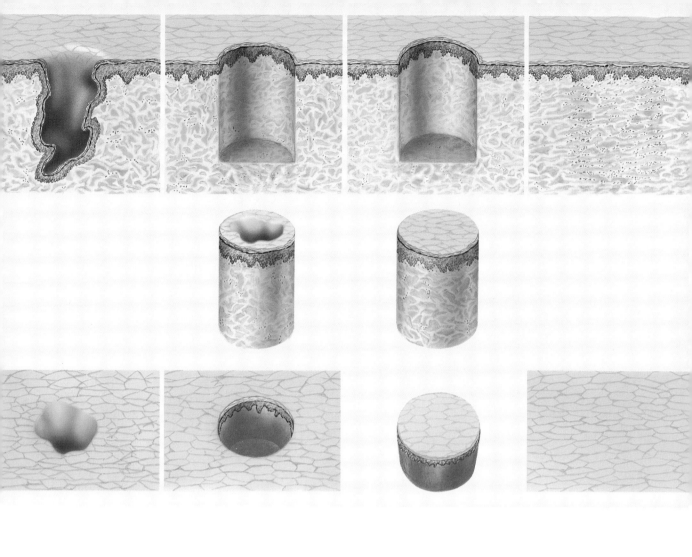

Collagen Injection

Injectable fibrillar bovine collagen has been used since 1976 as a biomedical device for augmentation of soft tissue. Indications for collagen implants range from acne scars, chickenpox scars, scars following accidents, surgical procedures, age-related atrophy, and wrinkles of facial skin. We will deal only with the correction of acne scars.

There is only one manufacturer worldwide (Collagen Corporation). Several implants are available:

Zyderm collagen implant test:
   0.1 ml suspension for injection containing 3.5 mg bovine collagen and 0.3 mg lidocaine

Zyderm collagen implant:
   1.0 ml suspension for injection containing 35 mg bovine collagen and 3.0 mg lidocaine

Zyderm II collagen implant:
   0.75 ml suspension for injection containing 48.75 mg bovine collagen (65 mg in the USA) and 2.25 mg lidocaine

Zyplast collagen implant:
   1.0 ml suspension for injection containing 35 mg bovine collagen, slightly cross-linked with glutaraldehyde

These solubilized collagens are provided in phosphate-buffered saline (pH 7.2).

Many patients require touch-up reinjections once or twice yearly since the implants are variably resorbed. Zyplast yields more lasting results.

Pharmacology

The collagen implant is a fibrillar suspension of highly purified pepsine-treated bovine dermal collagen. More than 95% of it is type I collagen, the remainder type III with no detectable noncollagen fragments. The collagen implant is a weak immunogen for humans, as roughly 3% of patients tested intradermally show an inflammatory reaction which is probably allergic in origin. A further 0.6% of patients develop an immune reaction during treatment despite a negative test. It is natural that neither increasing the injected volume nor increasing the number of injections is associated with an enhanced incidence of adverse reactions.

The immune response to collagen in patients tested or treated with this biomedical device is a hypersensitivity reaction directed to heterogenous sites from native and denatured collagen. The immune response is only directed against determinants specific for bovine collagen.

There is no evidence that collagen injections can induce autoimmune diseases such as lupus erythematosus or scleroderma. Law suits have arisen which claim that collagen implants can induce connective tissue disorders. Outside experts have concluded that there is no connection. Despite this clean bill of health, the manufacturer cautions that patients suffering from arthritis, lupus erythematosus, dermatomyositis, polymyositis, Hashimoto thyreoiditis, Basedow's disease, periarteritis nodosa, scleroderma, colitis ulcerosa, Crohn's disease, Sjögren's syndrome, and Reiter's disease should not receive collagen injections. Furthermore lidocaine hypersensitivity has to be ruled out. Finally, it is not administered in pregnancy, nursing mothers, and children, as there is no adequate information for these patients. Previous injections with silicone do not contraindicate collagen injection.

Indications

Collagen can be used to treat acne scars, mostly limited to the face: shallow, depressed, scars, crateriform scars, or linear types of scars. The best results are obtained in soft scars which can be elevated when pinched. Deep fibrotic ice-pick scars respond the least.

Complications

Local reactions present clinically erythema, induration, and pruritus, and histologically foreign body granulomas or necrobiotic granulomas. This is accompanied by a palisading infiltrate of lymphocytes, plasma cells, eosinophils, neutrophils, macrophages, and giant cells. Indurated inflammatory papules disappear very slowly with time. Intradermal corticosteroids hasten their disappearance.

Oral isotretinoin, in a low dose of about 0.2 mg/kg body weight per day for several months almost completely cleared the granulomatous infiltrations in the patients we have seen.

Injection in the eye area must be done with caution. Loss of vision has been reported. There was retrograde migration of collagen with occlusion of the retinal artery.

Another rare complication is a delayed tissue necrosis in the glabellar region.

Test Procedure

Zyderm collagen implant test 0.1 ml, is injected intracutaneously into the volar side of the forearm. An increasing number of physicians repeat the skin test 2–4 weeks later (double skin testing) to be on the safe side. The test sites are watched for about 1 month, mainly by the patients, for the development of an inflamed papule which lasts for more than 48 h. Other corrective techniques are advised for patients with positive tests.

Scar Treatment

As the implanted collagen shrinks to some extent, overcorrection of the scar is indicated.

Zyderm Collagen Implant shrinks by 60%–75% of its original volume. Therefore, an overcorrection of up to 200% is recommended. The manufacturer suggests 1–10 ml for a single session; the maximum amount for a single session is 30 ml. Likewise the maximal total dose per year is also set at 30 ml. Intervals between sessions are spaced at about 14 days.

Zyderm II Collagen Implant shrinks less than the above-mentioned preparation. Therefore an overcorrection of about 100% is recommended. Some experts prefer just to level but not to overcorrect the scar. Spacing the injections at 14-day intervals, up to three sessions with an average volume of 1.75 ml, is a standard procedure.

Zyplast Collagen Implant shrinks less than Zyderm or Zyderm II. Therefore only a modest overcorrection is recommended. The maximal dose per year is 30 ml. Injections are always made into the scarred tissue, not beneath it, and not into the subcutaneous fat.

One should not implant collagen without proper training. A lot of experience is required to learn the art of correction. Before using foreign implants physicians should be very well informed about indications, safety procedures, injection techniques, and interpretation of test results. Often the final result does not come up to the expectations of the patient.

Clark DP, Hanke CW, Swanson NA (1989) Dermal implants: safety of products injected for soft tissue augmentation. J Am Acad Dermatol 21:992–998

Cooperman L, Michaeli D (1984) The immunogenicity of injectable collagen. I. A 1-year prospective study. J Am Acad Dermatol 10:638–646

Cooperman L, Michaeli D (1984) The immunogenicity of injectable collagen. II. A retrospective review of seventy-two tested and treated patients. J Am Acad Dermatol 10:647–651

DeLustro F, Fries J, Kang A, Katz S, Kaye R, Reichlin M (1988) Immunity to injectable collagen and autoimmune disease: a summary of current understanding. J Dermatol Surg Oncol (Suppl 1) 14:57–65

Hanke CW, Higley HR, Jolivette DM, Swanson NA, Stegman SJ (1991) Abscess formation and local necrosis after treatment with Zyderm or Zyplast Collagen Imlant. J Am Acad Dermatol 25:319–326

Klein AW (1988) Indications and implantation techniques for the various formulations of injectable collagen. J Dermatol Surg Oncol (Suppl 1) 14:27–30

Klein AW, Rish DC (1984) Injectable collagen update. J Dermatol Surg Oncol 10:519–522

Knapp TR, Kaplan EN, Daniels JR (1977) Injectable collagen for soft tissue augmentation. Plast Reconstr Surg 60:398–405

Schurig V, Dorn M, Konz B (1986) Granulombildung an Test- und Behandlungsstellen durch intrakutan verabreichtes, injizierbares Kollagen. Hautarzt 37:42–45

Stegman SJ, Chu S, Bensch K, Armstrong R (1987) A light and electron microscopic evaluation of Zyderm collagen and Zyplast implants in aging human facial skin: a pilot study. Arch Dermatol 123:1644–1649

Tromovitch TA, Stegman SJ, Glogau RG (1984) Zyderm-collagen: implantation techniques. J Am Acad Dermatol 10:273–278

Watson W, Kaye RL, Klein A, Stegman SJ (1983) Injectable collagen: a clinical overview. Cutis 31:543–546

Correction of Facial Scars

Solubilized bovine collagen is helpful in correcting acne scars, providing that these are not fibrotic or of the deep ice-pick type. Shallow scars respond best after intradermal injections with overcorrection by 50%–100%. Resorption of the implant often requires touch-ups at 6- to 12-month intervals. Satisfactory results were obtained in this man, with multiple through-like scars on the cheek before (*above*) and after completion of treatment (*below*).

Courtesy of Collagen Corporation, Palo Alto, USA

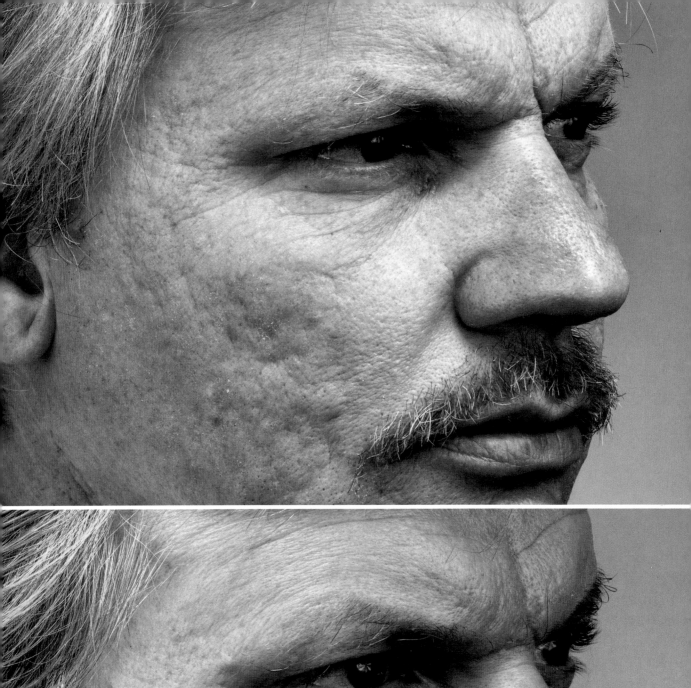
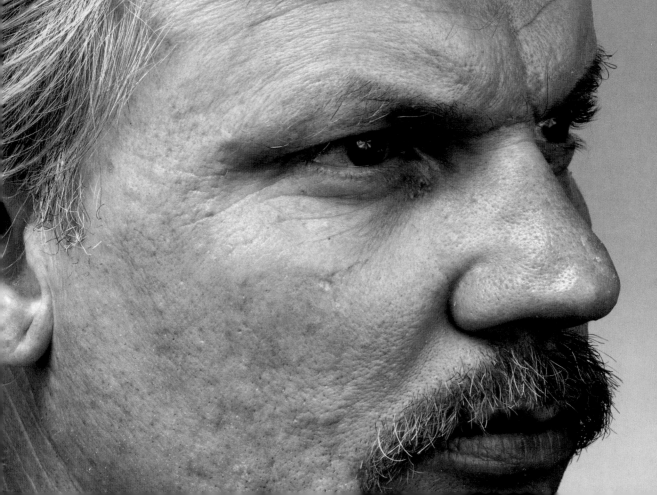

Silicone Injection

Silicone has been used for many decades to augment tissue. Plastic surgeons and gynecologists augmenting breasts in women sometimes insert silicone-filled closed systems into the breast. Unless these tightly sealed devices rupture or become leaky no silicone comes into direct contact with living tissue. The injection of medical-grade fluid silicone to improve scars has also a long tradition. Curiously only a few reports can be found in dermatologic journals, and then mostly in the dermatosurgical or cosmetologic literature. There is good reason for this. Silicone is not a registered pharmaceutic; no pharmaceutical company produces silicone approved for the correction of scars, originating from acne, trauma, accidents, or surgery. Still some dermatologists have outstanding personal experience with this compound, evidently for many years.

Indication and Selection of Lesions

Broad-based so-called valley scars which are wide but not steep and are remnants of previous inflammatory acne lesions can be permanently elevated with this technique. A pinch test tells what a valley lesion means. Pinching the lesion between thumb and index finger makes the scar float up and disappear completely. It would not elevate if there were a fibrous strand below, making the pit unyielding. Other scars, being traumatic or hereditary, are also eligible for this treatment, provided they lift up in the pinch test.

Injection Technique

Medical-grade silicone with a viscosity of 350° centistokes is autoclaved in small vials at 100° C for 20 min. Small syringes, e.g., 3 cm^3 of the Luer Lok type, without three-finger booster attachment are preferred. For injection a disposable 30-gauge needle is used. This is inserted outside the scar, moved into the center beneath it, and the silicone is injected into the dermis. All injections are made without pressure into the scar tissue. At any session only small amounts of silicone are injected, and the depressed scar is not fully elevated. Not more than 1–2 ml silicone is used during any treatment session. Avoid overcorrections. Reinjections are possible, approximately at monthly intervals, often requiring several sessions to elevate the scar completely.

Side Effects and Complications

Intolerance reactions seem to be rare, but they are of major concern if they occur. Pretreatment trials before going into facial scars, as is done with collagen injections, has not been recommended by the authors who are experts for silicone injection. Silicone granulomas are a feared, often very late sequel. Multiple granulomas, similar to paraffinomas, can appear months, years, or even decades after the silicone injection. Stone-hard, inflammatory, bulky infiltrates develop not only at the side of injection but in so-called drain-off areas, e.g., in the face below the jaw line. The induration persists, is extremely refractory to treatment, and can cause serious facial disfigurement, often followed by courtcases. The histology of silicone granulomas is of the Swiss-cheese type with large lipid-filled cells, surrounded by granulocytes and lymphocytes. This is best demonstrated in cryostate sections. An adjuvant general disease is the worst complication.

Another complication is a reddish or bluish discoloration of the skin if too much silicone is injected too superficially into the skin, silicone lakes, because of the Tyndall effect.

Some improvement of silicone granulomas by intralesional injection of diluted corticosteroid crystal suspensions was reported. In a personal case, which was referred to us for treating horrendous silicone granulomas of the face present for many years, orally given isotretinoin in low doses (10–30 mg total dose per day) resulted in a complete resolution. The anti-inflammatory action of isotretinoin was the reason for selecting this treatment modality.

We have no personal experience with silicone injection and do not recommend it in our training institutions, but are aware that others do so.

Apesos J, Pope TL (1985) Silicone granuloma following closed capsulotomy of mammary prosthesis rupture. Ann Plast Surg 14:403–406

Aronsohn RB (1984) A 22-year experience with the use of silicone injections. Am J Cosm Surg 1:21–28

Bronzena SJ, Fenske NA, Cruse CW, Espinoza CG, Vasey FB, Germain BF, Espinoza LR (1988) Human adjuvant disease following augmentation mammoplasty. Arch Dermatol 124:1383–1386

Clark DP, Hanke CW, Swanson NA (1989) Dermal implants: safety of products injected for soft tissue augmentation. J Am Acad Dermatol 21:992–998

Duffy DM (1990) Silicone: a critical review. Adv Dermatol 5:93–107

Fulton JE Jr (1990) The elevation of acne scars with injectable silicone. Am J Cosm Surg 7:99–105

Lazar AP, Lazar P (1991) Localized morphea after silicone gel breast implantation: more evidence for a cause-and-effect relationship. Arch Dermatol 127:263

Orentreich D, Orentreich N (1987) Acne scar revision update. Dermatol Clin 5:359–368

Orentreich DS, Orentreich NO (1988) Injectable fluid silicone. In: Roenigk RK, Roenigk HH Jr (eds) Dermatologic surgery: principles and practice. Decker, New York, pp 1349–1395

Pearl RM, Laub DR, Kaplan EN (1978) Comptreating following silicone injections for augmentation of the contours of the face. Plast Reconstr Surg 61:888–891

Selmanowitz VJ, Orentreich N (1977) Medical grade fluid silicone. J Dermatol Surg Oncol 3:597–611

Webster RC, Fuleihan NS, Hamdan US, Gaunt JM, Smith RC (1986) Injectable silicone: report of 17 000 facial treatments since 1962. Am J Cosm Surg 3:41–48

Webster RC, Hamdan VS, Fuleihan NS, Gaunt JM, Smith RC (1986) Injectable silicone: its history and its current status. Am J Cosm Surg 3:31–38

Therapeutic Pearls

A satisfactory way to improve depressed scar tissue is by soft tissue augmentation, which can be achieved with solubilized collagen, silicone, and lipoinjection (injection of suspended adipocytes from the same patient).

Above Silicone injection. Silicone injections have been used for decades, though it is not approved by federal agencies. Medical grade silicone is to be used, and proper guidelines must be followed. Proper indication and correct injection techniques are mandatory. The follow-up photograph to the right shows the final result

Below Intralesional corticosteroid. Hemorrhagic nodular abscesses, erroneously referred to as "cysts," may quickly respond to intralesional injection of a crystal suspension of corticosteroid. Triamcinolone acetonide suspension, 0.2 ml diluted to 2.5 mg/ml, were injected. Eight days later the nodule has completely flattened

Above: Courtesy of James E. Fulton, M.D., Ph.D., New Port Beach, California, USA

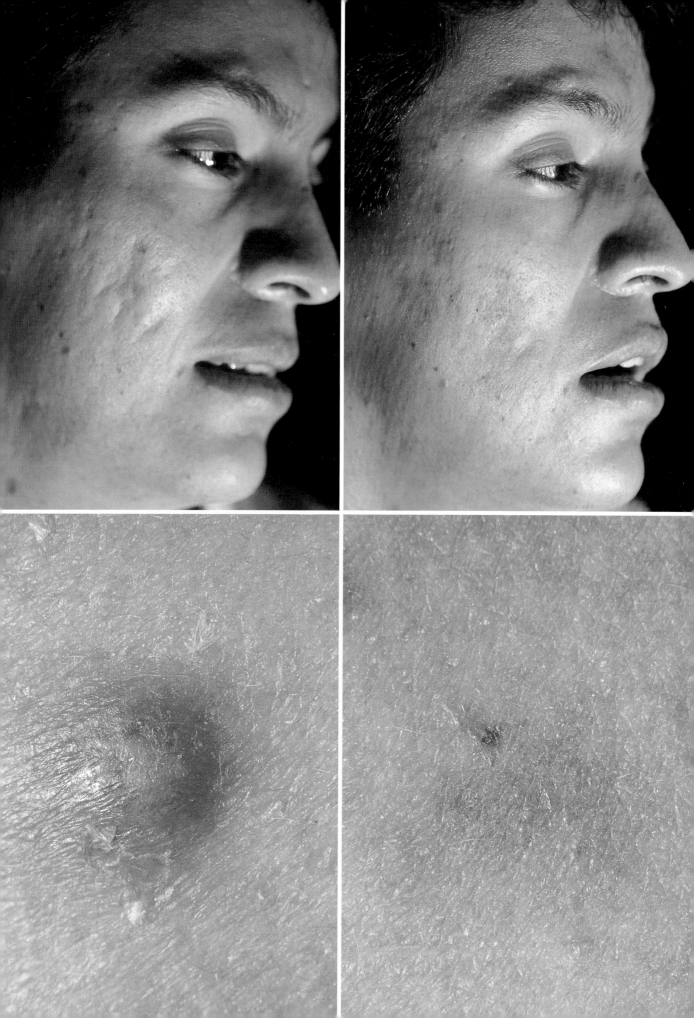

Camouflage

Acne is not only disfiguring but also discoloring. Healed papules may leave a red macule for many months. In dark-skinned people, postinflammatory hyperpigmentation creates long-lasting dark spots in bizarre patterns. Shallow scars are often hypopigmented. Papulopustules exhibit various shades of yellow, red, and purple. Physicians who traditionally devote their attention to the eradication of lesions are not sufficiently aware of the great psychologic benefits provided by camouflage cosmetics. Covering or camouflage cosmetics instantly improve the appearance and furnish the psychological boost which promotes self-confidence and socializing. Cosmetic treatment is a valuable adjunct to drug therapy. Dermatologists lag behind plastic surgeons in employing professional cosmeticians and aestheticians to conceal unsightly lesions. Moreover, there are make-up artists who in 10 min or so, using easily obtainable cosmetics, can create stunning transformations which not only conceal lesions but create a figure of beauty that banishes any hint of disease.

Boutique cosmetic counters employ cosmeticians who are expert in the art of camouflage therapy. The selection of the appropriate shades and textures from a large inventory of possibilities cannot be self-learned. Short training lessions in the application of well-selected cosmetics and their removal are exceedingly helpful. A few basic principles should be mentioned. For example, red and green are complementary colors. Thus, applying a green-tinted lotion to a red lesions instantly makes it invisible, a purely optical effect. Yellow and purple follow this rule, too. Foundation lotions containing opaque particles in a great variety of shades can be spotted onto practically any lesion. One needs only to select a tint that blends smoothly with the patient's complexion. In fact, many of the old fashioned pasty antiacne topicals did nothing more than provide comforting camouflage. This probably contributes to the popularity of formulations containing precipitated sulfur.

In the US, Covermark and Dermablend are frequently used by dermatologists. Some skill and knowledge is required for optimal use. The skin must be carefully cleared before the application.

Another problem which plagues acne patients is the disagreeable shine induced by excessive oiliness. Some cosmetic houses produce thin papers which absorb oil without the necessity of removing make-up. This is a quick and great convenience and can be repeated frequently during the day. A useful and inexpensive product is, for example, Kleenex.

Another way to conceal oiliness without affecting sebum production is the application of a lotion containing particulate acrylate copolymers. These form aggregates which attract and disperse oil droplets, making them invisible. When the polymer is placed near a droplet of sebum this migrates to the polymer and literally disappears. One such product is

Polytrap, an ultralight, free-flowing white polymer powder of highly cross-linked polymethacrylate (Dow Chemical Company, Owen). Its particles are capable of quickly and selectively adsorbing high amounts of lipophilic and certain hydrophilic liquids. The polymethacrylate consists of particles less than 1 μm in size; these fuse to agglomerates of 20 to 80 μm, which are clustered to macroparticles 200–1 200 μm in size. The powder is capable of taking up about four times its weight of lipids. Several cosmetic companies now produce these sophisticated preparations in make-up vehicles (Estée Lauder: Self-Forming Facewash System; and Allercreme Cosmetics: Oil Regulating Lotion).

Psychosocial Aspects

The role of emotions in the causation and course of acne is controversial. The literature is replete with extreme viewpoints. Substantive knowledge is lacking. We wish to make it clear that acne is not a psychosomatic disease. Referring patients to psychiatrists is generally futile. On the other hand, acne can sensibly be regarded as a somatopsychic disorder in which the clinical expressions of the disease generate secondary psychological disturbances. Acne frequently worsens when emotional stress is superimposed. Anxiety deeply colors the disease and can greatly aggravate its expression and contribute to resistance to therapy. Accordingly, one has to treat the whole person as well as the lesions. Depressive episodes speak for the seriousness of this pestilential disorder.

Pubertal acne arrives at the worst possible time in life when tremendous psychological and bodily transformations are taking place. Acne is a disfiguring disease and its victims are often derided and, worse yet, shunned by their peers. A common result is loss of confidence and self-esteem, probably ending in social isolation or extreme timidity. Sometimes the sufferers believe that their lesions are a punishment for various transgressions of social rules of conduct. They accept the disease as just retribution and irrationally resist treatment.

It is helpful to get these thoughts out into the open where they can be dealt with sympathetically. Body language will often alert the physicians to the overly tense and nervous person in deep emotional trouble. The physician should be able directly and comfortably to explore the patients' own views about the role of emotions, explicitly targeting subjects related to sex, menstrual periods, social interactions, school and job performance, sleeping habits, diet, and use of drugs, among others. In-depth psychoanalytical probing is not appropriate.

Dealing with false and irrational beliefs is often reassuring in itself. It is important to state categorically that acne is not contagious and is not an infection. Above all, taking the time to discuss these sensitive topics strengthens the physicians stature as a compassionate, caring doctor. When trust and respect have been established, anxious patients are more likely to follow the therapeutic regimen and will achieve a swifter and more beneficial outcome. Girls are understandingly more concerned than boys and are more likely to seek dermatologic help. Many are angry and hurt and are driven to masochistic self-attacks. They tend to become pickers and pressers who try by various manipulations to rid the skin of the unsightly lesions. Every patient should be asked about such self-manipulations, especially if there is evidence of excoriations. Often comedones are crushed and extruded into the tissue, provoking furious inflammatory granulomas.

The ability of emotions to aggravate the disease should be discussed without being overly stern or pessimistic. In patients who are emotionally devastated we prescribe anxiolytics or antidepressants as indicated along with antiacne medications. Psychiatric referral is appropriate for patients who fail to respond to dermatologic management.

Albers HJ (1985) Psychological dilemma and management of the acne patient. In. Cullen SI (ed) Focus on acne vulgaris. Royal Society of Medicine Services, London, pp 27–34

Arnetz BB (ed) (1991) Dermatological psychosomatics. Acta Derm Venereol [Suppl 156] (Stockh)

Macdonald Hull S, Cunliffe WJ, Hughes BR (1991) Treatment of the depressed and dysmorphophobic acne patient. Clin Exp Dermatol 16:210–211

Jowett S, Ryan T (1985) Skin disease and handicap: an analysis of the impact of skin conditions. Soc Sci Med 20:425–429

Koo JYM, Smith LL (1991) Psychologic aspects of acne. Pediatr Dermatol 8:185–188

Lim CCL, Tan TC (1991) Personality, disability and acne in college students. Clin Exp Dermatol 16:371–373

Lipowski ZJ (1986) Psychosomatic medicine: past and present. Part III. Current research. Can J Psych 31:14–21

Marks R (1985) Acne – social impact and health education. JR Soc Med (Suppl 10) 78:21–24

Motley RJ, Finlay AY (1989) How much disability is caused by acne? Clin Exp Dermatol 14:194–198

Myhill JE, Leichtman SR, Burnett JW (1988) Self-esteem and social assertiveness in patients receiving isotretinoin treatment for cystic acne. Cutis 41:171–173

Panconesi E (1984) Psychosomatic dermatology. In: Panconesi E (ed) Clinics in dermatology stress and skin diseases: psychosomatic dermatology. Lippincott, Philadelphia, pp 94–179

Rasmussen JE, Smith SB (1983) Patient concepts and misconceptions of acne. Arch Dermatol 119:570–572

Rubinow DR, Peck GL, Squillace KM, Gantt GG (1987) Reduced anxiety and depression in cystic acne patients after successful treatment with oral isotretinoin. J Am Acad Dermatol 17:25–32

Van der Meeren HLM, Van der Schaar WW, Van den Hurk CMAM (1985) The psychological impact of severe acne. Cutis 36:84–86

Wu SF, Kinder BN, Trunnell TN, Fulton JE (1988) Role of anxiety and anger in acne patients: a relationship with the severity of the disorder. J Am Acad Dermatol 18:325–333

Spontaneous Involution of Acne

The most agreeable feature of acne vulgaris is its spontaneous disappearance after adolescence in most patients. This phenomenon is unexplained.

Out of many observations we have developed a theory which, though speculative, is not without some factual foundation. It has to do with the slow maturation of the keratinizing epithelium of sebaceous follicles. The basic idea is that the sebaceous follicle does not suddenly acquire adult proportions at puberty. In normal persons, histologic study shows that its volume progressively increases during adolescence. We and others have found that the production of sebum continually increases during adolescence and, indeed, tends to keep increasing well into early adulthood. Enlargement is not limited to the glands; the dermis also thickens, and the size of the whole pilosebaceous unit increases. Terminal hairs become longer and thicker. What has struck us are anatomic changes in the keratinization patterns. In youngsters, the follicular epithelium produces fragile horny cells which slough soon after their formation. The follicle is not lined by an effective stratum corneum barrier. Therefore, all substances within the canal can easily diffuse across the epithelium. In adults, however, the infundibulum is lined by a sturdy horny layer which can act as an effective barrier and protects the epithelium against assaults of comedogenic substances in sebum and a host of toxic substances produced by a dense population of *Propionibacterium acnes*. It will be recalled that the *Propionibacterium acnes* count in adults is the same in both acne and nonacne subjects. By that time the latter have formed a horny layer barrier and the follicle can resist the potentially injurious compounds, e.g., enzymes produced by *Propionibacterium acnes*.

We have demonstrated that follicular reactivity decreases with age, especially after the age of 60 years. Pustules are not so easily elicited by topical potassium iodide, and application of topical corticosteroids results in a less severe acneiform eruption. It seems reasonable to attribute this reduced response to the presence of a well-developed stratum corneum within the sebaceous follicles.

Another indication comes from the successful treatment of severe inflammatory acne with isotretinoin. Many patients remain completely clear after one full course of isotretinoin, although their sebum output comes back to almost pretreatment levels, and *Propionibacterium acnes* colonizes follicles again. In these patients the stratum corneum layers in the infrainfundibulum have been completely restored.

Similarily astonishing is that boys, once afflicted with acne fulminans, virtually remain free of further acne lesions after successful treatment.

In summary, it is still a mystery why acne involutes spontaneously. We hypothesize that the development of an effective stratum corneum barrier may represent an essential step in this process.

Gebhart W (1989) Immunoglobulin A-mediated local immunity in the sebaceous follicle. In: Marks R, Plewig G (eds) Acne and related disorders. Dunitz, London, pp 23–26

Plewig G, Kligman AM (1972) Follikuläre Pusteln im Kaliumjodid-Epicutantest. Arch Dermatol Forsch 242:137–152

Subject Index